Anesthesia and Perioperative Care for Aortic Surgery

Kathirvel Subramaniam
Kyung W. Park
Balachundhar Subramaniam

Editors

Anesthesia and Perioperative Care for Aortic Surgery

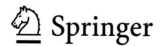

Editors

Kathirvel Subramaniam, MD
Clinical Assistant Professor
University of Pittsburgh Medical
Center - Presbyterian Hospital
Department of Anesthesiology
Pittsburgh, PA
USA
subramaniamk@upmc.edu

Kyung W. Park, MD, MBA
Departments of Anesthesia and
of Surgery
The Ohio State University Medical Center
Doan Hall 168, 450 W. 10th Avenue
Columbus, OH
USA
Tim.Park@osumc.edu

Balachundhar Subramaniam, MBBS, MD
Assistant Professor in Anesthesia
Harvard Medical School
Director
Division of Cardiovascular
Anesthesiology Research
Beth Israel Deaconess Medical Center
Boston, MA
USA
bsubrama@bidmc.harvard.edu

ISBN 978-0-387-85921-7   e-ISBN 978-0-387-85922-4
DOI 10.1007/978-0-387-85922-4
Springer New York Dordrecht Heidelberg London

Printed on acid-free paper

Humana Press is part of Springer Science+Business Media (www.springer.com)

I dedicate this textbook to my parents (Palaniammal & Subramaniam), my wife (Dalia), my children (Manav & Manas) and my teachers.

Kathirvel Subramaniam

This book would not have been posible without the support and patience of my family, for which I am most grateful

Kyung W. Park

I would like to dedicate this work to my wife (Kalpana), kids (Nirmal, Pavi and Amal) and my parents (Parimala and Subramaniam)

Balachundhar Subramaniam

Preface

Some 15 years ago, as the authors were all working at a high-volume vascular surgical center of the Beth Israel Deaconess Medical Center in Boston, there was a realization that patients undergoing vascular surgery present the anesthesiologist with a unique set of challenges. These patients are usually elderly with a host of cardiac, cerebrovascular, renal, and metabolic comorbidities, which are usually expected to get worse either transiently or permanently with the insult of the major vascular surgery. Meeting the challenges is not only a lofty goal for the anesthesiologists involved, but also is a requirement predicated on the covenant relationship that the anesthesiologists have with the patients. And doing so requires comprehensive understanding of the pathophysiology and anatomy of the disease processes, the surgical techniques used to address the ailments, and the spectrum of anesthetic medications and monitoring modalities.

This book represents our best attempt to bring together these components that need to be understood in order to properly meet the challenges of caring for a complex vascular patient with a disease of the aorta and its major branches. We have brought together the expertise and experience of some of the best surgical, medical, and anesthetic minds on the subject. This book is intended for cardiac anesthesiologists, cardiovascular surgeons, intensivists, nurse anesthetists, residents, and fellows of these respective specialties who are involved in the care of aortic surgical patients. Recent developments in aortic surgery such as endovascular surgery make the older textbooks on this subject obsolete.

Chapters include anatomical description of aorta, pathogenesis of acute aortic syndrome, preoperative evaluation, detailed description of aortic surgery and anesthesia for specific aortic procedures (ascending aorta, arch, descending aorta, endovascular surgery, trauma, and surgery for congenital aortic pathologies). Intraoperative echocardiography and cerebral monitoring have gained importance in cardiac surgery in recent years and separate chapters describe these monitoring techniques. Two chapters are devoted to specific organ protection (spinal cord and renal protection) since organ dysfunction is a major cause of mortality and morbidity after aortic surgery. The book ends with a concise description of postoperative care. Overall, this is a complete textbook on aortic anesthesia, which will serve as a reference for those involved in the care of aortic surgical patients.

This book would not have been possible without the support of the editors of Springer publishers, Brian Belval, Shelley Reinhardt, and Catherine Paduani, for which we are most grateful. We are also indebted to Joanna Perey, editorial assistant, and to Rebecca McArdle, our coach and development editor at Springer, for their undying support. We are thankful to all the authors for their significant contributions. We are thankful to Christopher Edwards and Shaw Kristin for their help with the artwork.

We hope that this book will help you to offer better care for aortic surgical patients.

Kathirvel Subramaniam
Kyung W. Park
Balachundhar Subramaniam

Contents

Contributors

Elnazeer O. Ahmed, MBBS, MD, FRCSI
Department of Cardiac Surgery, London Health Sciences Centre,
London, ON, Canada

John G.T. Augoustides, MD, FASE, FAHA
Department of Anesthesiology and Critical Care, University of
Pennsylvania Medical Center, Philadelphia, PA, USA

Jeffrey Balzer, PhD
Neurological Surgery, University of Pittsburgh Medical Center,
Pittsburgh PA, USA

Jay K. Bhama, MD
Division of Cardiac Surgery, Department of Cardiothoracic Surgery,
University of Pittsburgh Medical Center, Pittsburgh, PA, USA

John C. Caldwell, MD
Division of Cardiovascular Anesthesia, University of Pittsburgh Medical
Center – Presbyterian University Hospital, Pittsburgh, PA, USA

Davy C. Cheng, MD
Department of Anesthesia & Perioperative Medicine, London, ON, Canada

John R. Cooper, Jr, MD
Division of Cardiovascular Anesthesiology, Department of Surgery,
Baylor College of Medicine, and The Texas Heart Institute at St. Luke's
Episcopal Hospital, Houston, TX, USA

Joseph S. Coselli, MD
Division of Cardiothoracic Surgery, Michael E. DeBakey
Department of Surgery, Baylor College of Medicine,
and The Texas Heart Institute at St. Luke's Episcopal Hospital,
Houston, TX, USA

Donald J. Crammond, PhD
Department of Neurological Surgery,
University of Pittsburgh Medical Center, Pittsburgh, PA, USA

Jagan Devarajan, MD, FRCA
Clinical fellow in Anesthesiology, Department of Anesthesiology,
Cleveland Clinic, Cleveland, OH, USA

Fellery de Lange, MD, PhD
Department of Anesthesiology, Division of Cardiothoracic
Anesthesiology and Critical Care Medicine,
Duke University Medical Center, Durham, NC, USA

James A. DiNardo, MD
Department of Cardiac Anesthesia, Harvard Medical School,
Children's Hospital Boston, Boston, MA, USA

Tomas Drabek, MD
Department of Anesthesiology, University of Pittsburgh Medical Center,
Presbyterian Hospital, Pittsburgh, PA, USA

Theresa A. Gelzinis, MD
Department of Anesthesiology, University of Pittsburgh,
1 200 Lothrop Street, 15213, Pittsburgh, PA, USA

Thomas G. Gleason, M.D.
Department of Cardiothoracic Surgery,
Center for Thoracic Aortic Disease, University of Pittsburgh
Medical Center, Pittsburgh, PA, USA

Enrique Gongora, MD
Division of Cardiac Surgery, Department of Surgery,
Thoracic Transplantation and Mechanical Circulatory Support,
Heart Transplantation Program, Texas A&M Helath Science
Center College of Medicine, Scott & White Hospital and Clinics,
Temple, TX, USA

Miguel Habeych, MD, MPH
Department of Neurosurgical Surgery, University of Pittsburgh
Medical Center – Presbyterian University Hospital,
Pittsburgh, PA, USA

Richard C. Hsu, MD, PhD
Department of Vascular Surgery, Beth Israel Deaconess Medical Center,
110 Francis St Suite 5B, Boston 02215, MA, USA

Chad Hughes, MD
Division of Thoracic and Cardiovascular Surgery, Department of Surgery,
Aortic Surgery Program, Duke Heart Center, Duke University Medical
Center, Durham, NC, USA

Barry D. Kussman, MBBCh
Department of Anesthesiology, Perioperative and Pain Medicine,
Children's Hospital Boston and Harvard Medical School,
300 Longwood Avenue, Boston, MA, USA

Scott A. LeMaire, MD
Division of Cardiothoracic Surgery, Michael E. DeBakey
Department of Surgery, Baylor College of Medicine, and The Texas Heart
Institute at St. Luke's Episcopal Hospital, Houston, TX, USA

Adam B. Lerner, MD
Department of Anesthesia, Critical Care, and Pain Medicine,
Beth Israel Deaconess Medical Center, 330 Brookline Avenue,
Boston, MA 02215, USA; Department of Anesthesia, Harvard Medical
School, Boston, MA, USA

Donn Marciniak, MD
Department of Cardiothoracic Anesthesia, Cleveland Clinic Foundation,
Cleveland, OH, USA

G. Burkhard Mackensen, MD, PhD
Department of Anesthesiology, Duke University Medical Center,
Durham, NC, USA

John M. Murkin, MD, FRCPC
Department of Anesthesiology and Perioperative Medicine, University
Hospital – London Health Sciences Center, London, ON, Canada

Andrew W. Murray, MB. ChB
Department of Anesthesiology, University of Pittsburgh Medical
Center – Presbyterian and VA Hospital, Pittsburgh, PA, USA

Kyung W. Park, MD, MBA
Departments of Anesthesia and of Surgery, The Ohio State University
Medical Center, Doan Hall 168, 450 W. 10th Avenue,
Columbus, OH, USA

Joseph J. Quinlan, MD
University of Pittsburgh Medical Center – Presbyterian Hospital,
Pittsburgh, PA, USA

Marc Schermerhorn, MD
Department of Vascular Surgery, Beth Israel Deaconess Medical Center,
110 Francis St Suite 5B, Boston 02215, MA, USA

Andrew D. Shaw, MB, FRCA, FCCM
Department of Anesthesiology, Duke University, Medical Center,
Durham, NC, USA

Charles E. Smith, MD, FRCPC
Department of Anesthesia, MetroHealth Medical Center,
Case Western Reserve University, 2500 MetroHealth Drive,
Cleveland, OH 44109, USA

Mark Stafford-Smith, MD, CM, FRCPC, FASE
Department of Anesthesiology, Duke University Medical Center, Durham,
NC 27710, USA

Balachundhar Subramaniam, MBBS, MD
Assistant Professor in Anesthesia, Harvard Medical School,
Director of Cardiovascular Anesthesiology Research,
Beth Israel Deaconess Medical Center, Boston, MA, USA

Kathirvel Subramaniam, MD
Department of Anesthesiology, University of Pittsburgh Medical
Center – Presbyterian Hospital, Pittsburgh, PA, USA

Madhav Swaminathan, MD
Department of Anesthesiology, Duke University Medical Center,
Durham, NC, USA

Parthasarathy D. Thirumala, MD
Department of Neurosurgery, University of Pittsburgh Medical Center,
Pittsburgh, PA, USA

Cynthia M. Wells, MD
Department of Anesthesiology,
University of Pittsburgh Medical Center – Presbyterian Hospital,
Pittsburgh, PA, USA

Applied Anatomy of the Aorta

1

Jagan Devarajan and Balachundhar Subramaniam

A clear understanding of the functional anatomy of the aorta allows the anesthesiologist to provide optimal perioperative care to patients who undergo surgical procedures involving the aorta. This chapter describes the anatomy of the aorta with relevance to preoperative preparation, intraoperative surgical, anesthetic, and hemodynamic management, and maintenance of organ perfusion in the perioperative period.

Anatomy

The aorta is the major blood vessel that carries oxygen and metabolic nutrients to the entire body through its series of branches. The aorta originates from the base of the left ventricle and ascends for a short distance as the ascending aorta, which then arches toward the left forming the arch of aorta (Fig. 1.1). The arch of aorta then continues as the descending thoracic aorta, which runs in a relatively straight course anterior to the vertebral column (Fig. 1.2). The descending thoracic aorta becomes the abdominal aorta at the level of the aortic hiatus of the diaphragm anterior to the 12th vertebral body (T_{12}). The abdominal aorta terminates opposite the lower border of L_4 by dividing into the right and left common iliac arteries.[1]

The ascending aorta is about 3.2 cm in diameter and narrows slightly to 2.72–2.84 cm at the arch of aorta. It measures 2.51–2.55 cm in diameter at the level of the descending thoracic aorta and narrows down progressively as it gives rise to several branches and measures 1.75 cm in diameter at its terminal branching level. The aforementioned values are for males and are greater than corresponding values for females by 0.25–0.30 cm at all levels.[2] These diameters are important, as aneurysms are defined in relation to the normal size at corresponding levels.[3] An aortic aneurysm is a permanent aortic dilatation of at least 1.5 times the diameter of the expected normal value. Sixty-five percent of aneurysms affect the abdominal aorta, with the remaining 35% in the thoracic aorta.[3] In fact, abdominal aortic aneurysms are present in more than one in 20 men who are above 65 years of age when screened by ultrasound.[4] Ten percent of aortic aneurysms are present in both the thoracic and abdominal aorta.[5]

Ascending Aorta

The ascending aorta commences at the upper part of the base of left ventricle at the level of third costal cartilage and is about 5 cm in length. It courses upward, anteriorly and to the right, to continue as the arch of aorta and runs parallel to the axis of the heart. It has three small dilatations called the aortic sinuses or sinuses of Valsalva, which are situated opposite to the cusps of aortic valve (Fig. 1.3).

J. Devarajan (✉)
Clinical fellow in Anesthesiology, Department of
Anesthesiology, Cleveland Clinic, Cleveland, OH, USA
e-mail: drdjagan2000@yahoo.com

K. Subramaniam et al. (eds.), *Anesthesia and Perioperative Care for Aortic Surgery*,
DOI 10.1007/978-0-387-85922-4_1, © Springer Science+Business Media, LLC 2011

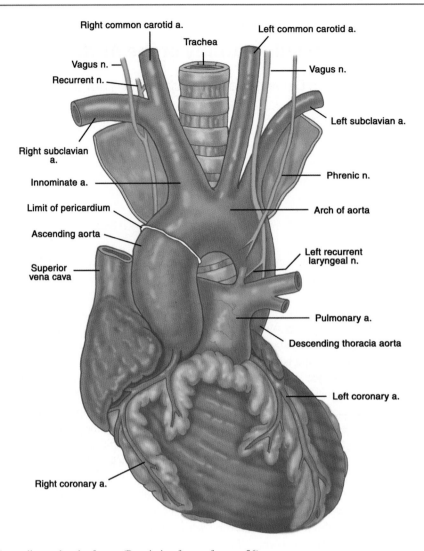

Fig. 1.1 Ascending and arch of aorta (Permission from reference 56)

The proximal half of the ascending aorta is situated within the pericardium along with the pulmonary artery (Fig. 1.1). The two coronary arteries arise from this part of aorta. The right coronary artery arises from the right anterior aortic sinus and the left coronary artery, which is larger than the right, from the left anterior aortic sinus and divides into the anterior descending and the circumflex branch. They both originate at the commencement of the aorta immediately above the attached margins of the semilunar valves.

The incidence of coronary artery anomalies varies from 0.46% to 5.64% in adults undergoing coronary angiography.[6] There are variations in the number, shape, and location of the ostia or origins of the coronary arteries. Some of these anomalies are benign variants while others could lead to myocardial ischemia/infarction, cardiac arrhythmias, and sudden death.[7] When they are identified during childhood in conditions such as the tetralogy of Fallot or transposition of great vessels, they may dictate varying surgical approaches. The left coronary artery can originate from the right coronary artery in children with tetralogy of Fallot. If the left coronary artery or the left anterior descending artery arises from the right sinus of Valsalva, its subsequent course between the aorta and pulmonary artery makes it more prone to compression causing myocardial ischemia or even sudden death in young individuals (Fig. 1.4).

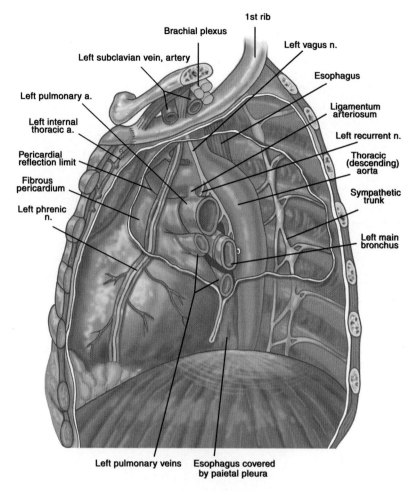

Fig. 1.2 Course of descending aorta in the mediastinum (Permission from reference 57)

They may originate higher in the sinus and, during root replacements, this could lead to potential obstruction or impedance. High takeoffs could lead to acute angles, ostial ridges, and an intramural course resulting in myocardial ischemia. The presence of a single coronary ostium poses additional challenges with the arterial switch repair. Arterial switch mortality has historically been increased in the presence of a single coronary ostium, possibly attributed to kinking, stretching, or thrombosis of the reimplanted artery.

Many of the clinical manifestations of aortic dissection can be explained by anatomy of the ascending aorta. If aortic dissection progresses in a retrograde manner and involves the aortic valve, it presents with acute aortic regurgitation,[8] and acute myocardial ischemia or infarction may result due to coronary occlusion.[9] The right coronary artery is most commonly involved, which can subsequently lead to complete heart block.[10] Because the initial part of the ascending aorta is surrounded by the pericardium (Fig. 1.1), complications such as hemopericardium[11], cardiac tamponade, and sudden death[12] can occur owing to rupture of the dissecting aorta or aneurysm into the pericardial space. If the pericardial sac is filled with blood, it can compress the right atrium, the pulmonary artery, and the adjoining part of the right ventricle.[13]

Arch of Aorta

The arch of aorta begins at the level of the second sternocostal joint on the right side as a continuation of the ascending aorta, and arches toward the

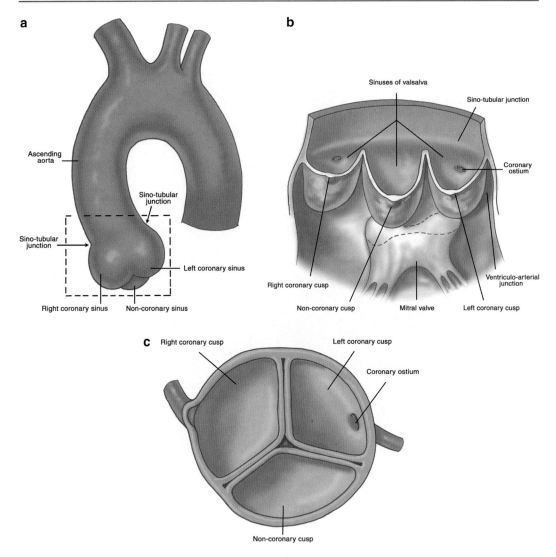

Fig. 1.3 Aortic root and components. Aortic sinuses of Valsalva seen from outside (**a**). Aortic sinuses seen from inside of the aorta (**b**). Aortic valve cusps in short axis orientation (**c**)

left in front of the trachea forming the descending thoracic aorta at the level of the body of the fourth thoracic vertebra. Its upper border is usually about 2.5 cm below the superior border of the manubrium sternum. There is narrowing of the lumen of aorta between the origin of the left sub-clavian artery and the attachment of ligamentum arteriosum known as aortic isthmus, which is fol-lowed by a dilatation known as aortic spindle. There are three branches given off by the arch of aorta: the innominate, the left common carotid, and the left subclavian artery (Fig. 1.1).

The incidence of aortic arch anomalies is approximately 1–3% of congenital cardiac defects, among which the double aortic arch and the right-sided aortic arch constitute 40% and 30%, respectively.[14] Usually the aorta arches toward the left side, but sometimes it passes over the root of the right lung and passes down on the right side of the vertebral column, a condition known as a right-sided aortic arch (Fig. 1.5).[15] In such cases, all the thoracic and abdominal viscera are trans-posed.[16] Occasionally, the aorta in patients with a right-sided aortic arch may cross over to the left

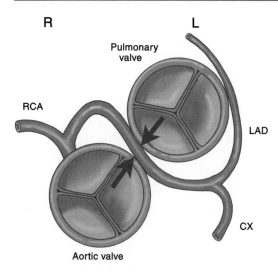

R   L

Pulmonary
valve

RCA

LAD

CX

Aortic valve

Fig. 1.4 Image of anomalous origin of the left coronary artery from the right coronary sinus. The artery courses between aorta and pulmonary artery, which can lead to compression and myocardial ischemia. RCA – Right coronary artery; LAD – Left anterior descending artery; CX – Circumflex artery (Redrawn with permission from www.radiologyassistant.nl, Date accessed 05/15/2010)

side in front of the vertebral column and descend on the left side; it is then known as a circumflex aortic arch. A right-sided aortic arch with mirror imaging of branches alone does not produce symptoms; however, a right-sided aortic arch is associated with a 98% incidence of congenital cardiac abnormalities, which dictate symptoms.[17] Rarely, a right-sided aortic arch may be associated with Kommerell diverticulum, which may cause compression of esophagus or trachea.[18]

Occasionally, there may be two aortic arches, one on each side, which may form a complete ring and encircle trachea and esophagus and can cause respiratory and/or feeding difficulties. There may be lack of luminal continuity between the ascending and descending thoracic aorta, and this condition is known as an interrupted aortic arch.[19] This discontinuity may be complete or it may be spanned by an atretic fibrous band[20] and is present in 1% of critically ill neonates with congenital heart disease.

Right Sided Aortic Arch with Anomalous Left Subclavian A.

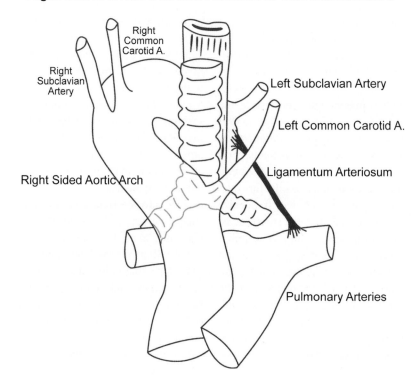

Right Common Carotid A.

Right Subclavian Artery

Left Subclavian Artery

Left Common Carotid A.

Ligamentum Arteriosum

Right Sided Aortic Arch

Pulmonary Arteries

Fig. 1.5 Right-sided aortic arch

Coarctation of the aorta is a congenital abnormality that is characterized by marked stenosis or complete obliteration of the lumen of the aorta at or just below the attachment of ligamentum arteriosum. It is important to know[21] the site of the coarctation in order to decide the site of invasive arterial blood pressure monitoring because the preductal and postductal arterial pressures can be very different.

Clinical manifestations of the above rare congenital anomalies vary from an asymptomatic incidental finding in adolescents and adults to respiratory stridor in neonates.[15,22] Less severe manifestations include recurrent nonspecific respiratory tract infections, wheezing, recurrent cough, or pneumonia. Esophageal symptoms such as dysphagia or vomiting are usually elicited rather than being reported.[23]

The arch of aorta is a common site for aneurysmal dilatation and knowledge of the anatomical relations of the arch helps to explain different clinical manifestations that may ensue. The sternum and rib cartilages can become eroded by the impingement of the aortic arch aneurysm as it projects forward. It can present as a pulsating mass on the front of the chest, above the manubrium. Aneurysms of arch of aorta can compress the adjacent trachea and bronchi, which may result in tracheal tugging, stridorous breathing, dyspnea, and platypnea.[24,25] Compression of the bronchus and lung may also result in atelectasis or compressive pneumonia. Very rarely the aneurysm can burst into the lung, trachea, and/or bronchi, causing hemoptysis.[26] Preoperative imaging should be reviewed in patients with symptoms for the safety of airway management. Involvement of the esophagus, producing dysphagia, is not uncommon and has frequently been mistaken for an esophageal stricture; or rarely the aneurysm may burst into the esophagus, resulting in a fatal hemetemesis. Compression of the superior vena cava or the innominate vein is possible, causing venous engorgement of the face, right arm, and anterior chest wall. Congestion of the brain can manifest as headache, vomiting, or vertigo. An aneurysm can perforate into the superior vena cava, resulting in an arteriovenous aneurysm. This condition manifests as sudden onset of dyspnea, intense congestion of the face and upper part of the body, and is accompanied by a palpable thrill and a continuous humming murmur over the sternum, loudest during systole. Similar symptoms may be seen when an aortic aneurysm erodes into the pulmonary artery.[27]

Several nerves can be injured during aortic surgical procedures or compressed by the pathologic diseases of aorta. While right recurrent laryngeal nerve is well away from the aorta lying close to right subclavian artery, the left recurrent laryngeal nerve winds closely around the arch (Fig. 1.1) and, when compressed[28] or injured, can give rise to hoarseness of voice.[29] Postoperative vocal card paralysis has been reported in 21–32% of patients after thoracic aortic surgery.[30–32] Other nerves that are likely to be at risk for injury during aortic surgery include phrenic nerve (diaphragmatic paralysis) and vagus nerve. The arch of aorta is also closely related to the superior cervical sympathetic ganglion, and Horner's syndrome may result from either dissection or aneurysmal dilatation compressing the nerves.[33]

Sometimes many of the physical signs of an aortic aneurysm may be simulated by a simple benign condition causing a hyperdynamic circulation due to the nature of highly distensible elastic aorta, without any true aneurysmal dilatation. This presentation is called a dynamic dilatation of the aorta and may be benign. Young people with aortic regurgitation and athletes with hypertrophied hearts, patients with Graves' disease or with marked anemia may have a throbbing pulsation above the suprasternal notch mimicking an aneurysm of the aortic arch.

The innominate artery is the largest branch of the arch of the aorta, and is 4–5 cm in length. It divides into the right common carotid and right subclavian arteries at the level of the right sternoclavicular joint. The subclavian arteries continue as the axillary arteries and supply the upper limbs. The close anatomical relationship between brachial plexus and axillary artery is important because this artery is increasingly used for arterial cannulation in aortic surgery. The common carotid arteries divide into the external and internal carotid arteries at the level of the upper border of the thyroid cartilage. The external carotid arteries supply the exterior of the head, the face, and the greater part of the neck, whereas the internal carotid system supplies the majority of structures within the cranial and orbital cavities. Though the branches of subclavian and carotid vessels are not encountered directly during aortic surgery, internal mammary artery should be preserved for current or future coronary bypass procedure.

It is also important to understand the blood supply of the brain, which comes from two sources: anterior circulation from internal carotid artery of both sides and posterior circulation (vertebrobasillar system) originating from subclavian artery on each side. They form a rich network of anastomoses called circle of Willis inside the cranium and supply the brain (Fig. 1.6). Circle of Willis may be incomplete in significant number of patients. During repair of aortic arch with hypothermic circulatory arrest, perfusion through both carotid arteries is advisable in such patients. In patients with dominant left vertebral artery, incomplete intracranial communications or occlusion of right vertebral artery, perfusion through left subclavian artery is also required.

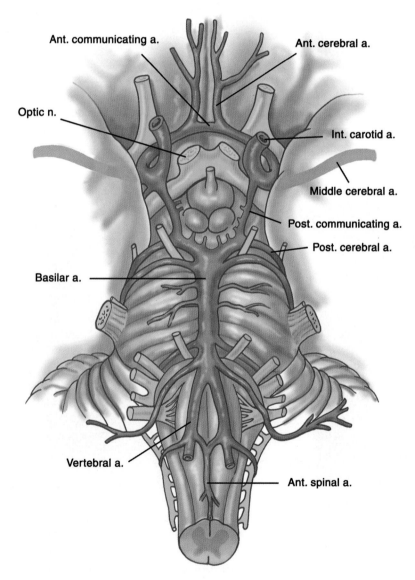

Fig. 1.6 Circle of Willis at the base of the brain (Permission from reference 57)

Endovascular aortic stents are commonly utilized in the treatment of aortic pathology involving proximal descending thoracic aorta. Left subclavian artery may be occluded by proximal end of endograft since it allows gain of proximal landing zone up to 2 cm. Left subclavian artery supply the left upper limb, contributes to the posterior circulation of the brain and circle of Willis, and also contributes to the spinal cord blood supply. Because of rich collateral circulation, occlusion of left subclavian artery may be well tolerated. However, in patients with dominant left vertebral artery, separate origin of vertebral artery from arch, left internal mammary artery pedicle graft, left upper limb dialysis access and in patients with documented post-endograft ischemia, subclavian–carotid artery bypass should be performed. Preoperative computerized tomographic angiographic scan or intraoperative angiography can be utilized to define the anatomy of arch vessels and branches.

Descending Aorta

The descending thoracic aorta is contained within the posterior mediastinum (Fig. 1.2). It begins at the lower border of the fourth thoracic vertebra where it is continuous with the arch of aorta. The junction of the relatively mobile aortic arch and relatively fixed descending aorta is the common site for traumatic rupture of aorta. Descending aorta starts on the left side of the vertebral column and becomes anterior to the vertebral column at its termination. The esophagus lies on the right side of the aorta in the upper part; but in the lower thorax, it is in front of the aorta and moves to the left side of the aorta closer to the diaphragm (Fig. 1.7). This anatomical relationship is important to understand, as this will dictate the imaging of the descending thoracic aorta with transesophageal echocardiography.

Branches from the descending aorta are mainly divided into parietal and visceral. Visceral branches are distributed to the pericardium, the

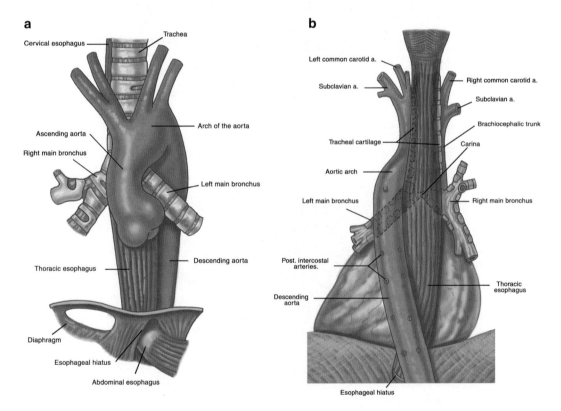

Fig. 1.7 Relationship of esophagus to thoracic aorta. Anterior view (**a**). Posterior view (**b**) (Permission from reference 58)

bronchi, the esophagus, and the mediastinum. The parietal branches are the intercostal, subcostal, and superior phrenic arteries. The intercostal arteries play a role in the reinforcement of blood supply to the spinal cord, which is considered in detail below.

There are usually nine pairs of intercostal arteries, which originate from the posterior aspect of the descending aorta corresponding to the lower nine intercostal spaces. A branch from the costocervical trunk of the subclavian artery supplies the first two spaces. Because the right intercostal arteries originate from left side of the thorax, they take a longer course and pass across the vertebral body posterior to the esophagus, the thoracic duct, and the vena azygos, and are covered by the right lung and pleura. The left intercostal arteries run backward on the sides of the vertebra and are covered by the left lung and pleura. The remainder of the course of the intercostal arteries is similar for both sides.

Each artery divides into an anterior and a posterior ramus. The anterior ramus gives rise to cutaneous, muscular, and mammary branches. The anterior ramus crosses the intercostal space medial to the angle of the rib. For this reason, when performing pleurocentesis, the procedure should never be performed near the midline posterior to the angle of rib. The posterior midscapular line is a common site for pleural aspiration. The intercostal artery along with the vein and nerve are located in the upper part of the intercostal space in the intercostal groove from axilla forward onto anterior chest wall (Fig. 1.2). Hence, the puncture site for an intercostal drain should be just above the upper border of rib to avoid injury to the neurovascular bundle. Intercostal nerve blocks are performed at the angle of the rib due to many advantages at this position. It avoids dural puncture and palpation of rib as the landmark is easier. Moreover, the subcostal groove at this location is wider thereby minimizing the chances for pleural injury. The lateral branch of the intercostal nerve will be effectively blocked at this point. The posterior ramus gives off a spinal branch, which enters the spinal cord through the intervertebral foramen and is distributed to the medulla spinalis and its membranes and the vertebra.

Complex symptoms may arise from aneurysmal dilatation of the descending thoracic aorta due to its inherent location and relation to different structures. Aneurysms generally enlarge backward toward the left side of the vertebral column, causing resorption of vertebral bodies and chronic back pain.[34,35] It can cause compression of the intercostal nerves causing pain, in the corresponding dermatomes. It can also compress or displace the heart causing arrhythmias. This part of the aorta also affects the esophagus and can cause dysphagia or hematemesis due to rupture or communication with the esophagus.[36] Aneurysms can burst into the pleural cavity causing hemothorax[37,38] or into the posterior mediastinum causing hemomediastinum resulting in exsanguinations and/or compression of mediastinal structures.[39,40] Aneurysms from the descending aorta can potentially compress the left main bronchi, which would result in coughing and/or bronchiectasis.[41] This should be kept in mind at the time of insertion of double lumen endotracheal tubes. Reviewing the preoperative imaging (e.g., computerized tomographic angiography) would be helpful in choosing the correct side of double lumen tube placement. Symptoms of asthma have been reported due to compression of left pulmonary plexus.

Abdominal Aorta

The abdominal aorta begins at the aortic hiatus of the diaphragm, in front of the lower border of the T12 vertebra, and ends at L4, dividing into the two common iliac arteries. It diminishes rapidly in size, due to many large branches coming off before termination, as mentioned above. Apart from the terminal branches, it gives rise to both parietal and visceral branches (Fig. 1.8). Visceral branches are unpaired and paired. The unpaired ones are the celiac, the superior mesenteric, and the inferior mesenteric arteries and the paired branches are the renal, the middle suprarenal, and the gonadal arteries. Parietal branches are the inferior phrenic, the lumbar, and the middle sacral arteries. It is important to know the territory and site of origin of these lateral lumbar branches during reimplantation in aortic surgery.

The celiac artery is a short thick trunk, about 1.25 cm in length, which arises from the front of

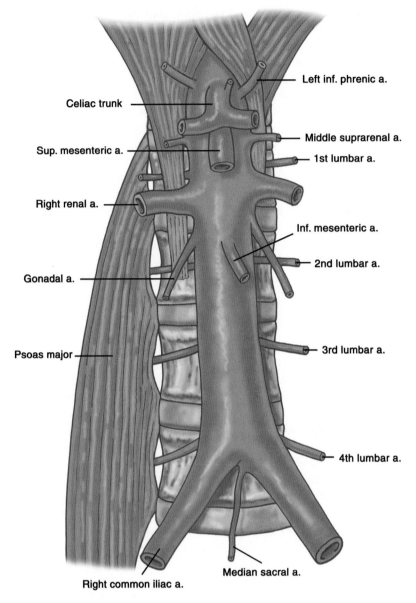

Celiac trunk

Sup. mesenteric a.

Right renal a.

Gonadal a.

Psoas major

Right common iliac a.

Left inf. phrenic a.

Middle suprarenal a.

1st lumbar a.

Inf. mesenteric a.

2nd lumbar a.

3rd lumbar a.

4th lumbar a.

Median sacral a.

Fig. 1.8 Branches of abdominal aorta. Adapted with permission from[57]

the aorta, just below the aortic hiatus of the diaphragm, and divides into three large branches, the left gastric, the hepatic, and the splenic, which supply the stomach, the liver, and the spleen, respectively. Celiac axis coverage may be necessary with endografts and is well tolerated if the celiac artery is small and superior mesenteric artery is large enough to provide collaterals to the celiac system. Just below the celiac branch, the superior mesenteric artery arises that supplies the whole length of the small intestine, except the superior part of the duodenum; it also supplies the cecum and the ascending part of the colon and about one-half of the transverse colon. The rest of the intestines and rectum are supplied by the inferior mesenteric artery, which is smaller than the superior mesenteric artery and is originating 3–4 cm above the terminal division of the aorta into the common iliac arteries. The above anatomical points help us to understand the risk of perioperative intestinal ischemia during aortic surgeries. The middle suprarenal arteries are lateral branches, which arise at L1 and supply suprarenal glands where they also anastomose with the renal and the inferior phrenic arteries. The renal arteries are also lateral branches, which arise at L1 and supply each kidney. The right renal artery is longer than the left, due to the left-sided position of the aorta, and the left renal artery is somewhat higher than the right. A pair of gonadal arteries arises from the aorta just below the renal arteries and supply testes or ovaries.

The abdominal aorta divides at the level of body of the fourth lumbar vertebra, into the two terminal common iliac arteries. Each is about 5 cm in length, passes downward and laterally, and divides opposite the intervertebral space between the L5 and S1 into two branches, the external iliac and hypogastric arteries, the former continuing as femoral artery nourishing the lower extremity and the latter supplying the viscera and parietes of the pelvis.

The abdominal aorta is closely related to the celiac plexus, splanchnic nerves, and lumbar nerves, which explains the different kinds of pain[42,43] experienced by patients with abdominal aortic aneurysm (AAA). It causes two types of pain:

1. Fixed constant back pain due to pressure or displacement of the celiac and splanchnic nerves
2. Sharp lancing, radicular pain in the loins, testes, lumbar areas, and lower limbs due to compression of the lumbar plexus

The aneurysm causing the latter type of pain stands more at risk of rupture into or behind the peritoneal cavity. Aneurysms of the abdominal aorta usually arise either at its upper part close to or involving the celiac arteries or at its lower part near the aortic bifurcation. When an aneurysm arises from the anterior aspect of the aorta near the celiac trunk, it forms a pulsating tumor in the left hypochondrium or epigastric regions, sometimes causing nonspecific symptoms of dyspepsia or constipation. It can compress the common bile duct causing jaundice.[44] Aortic aneurysm has been reported to rupture into the esophagus or stomach causing aortoesophageal or aortogastric fistula,[45–47] into the vena cava causing aortocaval fistula[48] and into the left renal vein causing aortorenal fistula.[49] The importance of knowing the extent of the aneurysm, involvement of the renal arteries, and the relation of the neck of the aneurysm cannot be overemphasized in planning for endovascular repair of aortic aneurysms.

Anatomy of the Blood Supply to the Spinal Cord

A thorough understanding of the anatomy of the blood supply to the spinal cord[50] is essential in order to be aware of and assess the risks of spinal cord ischemia and decide the ways to prevent potential neurological damage after aortic surgery.[51] The spinal cord is very finely balanced between its blood supply and metabolic demand. Any disturbance can lead to ischemia. The blood supply of the spinal cord is derived from three longitudinal arteries: one anterior and two posterolateral arising from vertebrobasillar system and reinforced by various segmental arteries at every level of spinal cord (Fig. 1.9).

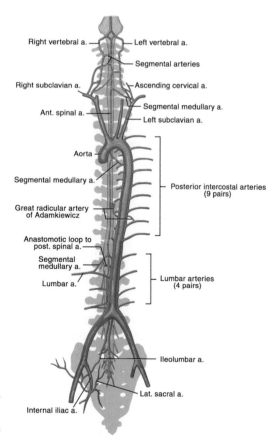

Fig. 1.9 Segmental blood supply of the spinal cord (Modified and reprinted with permission from reference 59)

Longitudinal Arteries

After giving rise to the anterior spinal branches, both vertebral arteries unite to form the basilar artery at the base of the medulla oblongata. The single anterior spinal artery formed by the union of two anterior spinal branches runs in the anterior median sulcus. The site of formation of the anterior spinal artery varies and is anywhere between C1 and C6. The posterior spinal arteries originate from the posterior inferior cerebellar artery and are duplicated through the entire spinal cord. There is usually a rich network of arborizing smaller arteries and arterioles interlinking these arteries across the midline along the posterior aspect of the spinal cord. Though there is an extensive linking between the two posterolateral spinal arteries, there is scarce communication between the posterior and the anterior spinal arteries. However, there is a constant cruciate anastomosis at the conus medullaris between the anterior and the posterior systems. The longitudinal arteries are the main source of blood supply for the upper cervical cord. Anterior spinal artery supplies anterior two-third and posterior spinal arteries supplies posterior one-third of the spinal cord. Beginning with lower cervical level, the above longitudinal spinal arterial system needs reinforcement by a varying number of segmental medullary and radicular arteries to supply the cord.

Segmental Arteries

Segmental arteries supplying the spinal cord originate from the subclavian or vertebral arteries (in the cervical region), intercostal and lumbar arteries (thoracolumbar region), and from the branches of hypogastric artery (internal iliac artery) in the sacral region. The intercostal and lumbar arteries arise in pairs from the posterolateral aspect of the aorta. Dorsal spinal branch of these paired arteries gives origin to radicular and medullary arteries, which supply the nerve roots, ganglion, and the spinal cord (Fig. 1.10). The human neonate has the greatest abundance of blood vessels. However, as a child grows and matures, many

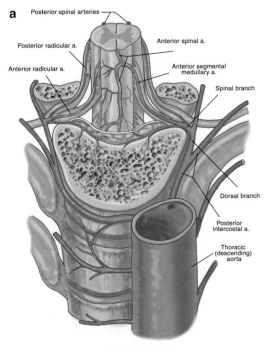
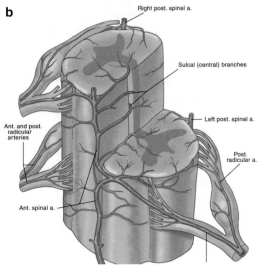

Fig. 1.10 Spinal cord blood supply. Spinal branch of posterior intercostal artery originates in pairs on the back of aorta, supplies the nerve roots, ganglion, and the spinal cord (**a**). Anterior segmental medullary artery is the main source of blood supply for anterior spinal cord at thoracolumbar spinal cord (**b**). Adapted with permission from[60]

paired radicular arteries at each vertebral level involute, and the adult is left with only a few radicular arteries that reinforce the blood supply to spinal cord. Between C8 and T9, there are very few intercostal arteries providing anterior segmental blood supply; therefore, this part of spinal cord is vulnerable to ischemic injury. Unlike anterior medullary branches, posterior segmental medullary branches that reinforce the posterior spinal arteries are small, numerous, and evenly distributed. The largest anterior segmental medullary branch of posterior intercostal artery (known as arteria radicularis magna (ARM) and the artery of Adamkiewicz) is the main source of blood supply for the lower two-thirds of the spinal cord and lumbar enlargement. It has a characteristic hairpin bend. The most common site of the origin of ARM is T10, usually on the left. In 15% of patients, it originates between T5 and T8, 75% between T9 and T12, and 10% between L1 and L2. Knowledge of the level of origin of the ARM and the other large radicular arteries is critical to help in the determination of perioperative strategies for the prevention of paraplegia[52] after open and endovascular aortic surgery. Advanced imaging techniques such as magnetic resonance angiography (MRA) can help in the visualization of collateral blood supply to the spinal cord preoperatively. Presence of collaterals is associated with stable spinal cord function intraoperatively and absence of collaterals increases the chances of neurologic dysfunction postoperatively.[53]

Pelvic Circulation

Pelvic blood supply to the distal spinal cord is derived from the lumbar, iliolumbar, and lateral sacral arteries, which anastomose with anterior spinal and other segmental vessels such as artery of Adamkiewicz. Iliolumbar and lateral sacral arteries are branches of posterior division of internal iliac artery (Fig. 1.9). Distal source of spinal cord is critical when the artery of Adamkiewickz is compromised by the disease or surgical procedure or if it arises high in the spinal cord.[54,55] Pelvic circulation is the main source of distal spinal cord blood supply intraoperatively with aortic cross clamping and distal aortic perfusion. Augmentation of blood pressure perioperatively preserves blood flow through these collaterals and prevents the development of neurological deficits.

Key Notes

1. Understanding the anatomical basis of the disease process of aorta is the primary step and essential for the anesthesiologists involved in the care of aortic surgical patients.
2. Aorta is anatomically divided into aortic root, ascending aorta, arch of aorta, descending thoracic, and abdominal aorta.
3. Congenital anomalies of coronary arteries and aortic arch may be detected as an accidental finding in the adults or can present in children as an associated anomaly with other congenital heart diseases.
4. Anatomical relationship of aorta with other intrathoracic contents dictates symptoms of the diseases of aorta such as aneurysms.
5. Brain is supplied by both internal carotid and vertebrobasillar circulation, which form a rich network of anastomosis inside the cranium (circle of Willis).
6. Proximal ascending aorta is contained in the pericardium. Bleeding originating from this portion may cause cardiac tamponade. Bleeding from arch of aorta and descending aorta may present as mediastinal hematoma or left pleural effusion.
7. The junction of arch and descending aorta is the site for many disease process: patent ductus arteriosus, coarctation of aorta, and traumatic rupture of aorta.
8. Anesthesiologists should be aware of the relationship of descending thoracic aorta and esophagus to accurately interpret the images obtained with transesophageal echocardiography.
9. Preoperative imaging and intraoperative angiography should be done to evaluate carotid, vertebral, left subclavian, major intercostal arteries and branches of abdominal aorta before endovascular stenting procedures.
10. Spinal cord blood supply is derived from longitudinal network (vertebrobasillar system) and segmental arteries (branches of subclavian, vertebral, intercostal, lumbar, and sacral arteries). Interruption by stenting, cross clamping, or embolization may result in paraplegia.

References

1. Gatzoulis MA. Heart and great vessels. In: Standring S, ed. *Gray's Anatomy: The Anatomical Basis of Clinical Practice*. 40th ed. New York: Churchill Livingstone; 2008:959–988.

2. Hager A, Kaemmerer H, Rapp-Bernhardt U, et al. Diameters of the thoracic aorta throughout life as measured with helical computed tomography. *J Thorac Cardiovasc Surg*. 2002;123:1060–1066.

3. Isselbacher EM. Thoracic and abdominal aortic aneurysms. *Circulation*. 2005;111:816–828.

4. Ernst CB. Abdominal aortic aneurysm. *N Engl J Med*. 1993;328:1167–1172.

5. Dobrin PB. Pathophysiology and pathogenesis of aortic aneurysms. Current concepts. *Surg Clin North Am*. 1989;69:687–703.

6. Angelini P. Coronary artery anomalies: an entity in search of an identity. *Circulation*. 2007;115:1296–1305.

7. Pasquali SK, Hasselblad V, Li JS, Kong DF, Sanders SP. Coronary artery pattern and outcome of arterial switch operation for transposition of the great arteries: a meta-analysis. *Circulation*. 2002;106:2575–2580.

8. Patel HJ, Deeb GM. Ascending and arch aorta: pathology, natural history, and treatment. *Circulation*. 2008;118:188–195.

9. Nienaber CA, Eagle KA. Aortic dissection: new frontiers in diagnosis and management: Part I: from etiology to diagnostic strategies. *Circulation*. 2003;108: 628–635.

10. Davis GG, ed. *Applied anatomy: the construction of the human body considered in relation to its functions, diseases and injuries*. 2nd ed. New York: JB Lippincott Company; 1913:208–210.

11. Bains SR, Kedia A, Roldan CA. Pericarditis as initial manifestation of proximal aortic dissection in young patients. *Am J Emerg Med*. 2008;26:379.e3–379.e5.

12. Spitzer S, Blanco G, Adam A, Spyrou PG, Mason D. Superior vena cava obstruction and dissecting aortic aneurysm. *JAMA*. 1975;233:164–165.

13. Schofield PM, Bray CL, Brooks N. Dissecting aneurysm of the thoracic aorta presenting as right atrial obstruction. *Br Heart J*. 1986;55:302–304.

14. Maddali MM, Valliattu J, al Delamie T, Zacharias S. Selection of monitoring site and outcome after neonatal coarctation repair. *Asian Cardiovasc Thorac Ann*. 2008;16:236–239.

15. McElhinney DB, Tworetzky W, Hanley FL, Rudolph AM. Congenital obstructive lesions of the right aortic arch. *Ann Thorac Surg*. 1999;67:1194–1202.

16. Brickner ME, Hillis LD, Lange RA. Congenital heart disease in adults. First of two parts. *N Engl J Med*. 2000;342:256–263.

17. Brickner ME, Hillis LD, Lange RA. Congenital heart disease in adults. Second of two parts. *N Engl J Med*. 2000;342:334–342.

18. Patiniotis TC, Mohajeri M, Hill DG. Right aortic arch with aberrant left subclavian artery: aneurysmal dilatation causing symptomatic compression of the right main bronchus in an adult. *Aust NZ J Surg*. 1995;65: 690–692.

19. McLaughlin RB Jr, Wetmore RF, Tavill MA, Gaynor JW, Spray TL. Vascular anomalies causing symptomatic tracheobronchial compression. *Laryngoscope*. 1999;109:312–319.

20. McLaren CA, Elliott MJ, Roebuck DJ. Vascular compression of the airway in children. *Paediatr Respir Rev*. 2008;9:85–94.

21. Friese KK, Dulce MC, Higgins CB. Airway obstruction by right aortic arch with right-sided patent ductus arteriosus: demonstration by MRI. *J Comput Assist Tomogr*. 1992;16:888–892.

22. Kumeda H, Tomita Y, Morita S, Yasui H. Compression of trachea and left main bronchus by arch aneurysm. *Ann Thorac Surg*. 2005;79:1038–1040.

23. Kussman BD, Geva T, McGowan FX. Cardiovascular causes of airway compression. *Paediatr Anaesth*. 2004;14:60–74.

24. Amirghofran AA, Mollazadeh R, Kojuri J. Hemoptysis due to aortic aneurysm at the site of coarctation repair. *Asian Cardiovasc Thorac Ann*. 2008;16:88–89.

25. Filston HC, Ferguson TB Jr, Oldham HN. Airway obstruction by vascular anomalies. Importance of telescopic bronchoscopy. *Ann Surg*. 1987;205:541–549.

26. Gulel O, Elmali M, Demir S, Tascanov B. Ortner's syndrome associated with aortic arch aneurysm. *Clin Res Cardiol*. 2007;96:49–50.

27. Lee SI, Pyun SB, Jang DH. Dysphagia and hoarseness associated with painless aortic dissection: a rare case of cardiovocal syndrome. *Dysphagia*. 2006;21:129–132.

28. Delabrousse E, Kastler B, Bernard Y, Couvreur M, Clair C. MR diagnosis of a congenital abnormality of the thoracic aorta with an aneurysm of the right subclavian artery presenting as a Horner's syndrome in an adult. *Eur Radiol*. 2000;10:650–652.

29. Dillman JR, Yarram SG, D'Amico AR, Hernandez RJ. Interrupted aortic arch: spectrum of MRI findings. *Am J Roentgenol*. 2008;190:1467–1474.

30. Ishimoto S, Ito K, Toyama M, et al. Vocal cord paralysis after surgery for thoracic aortic aneurysm. *Chest*. 2002;121:1911–1915.

31. Ohta N, Kuratani T, Hagihira S, Kazumi K, Kaneko M, Mori T. Vocal cord paralysis after aortic arch surgery: predictors and clinical outcome. *J Vasc Surg*. 2006;43:721–728.

32. Ohta N, Mori T. Vocal cord paralysis after surgery to the descending thoracic aorta via left posterolateral thoracotomy. *Ann Vasc Surg*. 2007;21:761–766.

33. Casati V, Barbato L, Spagnolo P, et al. Unexpected diagnosis and management of a type of interrupted aortic arch in an adult male scheduled for mitral valve surgery. *J Cardiothorac Vasc Anesth*. 2008;22: 263–266.

34. Cokluk C, Aydin K. Segmental artery pseudoaneurysm associated with thoracic spinal fracture. *Turk Neurosurg*. 2007;17:142–146.

35. Takahashi Y, Sasaki Y, Shibata T, Suehiro S. Descending thoracic aortic aneurysm complicated

with severe vertebral erosion. *Eur J Cardiothorac Surg.* 2007;31:941–943.

36. Amin S, Luketich J, Wald A. Aortoesophageal fistula: case report and review of the literature. *Dig Dis Sci.* 1998;43:1665–1671.

37. Lin YY, Hsu CW, Chu SJ, Tsai SH. Acute rupture of thoracic aorta aneurysm complicated with hemoptysis after EGD. *Gastrointest Endosc.* 2008;67:156–157.

38. Rahman HA, Sakurai A, Dong K, Setsu T, Umetani T, Yamadori T. The retroesophageal subclavian artery – a case report and review. *Kaibogaku Zasshi.* 1993;68:281–287.

39. Sengupta P, Mitra B, Saha K, Maitra S, Pal J, Sarkar N. Descending thoracic aortic aneurysm presenting as left sided hemorrhagic pleural effusion. *J Assoc Physicians India.* 2007;55:297–300.

40. Spiropoulos K, Petsas T, Lymberopoulos D, Solomou A, Spiliopoulou M, Haralambopoulou A. Orthopnea due to an aneurysm of the thoracic aorta. *Respiration.* 1995;62:174–176.

41. Penner C, Maycher B, Light RB. Compression of the left main bronchus between a descending thoracic aortic aneurysm and an enlarged right pulmonary artery. *Chest.* 1994;106:959–961.

42. Diekerhof CH, Reedt Dortland RW, Oner FC, Verbout AJ. Severe erosion of lumbar vertebral body because of abdominal aortic false aneurysm: report of two cases. *Spine.* 2002;27:E382–E384.

43. Galessiere PF, Downs AR, Greenberg HM. Chronic, contained rupture of aortic aneurysms associated with vertebral erosion. *Can J Surg.* 1994;37:23–28.

44. Dorrucci V, Dusi R, Rombola G, Cordiano C. Contained rupture of an abdominal aortic aneurysm presenting as obstructive jaundice: report of a case. *Surg Today.* 2001;31:331–332.

45. Katyal D, Jewell LD, Yakimets WW. Aorto-esophageal fistula secondary to benign Barrett's ulcer: a rare cause of massive gastrointestinal hemorrhage. *Can J Surg.* 1993;36:480–482.

46. Lau OJ. Acute aortogastric fistula following gastro-esophageal anastomosis. *Br J Surg.* 1983;70:504.

47. Lemos DW, Raffetto JD, Moore TC, Menzoian JO. Primary aortoduodenal fistula: a case report and review of the literature. *J Vasc Surg.* 2003;37:686–689.

48. Alexander JJ, Imbembo AL. Aorta-vena cava fistula. *Surgery.* 1989;105:1–12.

49. Thompson RW, Yee LF, Natuzzi ES, Stoney RJ. Aorta-left renal vein fistula syndrome caused by rupture of a juxtarenal abdominal aortic aneurysm: novel pathologic mechanism for a unique clinical entity. *J Vasc Surg.* 1993;18:310–315.

50. Wyss P, Stirnemann P, Mattle HP. Spinal lesions in surgery of the aorta. *Schweiz Rundsch Med Prax.* 1992;81:1105–1110.

51. Amabile P, Grisoli D, Giorgi R, Bartoli JM, Piquet P. Incidence and determinants of spinal cord ischaemia in stent-graft repair of the thoracic aorta. *Eur J Vasc Endovasc Surg.* 2008;35:455–461.

52. Acher CW, Wynn MM, Mell MW, Tefera G, Hoch JR. A quantitative assessment of the impact of intercostal artery reimplantation on paralysis risk in thoracoab-dominal aortic aneurysm repair. *Ann Surg.* 2008;248: 529–540.

53. Backes WH, Nijenhuis RJ, Mess WH, Wilmink MJ, Schurink GWH, Jacobs MJ. Magnetic resonance angiography of collateral blood supply to spinal cord in thoracic and thoracoabdominal aortic aneurysm patients. *J Vasc Surg.* 2008;48:261–271.

54. Rosenthal D. Risk factors for spinal cord ischemia after abdominal aortic operations. *J Vasc Surg.* 1999; 30:391–399.

55. Connolly JE, Ingegno M, Wilson SE. Preservation of the pelvic circulation during infrarenal aortic surgery. *Cardiovasc Surg.* 1996;4:65–70.

56. Henry G. *Anatomy of the Human Body.* 20th edn. Lewis, WH, re-ed. Philadelphia: Lea & Febiger; 1918.

57. Standring S ed. *Gray's Anatomy. The Anatomical Basis of Clinical Practice.* 40th edn. Philadelphia: Churchill Livingstone; 2008.

58. Putz R, Pabst R. *Sobotta – Atlas of Human Anatomy.* 14th edn. New York: Churchill Livingstone; 2008, Oct.

59. Yoshioka K, Niinuma H, Ohira A, et al. MR angiography and CT angiography of the artery of Adamkiewicz: noninvasive preoperative assessment of thoracoabdominal aortic aneurysm. *Radiographics.* 2003;23:15–25.

60. Saunders WB. *Netter's Atlas of Human Anatomy.* 4th edn. Philadelphia: Saunders; 2008 June.

Acute Aortic Syndrome

Cynthia M. Wells and Kathirvel Subramaniam

2

Acute aortic syndrome is a modern term that describes the acute presentation of patients with characteristic "aortic" pain caused by one of the life-threatening thoracic aortic conditions including aortic dissection, intramural hematoma, and penetrating atherosclerotic ulcer (Fig. 2.1). This entity involves acute lesions of the aorta involving the tunica media and can be distinguished by their etiopathogenesis and characteristic appearance using various diagnostic imaging modalities. Recent advances in imaging techniques and therapeutic interventions have increased awareness of these pathological conditions and emphasized the importance of early diagnosis and treatment.

Definition and Epidemiology

Acute aortic syndrome includes five classes of aortic disease (Table 2.1).[1] While being distinct pathological processes, there is the possibility of progression from one entity to another (Fig. 2.2). Each of these processes also shares the Stanford classification that defines the location and extent of aortic involvement. Stanford type A begins in the ascending aorta, while type B originates distal to the left subclavian artery to involve the descending thoracic aorta (Fig. 2.3). This classification system

C.M. Wells (✉)
Department of Anesthesiology, University of Pittsburgh Medical Center – Presbyterian Hospital,
Pittsburgh, PA, USA
e-mail: wellsc2@upmc.edu

is popular since it directs different management strategies and correlates with patient prognosis. Aortic dissections can also be classified as acute or chronic, depending on whether the dissection is less or greater than 2 weeks old.

Aortic Dissection

Classic aortic dissections (class I) are the most common cause of acute aortic syndromes (70%). Aortic dissection is the most common aortic catastrophe occurring two to three times more frequently than abdominal aortic rupture. The exact incidence is unknown but studies quote it to be 2.6–3.5 per 100,000 person-years.[2] Information gathered from the International Registry of Acute Aortic Dissection (IRAD) shows that two thirds of patients are male with a mean age of 63. Women are affected less often and present at a mean age of 67. Patients with dissections involving the ascending aorta tend to present at a younger age (50–55 years) than those with dissections of the descending aorta (60–70 years).

Table 2.2 outlines multiple risk factors for the development of aortic dissection with hypertension being the most common predisposing factor (72%). Following this is a history of atherosclerosis (31%), cardiac surgery (18%), and Marfan's syndrome (5%). Younger patients (<40 years of age) who present with aortic dissection most often have associated Marfan's syndrome, a bicuspid aortic valve or a history of aortic surgery.[3]

K. Subramaniam et al. (eds.), *Anesthesia and Perioperative Care for Aortic Surgery*,
DOI 10.1007/978-0-387-85922-4_2, © Springer Science+Business Media, LLC 2011

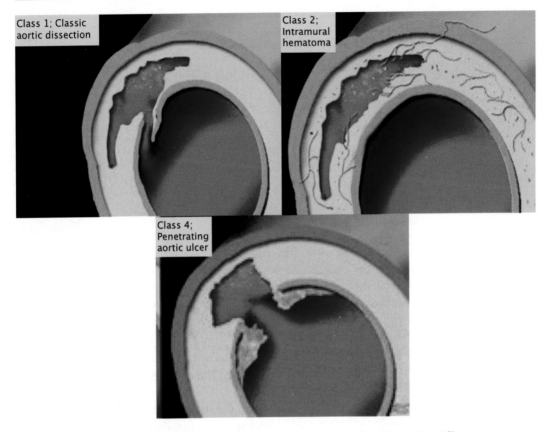

Fig. 2.1 Classification of acute aortic syndromes (Reprinted with permission from Berger F et al.[30])

Table 2.1 Classification of acute aortic syndrome

Class I – Classic aortic dissection
Class II – Intramural hematoma
Class III – Localized dissection, intimal tear without extensive intimal flap formation, localized bulge in the aortic wall
Class IV – Penetrating aortic ulcers
Class V – Iatrogenic or post-traumatic dissection

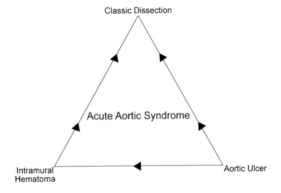

Fig. 2.2 Progression of one type of acute aortic syndrome to another type

Pathologically, classic aortic dissections (class I) are characterized by an intimal tear with separation of the aortic media into two layers, the inner two thirds and outer one third. This separation extends for a variable distance in both circumferential and longitudinal fashion. The vast majority of dissections originate from intimal tears in the ascending aorta within several centimeters of the sinuses of Valsalva where torsional movement of the aortic annulus provokes

additional downward traction in the aortic root and increases longitudinal stress in that segment of aorta. The other common site for an intimal tear to originate is in the descending aorta just distal to the origin of the subclavian artery at the

Fig. 2.3 Types of acute aortic syndromes based on the site of aortic involvement (Reprinted with permission from Springer[4])

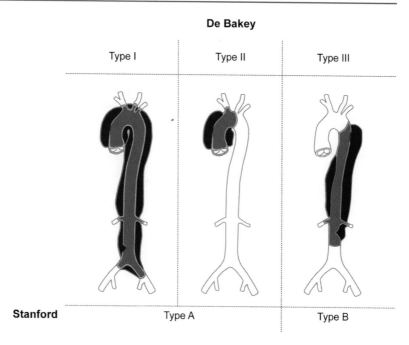

De Bakey

| Type I | Type II | Type III |

Stanford

| Type A | Type B |

Table 2.2 Risk factors for aortic dissection

Long-standing hypertension
Male
Advanced age
Prior cardiac surgery
Known aortic aneurysm or prior dissection
Cardiac catheterization/surgery
Connective tissue disorders
Marfan's syndrome
Ehlers–Danlos syndrome
Bicuspid aortic valve
Coarctation of the aorta
Hereditary thoracic aortic disease
Vascular inflammation
Deceleration injury
Cocaine
Peripartum

site of the ligamentum arteriosum. Tears occur in the isthmus area because of increased tension at the union of the relatively mobile aortic arch with the fixed descending thoracic aorta. From this point, blood under pressure extends the dissection in an antegrade direction although retrograde extension is also possible, thus forming a false lumen and double channel aorta. A further reentrance tear allows blood to circulate in the false lumen and communicate with the true lumen. Reentry tears are often located in the abdominal aorta, iliac arteries, or other aortic branches. These small communications, normally less than 2 mm in diameter, represent intercostal and lumbar arteries severed by the dissection process.[4] The true lumen is most often the smaller of the two and is surrounded by calcifications if present. The false lumen is located along the outer curve of the aortic arch and from the aortic isthmus, a dissection adopts a spiral route involving the left border of the descending thoracic aorta and the left posterior region of the infradiaphragmatic and infrarenal aorta (Fig. 2.4). From there, a dissection may involve any branches of aorta including the arch vessels, the left intercostal, renal, and iliac vessels, most often, it is the left renal and iliac artery which are involved. The celiac, superior mesenteric, and right renal arteries usually communicate with the true lumen. Dissections rarely extend to the common femoral arteries.

Class III dissections are characterized by the presence of an intimal tear without a flap or hematoma formation. Patients often present with the classic symptoms of dissection and may have associated aneurysms, aortic regurgitation, or

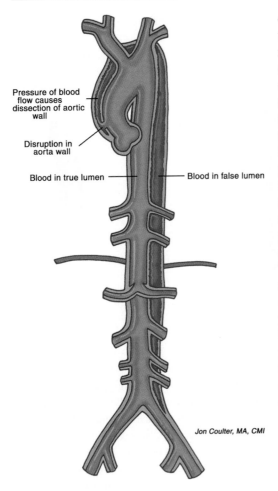

Pressure of blood
flow causes
dissection of aortic
wall

Disruption in
aorta wall

Blood in true lumen ——

—— Blood in false lumen

Jon Coulter, MA, CMI

Fig. 2.4 CT reconstruction of a type A dissection following graft placement in the ascending aorta. The dissection that extends into the descending aorta demonstrates how the defects spiral around the aorta

pericardial effusion. Imaging techniques such as CT, MRI, or TEE may fail to detect this type of dissection since each of these modalities depends on the presence and identification of an intimal flap or true and false lumen for diagnosis. Aortography may show an eccentric bulge in the aorta, which should raise the suspicion of this class of dissection. Treatment is similar to that for classic aortic dissection.[1]

Class V aortic dissections are caused by traumatic or iatrogenic injury. Traumatic dissections are described in detail in another chapter. Iatrogenic aortic dissections may result from

cardiac surgery, percutaneous coronary interventions, or endovascular procedures. Dissections resulting from cardiac surgical procedures may occur during the procedure, early in the postoperative period, or their presentation may be delayed for years.[5,6] The incidence varies between 0.12% and 0.35% of cardiac surgeries, but the mortality is high unless recognized early. Injury to the aorta can occur at the site of cross-clamp placement, cannulation and decannulation, aortotomy, cardioplegic cannulation, or aortocoronary anastomosis. Preexisting atherosclerotic or connective tissue disease, increased aortic diameter, previous heart surgery, a history of hypertension and elevated CPB pressures are all risk factors. There is a growing concern of an increased incidence of aortic dissection following off-pump coronary artery bypass grafting compared to on-pump CABG related to the application of a side-biting clamp under higher blood pressure and pulsatility.[7] Intraoperative TEE and epiaortic ultrasound may help in the prevention and early diagnosis of this potentially lethal complication. Type A dissections have been reported after diagnostic coronary angiography (0.01%) and other percutaneous interventions (0.03%).[8,9] Isolated coronary artery dissections and localized aortic dissections (less than 40 mm of ascending aortic involvement) can be treated with intracoronary or aortic stenting. However, a failed stenting procedure or progression of a dissection must be surgically treated. Retrograde type A dissections after endograft placement for type B dissections have been reported with an incidence of 10–27%.[10] The presentation may be acute or delayed for several months. Various etiological factors include wire and sheath manipulation in the arch, repeated balloon dilatations, oversizing of grafts, injury to a diseased aorta at the margin of inflexible grafts, and progression of disease unrelated to stent grafting. Surgical replacement with tube grafts is recommended in these patients and mortality is high (27%). Other procedures associated with an increased risk of aortic dissection include the insertion of intra-aortic balloon pumps, percutaneous angioplasty, and stenting for coarctation of the aorta.[11]

Intramural Hematoma

Aortic intramural hematomas (IMH) account for up to 20% of all cases of AAS and represent a variant of dissection characterized by the absence of an intimal flap, reentrant tear, or double channel with false lumen flow. IMH often occur in patients with severe atherosclerotic disease in which penetrating aortic ulcers or atherosclerotic plaques rupture causing intimal injury with blood entering the media. In patients with mild or no atherosclerosis, spontaneous rupture of the vasa vasorum may initiate aortic wall degeneration, which leads to hematoma formation in the aortic wall, splitting of the medial layer, and dissection formation without an intimal tear (Class II).[12] Patients in the first group tend to be older and have coexisting coronary and peripheral vascular disease. Absence of intimal tears is not mandatory in the diagnosis of IMH since small communications may be seen indicating rupture as a decompressing mechanism.[13] The presence of large intimal erosions or deep ulcer-like lesions in the intima is associated with a progressive disease course and poor outcome.[14]

IMH evolution is difficult to predict (Fig. 2.5). In some cases, the hematoma does not change in size. Resolution occurs in fewer than 10% of cases, but is more likely with less hematoma and aortic wall thickness.[2] When an IMH resolves, a localized aneurysm may develop because of a weakened media and remodeling, requiring close surveillance. Progression of IMH may lead to weakening and disruption of the intimal layer causing a classic dissection. Progression to dissection has been shown to occur in 16–47% of patients with IMH.[15] A few patients may demonstrate IMH and dissection in different segments of aorta, known as a hybrid case. Increasing aortic diameter (>50 mm) causing aneurysm formation is a poor prognostic factor associated with IMH.[16] In addition, increased permeability of the aortic wall may lead to pericardial or pleural effusions or a mediastinal hemorrhage. Most effusions will resolve. However, large and progressive fluid accumulations are an ominous signs. Weakening of the adventitial layer may lead to aortic rupture, while a contained rupture from disintegration of the outer medial layers with intact adventitia is not uncommon.[17] Similar to aortic dissections, the

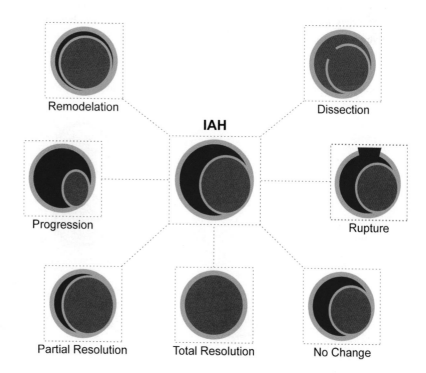

Fig. 2.5 Evolution of intramural hematoma (Reprinted with permission from Springer[4])

most common underlying condition associated with IMH is hypertension.

Penetrating Aortic Ulcer

The term penetrating atherosclerotic ulcer (PAU) describes a condition in which ulceration of an atherosclerotic lesion penetrates the intima and extends into the media, eroding the inner elastic layer of the aortic wall. The reason why most atherosclerotic ulcers do not penetrate the internal elastic lamina and few penetrate the media and adventitia is not clear. PAUs are focal lesions most often located in the descending thoracic aorta, which correlates with a greater disease burden in that region. These patients tend to be older with severe systemic atherosclerosis but without connective tissue diseases. Multiple PAUs are often found in a single patient. Imaging of PAU most often reveals extensive atherosclerosis with severe intimal calcification and plaque. A crater or extravasation of contrast is often visualized.[18]

Occasionally, PAU may progress (Fig. 2.6). This may precipitate a localized, intramural hemorrhage following progressive erosion and rupture of the vasa vasorum.[19] Further penetration to the adventitia may lead to the formation of a saccular aneurysm or pseudoaneurysm.[20] Symptomatic ulcers with signs of deep erosion are more prone to aortic rupture.[21] In rare cases, PAU may lead to aortic dissection, but those dissections arising from

a PAU tend to be less extensive and demonstrate a thick, calcified static flap in a location atypical for entrance tears. Longitudinal spread of aortic dissections arising from PAU is limited by medial fibrosis and calcification.[20]

Acute Expanding Aneurysms

Also included in many discussions of acute aortic pathology are symptomatic aortic aneurysms which may represent impending rupture. The acute expansion of an aortic aneurysm accounts for a significant number of patients who present with the sudden onset of chest pain. As aneurysms increase in size, the dilatation results in greater wall tension and a more rapid rate of expansion. In addition, aneurysms may be associated with progressive dissections, IMH, or PAU, all of which cause weakening of the aortic wall.

Etiopathogenesis

The physiopathological mechanism that precipitates the appearance of each of these entities varies somewhat; however, both acquired and genetic conditions share an underlying pathology that involves breakdown of the intimal layer and weakening of the aortic media, both of which lead to higher wall stress. In addition, it is common for there to be progression from one

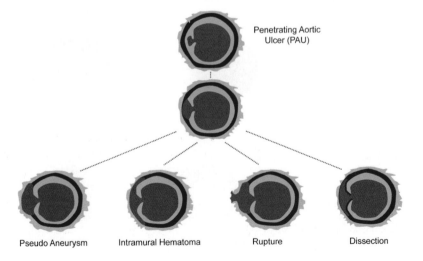

Fig. 2.6 Evolution of penetrating aortic ulcers (Reprinted with permission from Springer[4])

Penetrating Aortic Ulcer (PAU)

Pseudo Aneurysm   Intramural Hematoma   Rupture   Dissection type of lesion to another and some patients may concurrently manifest multiple types of lesions.

Hypertension and Mechanical Forces

The most common risk factor for aortic dissection is hypertension. Chronic exposure of the aorta to high pressures leads to intimal thickening, fibrosis, calcification, and extracellular fatty acid deposition. The extracellular matrix also undergoes accelerated degradation, apoptosis, and elastolysis. Both mechanisms lead to intimal weakening and medial degeneration.[22] At any site where there is tissue thickening and fibrosis, there is compromise of nutrient and oxygen supply to the arterial wall. Eventually, there is necrosis of smooth muscle cells and fibrosis of elastic tissue in the vessel wall. The resulting stiffness increases the risk of aortic pathology when exposed to the chronic trauma of arterial hypertension.

Genetic Predisposition

Marfan's syndrome, Ehlers–Danlos syndrome, familial forms of aortic aneurysm and dissection, as well as bicuspid aortic valve are genetic conditions that predispose patients to develop an acute aortic syndrome and correlate with earlier presentations. Among these, Marfan's syndrome is the most prevalent connective tissue disorder with an incidence of one in 7,000. The underlying defect is a mutation on the fibrillin-1 gene, which results in defective fibrillin in the extracellular matrix.[22]

Ehlers–Danlos syndrome is another inherited connective tissue disorder characterized by tissue fragility. The familial form of aortic disease has been localized to mutations on the fibrillin-1 gene, similar to Marfan's syndrome. Characteristic to each of the different genetic disorders is a similar pathophysiology that includes a dedifferentiation of vascular smooth muscle cells and enhanced elastolysis of aortic wall components. In addition, increased expression of metalloproteinases promotes fragmentation of elastic tissue in the medial layer.[22]

Matrix Metalloproteins

The matrix metalloproteins are a group of proteins whose primary function is to degrade extracellular matrix. Patients with thoracic aortic disease have been shown to have increased levels of these enzymes, which favor proteolysis within the aortic wall. There are still many unanswered questions related to the role these enzymes play in AAS; however, they may serve as a marker for aortic pathology or their inhibition may slow the progression of disease.[23]

Clinical Presentation

AAS is characterized clinically by "aortic pain," most often in a patient with a coexisting history of hypertension. The early recognition of pain associated with progressive aortic lesions is of paramount importance. Table 2.3 lists various presenting symptoms and signs of AAS and Table 2.4 lists the most common associated conditions. The characteristic findings listed may

Table 2.3 Presenting features of acute aortic syndrome

Chest pain – abrupt, severe, tearing, radiating
Anterior pain or radiation to neck – associated with ascending aorta
Radiation to back or abdomen – associated with descending aorta
Syncope or cerebrovascular accident
Hypertension – SBP > 150 mmHg
Shock or tamponade
Diastolic murmur
Pressure differential in upper extremities
Pulse deficits
End-organ ischemia

Table 2.4 Comorbid conditions associated with acute aortic syndrome

History of hypertension
Smoking
Known coronary artery disease
Thoracic or abdominal aortic aneurysm
Peripheral arterial disease
Prior stroke
Chronic renal insufficiency

Fig. 2.7 Types of visceral
organ malperfusion with
aortic dissections
(Reprinted with permis-
sion from Springer[4])

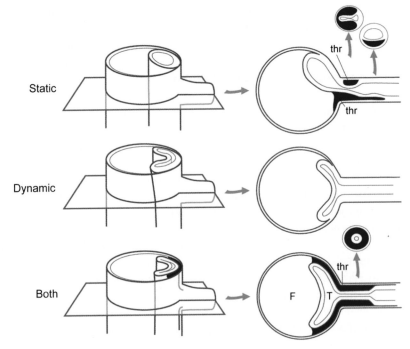

vary or be absent, emphasizing the necessity of a
high level of suspicion in order to avoid diagnostic delays and poor outcomes.

The pain caused by PAU and IMH is similar to
classic aortic dissection. The various types of
AAS cannot be reliably differentiated on clinical
grounds alone. Aortic pain is described as
severely intense, acute, tearing, throbbing, and
radiating.[24] In contrast to the increasing intensity
of dull cardiac pain, AAS is described as being
more abrupt and at maximal intensity from the
onset. In addition, 4.5% of patients deny having
any pain on presentation.[25] Pain located in the
anterior chest and neck is related to involvement
of the ascending aorta and may be easily confounded with that of ischemic syndromes. Back
and abdominal pain may indicate that there is
involvement of the descending aorta. Syncope
may be the presenting symptom in up to 20% of
cases and is associated with a proximal dissection. The onset of syncope or central neurological deficits indicates probable complications such
as obstruction of cerebral vessels, cardiac tamponade, or activation of cerebral baroreceptors.

Other presenting features of AAS may include
end-organ ischemia or pulse deficits.[3] Two types
of distal visceral organ malperfusion are described
(Fig. 2.7). In static obstruction, the dissection
flap enters the origin of the branch and encroaches
on the lumen. If there is no reentry, then the true
lumen will be narrowed to cause ischemia. In
dynamic obstruction, the flap prolapses and
obstructs the origin of the vessel without entering
the vessel. Static and dynamic obstruction may
be combined to contribute to branch obstruction.

Diagnostic Evaluation

As diagnostic modalities have improved over the
past 2 decades, the awareness of AAS has
increased significantly. PAU and IMH were virtually unknown in the prior era of aortic imaging by
aortography. These disorders were not classified
as being distinct entities until the mid-1980s.
In the current era of three-dimensional, high-
resolution imaging by computerized tomography
(CT), magnetic resonance (MR) imaging, and

transesophageal echocardiography (TEE), these two disorders have become increasingly recognized. The sensitivity and specificity of different imaging techniques and their comparison are given in Table 2.5.[26] The goals of diagnostic imaging in patients with suspected AAS are confirmation of the diagnosis, classification and type of aortic pathology, tear localization, and identification of signs indicating the need for emergent intervention (pericardial, mediastinal, or pleural hemorrhage).[2] Additional information includes arch and branch vessel involvement. Each imaging modality has distinct advantages (Table 2.6) and most patients require multiple imaging studies to diagnose and characterize the underlying aortic pathology.[27]

Electrocardiogram

An ECG is an important first diagnostic test performed for all patients presenting with acute chest pain, whether typical or atypical for an acute aortic syndrome. The differentiation of AAS from acute coronary syndrome (ACS) is important; however, it must be remembered the ACS may occur as a result of AAS.

Chest Radiography

While rapid imaging plays a crucial role in the diagnosis of AAS, the role of chest radiography has become limited, especially for conditions

Table 2.5 Results of meta-analysis – diagnostic accuracy of different imaging modalities for suspected aortic dissection (Reprinted with permission from American Medical Association[16])

Imaging technique	Number of studies	Sensitivity	Specificity	Positive likelihood ratio	Negative likelihood ratio
TEE	10	98 (95–99)	95 (92–97)	14.1 (6.0–33.2)	0.04 (0.02–0.08)
Helical CT	3	100 (96–100)	98 (87–99)	13.9 (4.2–46.0)	0.02 (0.01–0.11)
MRI	7	98 (95–99)	98 (95–100)	25.3(11.1–57.1)	0.05 (0.03–0.10)

Data reported with 95% confidence intervals. Likelihood ratios greater than 10 and less than 0.1 are considered strong evidence to confirm or ruling out the diagnosis of aortic dissection

Table 2.6 Comparison of imaging modalities (Reproduced with permission from Oxford University press and the primary author Professor Raimund Erbel[56])

	TTE/TEE	CT	MRI	Angiography	IVUS
Sensitivity	++	++	+++	++	+++
Specificity	+++	++	+++	++	+++
Classification	+++	++	++	+	++
Tear localization	+++	–	++	+	+
Aortic regurgitation	+++	–	++	++	–
Pericardial effusion	+++	++	++	–	–
Mediastinal hematoma	++	+++	+++	–	+
Side branch involvement	+	++	++	+++	+++
Coronary artery involvement	++	–	+	+++	++
X-ray exposure	–	++	–	+++	–
Patient comfort	+	++	+	+	+
Follow-up studies	++	++	+++	–	–
Intraoperative availability	+++	–	–	(+)	(+)

TTE/TEE – transthoracic/transoesophageal echocardiography; CT – computed tomography; MRI – magnetic resonance imaging; IVUS – intravascular ultrasound

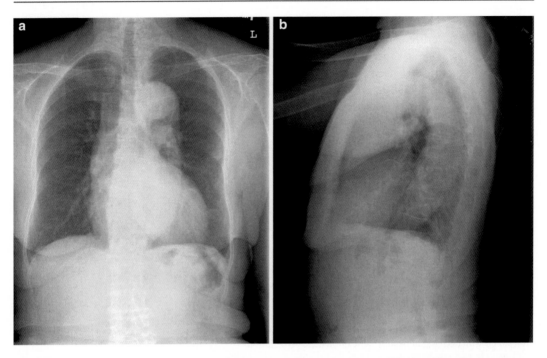

Fig. 2.8 PA (**a**) and lateral Chest X-Rays (**b**) demonstrating a dilated thoracic aorta and widened mediastinum

confined to the ascending aorta. In a study of 216 patients over a 6-year period, the sensitivity for aortic disease was 64%, with a specificity of 86%. The sensitivity for lesions of the ascending aorta was 47%, while that for disease involving distal aortic segments was 77%.[28] A chest X-ray may show widening of the aortic contour, displaced calcification, aortic kinking, or opacification of the aortopulmonary window (Fig. 2.8a and b).

Computerized Tomography (CT)

When AAS is suspected based on clinical presentation and an acute coronary syndrome has been excluded, cardiac-gated, contrast-enhanced multidetector CT angiography is nearly 100% sensitive and specific in the diagnosis, differentiation and staging of AAS.[29] Modern CT machines have up to 64 rows of detectors, and this enables them to generate multiple simultaneous images with a slice thickness of less than 1 mm. Multidetector CT is also extremely fast with spiral imaging of the entire thorax can be done in a single

breath-hold, which eliminates respiratory motion artifact. Cardiac gating is done to avoid artifacts produced because of the imaging being obtained during different phases of cardiac cycle. CT allows for a complete diagnostic evaluation of the thoracic aorta, including the lumen, aortic wall, and periaortic region. Both unenhanced and enhanced images are valuable. Unenhanced scans depict intramural hematoma (crescent shaped or circumferential wall thickening) and thrombosis of the false lumen. Contrast-enhanced imaging allows demonstration of an intimal flap, which is the most reliable finding in the diagnosis of dissection (Fig. 2.9a and b). Contrast differences between arterial and venous phase can help differentiate true and false lumens. Interestingly, it can be difficult to differentiate an aneurysm with thrombus from a dissection with a thrombosed false lumen. Intimal calcifications are displaced by a false lumen in the latter case.[30]

The diagnosis of IMH and PAU are also highly accurate with CT.[31,32] The diagnosis of PAU is made by the demonstration of an outpouching of the aortic wall with rough edges (Fig. 2.10).

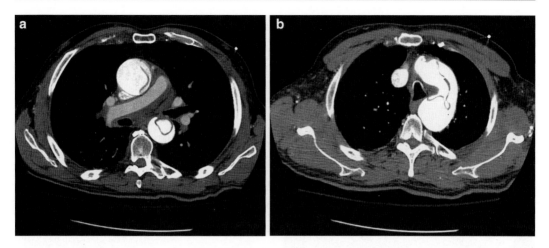

Fig. 2.9 Contrast-enhanced chest CT clearly depicting a type A dissection. The intimal flap is seen in the ascending and descending aorta (**a**) as well as the aortic arch (**b**)

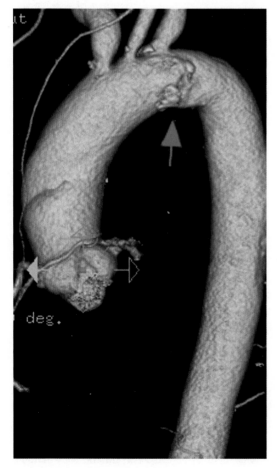

Fig. 2.10 CT reconstructions demonstrating PAU of the arch and descending aorta as indicated by arrows

The ulcer is usually surrounded by extensive atherosclerotic plaques. CT imaging of the aorta should include the iliac arteries for possible endovascular intervention and aortic arch branches to evaluate the extent of dissection and possible neurological complications. Other benefits of CT are its availability and noninvasiveness. The major drawbacks of CT are the exposure to large doses of ionizing radiation and contrast agents.[29] In addition, CT does not offer the capability to assess for aortic insufficiency or involvement of the coronary arteries.

Magnetic Resonance Imaging (MRI)

MRI is a valuable diagnostic tool for the diagnosis of acute aortic syndrome. MRI can be highly accurate even without the use of contrast. Although MRI has the highest sensitivity and specificity for the detection of all forms of aortic pathology and provides superior anatomic detail when compared to other imaging modalities, it is limited by availability, expense, and patient restrictions such as pacemakers, aneurysm clips, or other metal devices. Prolonged scanning time and limited access to unstable patients are other limitations. For these reasons, MRI is not a widely used tool (<5% of patients in IRAD)[3] (Fig. 2.11).

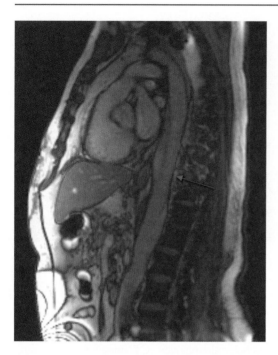

Fig. 2.11 MRI of the chest showing a descending aortic dissection

Echocardiography

Transthoracic echocardiography (TTE) can be used as screening tool for the diagnosis of AAS of the proximal aorta. TTE is useful in the rapid evaluation of aortic insufficiency, pericardial tamponade, arch vessel involvement, and left ventricular systolic function. Hemodynamically unstable patients in whom TTE has shown peri-cardial effusion to be present should be taken to the operating room for airway stabilization and further TEE evaluation. Thus, cardiac surgeons rely on echocardiography more than other imaging modalities including CTA in emer-gency situations.[33] A TEE can be done while the surgeon simultaneously prepares to open the chest.

Transesophageal echocardiography (TEE) is highly sensitive and specific in diagnosing tho-racic aortic pathologies. The only limitation is in the distal ascending aorta and proximal arch which are not clearly visualized by TEE in

most patients. Evaluation of the aortic valve and suitability for repair can be done with TEE. The diagnosis of an IMH is characterized by crescentric aortic wall thickening, the absence of an intimal flap and a lack of false lumen color flow typical of dissection. The primary limiting factor in the use of TEE is the requirement for a skilled echocardiographer to be immediately available to perform and interpret results in emer-gency situations.[29] A further detailed description of TEE examinations for aortic pathology is described elsewhere in this textbook.

Aortography

Since the development of newer, noninvasive imaging modalities, there has been a shift away from invasive techniques for imaging the aorta. Traditionally, aortography had been the gold standard for the diagnosis of aortic dissection. Its primary limitations include its invasive nature and further risk of intimal damage, the use of contrast agents, as well as limited visualization of thrombosed dissections, IMH, and occluded branch vessels. The specificity for diagnosing aortic dissection is >95%, but the sensitivity only averages 90%.[2] Intravascular ultrasound (IVUS) with high-frequency transducers (8–10 MHz) has been used to complement conventional angiogra-phy in the diagnosis of acute dissection. IVUS probes are advanced through guidewire and guid-ing catheters under fluoroscopy to evaluate the aorta from inside and provide useful information about the vessel wall and pathology.

Management

Once there is a suspicion of AAS, patients should be rapidly stabilized and transported to a tertiary care center with adequate aortic surgical and endovascular surgical expertise. It is there that further imaging and management should take place. Figure 2.12 provides an algorithm for the rapid evaluation and treatment of patients presenting with a suspected AAS.[29,34]

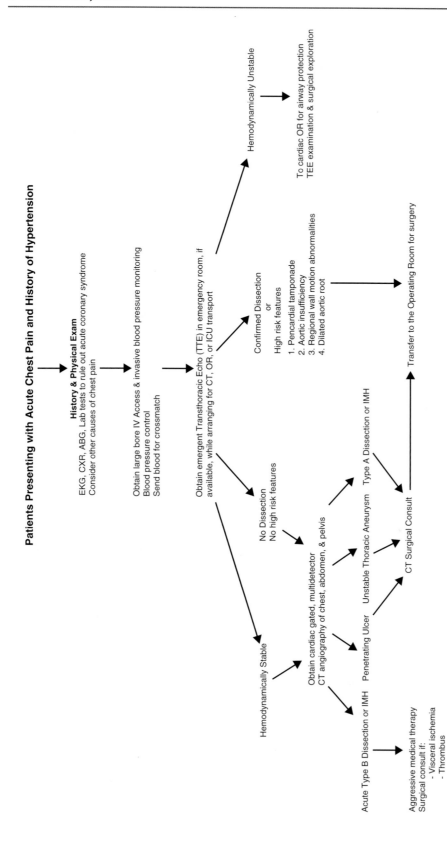

Fig. 2.12 Acute aortic syndrome management algorithm (Modified and reprinted with permission from the following resources[29,34])

Although the treatment of AAS remains a therapeutic challenge, diverse surgical and percutaneous strategies continue to evolve. There are many factors that affect management decision as listed in Table 2.7. One third of the mortality associated with AAS is the result of end-organ failure, which emphasizes the importance of early intervention. The goal of treatment is to prevent the progression of the disease and its lethal complications.

The initial management of all patients with AAS involves pain relief and aggressive blood pressure control. In normalizing the blood pressure, the goal is to reduce the force of left ventricular ejection (dP/dt), which is the primary cause of dissection extension and aortic rupture. Beta-blockers are the preferred agents because they not only reduce systemic pressure but also

lower heart rate. For most patients, the goal is a systolic pressure between 100 and 120 mmHg and heart rate <60 bpm or the lowest tolerable levels that provide adequate cerebral, coronary, and renal perfusion. Less is known about the role of calcium channel blockers for patients who are β-blocker intolerant, but they should reduce blood pressure without causing reflex tachycardia. If neither of the above agents is adequate to control the blood pressure, vasodilators may be added. However, they should never be used as an initial form of therapy before starting β-blockers because of the reflex tachycardia and increase in the force of left ventricular ejection leading to increased aortic wall stress.

Type A Aortic Dissection

Acute ascending aortic pathology (acute dissection, IMH, and PAU) should be treated as a surgical emergency because of the possible risk of life-threatening complications including aortic rupture, pericardial tamponade, and high early mortality (Fig. 2.13). Surgery is also aimed to relieve aortic regurgitation and reestablish coronary and branch vessel perfusion. Acute type A dissection has a mortality rate of 1–2% per hour during the first hours of symptom onset and without surgical treatment, the mortality rate is 20% by 24 h, 30% by 48 h, 40% at 1 week, and 50% at 1 month.[35] Even with surgical treatment,

Table 2.7 Patient factors affecting management decisions

| Disease location – type A or B |
| Retrograde extension into the arch and/or ascending aorta |
| Rupture or impending rupture |
| Site of entry and reentry |
| Involvement of side branches |
| Branch origin from true or false lumen |
| Risk of end-organ damage |
| Complications – rupture, coronary occlusion, aortic insufficiency, neurological |
| Diameters of the true and false lumens |
| Areas of normal vessel for stent-graft placement |
| Vessel tortuosity |

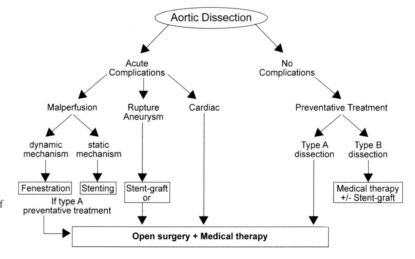

Fig. 2.13 Management of acute aortic dissection (Reprinted with permission from Springer[4])

the mortality rate is as high as 10% by 24 h and 20% at 1 month.[36,37]

Aortic arch and descending thoracic intimal tears are seen in 20–30% of patients with type A dissection and if left untreated predisposes to later distal reoperation.[38,39] Patients who require partial or total arch replacement with reconnection of supraaortic vessels to the graft must often undergo deep hypothermic circularoty arrest with antegrade or retrograde cerebral perfusion. If a dissection extends into the descending thoracic aorta, an elephant trunk extension of the arch graft is an option.[40] In a later procedure, the elephant trunk portion of the graft may be connected to the distal descending aorta, a tubular graft or endovascular graft. There are reports of endovascular repair of the ascending aorta in highly selected patients, but this has most often been for the purpose of temporizing symptoms and preventing disease progression before a more definitive open repair could be performed. It is most often not possible due to the anatomic restrictions of securing the graft in the ascending aorta. The placement of stent grafts has been applied to treat aortic branch occlusions in both type A and B acute aortic dissections. In type A dissections with visceral malperfusion, treatment of the leaking aorta and aortic valve take precedence over visceral malperfusion. However, patients with prolonged limb or bowel ischemia may be unsuitable for proximal aortic surgery, and endovascular treatment to restore perfusion to critical organs is recommended.

Type B Aortic Dissection

Uncomplicated Type B Dissection

Medical management (analgesics and antihypertensive therapy) still remains the main stay of therapy for patients with uncomplicated type B disease. It is safe to treat these patients medically with close follow-up for ischemic complications, disease progression, or aneurysmal enlargement. In a group of 384 patients with type B dissections, 73% were treated medically with a 10% in-hospital mortality. Long-term survival is 60–80% at 5 years.[3] Surgical repair has not been shown to improve outcomes in this group of patients. Recently, a completed randomized study (Investigation of stent grafts in patients with type B aortic dissection-INSTEAD) examined the use of endografts versus medical therapy in uncomplicated dissections. The results did not show any survival benefit at 2 years.[41]

Complicated Type B Dissections

Complicated type B aortic disease is differentiated by the presence of a distal malperfusion syndrome or rapid disease progression. Indications for intervention are similar to those for type A diseases; the prevention of life-threatening complications such as organ or limb ischemia, aneurysm expansion and risk of rupture, periaortic blood collection, intractable pain, aneurysm expansion or uncontrolled hypertension. The mortality rate for open surgical repair (graft replacement, fenestration, or bypass procedures) is 30–35% and even higher with the presence of visceral malperfusion.[42,43] Aortic endovascular grafting may be particularly beneficial in this group and has shown improved mortality rates (16%). The goals of endograft treatment include reconstruction of the aortic segment containing the entry tear, induction of thrombosis in the false lumen, and the reestablishment of flow in the true lumen and branches.[44] In one series, false lumen thrombosis was achieved in 85–100% of patients.

An additional benefit of stent grafts is the ability to relieve dynamic and combined static and dynamic obstructions successfully in complicated acute type B dissections.[45,46] Static obstructions are relieved by placing the graft in the branch vessel and dynamic obstructions may benefit from stents in the true lumen. Endografts have also been used in patients with retrograde type A dissection with intimal tear in the descending aorta to induce false lumen thrombosis.[47] Surgical treatment may be the only option in patients with failed endografts or patients unsuitable for this less-invasive technique.

With either surgical, endograft, or medical management, the risk of further dissection is never eliminated. Therefore, close, regular monitoring, most likely with CT imaging, is necessary to assess for progression or complications.

Intramural Hematoma

Type A Disease

The recommended treatment for patients with Type A IMH is prompt surgical intervention. Proximal IMH are independently associated with potential progression to dissection, aneurysm, and rupture as well as poor clinical outcomes.[17] The risk of a nonsurgical approach to type A IMH demonstrates an early mortality of 55% compared with 8% following surgical repair.[17] However, for patients with significant comorbidities and uncomplicated type A IMH (no dissection or intimal tear, thickness less than 11 mm, aortic diameter less than 50 mm), medical treatment with follow-up imaging and timed surgical intervention has been recommended.

Type B Disease

The management of IMH involving the descending aorta is similar to that recommended for type B dissections. The current literature supports medical management. However, if complications arise (ulceration, expansion, and dilatation), endograft placement may be considered although limited data exists. Endografts may cause erosion of the intima during the acute phase. IMH of the descending aorta have been associated with an in-hospital mortality rate of 10%, similar to that of type B aortic dissection, further emphasizing the importance of correct diagnosis and proper treatment.

Penetrating Aortic Ulcers

There are multiple important factors to identify when diagnosing PAU. One must determine the number (single or multiple), location (type A or B), and associated complications (IMH, dissection, pseudoaneurysm, and rupture). Type A PAU should be treated surgically. Medical therapy is indicated in stable patients with type B PAU.[48] Very few centers advocate any surgical intervention in uncomplicated type B patients because there is a high risk of organ failure and poor

prognosis due to the high likelihood of extensive atherosclerotic disease. For patients with symptomatic or progressive disease, focal PAU in the descending aorta are ideal targets for endograft placement. In a meta-analysis of 58 patients from 13 studies, complete sealing of the ulcer was possible in 94% of patients. Neurologic complications were present in 6% and the in-hospital mortality rate was 5%.[49] Long-term results are not known at this time.

Natural History and Prognosis

The outcomes of patients treated for AAS have improved significantly, although there still remains a high mortality rate in the acute phase. Table 2.8 lists predictors of in-hospital death.[50] Early clinical suspicion and greater surgical expertise appear to be the most important factors in reducing mortality.

Type A aortic dissections are highly lethal. Overall, mortality at 1 month is 20% with and 50% without surgical treatment for type A dissections. The risk of death is higher if there are complications of pericardial tamponade, involvement of the coronary arteries causing acute myocardial ischemia, or a malperfusion syndrome. Age greater than 70 has been identified as an independent risk factor for hospital death for acute type A dissection. Shock, hypotension, and tamponade are other risk factors for increased mortality.[37]

For type B dissections, the overall mortality rate is 10% with medical treatment. Circulatory shock and visceral ischemia predispose to a higher mortality in type B dissection.[51]

Table 2.8 Predictors of in-hospital death

Age >70
Abrupt onset of pain
Hypotension/cardiac tamponade/shock
Abnormal EKG
Kidney failure
Pulse deficits
Iatrogenic cause

Following the acute-phase, mid- to long-term survival depends not only on the underlying aortic disease but also other comorbidities. In patients with surgically corrected type A dissections, survival differences were based on the presence or absence of distal false lumen flow. In one study, the absence of a false lumen was achieved in 53% of patients compared to 10–20% in most series. In patients with absent false lumen flow, the survival was 85% at 6 years compared to 62% in patients with persistent false lumen flow.[37] At 10 years, the survival rate was 44% for corrected type A dissections compared to 32% in medically treated type B dissections.[51] The primary reasons for higher, long-term mortality in type B dissections were aneurysmal expansion and rupture. Dilatation in the descending aorta was greater in medically treated type B dissections compared to operated type A dissections. Dilatation occurs at a faster rate in patients with false lumen flow when compared to absent false lumen flow in type B dissections.[52] Junoven et al. described rupture in 18% and rapid expansion requiring surgery in 20% of patients with type B dissection at 3 years.[53] The impact of early endovascular treatment on the long-term survival of type B dissections is yet to be determined.

In patients with type A IMH, Kaji et al.[54] reported that surgery was required in 43% of patients during the acute phase and, among those discharged without surgery (57%), complete resolution occurred in 40% of patients. Type B IMH has a better long-term prognosis than type B dissections with 5-year survival reported between 43% and 90%.[17,55] Close follow-up with imaging techniques is recommended in patients undergoing medical treatment to look for complications (dilatation, pseudoaneurysm formation, and dissection).

Prevention and Follow-Up

At a time when there is an increasing elderly population, the awareness of such conditions as AAS is likely to continue to rise. This is due to improvements in diagnostic modalities, longer life expectancy, and longer exposure to elevated blood pressure. In order to best treat these patients, continued improvements in diagnostic imaging and therapeutic strategies are necessary, and a focus on surveillance and prevention will further reduce the morbidity and mortality associated with aortic pathology.

One possibility for the surveillance of patients at risk for the development or progression of AAS is the development of biomarkers, which would enable serum diagnosis. In addition, this would provide a fast and economic means of differentiating patients who present to the emergency room with chest pain. Possible markers currently include an assay for circulating smooth muscle myosin heavy chain protein, soluble elastin fragments and acute-phase reactants such as C-reactive protein, fibrinogen, and D-dimer.

All patients with a known aortic disease require close surveillance following discharge. Lifelong treatment of hypertension is required and regular assessments of the aorta should be performed at 1, 3, 6, 9, and 12 months as well as every 6–12 months thereafter, depending on the aortic size. The most important findings on imaging are aortic diameter, signs of aneurysm formation, and hemorrhage at surgical anastamosis or stent-graft sites. The close follow-up emphasizes the fact that aortic disease progression is not easy to predict. Repeated surgery is required in 12–30% of patients due to extension or recurrence of dissection, aneurysm formation, graft dehiscence, aortic insufficiency, or infection.[26]

Conclusion

Significant advances have been made in the diagnosis and management of acute aortic dissections over the past 2 decades. These advancements have led to a better understanding of aortic pathology and led to the discovery of variants that are collectively termed acute aortic syndrome. Despite a persistent level of uncertainty in the diagnosis and management of this lethal disorder, advances are being made and patient outcomes are improving.

Key Notes

1. The clinical progress of patients with AAS is unpredictable. A high level of suspicion is required for early diagnosis and crucial for patient survival.
2. The most common risk factor for AAS is hypertension, with men being affected more often.
3. Any mechanism that causes intimal damage and leads to weakening of the medial layers of the aortic wall can result in dissection, IMH, or PAU.
4. Acute aortic dissection, the most common etiology of AAS, is characterized by an intimal tear which is often preceded by medial wall degeneration or cystic medial necrosis.
5. IMH, a variant of aortic dissection, originates from a disruption of the vasa vasorum within the media. They are treated similar to dissections and have a similar prognosis.
6. PAU is associated with atherosclerotic disease and can lead to dissection or perforation. Both IMH and PAU are found most often in the descending aorta.
7. AAS may present in many ways. Most often there is the sudden onset of severe, sharp chest pain or back pain.
8. Type A aortic dissections are associated with high mortality rates and without surgery, 30-day mortality exceeds 50%.
9. Uncomplicated type B dissections have a 30-day mortality of 10% and may be managed medically. Complications require surgical intervention or endovascular stenting.
10. CT, MRI, and TEE are all accurate in the diagnosis of AAS.
11. The initial treatment of all patients with AAS is blood pressure control in order to decrease the force of left ventricular contraction and lower the risk of dissection extension or rupture. Beta-blockers are the preferred first-line agent to achieve a systolic pressure <120 mmHg and heart rate <60 bpm.
12. Surgery is the definitive treatment of type A acute aortic pathology. The goal is to prevent life-threatening complications such as aortic rupture or pericardial tamponade.
13. Medical therapy with β-blockers and antihypertensive agents is the recommended therapy for patients with uncomplicated type B aortic dissection, IMH, or PAU.
14. The advent and incorporation of less-invasive endovascular treatments has opened up new perspectives in the treatment of acute aortic disease and continued advances will result in improved patient outcomes.

References

1. Svensson LG, Labib SB, Eisenhauer AC, Butterly JR. Intimal tear without hematoma: an important variant of aortic dissection that can elude current imaging techniques. *Circulation*. 1999;99:1331–1336.
2. Tsai TT, Nienaber CA, Eagle KA. Acute aortic syndromes. *Circulation*. 2005;112:3802–3813.
3. Hagan PG, Nienaber CA, Isselbacher EM, et al. The International Registry of Acute Aortic Dissection (IRAD): new insights into an old disease. *JAMA*. 2000;283:897–903.
4. Evangelista A, Gonzalez-Alujas T. Pathophysiology of aortic dissection. In: Rousseau H, Verhoye JP, Heautot JF, eds. *Thoracic aortic Diseases*. 1st ed. Berlin Heidelberg, Germany: Springer; 2006:33–53.
5. Fleck T, Ehrlich M, Czerny M, et al. Intraoperative iatrogenic type A aortic dissection and perioperative outcome. *Interact Cardiovasc Thorac Surg*. 2006;5:11–14.
6. Elitz T, Kawohl M, Fritzsche D, et al. Aortic dissection after previous coronary artery bypass grafting. *J Card Surg*. 2003;18:519–523.
7. De Smet JM, Stefanidis C. Acute aortic dissection after off pump coronary artery surgery. *Eur J Cardiothorac Surg*. 2003;24:315–317.
8. Okamoto R, Makino K, Saito K, et al. Aorto-coronary dissection during angioplasty in a patient with myxedema. *Jpn Circ J*. 2000 Apr;64(4):316–320.
9. Wyss CA, Steffel J, Lüscher TF. Isolated acute iatrogenic aortic dissection during percutaneous coronary-intervention without involvement of the coronary arteries. *J Invasive Cardiol*. 2008 Jul;20(7):380–382.
10. Kpodonu J, Preventza O, Ramaiah VG, et al. Retrograde type A dissection after endovascular stenting of the descendingthoracic aorta. Is the risk real? *Eur J Cardiothorac Surg*. 2008 Jun;33(6):1014–1018. Epub 2008 Apr 21.
11. Panten RR, Harrison JK, Warner J, Grocott HP. Aortic dissection after angioplasty and stenting of an aortic coarctation:detection by intravascular ultrasonography but not transesophageal echocardiography. *J Am Soc Echocardiogr*. 2001 Jan;14(1):73–76.
12. Sheldon WS, Vandervoort PM, Black IW, Grimm RA, Stewart WJ. Aortic intramural hematoma in patients evaluated for aortic dissection: clinical,

echocardiographic, radiologic and pathologic findings. *Circulation*. 1994;90(Suppl I):I385.

13. Vilacosta I, de Dios RM, Pinto AG. Aortic intramural hematoma during coronary angioplasty: insights into the pathogenesis of intramedial hemorrhage. *J Am Soc Echocardiogr*. 2000;13:403–406.

14. Ganaha F, Miller DC, Sugimoto K, et al. Prognosis of aortic intramural hematoma with and without penetrating atherosclerotic ulcer: a clinical and radiological analysis. *Circulation*. 2002 Jul 16;106(3): 342–348.

15. Nienaber CA, Sievers HH. Intramural hematoma in acute aortic syndrome: more than on variant of dissection? *Circulation*. 2002;106:284–285.

16. Kaji S, Nishigami K, Akasaka T, et al. Prediction of progression or regression of type A aortic intramural hematoma bycomputed tomography. *Circulation*. 1999 Nov 9;100(19 Suppl):II281–II286.

17. Von Kodolitsch Y, Csösz SK, Koschyk DH, et al. Intramural hematoma of the aorta: predictors of progression to dissection and rupture. *Circulation*. 2003 Mar 4;107(8):1158–1163.

18. Hayashi J, Matsuoka Y, Sakamoto I, et al. Penetrating atherosclerotic ulcer of the aortoa: imaging features and disease concept. *RadioGraphics*. 2000;20: 995–1005.

19. Stanson AW, Kazmier FJ, Hollier LH, et al. Penetrating atherosclerotic ulcers of the thoracic aorta: natural history and clinicopathologic correlations. *Ann Vasc Surg*. 1986;1:15–23.

20. Vilacosta I, San Román JA, Aragoncillo P, et al. Penetrating atherosclerotic aortic ulcer: documentation by transesophagealechocardiography. *J Am Coll Cardiol*. 1998;32:83–89.

21. Ando Y, Minami H, Muramoto H, Narita M, Sakai S. Rupture of thoracic aorta caused by penetrating aortic ulcer. *Chest*. 1994;106:624–626.

22. Nienaber CA. Pathophysiology of acute aortic syndromes. In: Baliga RR, Nienaber CA, Isselbacher EM, Eagle KA, eds. *Aortic Dissection and Related Syndromes*. 1st ed. NewYork: Springer Science; 2007:17–44.

23. Botta DM, Elefteriades JA. Matrix metalloproteinases in aortic aneurysm and dissection. In: Elefteriades JA, ed. *Acute Aortic Disease*. 1st ed. NewYork: Informa Healthcare; 2007:131–146.

24. Wooley CF, Sparks EH, Boudoulas H. Aortic pain. *Prog Cardiovasc Dis*. 1998;40:563–589.

25. Ahmad F, Cheshire N, Hamady M. Acute aortic syndrome: pathology and therapeutic strategies. *Postgrad Med J*. 2006;82:305–312.

26. Shiga T, Wajima Z, Apfel CC, Inoue T, Ohe Y. Diagnostic accuracy of transesophageal echocardiography, helical computed tomography, and magnetic resonance imaging for suspected thoracic aortic dissection: systematic review and meta-analysis. *Arch Intern Med*. 2006;166:1350–1356.

27. Kapustin AJ, Litt HI. Diagnostic imaging for aortic dissection. *Semin Thorac Cardiovasc Surg*. 2005;17: 214–223.

28. Von Kodolitsch Y, Nienbar CA, Dieckmann C, et al. Chest radiography for the diagnosis of acute aortic syndrome. *Am J Med*. 2004;116:73–77.

29. Smith AD, Schoenhagen P. CT imaging for acute aortic syndrome. *Cleve Clin J Med*. 2008;75:7–9.

30. Berger F, Smithuis R, van Delden O. Thoracic Aorta – the Acute Aortic Syndrome. www.radiologyassistant. nl/en. Accessed May 25, 2009.

31. Reddy GP. Multidetector CT of acute aortic syndrome. *Imag Decision*. 2006;2:22–26.

32. Manghat NE, Morgan-Hughes GJ, Roobottom CA. Multi-detector row computed tomography: imaging in acute aortic syndrome. *Clin Radiol*. 2005;60:1256–1267.

33. Svensson LG. Acute aortic syndromes: time to talk of many things. *Cleve Clin J Med*. 2008;75:25–29.

34. Meredith EL, Masani ND. Echocardiography in the emergency assessment of acute aortic syndromes. *Eur J Echocardiogr*. 2009;10:i31–i39.

35. Hagan PG, Nienaber CA, Isselbacher EM, et al. The International Registry of Acute Aortic Dissection (IRAD): new insights into an old disease. *JAMA*. 2000;283:897–903.

36. Mehta RH, O'Gara PT, Bossone E, et al. Acute type A aortic dissection in the elderly: clinical characteristics, management, and outcomes in the current era. *J Am Coll Cardiol*. 2002;40:685–692.

37. Mehta RH, Suzuki T, Hagan PG, et al. Predicting death in patients with acute type A aortic dissection. *Circulation*. 2002;105:200–206.

38. Ergin MA, O'Connor J, Guinto R, Griepp RB. Experience with profound hypothermia and circulatory arrest in the treatment of aneurysms of the aortic arch. Aortic arch replacement for acute arch dissections. *J Thorac Cardiovasc Surg*. 1982;84:649–655.

39. Nguyen B, Müller M, Kipfer B, et al. Different techniques of distal aortic repair in acute type A dissection: impacton late aortic morphology and reoperation. *Eur J Cardiothorac Surg*. 1999;15:496–500.

40. Borst HG, Walterbusch G, Schaps D. Extensive aortic replacement using elephant trunk prosthesis. *Thorac Cardiovasc Surg*. 1983;31:37–40.

41. Isselbacher EM. Dissection of the descending thoracic aorta: looking into the future. *J Am Coll Cardiol*. 2007;50:805–807.

42. Heinemann MK, Buehner B, Schaefers HJ, Jurmann MJ, Laas J, Borst HG. Malperfusion of the thoracoabdominal vasculature in aortic dissection. *J Card Surg*. 1994;9:748–755.

43. Borst HG, Laas J, Heinemann M. Type A aortic dissection: diagnosis and management of malperfusion phenomena. *Semin Thorac Cardiovasc Surg*. 1991;3:238–241.

44. Ince H, Nienaber CA. The concept of interventional therapy in acute aortic syndrome. *J Card Surg*. 2002;17:135–142.

45. Slonim SM, Miller DC, Mitchell RS, Semba CP, Razavi MK, Dake MD. Percutaneous balloon fenestration and stenting for life-threatening ischemic complications in patients with acute aortic dissection. *J Thorac Cardiovasc Surg*. 1999;117:1118–1126.

46. Slonim SM, Nyman UR, Semba CP, Miller DC, Mitchell RS, Dake MD. True lumen obliteration in complicated aortic dissection: endovascular treatment. *Radiology*. 1996;201:161–166.

47. Kato N, Shimono T, Hirano T, Ishida M, Yada I, Takeda K. Transluminal placement of endovascular stent-grafts for the treatment of type A aortic dissection with an entry tear in the descending thoracic aorta. *J Vasc Surg*. 2001;34:1023–1028.

48. Tittle SL, Lynch RJ, Cole PE, et al. Midterm follow-up of penetrating ulcer and intramural hematoma of the aorta. *J Thorac Cardiovasc Surg*. 2002;123:1051–1059.

49. Eggebrecht H, Baumgart D, Schmermund A, et al. Penetrating atherosclerotic ulcer of the aorta: treatment by endovascular stent-graft placement. *Curr Opin Cardiol*. 2003;18:431–435.

50. Song JK, Kang SJ, Song JM, et al. Factors associated with in-hospital mortality in patients with acute aortic syndrome involving the ascending aorta. *Int J Cardiol*. 2007;115:14–18.

51. Nienaber CA, Eagle KA. Aortic dissection:new frontiers in diagnosis and management. *Circulation*. 2003;108:628–635.

52. Sueyoshi E, Sakamoto I, Hayashi K, Yamaguchi T, Imada T. Growth rate of aortic diameter in patients with type B aortic dissection during the chronic phase. *Circulation*. 2004;110(11 Suppl 1):II256–II261.

53. Junoven T, Ergin MA, Galla JD, et al. Risk factors for rupture of chronic type B dissections. *J Thoac Cardiovasc Surg*. 1999;117:776–786.

54. Kaji S, Akasaka T, Boribata Y, et al. Long term prognosis of patients with type A intramural hematoma. *Circulation*. 2002;106:248–252.

55. Kaji S, Akasaka T, Katayama M, et al. Long term prognosis of patients with type B intramural hematoma. *Circulation*. 2003;108:307–331.

56. Erbel R, Alfonso F, Boileau C, et al. Diagnosis and management of aortic dissection: task force on aortic dissection, European society of cardiology. *Eur Heart J*. 2001;22:1642–1681.

Preoperative Cardiac Evaluation Before Aortic Surgery

3

Kyung W. Park

Each year in the USA, nearly 30 million patients are estimated to undergo noncardiac surgery, and about one third of these patients have coronary artery disease (CAD) or risk factors for CAD.[1] About one million of those patients have perioperative cardiac complications that result in more than $20 billion in health-care expenditures.[1] The current standards for preoperative cardiac evaluation of these patients are the guidelines published by the American College of Cardiology (ACC) and the American Heart Association (AHA), initially in 1996[2] and updated in 2002[3] and again in 2007.[4] These guidelines were developed based on a review of the then-available literature and the opinions of experts from the disciplines of anesthesiology, cardiology, electrophysiology, vascular medicine, vascular surgery, and noninvasive cardiac testing.

The latest guidelines provide a five-step algorithm for stratifying patients' risks and triaging patients to surgery or cardiac evaluation. For aortic surgery, Step 3 of the algorithm, which asks whether the proposed surgery is a low-risk surgery, is irrelevant, so that the guidelines may be reduced to four steps. Aortic surgeries and other major vascular surgeries are classified as high risk for the purpose of the guidelines, meaning that these surgeries are generally associated

with 5% or greater risk of adverse cardiac events in the perioperative period.[4] The remaining four steps consider (1) whether the operation is emergent, (2) whether the patient has any acute cardiac conditions, (3) whether the patient has good functional capacity without symptoms, and (4) what clinical risk factors or comorbidities the patient brings to surgery. Consideration of how recently the patient has had a favorable cardiac evaluation or therapeutic cardiac intervention such as coronary revascularization is no longer deemed necessary in the latest guidelines.[3,4]

Step 1 of the guidelines is to consider if the surgery is emergent. If the proposed surgery is emergent, the patient should be taken to the operating room (OR) without any delay for preoperative cardiac evaluation. Any necessary cardiac evaluation may be performed either intraoperatively with, for instance, the use of transesophageal echocardiography or postoperatively, after the patient survives the emergent operation.

If the proposed surgery is not emergent, then in Step 2, one considers whether the patient has any acute cardiac conditions. These used to be called major clinical predictors in the earlier versions of the guidelines. Examples of acute cardiac conditions include unstable coronary syndromes, acute (<1 week) or recent (<1 month) myocardial infarction (MI), decompensated congestive heart failure (CHF), significant arrhythmias, and severe valvular diseases. Significant arrhythmias include a high-grade AV block, a newly recognized ventricular tachycardia, or atrial fibrillation with a

K.W. Park (✉)
Departments of Anesthesia and of Surgery,
The Ohio State University Medical Center,
Doan Hall 168, 450 W. 10th Avenue,
Columbus, OH, USA
e-mail: Tim.park@osumc.edu

K. Subramaniam et al. (eds.), *Anesthesia and Perioperative Care for Aortic Surgery*,
DOI 10.1007/978-0-387-85922-4_3, © Springer Science+Business Media, LLC 2011

rapid ventricular response. Severe valvular diseases are exemplified by severe aortic stenosis with a gradient >40 mmHg or aortic valve area <1.0 cm^2 or severe mitral stenosis symptomatic of progressive dyspnea on exertion, exertional presyncope or syncope or heart failure. If the patient has acute cardiac condition(s), then it is advised that they are managed or addressed before the patient is taken to the OR.

Step 4 of the guidelines considers whether the patient has good functional capacity without cardiac symptoms. A patient has poor functional capacity if he or she is unable to perform activities of greater than four metabolic equivalents (METs) without becoming symptomatic of chest pain or shortness of breath. One MET is the resting metabolic rate or the amount of oxygen consumed while sitting at rest, which is 3.5 mL/kg/min. Examples of activities that require less than four METs include driving (2 METs), cooking (2.5 METs), bowling (2–4 METs), walking for exercise at 5 km/h or less (<3.3 METs), raking leaves (3–4 METs), and golfing while riding a cart (2–3 METs).[5] Example of activities that require more than four METs include walking at 7 km/h (5.3 METs), walking up stairs (4.7 METs), snow shoveling (5.1 METs), and washing windows (4.9 METs).[5] If the patient does not have a poor functional capacity, then no further cardiac workup is recommended before taking the patient to the OR.

Step 5 considers the presence of clinical risk factors, which used to be called the intermediate clinical risk factors in earlier guidelines. These factors are stable angina, history of MI more than 1 month ago or Q waves on EKG, compensated CHF, diabetes mellitus, chronic renal insufficiency with serum creatinine greater than 2 mg/dL, and history of cerebrovascular disease. All other risk factors such as advanced age and hypertension do not figure into the triage decision. If the patient has none of the clinical risk factors, no further cardiac evaluation is indicated. If the patient has three or more clinical risk factors, noninvasive cardiac testing may be performed, if it will change management. When the patient has one or two clinical risk factors, it is up to the clinician to decide for or against any additional workup, if it will change management.

For aortic surgery, the entire guidelines on preoperative cardiac evaluation may be summarized as follows:

- If the operation is emergent, go to the OR.
- If the patient has an acute cardiac condition, manage it before going to the OR.
- If the patient has good functional capacity or has no clinical risk factors, go to the OR without further workup.
- If the patient has clinical risk factors, additional cardiac workup may be considered, but only if it will change management.

The key phrase in considering preoperative cardiac workup before aortic surgery is "if it will change management." The ACC/AHA guidelines do not specify how to change management. Rather the task is left up to the clinician to weigh the benefits and risks based on available literature and make clinical decisions. In the remaining chapter, we examine what value noninvasive cardiac testing may bring, what, if any, the role of prophylactic revascularization may be, and what changes in management may be considered perioperatively.

Noninvasive Cardiac Testing

Noninvasive cardiac tests assess myocardial function or perfusion. Tests of myocardial systolic function include transthoracic echocardiography and radionuclide scanning, in which the left ventricular ejection fraction (LVEF) is often reported as if it were the sine qua non of myocardial function. While a few small studies[6,7] have reported a correlation between preoperative LVEF and perioperative cardiac events, larger series have generally found that echocardiographic measurement of a low LVEF might be specific of cardiac complications, and thus, have a high negative predictive value (i.e., when the EF is not low, cardiac complications are unlikely), but is not a sensitive indicator, so it has a low positive predictive value (i.e., even when the EF is low, cardiac complications are still infrequent).[8] In a position paper, the American College of Physicians recommends against noninvasive assessment of resting LVEF by radionuclide angiography or transthoracic echocardiography to predict perioperative cardiac risk.[9]

Many patients who have a clinical diagnosis of CHF and normal systolic function might have diastolic dysfunction.[10] A detailed assessment of diastolic function can be provided by echocardiography, and a scoring system has been proposed.[11] But so far no studies have demonstrated the prognostic value of preoperative diastolic dysfunction in noncardiac surgical patients. Information obtained from preoperative echocardiography may change management in cases of (a) a murmur detected on preoperative physical examination that might indicate significant aortic or mitral stenosis, (b) a previously unrecognized pathologic murmur that might necessitate antibiotic prophylaxis, and (c) physical examination suggestive of previously unrecognized significant left ventricular dysfunction.[12]

Noninvasive tests of myocardial perfusion might be classified by the type of stress applied to elicit transient and reversible ischemia or by the mode of detecting the ischemic area.[13] Stress can be applied by exercise (e.g., treadmill, sitting or supine bicycle, or handgrip), by a pharmacologic agent that increases chronotropy and inotropy (e.g., dobutamine, atropine), or by a pharmacologic agent that can cause malredistribution of coronary blood flow (e.g., dipyridamole, adenosine). A significant fraction of the high-risk population cannot exercise to an adequate level and will require pharmacological stress testing. An ischemic event might be suggested or detected by the patient's reporting of symptoms, appropriate ECG changes (horizontal or downsloping ST segment depression of ≥ 0.1 mV or ST elevation of ≥ 0.15 mV in two contiguous leads[14]), reversible wall motion abnormalities on echocardiography, or reversible perfusion defects on radionuclide imaging with thallium or technetium.

Dobutamine stress echocardiography (DSE) and dipyridamole thallium imaging (DTI) have high negative predictive values that approach 100% but have low positive predictive values that are generally less than 20%.[15] The likelihood ratio of a positive test, which indicates how much the odds of a cardiac event increase when the test is positive, is computed as (1 − sensitivity) / specificity, whereas the likelihood ratio of a negative test, which indicates how much the odds of a cardiac event decrease when the test is negative, is computed

as (1−sensitivity)/specificity. For a test to be considered to be useful in risk stratification, the likelihood ratio of a positive or negative test should be greater than 10 or less than 0.2, respectively, because these numbers indicate a substantial change in risk from the pretest level.[15] While the likelihood ratios of negative DSE and DTI are often good, the likelihood ratios of positive tests are usually much less than 10, so these tests might not yield any useful information for risk stratification.[15]

Furthermore, in a review of 85 patients,[16] even when DSE was obtained in accordance with the ACC/AHA guidelines, the test was positive in only 4.7% of the patients. Thus, even when the guidelines are followed, not only is it unlikely that the stress test will be positive, but even when the test is positive, the likelihood of an adverse event is too low for the test to be considered to be discriminating in most circumstances.

Rather, the study by Lee et al.[17] suggests that simple consideration of clinical risk factors might be sufficient in risk stratification. Lee et al. first identified six clinical factors that predicted major cardiac complications in a derivation cohort of 2,893 patients undergoing elective noncardiac surgery. These factors were (1) high-risk surgery, (2) history of CAD, (3) history of cerebrovascular disease, (4) history of CHF, (5) preoperative use of insulin, and (6) preoperative serum creatinine greater than 2 mg/dL. The authors then validated the six factors in a validation cohort of 1,422 patients, in whom the cardiac event rates with 0, 1, 2, or ≥ 3 of the six risk factors were 0.4%, 0.9%, 7%, and 11%, respectively. Therefore, patients who have two or more risk factors can be considered to be at high risk. The key point is that these risk factors can usually be ascertained without subjecting the patient to any noninvasive or invasive cardiac testing.

Risk Modification by Perioperative Medical Therapy

Patients who have suspected or known CAD can undergo major noncardiac surgery with reduced cardiovascular complications when they are given β-adrenergic blockade perioperatively.[18–20] Poldermans et al.[20] studied 112 high-risk patients undergoing elective abdominal aortic or infrainguinal vascular surgeries who had new reversible wall motion abnormalities during preoperative DSE. The patients received bisoprolol or placebo perioperatively, starting at least a week before surgery. Bisoprolol was continued for 30 days, as long as the heart rate remained above 50 beats per minute and the systolic blood pressure was above 100 mmHg; additional doses of intravenous metoprolol was titrated perioperatively if the heart rate exceeded 80 beats per minute. Bisoprolol reduced 30-day mortality from 17% to 3.4% and nonfatal MI from 17% to 0%. The benefit of perioperative bisoprolol lasted until at least 2 years after surgery.[21] The beneficial effect of perioperative β-adrenergic blockade has been demonstrated not only with bisoprolol,[20,21] but also with atenolol,[18,19] esmolol,[22] labetalol,[23] oxprenolol,[23] and metoprolol,[24] so it might be a class effect rather than particular to a specific β-adrenergic blocking agent. More important than which agent is used might be how it is used. Raby et al.[22] advocated using a β-adrenergic blocking agent to keep the heart rate 20% below each patient's ischemic threshold (i.e., the lowest heart rate at which the patient has been demonstrated to experience myocardial ischemia). Such a regimen was shown to be beneficial in a small cohort ($n = 26$) of patients undergoing vascular surgery. Tailoring the dose of the β-adrenergic blocker to each patient might be logical, but no rationale for choosing a target rate 20% below the ischemic threshold has been presented. Furthermore, in many patients the ischemic threshold is not known. A reasonable rule of thumb might be that the anesthesiologist should use a β-adrenergic blocker perioperatively to achieve a heart rate that is lower than the known or suspected ischemic threshold without causing inadequate levels of coronary or cerebral perfusion pressure.

The importance of maintaining end-organ perfusion pressures during perioperative β-adrenergic blockade and titrating the dose to effect was highlighted during the recent POISE trial.[25] The POISE trial was a large international multicenter study that randomized 8,531 patients to receive extended-release metoprolol or a placebo, starting 2–4 h before a major noncardiac surgery and continued for 30 days. As might have been expected, the cardiovascular outcome was better in the study group, with reductions in the composite of cardiovascular death, MI, or cardiac arrest (5.8% vs. 6.9%, $P = 0.0399$) and MI (4.2% vs. 5.7%, $P = 0.0017$). However, all-cause mortality was increased in the metoprolol group (3.1% vs. 2.3%, $P = 0.0317$), as was the incidence of stroke (1.0% vs. 0.5%, $P = 0.0053$). Many of the strokes were ischemic and believed to be due to hypotension. In view of the POISE trial, recommendations regarding perioperative β-blockade may need to be revised.[26] Certainly, patients who have been on a β-blocker previously should be continued on the medication perioperatively, since the risk of withdrawal may be significant.[27] For patients with known CAD or at high risk for it, β-blockade may be indicated for long-term myocardial protection regardless of the surgery. However, in patients in whom CAD or its risk is recognized shortly before surgery, the POISE trial certainly brings to question the advisability of starting a β-blocker de novo immediately preoperatively. If a β-blocker is to be started, it needs to be started as much prior to surgery as possible, so that the clinician can titrate the dose up to the desired endpoint without adverse effects.

Reduction of perioperative cardiac complications with β-adrenergic blockade means that the positive predictive value and the likelihood ratio of a positive result for any preoperative cardiac test are also reduced. Boersma et al.[28] reanalyzed the patient population ($n = 1,351$) screened for Poldermans et al.'s study.[20] Important clinical predictors of adverse cardiac outcome in this population were age ≥70 years, current or prior angina pectoris, history of MI, history of CHF, or history of cerebrovascular accident. Among patients who had less than three clinical risk factors, β-adrenergic blockade lowered the perioperative cardiac complication rate from 2.3% to 0.8%; the results of DSE had no significant additional prognostic value. Among patients who had three or more clinical risk factors and perioperative β-adrenergic blockade, cardiac event rates differed significantly depending on the result of DSE (2% for a negative result vs. 10.6% for a positive result). This difference was mostly accounted for by those who had evidence of extensive ischemia (i.e., five or more ischemic segments), in whom the cardiac complication rate was 36%, whereas patients who had fewer ischemic segments (one to four) had a 2.8% complication rate, which is not significantly different from that of patients who had a negative test. Thus, with anticipated use of perioperative β-adrenergic blockade, a stress test such as DSE might be indicated if the patient has three or more clinical risk factors such as those identified by Boersma et al.[28] or Lee et al.,[17] but even then a positive result might have prognostic value only if it shows evidence of diffuse CAD.

Stain use has been shown to be beneficial in primary and secondary prevention of cardiovascular events in nonsurgical settings.[29] In addition, several retrospective and prospective studies demonstrated the beneficial effect of statins in reducing perioperative cardiovascular complications.[30–34] In a retrospective review of pharmacy records of 780,591 patients undergoing major noncardiac surgery and surviving at least into the second postoperative day, those who received a lipid-lowering agent had a lower postoperative mortality than the control group after propensity matching (2.18% vs. 3.15%, $P < 0.001$).[30] The number needed to treat with a statin to prevent one postoperative death ranged from only 30 for those with four or more of the clinical risk factors of Lee et al.[17] to 186 for those with none of the factors. Similar benefits of statins have been noted in retrospective reviews of vascular or aortic surgical patients.[31–33] In a prospective randomized trial of 100 vascular patients, of whom 56 were aortic surgical patients, the patients were randomized to receive either atorvastatin or a placebo for 45 days, regardless of their serum cholesterol levels.[34] They underwent the surgery an average of 30 days after randomization and were followed for 6 months for primary endpoints of cardiac death, MI, unstable angina, or stroke. The event rate was much lower in the statin group (8.0% vs. 26.0%, $P = 0.031$).

In addition to β-blockers and statins, there may be other classes of medications that may potentially lower perioperative cardiovascular complications.

Medications being investigated include those that act on the rennin–angiotensin– aldosterone (RAA) axis,[35] $Na^+–K^+$ exchange inhibitors,[36] or caspase inhibitors,[37] but definitive evidence of benefits from these is currently lacking. In a small study of 22 patients undergoing infrarenal aortic surgery, Licker et al. randomized them to receive either enalapril or a placebo immediately before aortic cross-clamping.[38] The treatment group experienced a smaller reduction in cardiac output and glomerular filtration rate with aortic cross-clamping and a significantly higher creatinine clearance on the first postoperative day. Such a study is suggestive of benefits of modulating the RAA axis, but larger studies are needed.

"Prophylactic" Coronary Revascularization?

The value of a positive preoperative stress test might lie in the identification of (a) prohibitively high-risk patients, leading to cancellation of the proposed noncardiac surgery; or (b) patients amenable to therapeutic maneuvers with reduction in risk of the noncardiac surgery. Revascularization by percutaneous transluminal coronary angioplasty (PTCA) with or without stenting or by coronary artery bypass graft surgery (CABG) might confer a long-term, symptom-free survival benefit in a subset of patients who have CAD[39–42]; however, the pathophysiology of perioperative MI differs somewhat from that of an MI in a nonoperative setting in that atherosclerotic plaque rupture and subsequent thrombus formation is not as important, and the significance of an imbalance in the myocardial oxygen supply:demand ratio (such as occurs with tachycardia) is greater in the perioperative period.[15] To triage the patient for coronary revascularization prior to noncardiac surgery to reduce the perioperative cardiac risk of the latter surgery, three conditions should be satisfied: (1) the combined risk of coronary angiography and coronary revascularization should not exceed the risk of the proposed noncardiac surgery performed without revascularization; (2) coronary revascularization should significantly lower the cardiac risk of the subsequently performed noncardiac surgery, with the magnitude of risk reduction preferably greater than the risk of coronary angiography and revascularization; and (3) the recovery time from coronary revascularization should be short enough that the proposed noncardiac surgery, especially if it is urgent, is not unduly delayed. When these conditions are not met, any indicated revascularization can be performed after the noncardiac surgery.

Regarding the first two conditions, Mason et al.[43] performed a decision analysis study in 1995 using the then-available literature data to compare the strategy of proceeding directly to major vascular surgery without any workup (strategy A) to that of coronary angiography followed by selective coronary revascularization before vascular surgery (strategy B). If CAD is found to be inoperable, cancellation of vascular surgery (strategy B-1) or proceeding with vascular surgery nonetheless (strategy B-2) were the options. They found that the overall mortality of strategy A (3.5%) would be lower than that of strategy B-2 (3.8%) and comparable to that of strategy B-1 (3.4%), and that the nonfatal MI or stroke rate as well as the cost of care would be lower with strategy A (5.0%) than with strategy B-1 (6.7%) or B-2 (7.0%).

Comparing more recent data, the national average mortality rate from CABG in the USA was about 2.5% in 2001.[44] The mortality rate was higher if the surgery was accompanied by valve replacement, emergent, non-primary surgeries (i.e., redo surgeries), in women, or in the elderly. Survivors of CABG who then underwent noncardiac surgery were reported to have a mortality of 1.7%.[45] These numbers can be compared with the data of Poldermans et al.,[20] which showed that patients who have positive preoperative DSE who undergo high-risk surgery could have a relatively low 30-day mortality rate of 3.4% and a nonfatal MI rate of 0% with the perioperative use of a β-adrenergic blocker in the absence of revascularization. These numbers would compare favorably to the sequential mortality of CABG and then noncardiac surgery in survivors of CABG. Thus, except possibly in patients who have three or more clinical risk factors and DSE (or a similar test)

showing extensive CAD, the strategy of proceeding with vascular surgery with optimal medical therapy might be favored over that of prophylactic coronary revascularization, unless there is some other reason for getting revascularization.

A direct comparison of different strategies was accomplished by McFalls et al.,[46] who randomized 510 vascular surgical patients with an angiogram-proven CAD and at an increased risk for cardiac complications to either prophylactic revascularization by angioplasty or coronary artery bypass surgery or medical therapy only. There was no significant difference in 30-day perioperative mortality or morbidity or in long-term mortality after a median follow-up of 2.7 years between the study groups. The main difference between the groups was that those who were revascularized had a delay from randomization to vascular surgery. At least for patients with stable cardiac symptoms, it appears that a strategy of revascularization is not supported prior to vascular surgery.

A third prerequisite for prophylactic coronary revascularization is that its benefit should be realized in such a time frame that the proposed noncardiac surgery is not unduly delayed. Posner et al.[47] reported that the risk of adverse cardiac outcomes after noncardiac surgery might be reduced by prior PTCA, but only if the interval between PTCA and the noncardiac surgery was more than 90 days. Furthermore, Kaluza et al.[48] noted that if noncardiac surgery is performed within 40 days of PTCA with a stent, the risk of stent thrombosis and death in the perioperative period might be prohibitively high (eight deaths [six from MI and two from major bleeding complications] in 40 patients, or 20% mortality in their report). Typically, ticlopidine and aspirin are started 3–5 days before PTCA with stenting and continued for 14–30 days depending on the risk of stent thrombosis. The risk of stent occlusion drops off sharply after the initial 30 days. Major surgery might be associated with activation of the procoagulant system, and the risk of stent occlusion might be increased by surgical stresses. What might have been adequate antiplatelet therapy in the nonsurgical period might not prove to be adequate during the perioperative period. Thus, undergoing a major noncardiac surgery during the early post-stenting period poses a significant dilemma in that discontinuation of the antiplatelet therapy increases the risk of stent thrombosis and MI, whereas its continuation (with or without an additional anticoagulant regimen such as heparin) increases the risk of major bleeding complications. If the patient gets a drug-eluting stent or intracoronary brachytherapy, the risk period for in-stent thrombosis may extend as long as a year or longer.[49] Thus, the available data suggest that if the proposed aortic surgery cannot be delayed for 30–40 days after PTCA with a bare metal stent or up to a year after a drug-eluting stent or intracoronary brachytherapy, prophylactic revascularization by PTCA might not be recommended to reduce the cardiac risk.

Regarding the early post-CABG period, Reul et al.[50] reported a 2.7% cardiac death rate (overall mortality 3.9%) in 255 patients who had simultaneous CABG and peripheral vascular surgery, a 2.2% cardiac death rate (overall mortality 3.6%) in 279 patients who had a CABG then peripheral vascular surgery 5 days to 3 weeks after CABG within the same hospitalization, and a 0% cardiac death rate (0.2% overall mortality) in 559 patients who had a CABG then a peripheral vascular surgery during a subsequent hospitalization 1 month to 10 years after CABG. In Breen et al.'s review, patients undergoing aortic or peripheral vascular bypass surgeries within 1 month of CABG ($n = 36$) had a much higher 30-day mortality rate that case-matched controls (20.6% vs. 3.9%, $P < 0.005$).[51] These data suggest that if the patient requires noncardiac surgery that cannot be delayed 30 days or longer and also has indications for coronary revascularization, performing coronary revascularization by PTCA or CABG might not result in improved short-term survival.

Patients with Valvular Stenosis

In the ACC/AHA guidelines,[4] a severe valvular stenosis is considered to be an acute cardiac condition and should lead to consideration of delay or cancellation of the proposed noncardiac surgery, so that the acute cardiac condition can be managed. One may consider echocardiography,

cardiac catheterization, or possible valve surgery. As in the case of patients who have CAD, the decision analysis for patients who have a significant valvular stenosis should consider the relative risks and benefits of the strategy of proceeding directly to noncardiac surgery versus the strategy of diagnostic workup and therapeutic interventions for the valvular abnormality followed by the noncardiac surgery. The initial diagnostic workup of transthoracic echocardiography carries negligible risks and might provide valuable information regarding the aortic valve and, to a lesser extent, the mitral valve. Better delineation of the mitral valve might require transesophageal echocardiography. Any additional intervention with angiography and valve surgery carries significant mortality and morbidity risks (mortality of about 6% for mitral valve replacement and 3.5% for aortic valve replacement in 2001[44]).

In the management of patients who have a significant valve disease who present for major vascular surgery, it is important that the clinician be aware of the pathophysiologic implications of the disease and manage the patient accordingly rather than necessarily subjecting the patient to corrective intervention before the vascular surgery. O'Keefe et al. reported on their experience with 48 patients who had severe aortic stenosis (AS; mean valve area 0.6 cm^2) who were not candidates for (or refused) aortic valve replacement and who needed noncardiac surgery.[52] There was only one cardiac event with no deaths for a complication rate of about 2%, which compares favorably with the 3.5% average mortality rate for aortic valve replacement reported for 2001 by the Society of Thoracic Surgeons.[44] More recently, Raymer and Yang compared 55 patients who had significant AS (mean valve area 0.9 cm^2) with case-matched controls who had similar preoperative risk profiles other than AS who were undergoing similar surgeries.[53] Cardiac complication rates were not significantly different between the groups. Thus, patients who have severe AS can undergo indicated noncardiac surgery safely provided that the presence of severe AS is recognized and they receive intensive intraoperative and perioperative care with full knowledge of the implications of AS.

Data are lacking regarding patients who have severe mitral stenosis or severe valvular regurgitation who undergo noncardiac surgery without prior valve surgery. In case reviews of patients who had severe idiopathic hypertrophic subaortic stenosis, there was a relatively high incidence of postoperative CHF (10–17%), but not MI or cardiac death.[54,55]

Key Notes

1. The American College of Cardiology (ACC) and the American Heart Association (AHA) have published guidelines for preoperative evaluation. As applied to aortic surgeries, the guideline effectively consists of four steps to consider the urgency of the operation, the presence of an acute cardiac condition, the patient's functional capacity, and comorbidities.
2. For emergent surgeries or for patients with good functional capacity or no clinical risk factors, no additional cardiac workup is needed preoperatively. If the patient has an acute cardiac condition, it should be managed preoperatively. With clinical risk factors and poor functional capacity, additional cardiac workup may be considered if it will change perioperative management.
3. Noninvasive cardiac tests assess myocardial function or perfusion. Both measurement of the systolic function (such as the left ventricular ejection fraction) and assessment of perfusion by stress testing have generally shown a high negative predictive value, but a low positive predictive value. While a negative test is highly predictive of a nonevent, a positive test does not necessarily imply a positive cardiac event with surgery. Simple consideration of clinical risk factors may identify patients at risk, without these tests. Rather than in simple risk stratification, certain noninvasive tests may have value in identification and quantification of stenotic valvular diseases and in identification of patients with prohibitive risks.
4. Perioperative cardiac risks may be modified by using β-adrenergic blockade and/or statins. β-adrenergic blockade must be titrated so that

perfusion pressures of end organs such as the brain are not compromised.
5. In patients with nonacute cardiac conditions, "prophylactic" revascularization by either bypass surgery or angioplasty with or without stenting does not appear to reduce the cardiac risk of a subsequent noncardiac vascular surgery, compared to maximal medical therapy alone.
6. Patients undergoing major vascular surgery after a recent coronary stenting may be at high risk for in-stent thrombosis or major hemorrhage, depending on how the antiplatelet therapy is managed perioperatively. This risk period may be 30–40 days after a bare metal stent and a year or longer after a drug-eluting stent or coronary brachytherapy. Similarly, the first month after coronary bypass surgery may represent a high-risk period.
7. Although severe aortic stenosis is considered an acute cardiac condition warranting preoperative management according to the ACC/AHA guidelines, retrospective data suggest that patients with severe aortic stenosis can undergo noncardiac surgery with comparable risks to those without it.

References

1. Mangano DT, Goldman L. Preoperative assessment of patients with known or suspected coronary disease. *N Engl J Med*. 1995;333:1750–1756.
2. ACC/AHA Task Force Report. Special report: guidelines for perioperative cardiovascular evaluation for noncardiac surgery. *Circulation*. 1996;93:1278–1317.
3. Eagle KA, Berger PB, Calkins H, et al. ACC/AHA guideline update for perioperative cardiovascular evaluation for noncardiac surgery – executive summary: a report of the ACC/AHA task force on practice guidelines (Committee to Update the 1996 Guidelines on Perioperative Cardiovascular Evaluation for Noncardiac Surgery). *J Am Coll Cardiol*. 2002;39:542–553.
4. Fleisher LA, Beckman JA, Brown KA, et al. ACC/AHA 2007 guidelines on perioperative cardiovascular evaluation and care for noncardiac surgery: executive summary: a report of the American College of Cardiology/American Heart Association Task Force on Practice Guidelines (Writing Committee to Revise the 2002 Guidelines on Perioperative Cardiovascular Evaluation for Noncardiac Surgery): developed in collaboration with the American Society

of Echocardiography, American Society of Nuclear Cardiology, Heart Rhythm Society, Society of Cardiovascular Anesthesiologists, Society for Cardiovascular Angiography and Interventions, Society for Vascular Medicine and Biology, and Society for Vascular Surgery. *Circulation*. 2007 Oct 23;116(17):1971–1996.

5. Jette M, Sidney K, Blumchen G. Metabolic equivalents (METS) in exercise testing, exercise prescription, and evaluation of functional capacity. *Clin Cardiol*. 1990;13:555–565.

6. Rossi E, Citterio F, Vescio MF, et al. Risk stratification of patients undergoing peripheral vascular revascularization by combined resting and dipyridamole echocardiography. *Am J Cardiol*. 1998;82:306–310.

7. Kontos MC, Brath LK, Akosah KP, Mohanty PK. Cardiac complications in noncardiac surgery: relative value of resting two-dimensional echocardiography and dipyridamole thallium imaging. *Am Heart J*. 1996;132:559–566.

8. Halm EA, Browner WS, Tubau JF, Tateo IM, Mangano DT. Echocardiography for assessing cardiac risk in patients having noncardiac surgery. *Ann Intern Med*. 1996;125:433–441.

9. Guidelines for assessing and managing the perioperative risk from coronary artery disease associated with major noncardiac surgery. Ann Intern Med 1997; 127:309–12.

10. Soufer R, Wohlgelernter D, Vita NA, et al. Intact systolic left ventricular function in clinical congestive heart failure. *Am J Cardiol*. 1985;55:1032–1036.

11. Rakowski H, Appleton CP, Chan KL, et al. Canadian consensus recommendations for the measurement and reporting of diastolic dysfunction by echocardiography: from the investigators of consensus on diastolic dysfunction by echocardiography. *J Am Soc Echocardiogr*. 1996;9:736–760.

12. O'Halloran TD, Kannam JP. Preoperative transthoracic echocardiography: when is it useful? *Int Anesthesiol Clin*. 2008;46:1–10.

13. Liao T, Park KW. Noninvasive tests of myocardial perfusion: stress tests and their values. *Int Anesth Clin*. 2001;39(4):1–10.

14. Selbst J, Comunale ME. Myocardial ischemia monitoring. *Int Anesthesiol Clin*. 2002;40(1):133–146.

15. Grayburn PA, Hillis LD. Cardiac events in patients undergoing noncardiac surgery: shifting the paradigm from noninvasive risk stratification to therapy. *Ann Intern Med*. 2003;138:506–511.

16. Morgan PB, Panomitros GE, Nelson AC, Smith DF, Solanki DR, Zornow MH. Low utility of dobutamine stress echocardiograms in the preoperative evaluation of patients scheduled for noncardiac surgery. *Anesth Analg*. 2002;95:512–516.

17. Lee TH, Marcantonio ER, Mangione CM, et al. Derivation and prospective validation of a simple index for prediction of cardiac risk of major noncardiac surgery. *Circulation*. 1999;100:1043–1049.

18. Mangano DT, Layug EI, Wallace A, Tateo I, Multicenter study of perioperative ischemia research group. Effect of atenolol on mortality and cardiovascular morbidity after noncardiac surgery. *N Engl J Med*. 1996;335:1713–1720.

19. Wallace A, Layug B, Tateo I, et al. Prophylactic atenolol reduces postoperative myocardial ischemia. *Anesthesiology*. 1998;88:7–17.

20. Poldermans D, Boersma E, Bax JJ, et al. The effect of bisoprolol on perioperative mortality and myocardial infarction in high-risk patients undergoing vascular surgery. *N Engl J Med*. 1999;341: 1789–1794.

21. Poldermans D, Boersma E, Bax JJ, et al. Bisoprolol reduces cardiac death and myocardial infarction in high-risk patients as long as 2 years after successful major vascular surgery. *Eur Heart J*. 2001;22:1353–1358.

22. Raby KE, Brull SJ, Timimi F, et al. The effect of heart rate control on myocardial ischemia among high-risk patients after vascular surgery. *Anesth Analg*. 1999;88:477–482.

23. Stone JG, Foex P, Sear JW, Johnson LL, Khambatta HJ, Triner L. Myocardial ischemia in untreated hypertensive patients: effect of a single small oral dose of a beta-adrenergic blocking agent. *Anesthesiology*. 1988;68:495–500.

24. Urban MK, Markowitz SM, Gordon MA, Urquhart BL, Kligfield P. Postoperative prophylactic administration of b-adrenergic blockers in patients at risk for myocardial ischemia. *Anesth Analg*. 2000;90:1257–1261.

25. POISE Study Group, Devereaux PJ, Yang H, et al. Effects of extended-release metoprolol succinate in patients undergoing non-cardiac surgery (POISE trial): a randomised controlled trial. *Lancet*. 2008; 371:1839–1847.

26. Sear JW, Giles JW, Howard-Alpe G, Foex P. Perioperative beta-blockade, 2008: what does POISE tell us, and was our earlier caution justified? *Br J Anaesth*. 2008;101:135–138.

27. Shammash JB, Trost JC, Gold JM, Berlin JA, Golden MA, Kimmel SE. Perioperative beta-blocker withdrawal and mortality in vascular surgical patients. *Am Heart J*. 2001;141:148–153.

28. Boersma E, Poldermans D, Bax JJ, et al. Predictors of cardiac events after major vascular surgery. *JAMA*. 2001;285:1865–1873.

29. Lee JW. Statins and cardiovascular risks. *Int Anesthesiol Clin*. 2005;43:55–68.

30. Lindenauer PK, Pekow P, Wang K, Gutierrez B, Benjamin E. Lipid-lowering therapy and in-hospital mortality following major noncardiac surgery. *JAMA*. 2004;291:2092–2099.

31. Poldermans D, Bax JJ, Kertai MD, et al. Statins are associated with a reduced incidence of perioperative mortality in patients undergoing major noncardiac vascular surgery. *Circulation*. 2003;107:1848–1851.

32. Kertai MD, Boersma E, Westerhout CM, et al. A combination of statins and beta-blockers is independently associated with a reduction in the incidence of perioperative mortality and nonfatal myocardial infarction in patients undergoing abdominal aortic aneurysm surgery. *Eur J Vasc Endovasc Surg*. 2004;28:343–352.

33. Kertai MD, Boersma E, Westerhout CM, et al. Association between long-term statin use and mortality after successful abdominal aortic aneurysm surgery. *Am J Med.* 2004;116:96–103.

34. Durazzo AES, Machado FS, Ikeoka DT, et al. Reduction in cardiovascular events after vascular surgery with atorvastatin: a randomized trial. *J Vasc Surg.* 2004;39:967–976.

35. Park KW. Angiotensin converting enzyme inhibitors, AG receptor blockers, and aldosterone receptor antagonists. *Int Anesthesiol Clin.* 2005;43:23–37.

36. Park KW. Na+-K+ exchange inhibitors. *Int Anesthesiol Clin.* 2005;43:69–75.

37. Li Y, Cohen R. Caspase inhibitors and myocardial apoptosis. *Int Anesthesiol Clin.* 2005;43:77–89.

38. Licker M, Bednarkiewicz M, Neidhart P, et al. Preoperative inhibition of angiotensin-converting enzyme improves systemic and renal haemodynamic changes during aortic abdominal surgery. *Br J Anaesth.* 1996;76:632–639.

39. Bonow RO, Epstein SE. Indications for coronary artery bypass surgery in patients with chronic angina pectoris: implications of the multicenter randomized trials. *Circulation.* 1985;72:V23–V30.

40. Hueb WA, Bellotti G, de Oliveira SA, et al. The Medicine, Angioplasty or Surgery Study (MASS): a prospective, randomized trial of medical therapy, balloon angioplasty or bypass surgery for single proximal left anterior descending artery stenosis. *J Am Coll Cardiol.* 1995;26:1600–1605.

41. Parisi AF, Folland ED, Hartigan P, Veterans Affairs ACME Investigators. A comparison of angioplasty with medical therapy in the treatment of single-vessel coronary artery disease. *N Engl J Med.* 1992;326:10–16.

42. Coronary angioplasty versus medical therapy for angina: the second Randomised Intervention Treatment of Angina (RITA-2) trial. Lancet 1997;350:461–468.

43. Mason JJ, Owens DK, Harris RA, Cooke JP, Hlatky MA. The role of coronary angiography and coronary revascularization before noncardiac vascular surgery. *JAMA.* 1995;273:1919–1925.

44. The Society of Thoracic Surgeons national database. Available at: http://www.sts.org/section/stsdatabase. Accessed November 14, 2008.

45. Eagle KA, Rihal CS, Mickel MC, Holmes DR, Foster ED, Gersh BJ. Cardiac risk of noncardiac surgery: influence of coronary disease and type of surgery in 3368 operations. *Circulation.* 1997;96:1882–1887.

46. McFalls EO, Ward HB, Moritz TE, et al. Coronary-artery revascularization before elective major vascular surgery. *N Engl J Med.* 2004;351:2795–2804.

47. Posner KL, van Norman GA, Chan V. Adverse cardiac outcomes after noncardiac surgery in patients with prior percutaneous transluminal coronary angioplasty. *Anesth Analg.* 1999;89:553–560.

48. Kaluza GL, Joseph J, Lee JR, Raizner ME, Raizner AE. Catastrophic outcomes of noncardiac surgery soon after coronary stenting. *J Am Coll Cardiol.* 2000;35:1288–1294.

49. Park KW. Intracoronary brachytherapy and drug-eluting coronary stents. *Int Anesthesiol Clin.* 2005;43:91–100.

50. Reul GJ Jr, Cooley DA, Duncan JM, et al. The effect of coronary bypass on the outcome of peripheral vascular operations in 1093 patients. *J Vasc Surg.* 1986;3:788–798.

51. Breen P, Lee JW, Pomposelli F, Park KW. Timing of high-risk vascular surgery following coronary artery bypass surgery: a 10-year experience from an academic medical centre. *Anaesthesia.* 2004;59:422–427.

52. O'Keefe JH Jr, Shub C, Rettke SR. Risk of noncardiac surgical procedures in patients with aortic stenosis. *Mayo Clin Proc.* 1989;64:400–405.

53. Raymer K, Yang H. Patients with aortic stenosis: cardiac complications in noncardiac surgery. *Can J Anaesth.* 1998;45:855–859.

54. Haering JM, Comunale ME, Parker RA, et al. Cardiac risk of noncardiac surgery in patients with asymmetric septal hypertrophy. *Anesthesiology.* 1996;85:254–259.

55. Kuroiwa M, Arai M, Ueno T, Takenaka T, Okamoto H, Hoka S. Perioperative cardiovascular complications in patients with hypertrophic cardiomyopathy. *Masui.* 2003;52:733–739.

Role of Echocardiography in Aortic Surgery

4

Kathirvel Subramaniam and Balachundhar Subramaniam

Introduction

An ideal imaging technique should be able to confirm the diagnosis of aortic disease, classify the nature of aortic pathology [classic dissection versus intramural hematoma (IMH)], define the extent of aortic involvement (ascending, arch, and descending), and evaluate for associated complications. The diagnostic test should be sensitive, specific, and highly accurate. Diagnostic testing should be readily available to be done as quickly as possible considering the early high mortality of acute aortic disease (1% per hour in the first 48 h). It should also be able to provide additional information, which impacts the patient's immediate management and long-term outcome such as myocardial ischemia, aortic valve (AV) regurgitation, cardiac tamponade, reentry tears, and aortic branch vessel involvement.

Echocardiography is readily available, accurate, and provides additional useful information about aortic valve, coronary artery, and branch vessel involvement. The aorta can be imaged using four different ultrasound approaches, namely, transsthoracic echocardiography (TTE), transesophageal echocardiography (TEE), epiaortic ultrasound (EUS), and intravascular ultrasound (IVUS). Each has its utility in the perioperative period.

K. Subramaniam (✉)
Department of Anesthesiology, University of Pittsburgh
Medical Center – Presbyterian Hospital, Pittsburgh,
PA, USA
e-mail: subramaniamk@upmc.edu

TTE

TTE is performed with a handheld transducer held against the surface of the chest. TTE images the aortic root and ascending aorta in the parasternal long-axis imaging plane from the intercostal spaces on the left and right side of the sternum (Figs. 4.1 and 4.2). The ascending aorta and arch are imaged in the suprasternal long axis by placing the transducer above the sternal notch or clavicle (Fig. 4.3). Apical views and subcostal windows are used to image aortic root and descending aorta (Figs. 4.4–4.6).

TTE is completely a noninvasive procedure. Patients suspected of having aortic pathology should undergo TTE first, and all possible data should be obtained. This often provides important clues to the diagnosis.[1-3] TEE exam can then be focused to confirm and assess the extent of the pathology along with the morphological features that impact management. TTE and TEE should be used in complementary manner. TTE can be used to diagnose dissection (Fig. 4.7), provide information on the extent of dissection (descending aorta, arch, and ascending aorta), aortic valve morphology, and regurgitation (Fig. 4.8), and identify the signs of leaking and ruptured aneurysm (pericardial and pleural effusion). Regional wall motion abnormalities (RWMA) can be evaluated by TTE, which will indirectly point to coronary artery involvement by dissection. TTE also provides important clues to the involvement of innominate and left carotid vessels in selected patients, which are difficult to assess by TEE.

K. Subramaniam et al. (eds.), *Anesthesia and Perioperative Care for Aortic Surgery*,
DOI 10.1007/978-0-387-85922-4_4, © Springer Science+Business Media, LLC 2011

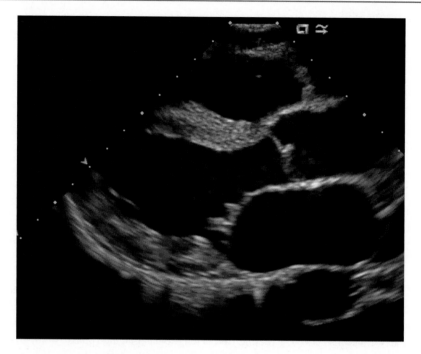

Fig. 4.1 Transthoracic parasternal long axis view

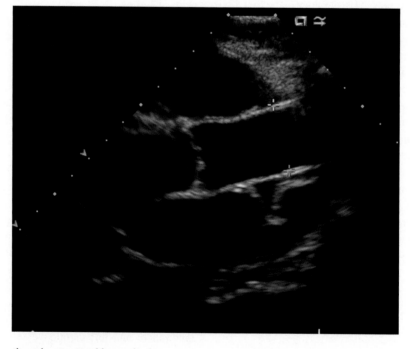

Fig. 4.2 Transthoracic parasternal long axis view

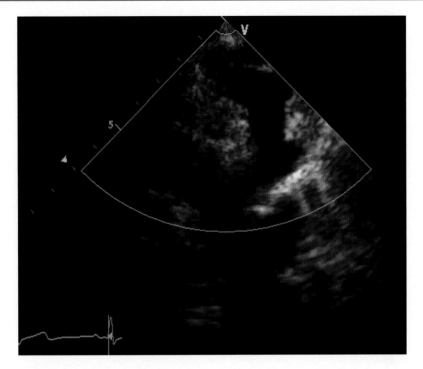

Fig. 4.3 Suprasternal long axis showing the arch vessels

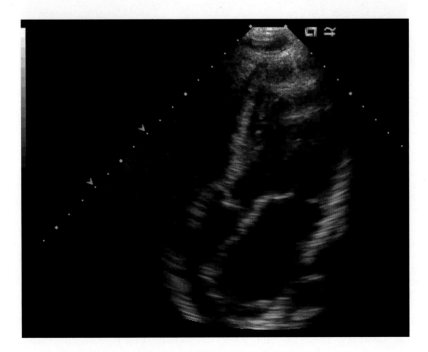

Fig. 4.4 Apical and subcostal windows imaging aortic root and descending aorta

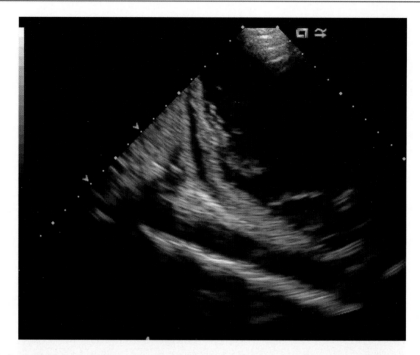

Fig. 4.5 Apical and subcostal windows imaging aortic root and descending aorta

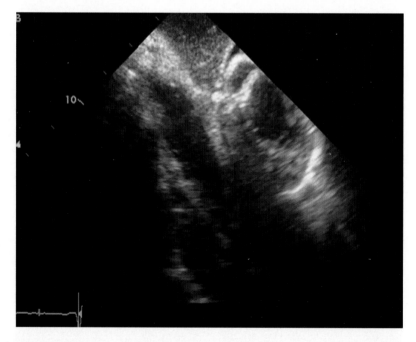

Fig. 4.6 Apical and subcostal windows imaging aortic root and descending aorta

The sensitivity and specificity of TTE for detecting aortic dissection are 75% and 90%, respectively, when adequate images are obtained.[4] The sensitivity is 78–100% for ascending aortic dis-section and 31–50% for descending thoracic aortic dissection.[5] TTE is technically difficult because of the ultrasound impedance induced by chest wall and lungs. Imaging is of poor quality in patients with

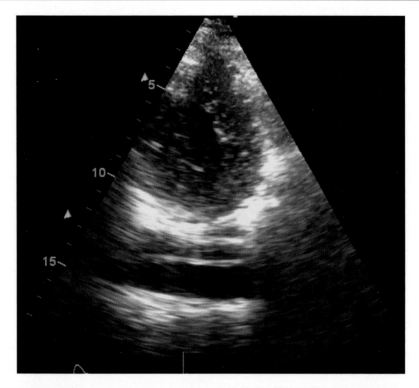

Fig. 4.7   TTE images with *arrows* showing descending aortic dissection and aortic regurgitation

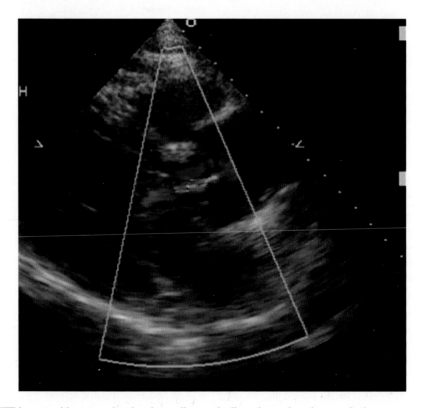

Fig. 4.8   TTE images with *arrows* showing descending aortic dissection and aortic regurgitation

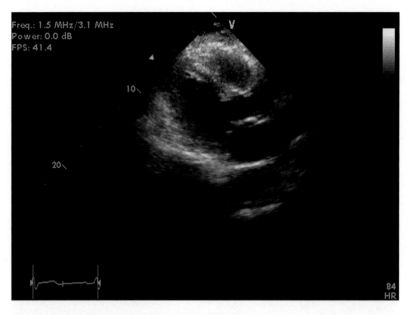

Fig. 4.9 Poor quality of TTE imaging in a patient with morbid obesity

obesity, chest deformity, and emphysema (Fig. 4.9).[1] Intimal flap may be difficult to differentiate from fluid in transverse sinus, catheter in right ventricular outflow tract, and calcified aortic root by TTE.[6] In older patients and in patients with atherosclerotic disease, the aorta becomes increasingly tortuous, displacing the aorta deeper into the chest cavity to prevent optimal imaging from the anterior chest wall.[7] Therefore, TTE alone may not provide a definitive diagnosis in aortic diseases.

TEE

Owing to the closeness of the esophagus to the aorta, the use of multiplane high-frequency TEE transducers can produce excellent high-resolution images of the entire aorta through multiple unobstructed windows. Multiple studies[8–23] have documented the accuracy, sensitivity, and specificity of TEE in the diagnosis of aortic pathology (>97%) (Table 4.1). Indications for the use of TEE in aortic pathology and procedures are defined by American Society of Echocardiography/ Society of Cardiovascular Anesthesiologists (Table 4.2). The most important limitation of TEE is the blind spot of distal ascending and proximal arch visualization, where the trachea

Table 4.1 Sensitivity and specificity for transesophageal echocardiography in diagnosis of aortic dissection

Study	Sensitivity	Specificity
Moore et al.[9]	88	N/A
Hashimoto et al.[10]	100	100
Ballal et al.[11]	97	100
Adachi et al.[12]	98	N/A
Simon et al.[13]	100	100
Erbel et al.[14]	99	N/A
Nienaber et al.[15]	98	77
Laissy et al.[16]	86	94
Bansal et al.[17]	97	N/A
Keren et al.[18]	98	95
Vignon et al.[19]	91	100
Pepi et al.[20]	100	100
Nishino et al.[21]	86	75
Sommer et al.[22]	100	94
Evangelista et al.[23]	99	100
Chirillo et al.[24]	98	97

and left main stem bronchus pass in between the esophagus and aorta (Fig. 4.10). As a result, a dissection limited to these areas could be missed by TEE alone, but fortunately occurrence of such a localized dissection is rare.[24] Positive computerized tomographic (CT) diagnosis of aortic dissection is rare when initial TEE examination ruled out the dissection.

Table 4.2 Indications for TEE during aortic surgery

Category I indications; Supported by strongest evidence or expert opinion: TEE is frequently useful in improving clinical outcomes in these settings and is often indicated depending on individual circumstances (e.g., patient risk and practice settings)
- Preoperative use in unstable patients with suspected thoracic aortic aneurysm, dissection, or disruption who needs to be evaluated quickly
- Intraoperative evaluation of acute persistent and life-threatening hemodynamic disturbances in which ventricular function and its determinants are uncertain and have not responded to treatment (can occur with aortic cross clamping, rupture of the aneurysm, dissection, etc.)
- Intraoperative assessment of aortic valve involvement in repair of aortic dissection with possible aortic valve involvement
- Intraoperative use in aortic valve repair (valve sparing aortic surgery)

Category II indications; Supported by weaker evidence and expert consensus: TEE may be useful in improving clinical outcomes in these settings and is often indicated depending on individual circumstances, but appropriate indications are less certain
- Preoperative assessment of patients with suspected acute thoracic dissections, aneurysms, or disruption
- Perioperative use in patients with hemodynamic disturbances
- Surgical procedures in patients with increased risk of myocardial ischemia, infarction, and hemodynamic disturbances
- Evaluation of regional myocardial function
- Intraoperative assessment of aortic valve replacement
- Intraoperative detection of air emboli
- Intraoperative detection of aortic atheromatous disease or other sources of aortic emboli
- Intraoperative use during repair of aortic dissections without aortic valve involvement

Category III indications; Little current scientific or expert support: TEE is infrequently useful in improving clinical outcomes in these settings and appropriate indications are uncertain; Intraoperative assessment of repair of thoracic aortic injuries

Reprinted with permission from American Society of Anesthesiologists and Lippincott Williams and Wilkins (Reference [104]).

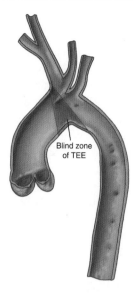

Fig. 4.10 Relationship of distal ascending aorta and proximal arch to esophagus and trachea/left main bronchus (Reprinted with permission from Taylor & Francis group (Reference [7]))

Localized dissection of the TEE blind spot can occur due to iatrogenic reasons such as aortic cross clamping and cannulation. Demertzis et al.[25] reported an intraoperative localized dissection of distal ascending aorta and aortic arch diagnosed by EUS but missed in post-bypass TEE examination after ascending aortic replacement.

An important advantage of TEE is its rapid performance in a wide variety of clinical environments such as emergency department, intensive care units, and operating rooms. In acutely ill patients at risk for hemodynamic collapse with needs for hemodynamic monitoring and infusion of medications, a bedside TEE is preferable to other imaging methods. TEE also eliminates the need for contrast agent and x-ray exposure required for CT and aortography and avoids the time delays and practical difficulties associated with magnetic resonance imaging (MRI).

At the University of Pittsburgh medical center, patients with suspected acute aortic syndromes arriving at the emergency department are initially evaluated, and the choice of the diagnostic test is decided based on the clinical condition and hemodynamic stability of the patient. Patients who are hemodynamically unstable or with a full stomach

Detailed TEE examination after anesthesia induction and muscle relaxation is helpful to rule out aortic dissection when preoperative CT and TTE were inconclusive. If the diagnosis is still doubtful, EUS can be utilized after sternotomy to rule out the diagnosis of dissection. EUS imaging also provides information of the TEE blind spot.

undergo TEE examination in the operating room after safe induction of general anesthesia and airway protected with the endotracheal tube. Topical anesthesia and intravenous sedation are utilized in a small number of stable patients with suspected dissection. This can be done either in the emergency room or in the intensive care unit. In many of these stable patients, CT angiography has replaced TEE as the diagnostic test of choice nowadays.

TEE in Conscious Subjects

Though institutional practices may vary, anesthesiology consultation is occasionally requested to perform TEE in conscious patients with suspected aortic dissection. Anesthesiologists should be aware of the safety precautions, preparation, and performance of TEE in conscious subjects.

Preparation

Informed consent explaining the risks and benefits of the procedure is obtained. Patients are explained about the mild abdominal discomfort and sensation of gagging during the procedure. Airway and suction equipment, induction medications, muscle relaxants, and emergency medications such as vasodilators, beta-blockers, vagolytics, and antiarrhythmics should be available. IV access and monitoring devices (EKG, invasive or noninvasive blood pressure, and pulse oximetry) are established. Nasal oxygen is administered. Midazolam 2 mg IV can be given in young, anxious, and hypertensive patients with dissection.

Procedure

Adequate topical anesthesia cannot be overemphasized since it is usually the deciding factor in patient discomfort that determines the success in passing the transducer. Patients are positioned in left lateral decubitus position with head flexed for the procedure. Bite block is required, and TEE probe is unlocked and tip should be straight during insertion. TEE probe is inserted in the midline

over the back of the tongue into the throat, and patient is instructed to swallow which will usually allow smooth passage of the probe. Procedure should be stopped if there is any resistance or severe gagging is encountered. Esophageal examination is done before advancing the probe gently through the gastroesophageal sphincter (usually 40 cm from teeth) for transgastric imaging. Upper esophageal views are done at the end because of the discomfort associated with the probe location.

In intubated patients, the TEE probe insertion is done in the supine position. The probe is positioned behind the endotracheal tube and gently advanced. Slight resistance is always encountered at upper esophageal sphincter level. Head flexion, movement of the head toward side, and forward pull of the mandible are helpful maneuvers to assist in the passage of the probe. In difficult cases, direct laryngoscopy and esophageal intubation can be achieved.

Precautions and Complications

TEE is minimally invasive and complications are very infrequent. Cardiac arrhythmias (atrial and ventricular arrhythmias, bradycardia, or heart block) and airway complications (vomiting, aspiration of gastric contents in unintubated patients, laryngospasm, and bronchospasm) can happen during the procedure. Hemodynamic response to probe insertion and manipulation should be prevented in patients with aortic disease. A hypertensive response leading to rupture of the aneurysm and dissection can be lethal.[26,27] Adequate local anesthesia, intravenous sedation, and drugs (vasodilators and beta-blockers) prevent catastrophic events in awake subjects. Adequate depth of anesthesia should be ensured in intubated patients to prevent the hypertensive response to probe insertion. Compression of esophagus and weakening of its wall by thoracic aneurysms may predispose to injury, perforation, and fistula formation during TEE examination. Preoperative imaging studies should be reviewed to look for compression of esophagus before TEE probe insertion. If resistance is encountered, procedure should be abandoned. EUS can be utilized in such patients. Rarely, insertion of the TEE probe in patients with giant thoracic aortic aneurysms may cause compression of mediastinal structures. Tracheal compression and airway obstruction from insertion of the TEE probe has been reported in patients with giant aortic pseudoaneurysm and dissection of ascending aorta.[28]

Echocardiographic Anatomy

The thoracic aorta is divided into three segments by specific anatomic landmarks. The ascending aorta originates with the aortic valve and ends at the origin of the innominate artery. The ascending aorta is further divided into the aortic root and the tubular ascending aorta. The aortic root is comprised of the aortic annulus, the aortic valve leaflets, and the sinus of Valsalva and is referred to as the aortic valve complex. A discrete area of narrowing, known as the sinotubular (ST) junction, marks the end of the aortic root. The normal dimensions are given in Table 4.3.[29] ST junction effacement occurs with age. The tubular ascending aorta can be described as proximal and distal using the pulmonary artery crossover as the reference. The aortic arch begins at the origin of the innominate artery and ends at the aortic isthmus directly opposite to the origin of the left subclavian artery. The arch gives rise to the great vessels at its superior margin. The descending thoracic aorta begins at the ligamentum arteriosum and ends at the aortic hiatus at the diaphragm. The descending thoracic aorta is loosely defined by its relationship to the esophagus. The esophagus and the aorta change positions in the chest in a twisting and turning fashion, which influences the optimal imaging of the aorta (Fig. 4.11). The proximal descending aorta lies anterior to the esophagus in the chest (probe 15–20 cm from the incisors), the mid descending

aorta is directly lateral to the esophagus (probe 30–35 cm from incisors), and the distal descending aorta is directly posterior to the esophagus (probe 45 cm from incisors). The echocardiographer should take this into consideration while designating the aortic wall as anterior, posterior, medial, and lateral to locate the pathology. In lower esophageal views, the anterior wall will be shown in the superior aspect of the image close to the transducer and the posterior wall away from the transducer. In the upper esophageal views, the wall close to the transducer will be posterior and the wall away from the transducer will be the anterior wall. It is important to label and document the transducer depth with the images taken in the echocardiographic examination of the aorta. The improper registration of depth is an obvious disadvantage compared to other imaging modalities such as CT and MRI.

Aortic Dimensions

The aortic diameter is largest at its origin and tapers in size at the descending level till bifurcation in the abdomen.[29,30] The overall dimensions (length and diameter) of the aorta are dependent on the body habitus (Table 4.4). Intima and media are combined as the inner layer and adventitia as the outer layer, represented as two rings in short axis. The inner layer is homogenous and moderately echogenic. Adventitia is thick, most echogenic, and is less homogenous and blends into adjacent chest structures. Measurements should be done from inner edge to inner edge. The aorta expands slightly during systole and measurements should be done at the same point in the cardiac cycle. The aorta is circular in the short axis, and the diameter is measured anteroposterior and right to left direction. Anteroposterior and superoinferior dimensions are measured in longitudinal planes. Inaccuracy in dimensions can arise from oblique or off-axis imaging. In the short axis, an oblique view may make the aorta oval leading to overestimation of the diameter. In the long axis, the diameter may be underestimated by off-axis imaging failing to cut through the center of aorta.

Table 4.3 Aortic root dimensions (cm) at end-diastole

Aorta	Mean (SD)	Range
Annulus	1.9 (0.2)	1.4–2.6
Sinus of Valsalva	2.8 (0.3)	2.1–3.5
Sinotubular junction	2.4 (0.4)	1.7–3.4
Ascending aorta	2.6 (0.3)	2.1–3.4

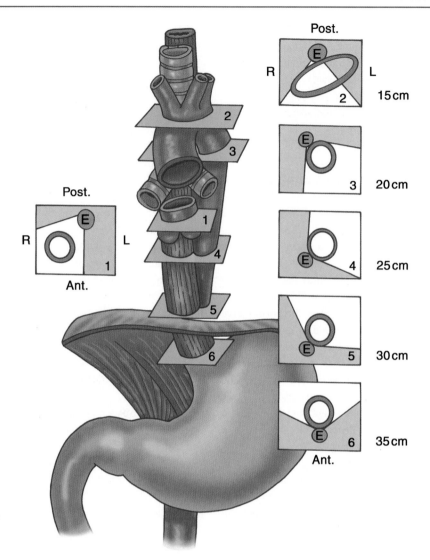

Fig. 4.11 Relation of esophagus and thoracic aorta from thoracic inlet to diaphragmatic hiatus (Modified from Freeman[103] with permission from Mayo Foundation for Medical Education and Research. All rights reserved)

Table 4.4 Aortic average diameter (mm) according to body image

Aortic segment	Small	Medium	Large
Ascending	28	32	39
Aortic arch	28	32	39
Descending	21	27	33
Diaphragmatic	20	26	33
Suprarenal	16	22	29

TEE Views of the Thoracic Aorta

TEE examination of the aorta starts with the probe in the midesophageal position and multiplane rotation to 30–60° to image aortic valve in short axis (Fig. 4.12). All three aortic valve cusps are examined for mobility and abnormalities (fusion of cusps, coaptation defects, calcification, and bicuspid and unicuspid valves). Intimal dissection flap involving the aortic valve cusps can also be appreciated. Slight anteflexion of the probe tip brings the imaging plane through the sinuses of Valsalva and the ostia of both coronary arteries. Color Doppler flow in short axis is used to detect the presence and location of aortic regurgitation jet in relation to the aortic valve cusps. Coronary artery flows should also be assessed by color flow.

From the midesophageal aortic valve short axis (ME AV SAX), rotate the multi-plane angle

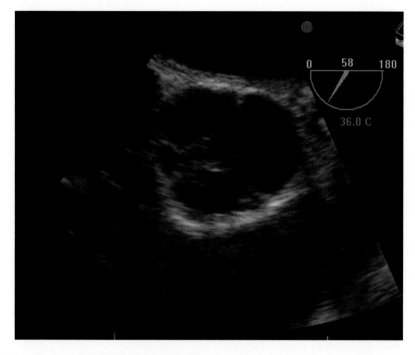

Fig. 4.12 Midesophageal aortic valve short axis and ME long axis

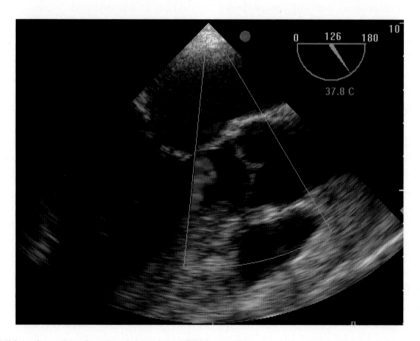

Fig. 4.13 Midesophageal aortic valve short axis and ME long axis

to between 120° and 160° until the long axis view (ME AV LAX) of the aortic valve develops (Fig. 4.13). The aortic root (aortic annulus, sinus of Valsalva, and sinotubular junction) and the proximal ascending aorta appear on the right side of the image. Aortic valve cusps (the right cusp in the bottom, left or noncoronary cusp above) are once again examined for calcification, restricted

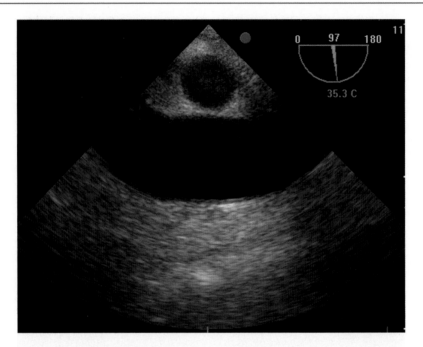

Fig. 4.14 ME ascending aorta long axis and short axis

mobility, and excessive mobility or prolapse. Intimal flap, its origin, extension, and its relation to the aortic valve cusps and the coronary ostia should be documented. Color flow Doppler can also be used to assess the severity of aortic regurgitation in this view. Aortic root dimensions are measured and compared with the table of normal values.

From ME AV LAX, reduce the multiplane angle to 100–120° and pull the probe out slightly. A long axis of the ascending aorta is obtained, and a short axis view of the right PA is also seen posterior to the aorta (Fig. 4.14). Both walls of the aorta are examined for calcification, atheromas, and dissection flaps. Ascending aortic diameter is also measured at the level of PA and compared with the normal values.

From ME ascending aortic LAX, the probe is rotated to 30° to obtain the ascending aorta in short axis (Fig. 4.15). An upright view of the main pulmonary artery with the right PA and the SVC can also be seen in this view. The probe is moved up and down to scan the short axis of different segments of the ascending aorta. As a rough guide, the aortic diameter should be the same as that of the pulmonary artery.

After midesophageal views, the probe is advanced into the stomach and the deep transgastric long axis view is obtained (Fig. 4.16). In this view, the whole ascending aorta and aortic arch coursing around the pulmonary artery may be visualized at the depth of 24 cm. With minor manipulations (extreme anteflexion and rotating the transducer between 0° and 15°) of the probe, the takeoff of the innominate artery can be visualized. To improve image quality, it may be necessary to increase the overall gain and frequency.

Rotation of the probe through 180° so that the transducer faces the posterior aspect of the esophagus at a depth of field between 4 and 6 cm enables visualization of the descending thoracic aorta. Reducing the gain and sector depth enables the detailed imaging of the wall of the aorta. The probe is withdrawn into the lower esophagus with the probe at 0°. Aorta is seen in short axis at 0° and in longitudinal axis at 90° (Fig. 4.17a & b). In the longitudinal view, the proximal segment is on the right, and the distal segment is on the left. The probe is withdrawn in 3–5 cm increments with a slight clockwise rotation to keep the aorta in the center of

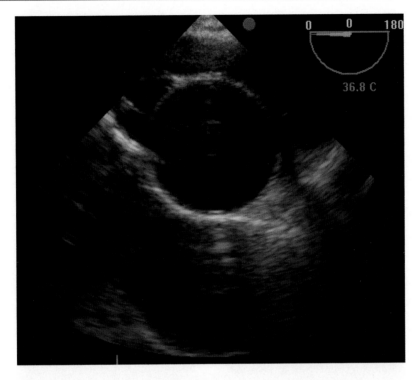

Fig. 4.15 ME ascending aorta long axis and short axis

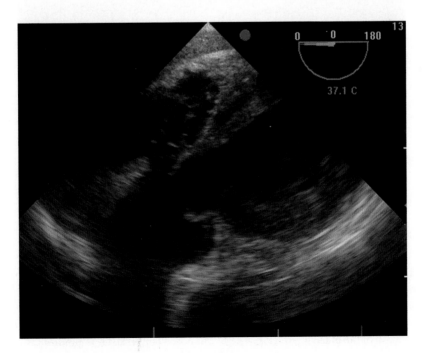

Fig. 4.16 Deep transgastric long axis view

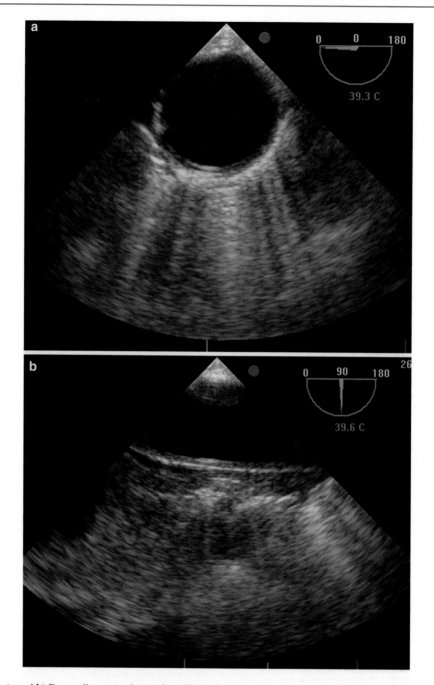

Fig. 4.17 (**a** and **b**) Descending aorta short axis and long axis

the image. The probe is withdrawn till the aortic arch appears in the long axis with the distal arch to the right and the proximal arch to the left (Fig. 4.18). The left subclavian artery can be easily seen by rotation of the plane to 90° (Fig. 4.19). With further counterclockwise rotation of the probe, two other brachiocephalic vessels can be visualized. Visualization of the innominate artery is the most difficult because of its location in the blind spot. Even in experienced hands, visualization is possible in only 40% of patients.[7]

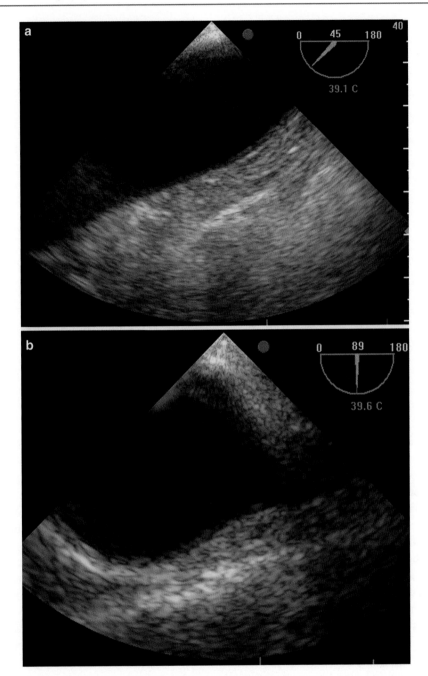

Fig. 4.18 (**a** and **b**) Upper esophageal aortic arch long axis and short axis

Patients with aortic disease have frequent coexistence of other valvular disease or coronary artery disease. It is important to perform a comprehensive TEE examination to scan for associated abnormalities. For example, regional wall motion changes may indicate associated coronary artery disease. Mitral valve disease is frequently associated with aortic disease of Marfan syndrome (MS).

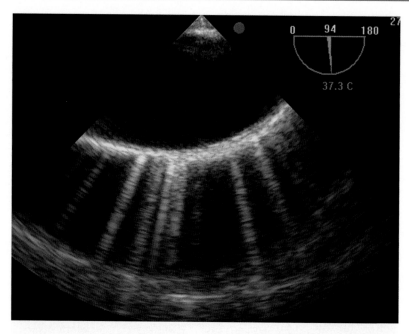

Fig. 4.19 Double barrel aorta and reverberation artifact

Artifacts in Aortic TEE

Reverberations are secondary reflections that occur along the path of a sound pulse and are a result of the ultrasound bouncing in between the structure and another reflecting surface. Reverberations appear as multiple equally spaced echoes on the display. These closely spaced reverberations merge and appear as a solid line directed away from the transducer. This is known as a comet tail or ring down artifact. Descending thoracic aorta is the common site for reverberation artifacts (Fig. 4.20).

A mirror image (Fig. 4.20) is a refraction artifact and is created when the sound reflects off a strong reflector and redirected toward a second structure. This redirection causes a replica or second copy of the structure to incorrectly appear on the image. Mirror artifact is always located deeper than real structure. A commonplace again is the descending aorta and is referred to as a double barrel aorta. A mirror image artifact may also appear in color Doppler.

Ultrasound beams projected by the transducer in a divergent manner (other than the central beam) can result in images when they encounter a strong specular reflector. Side lobe artifacts are commonly caused by calcification of the aortic root, the aortic valve, and the sinotubular junction (Fig. 4.21), but can also arise from fatty infiltration of the crista terminalis or an infusion catheter in the superior vena cava. In the ascending aorta, this creates an impression of false dissection. False dissections in the ascending aorta can also be caused by linear artifacts related to aorta–lung interface, anterior wall of left atrium, and a pulmonary artery catheter. Linear artifacts are more common when the aortic diameter is larger than the left atrial diameter. Color Doppler with normal homogenous color on both sides of the linear echo and artifact movement with motion of the originating structure on M-mode can be used to recognize these linear artifacts.

Near-field clutter arises from complex and nonuniform energy distribution in the portion of

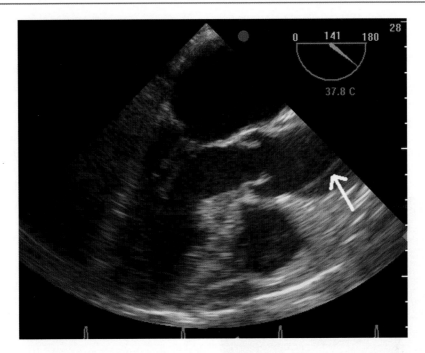

Fig. 4.20 Side lobe artifact (*arrow*)

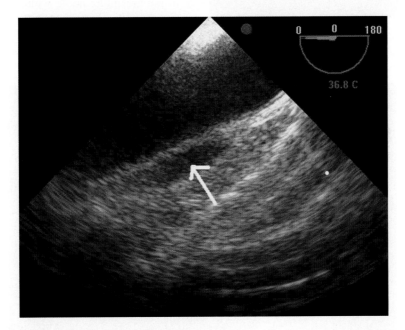

Fig. 4.21 Pericardial effusion (*arrow*) mimicking dissection

the sector adjacent to the transducer. This leads to limited visualization of structures adjacent to the probe as commonly encountered with the descending aortic wall close to the probe. This can also be encountered with epiaortic imaging without fluid interface (Fig. 4.22). High-frequency probes improve the visualization close to the probe.

Utility of TEE in the Diagnosis of Classic Aortic Dissection

Aortic dissections are classified into two types: Type A involves the ascending aorta, whatever the extension or the site of intimal tear. Type B involves the descending aorta with extension into the abdominal aorta or the aortic arch.

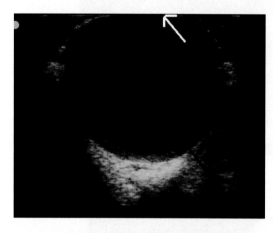

Fig. 4.22 Near-field clutter (*arrow*) with epiaortic imaging. Anterior wall of aorta is not seen

Intimomedial Flap

Dissection results in cleavage of medial layer into the inner two-third and the outer one-third. An intimal flap consists of the inner two-third of the media with the intimal layer. An intimal flap is linear, thin and intraluminal, mobile, and echogenic. It divides the aortic lumen into true and false lumens (Fig. 4.23). Mobility is correlated with mortality.[31] Increased mobility is also observed around the site of intimal tear.

Intimal Tear

The dissection begins at the intimal tear. Tear appears as a discontinuity in the intimal flap (Fig. 4.24). Sixty-five percent of dissections originate in the ascending aorta, 20% in the descending thoracic aorta, and 10% in the aortic arch.[32] The vast majority of dissections originate from the ascending aorta, within several centimeters above the sinuses of Valsalva, since torsion movement of aortic annulus provokes additional downward traction in the aortic root and

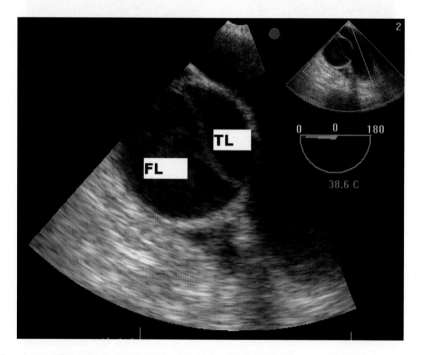

Fig. 4.23 True lumen (TL) and false lumen (FL) of ascending aortic dissection

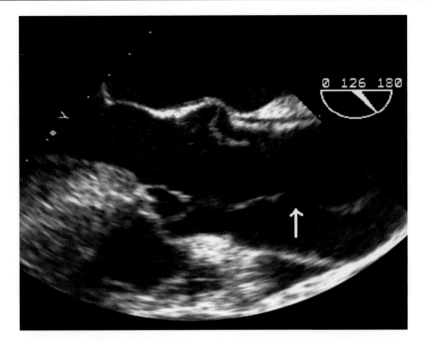

Fig. 4.24 Intimal tear (*arrow*) of ascending aorta

increases the longitudinal stress in the segment of the aorta. The other common site for the intimal tear is in the descending aorta just distal to the origin of the subclavian artery at the site of the ligamentum arteriosum. Tears occur in the isthmus area because of increased tension at the union of mobile aortic arch with the descending thoracic aorta, which is quite fixed. From this point, the dissection usually proceeds in antegrade direction, though retrograde extension is possible. Color flow will indicate flow through the intimal tear between true and false lumens. Flow can be bidirectional in 75% of patients.[33] Pulse wave Doppler may show the pressure gradient of 10–25 mmHg between the true and false lumens.[34] Primary entry tear identification is important since the resection of primary tear during surgical repair and inclusion of primary tears in the endograft exclusion procedures reduces the incidence of late reoperation. Primary tears could be multiple or in some cases may be located in the TEE blind spot. Successful identification of the primary tear is more successful in type B dissections (90%) than type A dissections (83%).[35]

Reentry Tears

Multiple communications between true and false lumen exists on careful screening of the entire aorta. Some represent entry sites with flow from the true toward false channel and others will be exit sites or have bidirectional flow. The reentry tear is usually located in the abdominal aorta, iliac arteries, or other aortic branches. These small communications, less than 2 mm in diameter, could represent the ostia of the intercostal or lumbar arteries that have been severed by the dissecting hematoma.[36] Color flow will also identify these multiple small communications in the descending aorta between true and false lumens (Fig. 4.25). Location of reentry tears can be documented with the probe depth from incisors, which will be useful for postoperative follow-up. Reentry of the dissection is a predisposition for chronic false lumen perfusion with no tendency to thrombus formation. Absent flow, spontaneous echo contrast, and thrombus formation in the false lumen after surgical or endovascular aortic

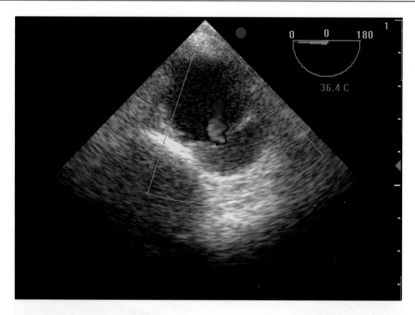

Fig. 4.25 Color flow through reentry tear in the descending aorta

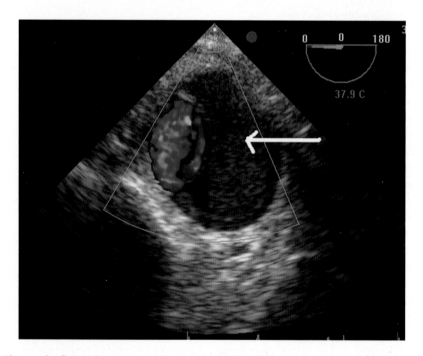

Fig. 4.26 Absent color flow and spontaneous echo contrast in false lumen (*arrow*)

repair (EVAR) are good prognostic factors (Fig. 4.26).[33,37,38] Ergin et al.[37] reported absence of false lumen flow distal to operated type A dissection in 53% of patients while other studies achieved obliteration of flow in false lumen in only 10–30% of patients.[39,40] Mohr-Kahaly et al. found persistence of flow in the false lumen in 71% of postoperative patients versus 82% of their medically treated patients in all types of dissection.[34]

Table 4.5 Echocardiographic differentiation of true and false lumens

	True lumen	False lumen
Size	Smaller	Large
Cardiac cycle	Expands during systole	Flap moves toward false lumen during systole
Velocity of blood flow	High and aliasing	Low
Direction of flow	Systolic antegrade	Antegrade systolic, delayed late peak or retrograde
Spontaneous echo contrast/thrombus	Absent	Thrombus/spontaneous echo contrast may be present
IV echo contrast washout	Faster	Slower
Thin cobweb like echos	Absent	Indicate residual strands of media joining intimal flap to outer wall of the false lumen especially in descending aorta

True and False Lumens

Echocardiographic differentiation is given in Table 4.5 (Figs. 4.23 and 4.24). Intimal flap and the flow in true and false lumens on either side of the flap are highly sensitive features of dissection. With large entry tears, flow in the nearby segments of the false lumen may have the same direction and timing as the true lumen flow.[41] With small or more distal entry tears, false lumen flow is less similar to true lumen flow and peak velocity may occur later in the cardiac cycle representing delay of flow into the false lumen. On occasions, when the dissecting canal has no reentry tear and ends in a cul-de-sac, the flow in the false channel can be antegrade and retrograde.[42] Spontaneous echo contrast and partial thrombosis are seen in sites away from entry or reentry tears where the high velocity flow keeps these changes from occurring.

A thickening of the aortic wall in excess of 15 mm has also been used as a sign of dissection, suggesting thrombosis of a false channel, which makes intimal flap difficult to recognize. Strict adherence to this criterion will minimize false-positive results.[43] False lumen thrombosis should be differentiated from aneurysm with thrombus formation, IMH, atherosclerotic ulcer with thrombosis, vascular mass, and finally coarctation or prior surgical repair. It is not uncommon for patients suspected of dissection to have these vascular pathologies involving thoracic aorta.[44] False lumen thrombosis will have a smooth intimal border or displaced intimal calcification compared to aneurysmal thrombus, which will have irregular border.[13]

Aortic Valve Involvement in Aortic Dissection (Fig. 4.27)

Aortic valve (AV) involvement is common in aortic dissection (40–76%). There are several mechanisms by which aortic valve can be affected by the dissection process: aortic dilatation leading to incomplete valve closure, abnormal aortic annulus because of MS or annuloaortic ectasia, diseased aortic valve (degenerative or bicuspid valve), prolapse of valve leaflets caused by extension of dissection to valve attachment, and prolapse of the intimal flap into the aortic annulus (Figs. 4.28 and 4.29). Various degrees of aortic incompetence may be associated (Fig. 4.30).

Defining the mechanism of AV involvement by TEE is important in devising the surgical plan.[45] Valve replacement is required in diseased valves (e.g., bicuspid valve with calcification). Valve replacement is also preferred in MS with diseased annulus or annuloaortic ectasia because of limited durability of valve repair in these patients. A valve-sparing operation is possible in all other mechanisms of valve involvement. In one series, preservation of the native aortic valve was possible in 86% of type A dissections with excellent results.[46]

TEE is superior to all other modalities in the assessment of aortic valve in dissections. TEE is

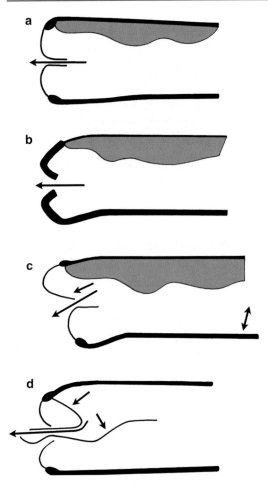

Fig. 4.27 Various mechanisms of aortic valve involvement and regurgitation in aortic dissection: (**a**) dilatation of aortic root and sinotubular junction, (**b**) diseased aortic valve, (**c**) flap causing prolapse of the aortic valve, and (**d**) prolapsing intimal flap into the valve (Reprinted with permission from Taylor & Francis Group (Reference [7]))

also utilized to assess the severity of residual aortic regurgitation in the post-bypass period if a valve repair is attempted (Figs. 4.31 and 4.32).

Coronary Artery Involvement

TEE can be used to diagnose occlusion of coronary artery by intimal flap or extension of dissection into the coronary artery (Fig. 4.33). Right coronary artery involvement is more common because of the common location of intimal

tear in the ascending aorta on the right side and progression of the dissection along the right lateral region of the ascending aorta. Left coronary artery involvement indicates extensive dissection.

In one series, one or both coronary arteries were noted to be involved in 21% of patients with dissection by surgical documentation.[10] An adequate view of the proximal coronary artery and ostia was obtained in 88% of the left main and 50% of the right coronary artery in these patients. TEE identified the involvement of coronary arteries in 86% of cases, while EKG changes were seen only in 33% of patients. Only 29% of patients with coronary artery involvement develop clinical myocardial infarction.

Development of new regional wall motion abnormalities on TEE can point to the involvement of coronary arteries in aortic dissection. RWMA may also be caused by coronary artery disease, which has been found to be associated with 43% of patients of aortic dissection in one series. Delaying the aortic repair for obtaining coronary angiography has not been shown to be beneficial. Three-fourths of patients underwent a bypass procedure for coronary artery involvement in dissections rather than for associated CAD.[47] On the other hand, patients presenting with chest pain and undergoing coronary arteriography for acute coronary syndrome actually can have acute aortic syndrome. TEE is also used to confirm flows through proximal coronary arteries in the post-bypass period (Fig. 4.34).

Branch Vessel Involvement

Aortic Arch

Progression of dissection from the ascending aorta to the arch occurs in the larger curvature of the arch where the arch branches originate. Arch vessels can be involved with dissection, disinsertion, obstruction of the artery ostium, or compression by false lumen. The innominate and the left common carotid arteries are more frequently involved than the left subclavian artery. TEE can localize the left subclavian arteries in

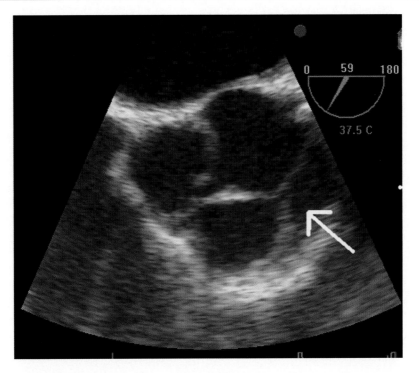

Fig. 4.28 Type C aortic valve involvement by intimal flap (*arrow*)

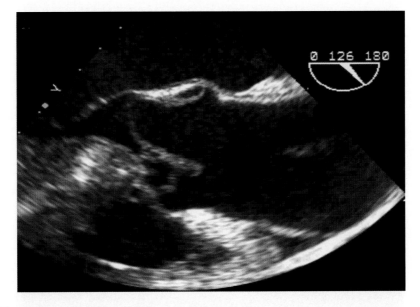

Fig. 4.29 Type D aortic valve involvement by aortic dissection

100% of patients (Fig. 4.35). With an experienced echocardiographer and multiplane probes, TEE can rule out involvement of the innominate and left carotid arteries in some patients.[33] The knowl- edge of great vessel involvement may not modify the surgical approach and the arch and branch vessels can be examined during the operation.[44] TTE and EUS can be utilized to evaluate the arch

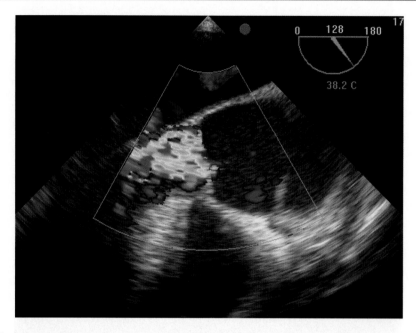

Fig. 4.30 Severe aortic regurgitation with aortic dissection demonstrated by color flow Doppler

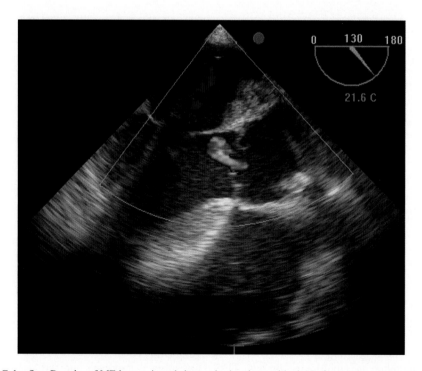

Fig. 4.31 Color flow Doppler of ME long axis and short axis showing residual AI after aortic valve repair

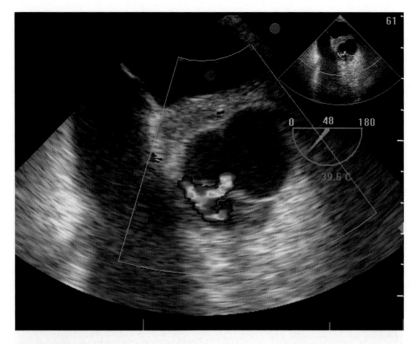

Fig. 4.32   Color flow Doppler of ME long axis and short axis showing residual AI after aortic valve repair

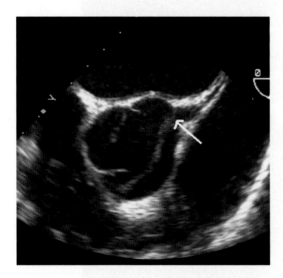

Fig. 4.33   Coronary artery involvement by dissection flap

vessel involvement and identify the intimal tears in the blind spot of TEE. Missing the intimal tears in the arch and replacing only the ascending aorta will result in continuous flow into the false lumen (Fig. 4.36).

Visceral Ischemia

Intraoperative TEE is not usually used to evaluate the abdominal organ ischemia because of obvious limited visualization of branch vessels. CT angiography is typically done preoperatively to evaluate the renal and mesenteric arteries. Intraoperative assessment of renal and spinal cord blood flow has been evaluated in isolated clinical trials.[48,49] This is very insensitive, time consuming, difficult, and impractical in the busy operating environment.

TEE assessment of celiac and superior mesenteric blood flow has been studied by Orihashi et al.[48,50] TEE provided real-time dynamic and continuous intraoperative information in their case series of 24 patients. It is technically challenging to diagnose mesenteric ischemia by TEE, but may be a promising tool. This may be useful in patients undergoing emergency surgery without preoperative imaging studies and in patients with unexplained metabolic acidosis complicating intraoperative management of both type A and B dissections.

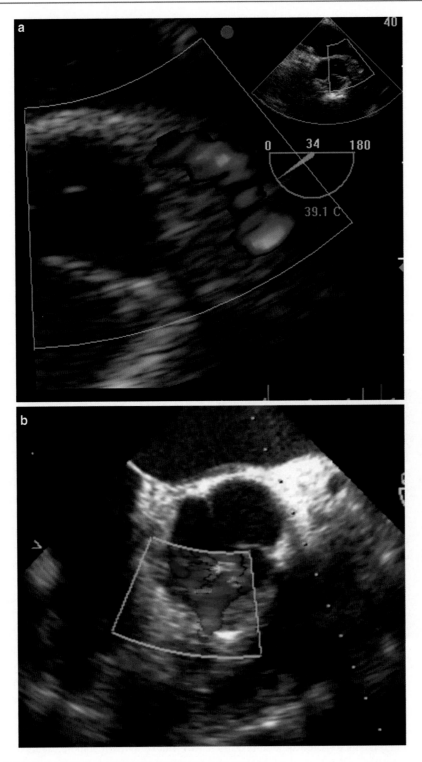

Fig. 4.34 Color flow of proximal *left* (**a**) and *right* (**b**) coronary arteries

Ruptured and Leaking Dissections

Rupture of intrapericardial portion of the aorta (the ascending aorta till the origin of the main pulmonary artery) will result in rapid deterioration from cardiac tamponade. For type A dissections, death is caused by intrapericardial rupture and cardiac tamponade in 80–90% of cases. For type B dissections, rupture causes 60–70% of deaths. Hemomediastinum is produced in cases of aortic arch rupture and a left hemothorax in rupture of the descending thoracic aorta. Echocardiographic signs of bleeding include pericardial and pleural effusions (left), widening of the oblique sinus with soft tissue echoes indicating hematoma, hazy echoes in the transverse sinus, and compression of right pulmonary artery and superior vena cava.[51] Increased blood flow velocity or color flow turbulence in the pulmonary artery may indicate compression by a hematoma. Mediastinal hematoma is characterized by an increased distance between the esophagus and the anteromedial wall of the aorta or increased distance between the posterolateral wall and the left visceral pleura measured at the level of the isthmus (Fig. 4.37).[52]

Pericardial collection can be readily recognized by external apical views on TTE and may obviate the need for TEE in the interest of moving the patient emergently to the operating room. TEE can then be done for detailed

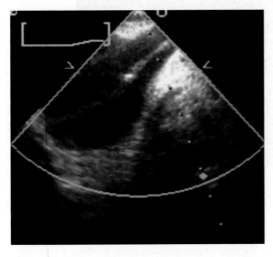

Fig. 4.35 Involvement of subclavian artery by dissection (*arrow*)

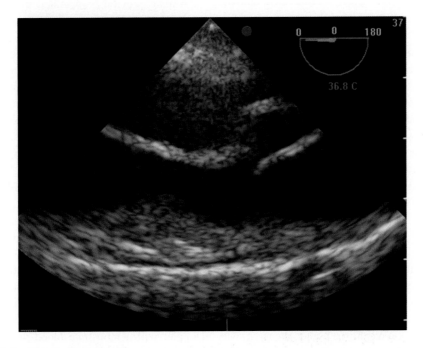

Fig. 4.36 Intimal tear in the aortic arch

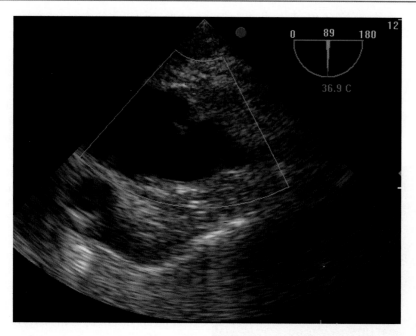

Fig. 4.37 Mediastinal hematoma (*arrow*)

evaluation of dissection process after the patient arrives in the operating room and is hemodynamically stabilized.

Late Complications

Patients with previously operated type A dissections and medically treated type B dissections can present to the operating room with complications. Progressive dilatations are more common in nonoperated type B dissections than operated type A dissections.[36] Enlargement of the false lumen leads to a dissecting aneurysm and makes the definition of the outer boundary difficult. Aneurysmal enlargement should be dealt with urgently, as the chances of rupture are very high. In a series of 50 type B medically managed dissections, 20% had rapid expansion and 18% had rupture at 3 years. Complications are more common with aortic diameter more than 40 mm and persistent false lumen flow.[53] Uncontained rupture into the pleural space and the mediastinum causes sudden death. Ruptures contained by aortic adventitia result in a pseudoaneurysm and hematoma formation. Both dissecting aneurysms and pseudoaneurysms can be identified by TEE. Contrast injection is helpful in diagnosing rupture and extravasation into the surrounding tissues.

Among previously operated type A dissections, abnormalities may develop in both operated and nonoperated segments. Dilation of noncontiguous, nonoperated aortic segments develops in 17% of patients with prior acute type A dissections.[54] Screening of progressive disease by imaging can potentially prevent rupture and redissection. When recurrent chest pain and hemodynamic instability occurs, redissection should be considered, and TEE can define new pathologic abnormality and extent. The images should be compared with previous TEE images at the time of surgery and discharge.

Pseudoaneurysm formation can occur in 7–25% of patients with composite grafts such as Bentall procedure secondary to hemorrhage at a suture line dehiscence (Fig. 4.38). Blood between the graft and aortic wall can create supravalvular aortic stenosis. Both of these complications can be detected and delineated by TEE.[55] Color flow Doppler will demonstrate blood flow into echo free space between graft and aortic wall.

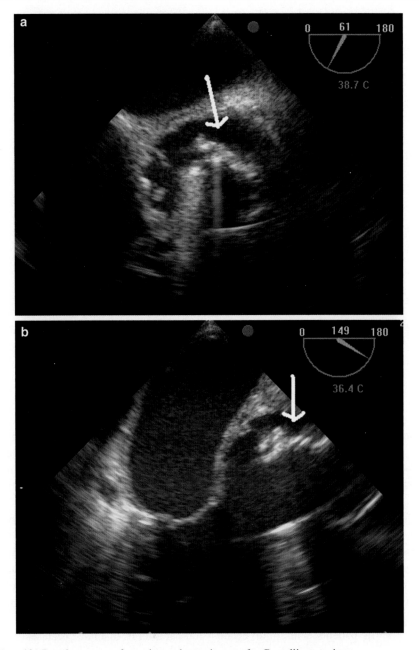

Fig. 4.38 (**a** and **b**) Pseudoaneurysm formation at the aortic root after Bentall's procedure

Mitral Regurgitation

Mitral regurgitation (MR) in aortic disease could be the result of wall motion changes related to coronary artery involvement, ventricular dilatation induced by aortic insufficiency, or a result of an underlying disorder such as MS (Fig. 4.39). Mitral valve involvement in MS (annular dilatation, annular calcification, and prolapse) is either isolated or associated with fusiform aneurysms.[56] Evaluation of the mechanism of MR is important in planning for surgical repair/replacement versus no intervention.

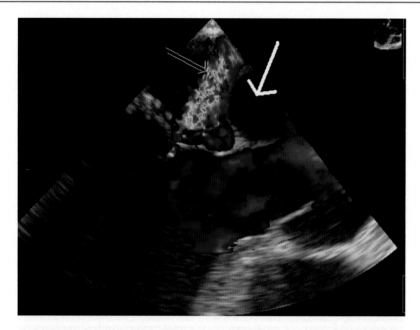

Fig. 4.39 ME long axis view showing aneurysm of sinus of Valsalva (*arrow*) with mitral disease and regurgitation in a patient with Marfan syndrome (*double arrow*)

Post-bypass evaluation is equally important after repair or if the decision was made to leave the MR alone.

Intramural Hematoma

Intramural hematoma (IMH) represents 15–30% of all aortic syndromes. In one series, IMH involved the ascending aorta in 48%, the aortic arch in 8%, and the descending aorta in 44% of patients.[57] IMH can occur in patients with severe atherosclerosis in whom penetrating aortic ulcers or atherosclerotic plaque rupture could be the initiating factor. In patients with mild or no atherosclerosis, spontaneous rupture of vasavasorum may initiate aortic wall degeneration, which eventually leads to a hematoma in the aortic wall and splitting of aortic wall layers and dissection formation without intimal tear.[58] Patients in the first group tend to be older and associated with coronary and peripheral vascular disease. Aortic insufficiency is rare. By TEE, intimal flap, reentry tears, or false lumen flows are not detectable unlike classic dissection

(Fig. 4.40).[59] There is a controversy regarding intimal tears in IMH. Some consider that finding an intimal tear precludes the diagnosis while others feel that IMH may be associated with intimal tears (small communications representing intimal rupture). Aortic wall normally measures 3–4 mm in thickness. Crescentric or circular thickening more than 5 mm with symptoms suffices for the diagnosis of IMH.[60] Echolucent areas or echo free space within the thickened aortic wall can also be demonstrated in some patients. This may represent a pool of low blood flow that comes from the aortic lumen through tiny intimal ruptures or the ostia of intercostal or lumbar arteries that have been severed by hematoma. Echolucency is not a poor prognostic sign.[61] The presence of fluid extravasation (pericardial and pleural effusion and periaortic mediastinal hemorrhage) is a frequent finding in IMH compared to classic dissections.[62] Large and progressive increases in effusion are ominous signs. IMH should be differentiated from dissection with false lumen thrombus, atherosclerotic aortic wall thickening, and aneurysmal dilatation with intramural thrombus. TEE is superior to

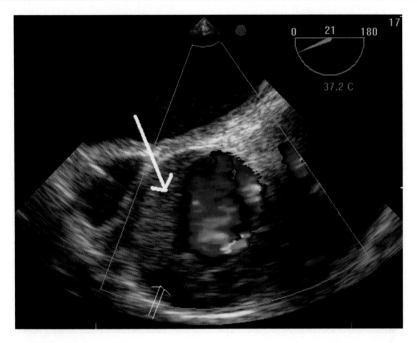

Fig. 4.40 Intramural hematoma with echolucency (*double arrow*) of ascending aorta

other techniques in demonstrating smooth intimal wall in IMH compared to all other disease processes.[60,61] The sensitivity and specificity of TEE in diagnosing IMH is 90% and 99%, respectively.[63] Although the studies that compare the diagnostic sensitivity and specificity of imaging techniques do not exist, their diagnostic accuracy does not appear to be significantly different. Surgical intervention is recommended in patients with type A IMH because ascending aortic involvement is an indicator of disease progression. Localized dissection, aneurysm formation, and rupture are sequel of IMH. Predictors of disease progression include maximum aortic diameter greater than 50 mm, rapid aortic enlargement, aortic wall thickness > 11 mm, large and repetitive fluid collection in the chest, localized dissection (Fig. 4.41), and presence of an associated penetrating ulcer or an ulcer-like projection in the involved segment.[64-66] All these should be looked for when you are presented with IMH and other imaging techniques like CT and MRI should be utilized in the decision-making process.

Penetrating Aortic Ulcers

This term describes the condition in which ulceration of an aortic atherosclerotic lesion penetrates the internal elastic lamina into media (Fig. 4.42). Patients are older and usually do not have connective tissue diseases. Most of the PAU occur in the descending aorta. The main handicap is that there is no imaging diagnostic technique that can document the disruption of internal elastic lamina. Vilacosta et al. evaluated the role of TEE in the diagnosis of PAU and concluded that TEE can recognize these ulcers and complications associated with them.[67] TEE may reveal an ulcerative plaque that projects deep into the medial wall layer, frequently with spontaneous contrast at the site. Color flow may demonstrate flow into the ulcer. PAU can be the precursor for IMH, dissection, adventitial rupture, or contained rupture with pseudoaneurysm formation, and all of these can be demonstrated by TEE.[67] They do not develop pericardial effusion, valvular insufficiency, or cardiovascular compromise but

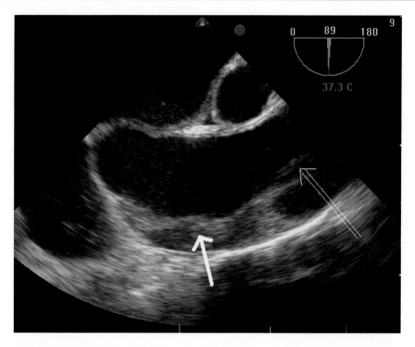

Fig. 4.41 Intramural hematoma progressing to dissection (*double arrow*) in the ascending aorta

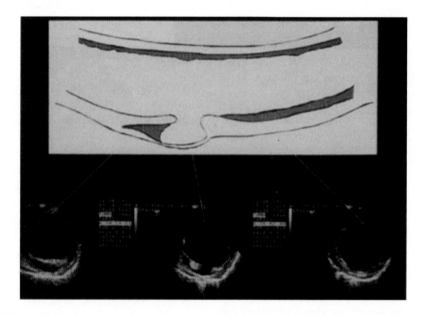

Fig. 4.42 Figure illustrating penetrating aortic ulcers (Reprinted with permission from [Springer publishers] reference [31])

may accumulate blood in the mediastinal and pleural space.

TEE features of dissections secondary to PAU have distinctive features from classic dissections; the dissections are short, being limited by the fibrosis and calcification of atherosclerosis. They occur commonly at the mid or distal descending aorta unlike classic dissections. The intimomedial

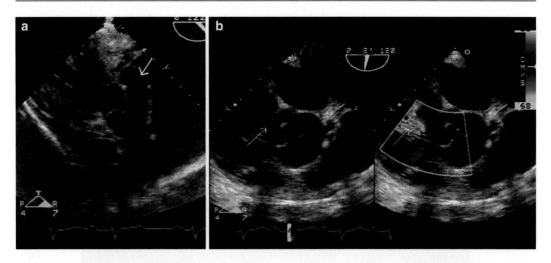

Fig. 4.43 (**a**) Congenital sinus of Valsalva aneurysm (*arrow*) shown in transgastric long axis view (**b**) Rupture (*arrow*) of noncoronary sinus of Valsalva into the right atrium with turbulent color flow through the rupture (*arrow*) *Acknowledgement*: Dr. Wilfred Lewis MD, Department of Anesthesiology, North share Medical center, Salem Hospital, Salem, MA

flap is thick, calcific, and static. The true lumen is larger than the false lumen and the dissection can take retrograde direction.[67] Medical therapy may be indicated in stable patients. Few centers advocate surgical therapy because of the frequent late complications.

Echocardiographic Evaluation of Aneurysms

Sinus of Valsalva Aneurysms

The etiology is usually congenital but can occur with cystic medial degeneration, MS, endocarditis, or a penetrating injury. A weakness in the aortic media at its junction with annulus fibrosis is thought to be the cause of the congenital aneurysms of the sinus of Valsalva. Abnormal dilatation of one or more of the sinuses gives windsock appearance in the midesophageal aortic valve short axis view. This typical appearance of an extended aneurysm channel is not seen in acquired aortic fistulas. They occur most commonly in the right coronary sinus (69%) and the noncoronary sinus (26%) (Fig. 4.43a) but can be seen in the left coronary sinus (5%). Other congenital cardiac diseases may be associated (bicuspid valve, VSD, ASD, pulmonic stenosis, and PDA). Patients are asymptomatic until the aneurysm ruptures into the right atrium or the right ventricle. Rupture will result in echocardiographic evidence of RV overload. Color Doppler will show a swirling flow pattern in an intact aneurysm and a high-velocity turbulent flow pattern in the ruptured aneurysm (Fig. 4.43b). The aortic valve is morphologically normal. Aortic valve prolapse and aortic incompetence may be associated. Compression of adjacent structures like RVOT, LVOT, and tricuspid valve (with varying degrees of tricuspid regurgitation) may be seen. A ventricular septal defect and conduction abnormalities may result.

Acquired aneurysms differ from congenital aneurysms in that they are often associated with dilatation of the ascending aorta, involve more than one sinus, may rupture into the pericardium or other cardiac chambers (endocarditis).[7] ME LAX view is especially useful in the diagnosis (Fig. 4.39).

Role of Intraoperative TEE in Aortic Aneurysm Surgery

The threshold for operations in asymptomatic patients includes an aortic diameter twice normal or an absolute aortic diameter of more than 5.5 cm and rapid growth (growth rate>5 mm/year).

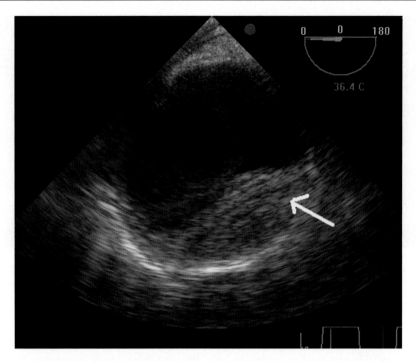

Fig. 4.44 Aneurysm of the aorta with mural thrombus formation (*arrow*)

Surgery is indicated for lower aortic diameters (4.5–5 cm) in patients with MFS, bicuspid aortic valve and in patients presenting for aortic valve surgery because of aortic stenosis or regurgitation.[68,69]

Intraoperative TEE can confirm the nature (true vs. false), location, extent, shape, size, and etiopathogenesis of aortic aneurysms and the presence of associated complications such as dissection and mural thrombus (Fig. 4.44). All this information may be available to the surgeon by preoperative imaging (CT/MRI or aortography) in elective surgical patients. There could be a variation in the measurements between CT imaging and TEE with TEE being less than CT measurements and variability increases with an increase in the diameter of the aneurysms. In few patients, aortic aneurysm may be an accidental finding detected by intraoperative TEE during another cardiac surgery such as coronary artery bypass grafting. Most surgeons will replace the aorta more than 4.5 cm in diameter. Between 4 and 4.5 cm, several factors such as age, expected survival, prolongation of CPB time, and requirement of DHCA with associated morbidity and mortality have to be considered for surgical decision-making. This finding also influences

the site of aortic cannulation even if the surgeon decides to leave the aneurysm alone. In recipients of heart transplantations, a finding of ascending aneurysms may influence the donor surgeon to take extra length of the ascending aorta along with the donor heart.

However, the most important use of intraoperative TEE is the assessment of the aortic valve and the aortic root to evaluate the feasibility of aortic valve repair and perform post-bypass assessment of the repaired valve for residual regurgitation.

In case of aortic pseudoaneurysms, TEE can further define the origin, etiology, extent and contents in the pseudoaneurysms. TEE can distinguish pseudo from true aneurysms by defining the narrow neck of the pseudoaneurysm by two-dimensional and Doppler technology (bidirectional blood flow through the connecting neck between the aorta and the pseudoaneurysm). The pseudoaneurysmal sac may expand during systole and collapse during diastole. Intraluminal spontaneous echo contrast, thrombus, or infective vegetations (mycotic aneurysms; Fig. 4.45) can be observed in the pseudoaneurysms. Pseudoaneurysms arising from the anterior or posterior wall should be defined, as the

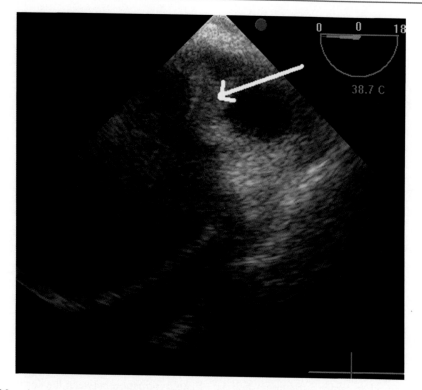

Fig. 4.45 Mycotic aneurysm of the ascending aorta filled with infective material (*arrow*)

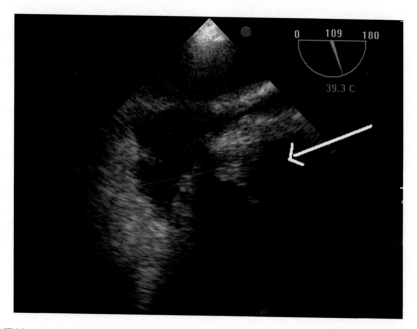

Fig. 4.46 ME bicaval view showing compression of right atrium and superior vena cava by huge pseudoaneurysm of ascending aorta (*arrow*)

anterior pathology is more prone for rupture dur-ing sternotomy. Compression of the surrounding structures such as the pulmonary artery, the right ventricular outflow tract, and the superior vena cava by a huge pseudoaneurysm can be noticed by TEE (Fig. 4.46).[70,71] Free rupture into the mediastinum

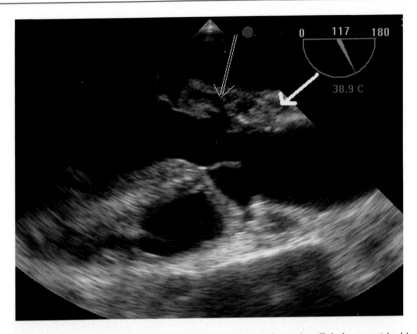

Fig. 4.47 Infective endocarditis with periannular aortic abscess (*arrow*) formation. Echolucency (*double arrows*) indicate cavity formation in the abscess

and fistula with other cardiac structures such as the right atrium, the right ventricle, and the pulmonary artery may be seen.[72–74] It may be difficult to obtain regular TEE views in cases of a huge pseudoaneurysm displacing the cardiac structures. Associated findings such as dissection, atherosclerotic ulcer, and infective endocarditis of the valves and vegetations will help in the identification of the etiology. Finally, TEE is a helpful tool to guide catheter-based treatments such as endograft and Amplatzer® septal occluder device for aortic pseudoaneurysms.[75]

Infectious Endocarditis Involvement in Aortic Root

Infections from the aortic and mitral valve may be associated with periannular thickening indicating abscess formation (thickness > 10 mm). Mitral aortic intervalvular fibrosa may be involved. Abscesses appear as homogenous echodense thickening by TEE (Fig. 4.47). Cavitation and echolucency occur later (Fig. 4.47). Rupture into the aortic root causes pseudoaneurysm with to and fro Doppler color flow signals (Fig. 4.48).

Fistula formation between the aortic root and the left atrium should be looked for by TEE in such cases (Fig. 4.48). TEE is more sensitive and specific than TTE for detection of periaortic complications with infective aortic valves. Perivalvular echo findings are associated with higher perioperative and long-term morbidity and mortality.

Traumatic Aortic Injuries

Thoracic aortic trauma is common after severe deceleration injuries. Aortic isthmus is involved in 90% of cases presenting to the operating room. TEE is highly sensitive (91%) and specific (100%).[76,77] TEE findings are important in planning management. Intimal tears and intramural localized hematoma can be managed medically. Subadventitial disruption and pseudoaneurysm formation should be treated either by endovascular or surgical management as appropriate. Active bleeding with increasing mediastinal hematoma or obstruction by thick flap (pseudo-coarctation) requires immediate surgery or endovascular surgery. TEE characteristics of traumatic subadventitial disruption differ from aortic dissection (Table 4.6)

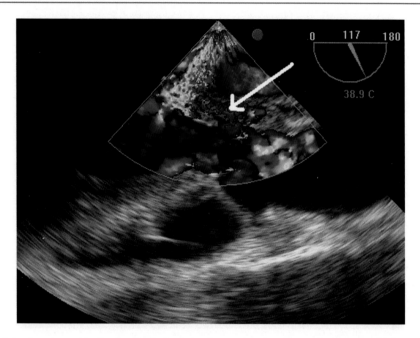

Fig. 4.48 Color flow (*arrow*) indicating fistula formation between periannular aortic abscess and left atrium

Table 4.6 TEE Characteristics of traumatic aortic injury

	Aortic trauma	Dissection
Site	Isthmus	Ascending, arch, descending any site
Flap	Highly mobile, contains both intima and media (3–5 mm)	Thin (intima + 1/3 media), less mobile
Flap	Runs oblique and vertical through the lumen	Runs parallel to the lumen
Aortic contour	Deformed, asymmetric	None
Aortic diameter	Preserved	Symmetrically enlarged
Entry, reentry tears	Absent	Present
Thrombus in false lumen	Absent	May be present
Mediastinal hematoma	Present	May be present
Flow velocities	Similar on either side of the flap	Differential velocities
Mosaic pattern around the lesion	Present	Absent

(Fig. 4.49). TEE cannot be utilized in patients with severe edema from facial and mandibular fractures and in patients with unstable neck trauma.

Coarcation of Aorta

Coarctation presents as the narrowed segment of the aorta below the origin of the subclavian artery in TEE with color flow turbulence and increased velocity at the stenotic level (Fig. 4.50). It is difficult to align the continuous wave Doppler to stenotic segment and measure the pressure gradient across the stenosis in TEE views. TTE suprasternal views can estimate pressure gradient reliably. It is also possible to observe collateral flow by TEE. Associated cardiac anomalies should be looked for in the perioperative TEE examination (ventricular septal defect, bicuspid aortic valve, patent ductus arteriosus, mitral stenosis, or regurgitation). Patent

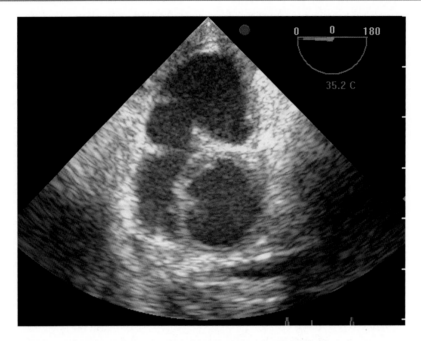

Fig. 4.49 Traumatic aortic disruption. Note the thick flap running vertically inside aortic lumen

ductus arteriosus can be diagnosed by TEE and its size and blood flow can be assessed. Systemic blood flow to pulmonary blood flow ratio can be calculated. Persistent distension of the left side of the heart during bypass may be an indication to look for and rule out patent ductus arteriosus.

Iatrogenic Aortic Injury

Iatrogenic injuries to the aorta can be caused by intraluminal balloon pump insertion, stenting, and aortic cannulation and decannulation for cardiopulmonary bypass (Fig. 4.51). TEE guided instrumentation can prevent these injuries. Routine examination of the aortic wall and lumina after any instrumentation should be done to detect these injuries early. Localized dissection and embolization are the main injuries. TEE is used as guide to cannulate the true lumen in patients with dissection either from the femoral artery or from the ascending aorta. Flow in true lumen is observed by TEE after cannulation to confirm the position of the arterial cannula.

Echocardiography for Endovascular Aortic Surgery

TEE

Intraoperative TEE is a very useful adjunct in patients undergoing thoracic aortic endoluminal surgery. TEE is an attractive intraoperative imaging modality in addition to the standard imaging technique of "angiography" used to deploy the stents.[78–80] TEE helps minimize contrast exposure for fluoroscopy. TEE has been shown to be useful in deployment of stents for various types of lesions (dissections, aneurysms, and traumatic aortic injury) located in the descending thoracic aorta, the aortic arch, and the ascending aorta.[81,82] Visualization of lesions in the blind spot (distal ascending aorta and proximal arch) is limited (Fig. 4.52). Other disadvantages are possible discomfort due to the continuous esophageal imaging and thereby necessitating general anesthesia, which could have been avoided in some if not all. The associated complications with TEE placement should be recognized and cared for. Although TEE probe by

Fig. 4.50 Coarctation of aorta (**a**) with turbulent flow across the coarctation (**b**)

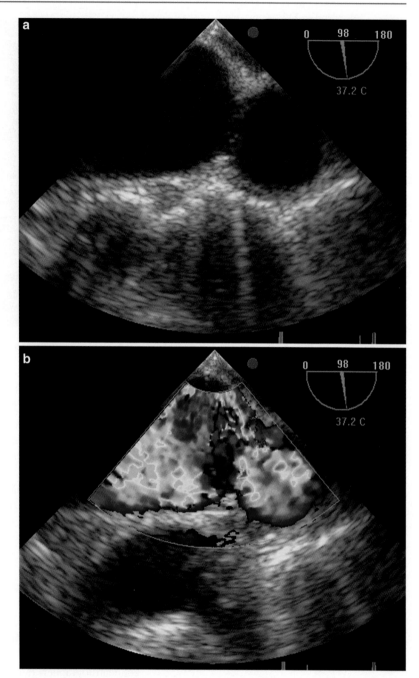

itself could play the role of a landmark and help the surgeon to optimize stent position and deployment, it interferes with fluoroscopic examinations (Fig. 4.53). Therefore, TEE is used in between fluoroscopic imaging to avoid interference.

IVUS

Intravascular ultrasound (IVUS) is used by the endovascular surgeons to aid fluoroscopy in endograft procedures for aneurysms, dissections,

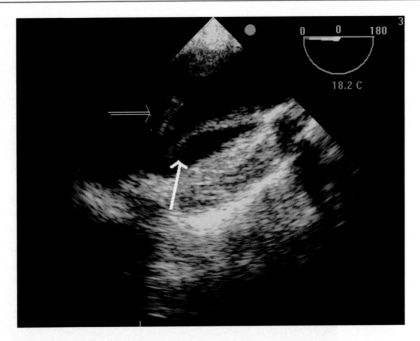

Fig. 4.51 Iatrogenic dissection of proximal aortic arch (*arrow*) by aortic cannulation (*double arrow*)

and traumatic disruptions. An IVUS probe (8–10 MHz probe for aorta) is introduced through the endovascular sheath to study the endoluminal aspect of the aorta (Fig. 4.54a and b). Imaging is displayed in the fluoroscopy screen and used to compare and correlate the findings of fluoroscopy (Fig. 4.55). IVUS can delineate intraluminal pathology, assess landing zones, locate branch vessels, and allow measurements for stent size selection[83] (Fig. 4.56a). IVUS can also assess the accuracy of endograft deployment, degree of device expansion, and stent apposition of the prosthesis to the vessel wall[83] (Fig. 4.56b).

TEE and Pre-stent Deployment Phase

The first purpose of TEE examination is to confirm the diagnosis of thoracic aortic disease (aneurysm, dissection, and traumatic aortic injury) for which endovascular therapy is planned. TEE also helps with exact lesion localization, sizing of the lesion, and the choice of the landing zones as it can delineate the presence of calcifications, complex atheromatous plaques, and intraluminal

thrombus.[31] TEE also has the ability to locate large intercostal arteries so that their exclusion by the graft can be avoided and occlusion can be detected early if it occurs. However, their visualization is not consistent. Finally, a comprehensive cardiac and valvular function can be evaluated and monitored continuously during the procedure since most of these patients have severe concomitant cardiac disease.

Stent Deployment Phase

TEE can help place guidewires and endovascular delivery sheath. This is an extension of skills routinely used by the intraoperative echocardiographer during the management of minimally invasive cardiac surgery. In the longitudinal view, the catheter delivery device can be visualized only in precise planes. The short axis view is more useful to visualize positioning of these devices. The stent-graft delivery system is distinguished from the guidewire by differences in echogenicity and thickness.[80] The stent-graft can be differentiated from the delivery system by

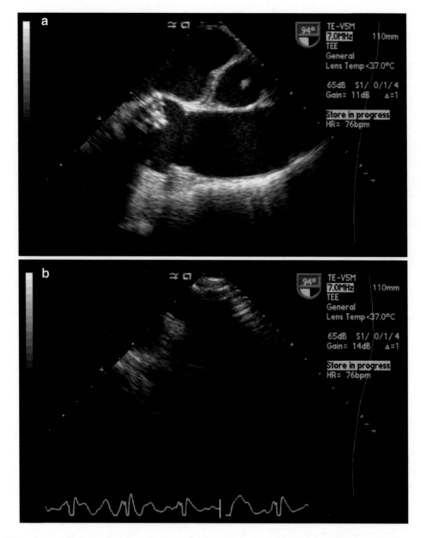

Fig. 4.52 TEE views of distal ascending aorta and proximal arch are limited by interposition of trachea and left bronchus

the unique echogenic pattern and shadow from the metallic stent.[80] TEE has the ability to visualize the undeployed stent-graft in relation to the normal and diseased aorta and ensure that the endograft bridges the diseased aortic segment (Fig. 4.57a–d).

Several complications due to intraaortic manipulations can happen during this phase. Extensive instrumentation in the aorta can lead to disruption of atherosclerotic plaques or intraluminal thrombus resulting in stroke. TEE helps in avoidance of such complications during instrumentation.

TEE guidance prevents the unintentional entry of the wires and stent introducer into the pseudoaneurysm and false lumen of dissections.[84,85] Intimal dehiscence and iatrogenic dissections can be diagnosed early by TEE.[86,87]

Post-deployment Phase

Immediately after stent deployment, TEE confirms the placement of endograft across the diseased aorta. Both proximal and distal ends and

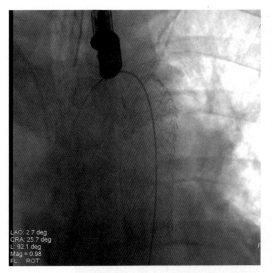

Fig. 4.53 Fluoroscopic image of endovascular stent deployment. TEE may interfere with fluoroscopy so the probe has to be withdrawn intermittently

Table 4.7 Classification of endoleaks

Type	Description
I	Attachment site leak
	A Proximal leak
	B Distal leak
	C Iliac occluder (seen with abdominal aneurysms)
II	Branch leaks
	A To and fro simple flow from branch vessel into the aneurismal sac
	B Complex flow through two or more branch vessels into aneurismal sac
III	Graft defect
	A Midgraft hole
	B Junctional leak or graft disconnection
	C Other mechanism (failure from suture holes)
IV	Graft wall porosity

Classification of endoleaks (From Swaminathan,[105] with permission.)
EVAR endovascular aortic repair, *AAA* abdominal aortic aneurysm

the endoluminal side of the graft should be inspected. It is not uncommon to see some debris, small clots, or spontaneous echo contrast on the endoluminal side, and these are the consequence of decreased aortic flow due to induced hypotension during deployment. Malpositioning of the endograft with the aorta and mal-alignment of the two endografts diagnosed with TEE can lead to early interventions.[88,89] Color flow is utilized to detect endoleaks. Balloon inflation to optimize the degree of contact between the stent and aortic wall or to treat the mal-aligned grafts is done using TEE guidance.[31]

Detection of Endoleaks

An endoleak occurs when there is persistent blood flow into the aneurysmal sac or the excluded portion of the aorta.[90] Color flow Doppler helps detect the leaks from the central aorta into the excluded diseased aorta.[80] Device migration, malposition, or mal-alignment is associated with endoleaks. A persistent leak into the aneurysmal sac causes endotension and has the potential to expand and rupture.[91] Leaks can be antegrade (from the proximal and distal ends of the aortic endograft) or retrograde (aneurysmal sacs can fill

via the branches such as the intercostal arteries). Endoleaks are not always visualized by CT or angiography.[92]

Definition of Endoleaks and Endotension

The definitions and the management of endoleaks and endotensions were agreed upon (103) in a multidisciplinary consensus conference. Endoleaks and endotensions were classified in this consensus conference (Table 4.7).[93] A type I endoleak is usually treated with an additional graft in the proximal or the distal end. It potentially leads to persistent blood flow and increased endotension. Not all endoleaks lead to endotension. However, there is no clinical way to measure endotension. A retrograde flow into the aneurysmal sac from a patent collateral branch vessel leads to type II endoleaks. These leaks tend to resolve spontaneously. Type III leaks which result from graft defects are usually treated with a covered stent. Graft porosity, otherwise known as type IV, is a diagnosis by exclusion of an identifiable source of leaks. Pulse wave Doppler-aided quantification of endoleak velocity helps to discriminate true leaks from porosity. A minimum peak velocity of 50 cm/s is the suggested cutoff.[94] Endoleaks are termed primary if

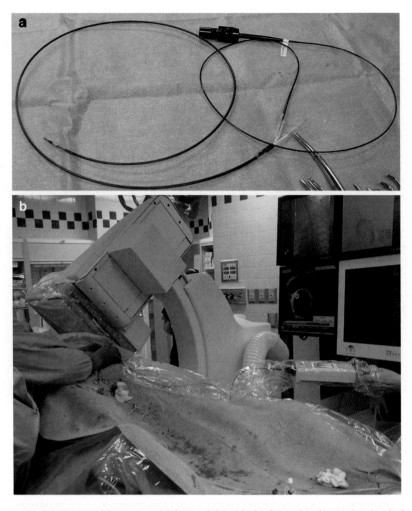

Fig. 4.54 Intravascular ultrasound instrument (**a**) inserted through the femoral endovascular sheath (**b**) to study the aortic intraluminal pathology

occurring within 30 days of stent deployment as opposed to secondary leaks, which are seen later.[95]

Utility of TEE in Endoleak Detection

The importance of TEE in evaluating endoleaks has been described.[78,79] Color flow Doppler has been found to be sensitive in detecting endoleaks even when angiography fails to detect the smaller ones. Angiography may miss the small dye quantity or may be at an off angle. Presence of spontaneous echo contrast within the aneurysmal sac may also be the first suggestion of an endoleak. Presence of a dynamic echocardiographic "smoke"

is very different from the static one. A dynamic smoke often implies a leak. In 22 consecutive patients undergoing thoracic aortic stent placements, TEE has been shown to have increased sensitivity and specificity in identifying endoleaks.[79] Intraoperative TEE provides additional information and improves immediate and late procedural results by detecting endoleaks.[96] TEE has also been shown to detect perigraft leakage, which was not previously identified during the intraoperative fluoroscopy.[97] Contrast-enhanced ultrasound has been shown to detect endoleaks, particularly when other modalities fail.[98]

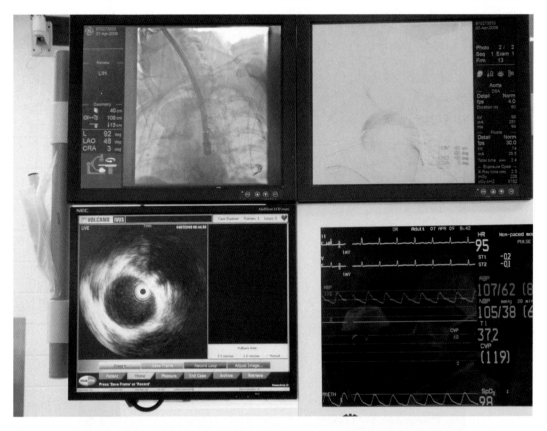

Fig. 4.55 Endovascular suite screens showing fluoroscopic images, intravascular ultrasound, and vitals monitor

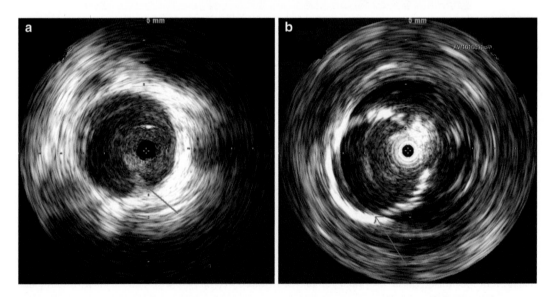

Fig. 4.56 (**a** and **b**) Intravascular ultrasound image of traumatic intimal flap (*arrow*) and the image after endovascular stenting (**b**)

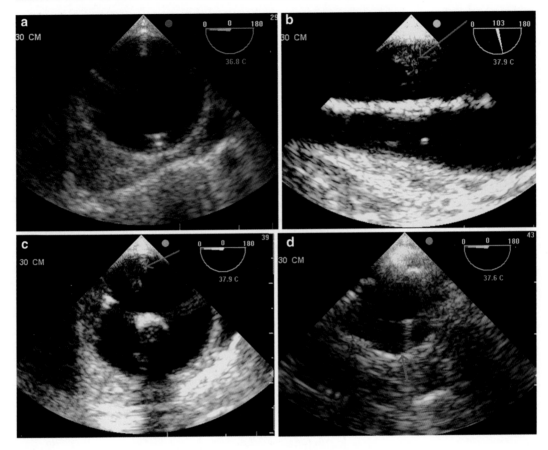

Fig. 4.57 The use of TEE in endovascular stenting. (**a**) Guidewire within aortic lumen. Descending aortic long axis (**b**) and short axis (**c**) showing the endovascular stent bridging the traumatic intimal flap (*arrow*) of thoracic aorta (**d**) shows TEE image after endovascular stent deployment (*arrow*)

Comparison of TEE with Other Modalities for Endoleak Detection

A comparison of angiography, TEE and intravascular ultrasound (IVUS) was done to evaluate their ability to guide stent-graft implantation. TEE was superior to IVUS and angiography in endoleak detection.[99] Guidewire position over the entire length of the disease aorta was documented more frequently by TEE and IVUS compared to angiography.[100] The entry site of dissection was better identified with TEE and IVUS. The proximal leaks were identified well by TEE leading to additional graft placement. TEE, by its multiplane visualization and versatility, was superior to angiography in detection of endoleaks especially at the left carotid and the left subclavian branch takeoffs. TEE provides additional incremental information to angiography in safe placement of stent-grafts.[99] In patients with extension of aneurysm/dissection into the abdominal aorta, IVUS was found to improve stent-graft placement along with angiography. TEE has a limited role in abdominal aortic aneurysm (AAA)/dissection management with stent/grafts.[100] TEE assessment of endoleak and thromboexclusion had a sensitivity of 100% and specificity of 100% and was identical to that of postoperative computed tomography or angiography.[101]

TEE Guided Algorithm for Stent Placement in Aortic Dissection

Rocchi et al.[102] developed a TEE-based algorithm (Fig. 4.58) to assess the outcome and guide intraoperative decision-making in patients

Fig. 4.58 TEE-based
algorithm for evaluation of
outcome after endovascular
surgery for aortic dissections
(Reprinted from reference
(102) with permission from
Elsevier)

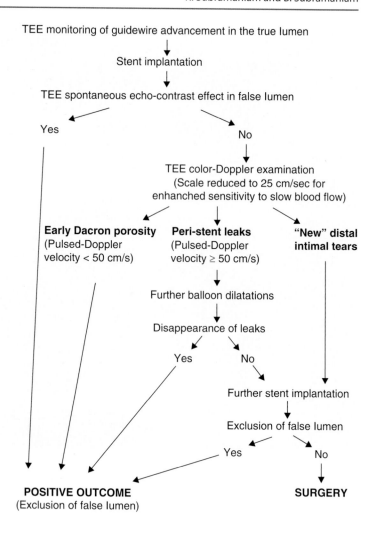

undergoing endovascular surgery for aortic dissection. TEE was used to identify the guidewire in the true lumen first. Following the stent implantation, TEE was used to check stent expansion and false lumen exclusion. Presence of a smoke in the excluded portion of the aorta was the initial marker of good outcome. If there was no smoke, color Doppler examination was done at a low scale of 25 cm/s (enhanced sensitivity to low velocity blood flow). Presence of endoleaks and new additional intimal tears were treated with additional stents. Peri-stent leaks with pulsed Doppler velocity ≥ 50 cm/s were treated with further balloon dilatations. If they did not disappear, further stent implantation was done. Flows with pulsed-wave Doppler velocity less than 50 cm/s were designated as Early Dacron porosity and identified as a positive outcome. In patients with entry intimal tears close to the left subclavian artery, the artery was visualized before and after stent placement with aortic arch imaging at 70°; pulsed-wave Doppler and color Doppler were used to ensure patency of the left subclavian artery. Procedural success was defined by predischarge spiral CT showing a complete exclusion of the false lumen with thrombosis and absence of antegrade flow. Persistent of flow in the false lumen in the abdominal aorta was not considered as a procedural failure.

TEE and IVUS cannot completely replace fluoroscopy. They are useful adjuvants for thoracic endoaortic surgery as they can confirm the diagnosis, assist in the stent-graft placement, assess the adequacy of isolation of pathology, and detect endoleaks.

Key Notes

1. Echocardiography is invaluable in the preoperative assessment, intraoperative management, and postoperative follow-up of aortic diseases.
2. Sensitivity and specificity of transesophageal echocardiography is comparable to other modern imaging modalities (CT angiography and MRI scanning).
3. Echocardiography is the modality of choice for the evaluation of hemodynamically unstable aortic surgical patient.
4. Echocardiography is the method of choice for the evaluation of aortic valve in aortic pathologies and assessment of aortic valve after repair of aortic valve is a category 1 indication for intraoperative TEE.
5. Echocardiography is also helpful in the evaluation of coronary arteries, branch vessels, and other complications such as tamponade or leaking aneurysms.
6. TEE and IVUS are very useful in defining intimal pathology, guiding the endograft placement and also evaluation for endoleaks when used in combination with fluoroscopy during endovascular aortic surgery.

References

1. Victor MR, Mintz GS, Kotler MN, Wilson AR, Segal BL. Two-dimensional echocardiographic diagnosis of aortic dissection. *Am J Cardiol.* 1981;48:1155–1159.
2. Mathew T, Nanda NC. Two-dimensional and Doppler echocardiographic evaluation of aortic aneurysm and dissection. *Am J Cardiol.* 1984;54: 379–385.
3. Khandheria BK, Tajik AJ, Taylor CL, et al. Aortic dissection: review of value and limitations of two-dimensional echocardiography in a six year experience. *J Am Soc Echocardiogr.* 1989;2:17–25.
4. Granato JE, Dee P, Gibson RS. Utility of two-dimensional echocardiography in suspected ascend-

5. Evangelista A, Avegliano G, Elorz C, González-Alujas T, Garcia del Castillo H, Soler-Soler J. Transesophageal echocardiography in the diagnosis of acute aortic syndrome. *J Card Surg.* March–April 2002;17(2):95–106.
6. Chandrasekaran K, Currie PJ. Transesophageal echocardiography in aortic dissection. *J Inv Card.* 1989;1:328–338.
7. St John Sutton MG, Maniet AR. Diseases of the thoracic aorta. In: St John Sutton MG, Maniet AR, eds. *Atlas of multiplane transesophageal echocardiography.* 1st ed. New York: Taylor & Francis; 2003:333–468.
8. Moore AG, Eagle KA, Bruckman D, et al. Choice of computed tomography, transesophageal echocardiography, magnetic resonance imaging, and aortography in acute aortic dissection: International Registry of Acute Aortic Dissection (IRAD). *Am J Cardiol.* May 15, 2002;89(10):1235–1238.
9. Hashimoto S, Kumada T, Osakada G, et al. Assessment of transesophageal Doppler echography in dissecting aortic aneurysm. *J Am Coll Cardiol.* November 1, 1989;14(5):1253–1262.
10. Ballal RS, Nanda NC, Gatewood R, et al. Usefulness of transesophageal echocardiography in assessment of aortic dissection. *Circulation.* 1991;84: 1903–1914.
11. Adachi H, Omoto R, Kyo S, et al. Emergency surgical intervention of acute aortic dissection with the rapid diagnosis by transesophageal echocardiography. *Circulation.* November 1991;84:14–19.
12. Simon P, Owen AN, Havel M, et al. Transesophageal echocardiography in the emergency surgical management of patients with aortic dissection. *J Thorac Cardiovasc Surg.* 1992;103:1113–1117.
13. Erbel R, Engberding R, Daniel W, Roelandt J, Visser C, Rennollet H. Echocardiography in diagnosis of aortic dissection. *Lancet.* March 4, 1989;1(8636): 457–461.
14. Nienaber CA, von Kodolitsch Y, Nicolas V, et al. The diagnosis of thoracic aortic dissection by noninvasive imaging procedures. *N Engl J Med.* 1993;328:1–9.
15. Laissy JP, Blanc F, Soyer P, et al. Thoracic aortic dissection: diagnosis with transesophageal echocardiography versus MR imaging. *Radiology.* 1995;194: 331–336.
16. Bansal RC, Chandrasekaran K, Ayala K, Smith DC. Frequency and explanation of false negative diagnosis of aortic dissection by aortography and transesophageal echocardiography. *J Am Coll Cardiol.* May 1995;25(6):1393–1401.
17. Keren A, Kim CB, Hu BS, et al. Accuracy of biplane and multiplane transesophageal echocardiography in diagnosis of typical acute aortic dissection and intramural hematoma. *J Am Coll Cardiol.* September 1996;28(3):627–636.
18. Vignon P, Guéret P, Vedrinne JM, et al. Role of transesophageal echocardiography in the diagnosis

ing aortic dissection. *Am J Cardiol.* July 1, 1985;56(1): 123–129.

and management of traumatic aortic disruption. *Circulation*. November 15, 1995;92(10):2959–2968.

19. Pepi M, Campodonico J, Galli C, et al. Rapid diagnosis and management of thoracic aortic dissection and intramural haematoma: a prospective study of advantages of multiplane vs. biplane transoesophageal echocardiography. *Eur J Echocardiogr*. 2000;1: 72–79.

20. Nishino M, Tanouchi J, Tanaka K, et al. Transesophageal echocardiographic diagnosis of thoracic aortic dissection with the completely thrombosed false lumen: differentiation from true aortic aneurysm with mural thrombus. *J Am Soc Echocardiogr*. 1996;9:79–85.

21. Sommer T, Fehske W, Holzknecht N, et al. Aortic dissection: a comparative study of diagnosis with spiral CT, multiplanar transesophageal echocardiography, and MR imaging. *Radiology*. 1996;199: 347–352.

22. Evangelista A, Garcia-del-Castillo H, Gonzalez-Alujas T, et al. Diagnosis of ascending aortic dissection by transesophageal echocardiography: utility of M-mode in recognizing artifacts. *J Am Coll Cardiol*. 1996;27:102–107.

23. Chirillo F, Cavallini C, Longhini C, et al. Comparative diagnostic value of transesophageal echocardiography and retrograde aortography in the evaluation of thoracic aortic dissection. *Am J Cardiol*. 1994;74: 590–595.

24. Grossman CM, D'Augostino AN. Advanced atherosclerosis in false channels of chronic aortic dissection. *Lancet*. 1993;342:1428–1429.

25. Demertzis S, Casso G, Torre T, Siclari F. Direct epi-aortic ultrasound scanning for the rapid confirmation of intraoperative aortic dissection. *Interact Cardiovasc Thorac Surg*. August 2008;7(4):725–726.

26. Kim CM, Yu SC, Hong SJ. Cardiac tamponade during transesophageal echocardiography in the patient of circumferential aortic dissection. *J Korean Med Sci*. June 1997;12(3):266–268.

27. Dalby Kristensen S, Ramlov Ivarsen H, Egeblad H. Rupture of aortic dissection during attempted transesophageal echocardiography. *Echocardiography*. July 1996;13(4):405–406.

28. Arima H, Sobue K, Tanaka S, Morishima T, Ando H, Katsuya H. Airway obstruction associated with transesophageal echocardiography in a patient with a giant aortic pseudoaneurysm. *Anesth Analg*. September 2002;95(3):558–560.

29. Triulzi M, Gilliam LD, Gentile F, et al. Normal cross sectional echocardiographic values: linear dimensions and chamber areas. *Echocardiography*. 1984;1: 403–426.

30. Fossier AE. Size of the normal aorta. *Ann Clin Med*. 1924;3:525.

31. Massabuau P. Transesophageal echocardiography for diagnosis and treatment of aortic diseases. In: Rousseau H, Verhoye JP, Heautot JF, eds. *Thoracic Aortic Diseases*. 1st ed. Berlin/Heidelberg: Springer; 2006:33–53.

32. Roberts WC, Honing HS. The spectrum of cardiovascular disease in Marfan syndrome: a clinico-

morphologic study of 18 necropsy patients and comparison to 151 previously reported necropsy patients. *Am Heart J*. 1982;104:115–135.

33. Erbel R, Alfonso F, Boileau C, et al. Diagnosis and management of aortic dissection. *Eur Heart J*. September 2001;22(18):1642–1681.

34. Mohr-Kahaly S, Erbel R, Rennollet H, et al. Ambulatory follow-up of aortic dissection by transesophageal two-dimensional and color-coded Doppler echocardiography. *Circulation*. July 1989;80(1): 24–33.

35. Adachi H, Kyo S, Takamoto S, Kimura S, Yokote Y, Omoto R. Early diagnosis and surgical intervention of acute aortic dissection by transesophageal color flow mapping. *Circulation*. November 1990;82(Suppl 4):19–23.

36. Evangelista A, Gonzalez-Alujas T. Pathophysiology of aortic dissection. In: Rousseau H, Verhoye JP, Heautot JF, eds. *Thoracic Aortic Diseases*. 1st ed. Berlin/Heidelberg: Springer; 2006:33–53.

37. Ergin MA, Phillips RA, Galla JD, et al. Significance of distal false lumen after type A dissection repair. *Ann Thorac Surg*. April 1994;57(4): 820–824.

38. Erbel R, Oelert H, Meyer J, et al. Effect of medical and surgical therapy on aortic dissection evaluated by transesophageal echocardiography. Implications for prognosis and therapy. The European Cooperative Study Group on Echocardiography. *Circulation*. May 1993;87(5):1604–1615.

39. Moore NR, Parry AJ, Trottman-Dickenson B, Pillai R, Westaby S. Fate of the native aorta after repair of acute type A dissection: a magnetic resonance imaging study. *Heart*. 1996 Jan;75(1):62–66.

40. Barron DJ, Livesey SA, Brown IW, Delaney DJ, Lamb RK, Monro JL. Twenty-year follow-up of acute type a dissection: the incidence and extent of distal aortic disease using magnetic resonance imaging. *J Card Surg*. May–June 1997;12(3):147–159.

41. Erbel R, Mohr-Kahaly S, Rennollet H, et al. Diagnosis of aortic dissection: the value of transesophageal echocardiography. *Thorac Cardiovasc Surg*. November 1987;35(Spec No 2): 126–133.

42. Roberts WC. Aortic dissection: anatomy, consequences and causes. *Am Heart J*. 1981;101:195-214.

43. Iliceto S, Nanda NC, Rizzon P, et al. Color Doppler evaluation of aortic dissection. *Circulation*. April 1987;75(4):748–755.

44. Chan KL. Usefulness of transesophageal echocardiography in the diagnosis of conditions mimicking aortic dissection. *Am Heart J*. August 1991;122(2): 495–504.

45. Movsowitz HD, Levine RA, Hilgenberg AD, Isselbacher EM. Transesophageal echocardiographic description of the mechanisms of aortic regurgitation in acute type A aortic dissection: implications for aortic valve repair. *J Am Coll Cardiol*. September 2000;36(3):884–890.

46. Mazzucotelli JP, Deleuze PH, Baufreton C, et al. Preservation of the aortic valve in acute aortic

dissection: long-term echocardiographic assessment and clinical outcome. *Ann Thorac Surg*. June 1993; 55(6): 1513–1517.

47. Penn MS, Smedira N, Lytle B, Brener SJ. Does coronary angiography before emergency aortic surgery affect in-hospital mortality? *J Am Coll Cardiol*. March 15, 2000;35(4):889–894.

48. Orihashi K, Matsuura Y, Sueda T, et al. Abdominal aorta and visceral arteries visualized with transesophageal echocardiography during operations on the aorta. *J Thorac Cardiovasc Surg*. April 1998;115(4): 945–947.

49. Voci P, Tritapepe L, Testa G, Caretta Q. Imaging of the anterior spinal artery by transesophageal color Doppler ultrasonography. *J Cardiothorac Vasc Anesth*. October 1999;13(5):586–587.

50. Orihashi K, Sueda T, Okada K, Imai K. Perioperative diagnosis of mesenteric ischemia in acute aortic dissection by transesophageal echocardiography. *Eur J Cardiothorac Surg*. December 2005;28(6): 871–876.

51. Chandrasekaran K, Edwards WD, Malouf JF, Gillman G, Oh JK. Role of echocardiography in the diagnosis of aortic dissection. In: Baliga RR, Nienaber CA, Isselbacher EM, Eagle KA, eds. *Aortic Dissection and Related Syndromes*. 1st ed. New York: Springer; 2007:61–85.

52. Vignon P, Rambaud G, François B, Preux PM, Lang RM, Gastinne H. Quantification of traumatic hemomediastinum using transesophageal echocardiography: impact on patient management. *Chest*. June 1998;113(6):1475–1480.

53. Juvonen T, Ergin MA, Galla JD, et al. Risk factors for rupture of chronic type B dissections. *J Thorac Cardiovasc Surg*. April 1999;117(4):776–786.

54. Heinemann M, Laas J, Karck M, Borst HG. Thoracic aortic aneurysms after acute type A aortic dissection: necessity for follow-up. *Ann Thorac Surg*. April 1990;49(4):580–584.

55. San Román JA, Vilacosta I, Castillo JA, Rollán MJ, Sánchez-Harguindey L. Role of transesophageal echocardiography in the assessment of patients with composite aortic grafts for therapy in acute aortic dissection. *Am J Cardiol*. March 1, 1994;73(7):519–521.

56. Roberts WC, Honig HS. The spectrum of cardiovascular disease in the Marfan syndrome: a clinico-morphologic study of 18 necropsy patients and comparison to 151 previously reported necropsy patients. *Am Heart J*. July 1982;104(1):115–135.

57. Nienaber CA, von Kodolitsch Y, Petersen B, et al. Intramural hemorrhage of the thoracic aorta. Diagnostic and therapeutic implications. *Circulation*. September 15, 1995;92(6):1465–1472.

58. Sheldon WS, Vandervoort PM, Black IW, Grimm RA, Stewart WJ. Aortic intramural hematoma in patients evaluated for aortic dissection: clinical, echocardiographic, radiologic and pathologic findings. *Circulation*. 1994;90(Suppl I):I385.

59. Vilacosta I, de Dios RM, Pinto AG. Aortic intramural hematoma during coronary angioplasty: insights into the pathogenesis of intramedial hemorrhage. *J Am Soc Echocardiogr*. 2000;13:403–406.

60. Song J-K. Diagnosis of intramural hematoma. *Heart*. 2004;90:368–371.

61. Song JM, Kang DH, Song JK, et al. Clinical significance of echo-free space detected by transesophageal echocardiography in patients with type B aortic intramural hematoma. *Am J Cardiol*. March 1, 2002;89(5): 548–551.

62. Evangelista A, Dominguez R, Sebastia C, et al. Prognostic value of clinical and morphologic findings in short-term evolution of aortic intramural haematoma. Therapeutic implications. *Eur Heart J*. January 2004;25(1):81–87.

63. Keren A, Kim CB, Hu BS, et al. Accuracy of biplane and multiplane transesophageal echocardiography in diagnosis of typical acute aortic dissection and intramural hematoma. *J Am Coll Cardiol*. September 1996;28(3):627–636.

64. Ganaha F, Miller DC, Sugimoto K, et al. Prognosis of aortic intramural hematoma with and without penetrating atherosclerotic ulcer: a clinical and radiological analysis. *Circulation*. July 16, 2002;106(3): 342–348.

65. Kaji S, Nishigami K, Akasaka T, et al. Prediction of progression or regression of type A aortic intramural hematoma by computed tomography. *Circulation*. November 9, 1999;100(19 Suppl):II281–II286.

66. Song JM, Kim HS, Song JK, et al. Usefulness of the initial noninvasive imaging study to predict the adverse outcomes in the medical treatment of acute type A aortic intramural hematoma. *Circulation*. September 9, 2003;108(Suppl 1):II324–II328.

67. Vilacosta I, San Román JA, Aragoncillo P, et al. Penetrating atherosclerotic aortic ulcer: documentation by transesophageal echocardiography. *J Am Coll Cardiol*. July 1998;32(1):83–89.

68. Bickerstaff LK, Pairolero PC, Hollier LH, et al. Thoracic aortic aneurysms: a population based study. *Surgery*. 1982;92:1103–1109.

69. Iung B, Gohlke-Barwolf C, Tornos P, et al. Recommendations on the management of the asymptomatic patient with valvular heart disease. *Eur Heart J*. 2002;23:1253–1266.

70. Baldari D, Chiu S, Salciccioli L. Aortic pseudoaneurysm as a rare cause of superior vena cava syndrome – a case report. *Angiology*. May–June 2006;57(3):363–366.

71. Deng YB, Li CL, Chang Q. Chronic traumatic pseudoaneurysm of the ascending aorta causing right ventricular inflow obstruction. *Circ J*. April 2003;67(4): 359–361.

72. Revilla A, San Román JA, Fernández-Avilés F. Images in cardiology. Aortopulmonary fistula in an acute aortic syndrome. *Heart*. March 2006; 92(3):360.

73. Rognoni A, Iorio S, Leverone M, Marino P. Aortic pseudoaneurysm and aorta-right atrium fistula: a case report. *G Ital Cardiol (Rome)*. March 2006;7(3): 234–237.

74. Yokote Y, Kyo S, Matsumura M, Asano H, Tanabe H, Omoto R. Aortobiventricular fistulas associated

with pseudoaneurysm of the ascending aorta 12 years after patch repair of supravalvular aortic stenosis. *Jpn J Thorac Cardiovasc Surg*. February 2001;49(2): 132–134.

75. Kanani RS, Neilan TG, Palacios IF, Garasic JM. Novel use of the Amplatzer septal occluder device in the percutaneous closure of ascending aortic pseudoaneurysms: a case series. *Catheter Cardiovasc Interv*. January 2007;69(1):146–153.

76. Smith MD, Cassidy JM, Souther S, et al. Transesophageal echocardiography in the diagnosis of traumatic rupture of the aorta. *N Engl J Med*. 1995;332:356–362.

77. Vignon P, Gueret P, Vedrinne JM, et al. Role of transesophageal echocardiography in the management of traumatic aortic disruption. *Circulation*. 1995;92: 2959–2968.

78. Swaminathan M, Lineberger CK, McCann RL, Mathew JP. The importance of intraoperative transesophageal echocardiography in endovascular repair of thoracic aortic aneurysms. *Anesth Analg*. 2003;97(6):1566–1572.

79. Rapezzi C, Rocchi G, Fattori R, et al. Usefulness of transesophageal echocardiographic monitoring to improve the outcome of stent-graft treatment of thoracic aortic aneurysms. *Am J Cardiol*. 2001;87(3): 315–319.

80. Moskowitz DM, Kahn RA, Konstadt SN, Mitty H, Hollier LH, Marin ML. Intraoperative transoesophageal echocardiography as an adjuvant to fluoroscopy during endovascular thoracic aortic repair. *Eur J Vasc Endovasc Surg*. 1999;17(1):22–27.

81. Dake MD, Miller DC, Semba CP, Mitchell RS, Walker PJ, Liddell RP. Transluminal placement of endovascular stent-grafts for the treatment of descending thoracic aortic aneurysms. *N Engl J Med*. 1994;331(26): 1729–1734.

82. Van der Starre P, Guta C, Dake M, Ihnken K, Robbins R. The value of transesophageal echocardiography for endovascular graft stenting of the ascending aorta. *J Cardiothorac Vasc Anesth*. 2004;18(4):466–468.

83. Song TK, Donayre CE, Kopchok GE, White RA. Intravascular ultrasound use in the treatment of thoracoabdominal dissections, aneurysms and transactions. *Semin Vasc Surg*. 2006;19:145–149.

84. Fayed A. Images in anesthesia; a misplaced guide wire in the false lumen during endovascular repair of a type B aortic dissection. *Can J Anesth*. 2007;54: 947–948.

85. Dobson G, Petrasek P, Alvarez N. Images in anesthesia: transesophageal echocardiography enhances endovascular stent placement in traumatic transsection of the thoracic aorta. *Can J Anaesth*. 2004;51(9):931.

86. Martin M, Moris C, Hevia S, et al. Intimal dehiscence during endovascular treatment of thoracic aortic dissection. *Int J Cardiol*. 2006;114:e1–e2.

87. Misfeld M, Notzold A, Geist V, Richardt G, Sievers HH. Retrograde type A dissection after endovascular

stent grafting of type B dissection. *Z Kardiol*. 2002;91:274–277.

88. Fayed A. Thoracic endovascular stent graft with a bird's beak sign. *Can J Anaesth*. 2008;55:785-786.

89. Fayed A. Echocardiography images of endovascular mal-aligned stent grafts. *Can J Anesth*. 2008;55: 306–307.

90. White GH, Yu W, May J, Chaufour X, Stephen MS. Endoleak as a complication of endoluminal grafting of abdominal aortic aneurysms: classification, incidence, diagnosis, and management. *J Endovasc Surg*. 1997;4(2):152–168.

91. Malina M, Lanne T, Ivancev K, Lindblad B, Brunkwall J. Reduced pulsatile wall motion of abdominal aortic aneurysms after endovascular repair. *J Vasc Surg*. 1998;27(4):624–631.

92. Alimi YS, Chakfe N, Rivoal E, et al. Rupture of an abdominal aortic aneurysm after endovascular graft placement and aneurysm size reduction. *J Vasc Surg*. 1998;28(1):178–183.

93. Veith FJ, Baum RA, Ohki T, et al. Nature and significance of endoleaks and endotension: summary of opinions expressed at an international conference. *J Vasc Surg*. 2002;35(5):1029–1035.

94. Dobson G, Maher N, Ball M, Kryski A, Moore R. Images in anesthesia: echo contrast as an adjunct to intraoperative angiography in the detection of endoleaks. *Can J Anaesth*. 2006;53(5):516–517.

95. Hughes GC, Sulzer CF, McCann RL, Swaminathan M. Endovascular Approaches to Complex Thoracic Aortic Disease. *Semin Cardiothorac Vasc Anesth*. 2008;12:298–319.

96. Fattori R, Caldarera I, Rapezzi C, et al. Primary endoleakage in endovascular treatment of the thoracic aorta: importance of intraoperative transesophageal echocardiography. *J Thorac Cardiovasc Surg*. 2000;120(3):490–495.

97. Gonzalez-Fajardo JA, Gutierrez V, San Roman JA, et al. Utility of intraoperative transesophageal echocardiography during endovascular stent-graft repair of acute thoracic aortic dissection. *Ann Vasc Surg*. 2002;16(3):297–303.

98. Napoli V, Bargellini I, Sardella SG, et al. Abdominal aortic aneurysm: contrast-enhanced US for missed endoleaks after endoluminal repair. *Radiology*. 2004;233(1):217–225.

99. Koschyk DH, Nienaber CA, Knap M, et al. How to guide stent-graft implantation in type B aortic dissection? Comparison of angiography, transesophageal echocardiography, and intravascular ultrasound. *Circulation*. 2005;112(9 Suppl):I260–I264.

100. Koschyk DH, Meinertz T, Hofmann T, et al. Value of intravascular ultrasound for endovascular stent-graft placement in aortic dissection and aneurysm. *J Card Surg*. 2003;18(5):471–477.

101. Orihashi K, Matsuura Y, Sueda T, et al. Echocardiography-assisted surgery in transaortic endovascular stent grafting: role of transesophageal echocardiography. *J Thorac Cardiovasc Surg*. 2000;120(4):672–678.

102. Rocchi G, Lofiego C, Biagini E, et al. Transesophageal echocardiography-guided algorithm for stent-graft implantation in aortic dissection. *J Vasc Surg.* 2004;40(5):880–885.

103. Freeman WK. Diseases of the thoracic aorta: assessment by transesophageal echocardiography. In: Freeman WK, Seward JB, Khandheria BK, Tajik AJ, eds. *Transesophageal Echocardiography.* Boston, MA: Little, Brown and Co; 1994.

104. Practice guidelines for perioperative transesophageal echocardiography. A report by the American Society of Anesathesiologists and the Society of Cardiovascular Anesthesiologists Task force on Transesophageal Echocardiography. *Anesthesiology.* 1996;84:986.

105. Swaminathan M et al. The importance of intraoperative transesophageal echocardiography in endovascular repair of thoracic aortic aneurysms. *Anesth Analg.* 2003;97:1566–1572.

Operative Techniques in Surgery of the Proximal Thoracic Aorta and Aortic Arch

5

Enrique Gongora and Thomas G. Gleason

Introduction

There is a strikingly uniform histopathology (cystic medial degeneration) inherent to most all diseases affecting the proximal thoracic aorta, and this pathology imparts a disruption of the structural integrity of the aortic wall giving rise to aneurysm formation, dissection, or rupture – the final common pathway of untreated proximal thoracic aortic disease. It is important to fully understand the clinical modes of presentation of proximal thoracic aortic disease as the surgical management and timing of intervention vary accordingly. Patient comorbidity, extent of thoracic aortic reconstruction required, and timing of surgery, all impact morbidity and mortality following proximal thoracic aortic surgery. The extent of reconstruction is predicated on the condition of the aortic root and the aortic valve, the presence of an underlying connective tissue disorder, the life expectancy of the patient, the desired anticoagulation status, the need for associated cardiac procedures, as well as surgeon experience. The ultimate outcome of patients undergoing these procedures depends on thorough preoperative surgical planning; meticulous myocardial, cerebral, and spinal cord protection; precise operative technique; and dutiful postoperative care. Thoracic aortic surgery is complex and mandates a seamless interaction between surgeons and cardiac anesthesiologists to ensure optimal patient outcomes.

History

Abnormal dilatation of arteries was observed by Egyptian physicians dating back to 1550 BC, as illustrated in the Ebers Papyrus. Galen in the second century AD presented a detailed description and coined the term "aneurysm." Later, Antyllus differentiated between traumatic and degenerative aneurysms.[1] Ambrose Pare described a ruptured thoracic aortic aneurysm and concluded that "the aneurysms which happen in the internal parts are incurable".[2]

Surgical repair of aneurysmal disease of the thoracic aorta began after Oschner's report of a successfully resected aneurysm of the descending aorta in 1944.[3] Cooley performed the first repair of an ascending aortic aneurysm in 1950.[4] Initially, repair of thoracic aneurysms was limited to select saccular aneurysms that were amenable to clamping at the base of the aneurysm followed by resection and lateral aortorrhaphy. Crafoord described the first resection of an aortic coarctation with end-to-end anastomosis in 1945.[5] The introduction of aortic homografts allowed excision of fusiform and large saccular aneurysms not amenable to lateral resection. Gross

E. Gongora (✉)
Division of Cardiac Surgery, Department of Surgery, Thoracic Transplantation and Mechanical Circulatory Support, Heart Transplantation Program, Scott & White Clinic, Texas A&M Helath Science Center College of Medicine, Scott & White Hospital and Clinics, Temple, TX, USA
e-mail: egongora@swmail.sw.org

K. Subramaniam et al. (eds.), *Anesthesia and Perioperative Care for Aortic Surgery*, DOI 10.1007/978-0-387-85922-4_5, © Springer Science+Business Media, LLC 2011

pioneered the use of homografts to restore aortic continuity after resection of aortic coarctation.[6] Cooley and DeBakey later reported the first use of an allograft for replacement of the thoracic aorta for aneurysmal disease.[7]

The modern era of thoracic aneurysm surgery was ushered by the development of cardiopulmonary bypass (CPB) and synthetic prosthesis for vascular replacement. The first successful replacement of the ascending aorta with the use of extracorporeal circulation was reported by Cooley and DeBakey using an aortic allograft in 1956.[8] The development of the knitted Dacron prosthesis for vascular replacement by DeBakey and colleagues allowed easier access to a usable graft for aortic replacement.[9]

As materials and techniques improved, more extensive repairs became possible. Starr in 1963 performed the first replacement of the supracoronary ascending aorta with separate mechanical aortic valve replacement.[10] This was followed by replacement of the aortic root and ascending aorta with a composite valved-graft conduit by Bentall and De Bono in 1968.[11] New surgical approaches and the development of cerebral and spinal cord protective strategies now allow routine replacement of the aortic arch and thoracoabdominal aorta with good outcomes.[12]

Spectrum of Aortic Disease and Clinical Presentation

A true aortic aneurysm is defined as vascular dilation of 50% or greater relative to normal diameter when all three layers of the aortic wall (intima, media, and adventitia) remain intact. In contrast, a pseudoaneurysm (false aneurysm) is a contained vascular disruption – contained by tissues or scar that surrounds the vessel – such that a contained vascular outpouching is present that does not contain all three of the normal layers of the vessel wall.[13] It is reported that isolated thoracic aortic aneurysms are more common in the ascending thoracic aorta and aortic arch (40%) than in the descending thoracic aorta (31%), but patients frequently have aneurysms in both locations (29%).[14] The mean age at the time of diagnosis

ranges from 59 to 69 years. Men are typically diagnosed at a younger age, and there is a 2:1 to 4:1 male predominance.[15] Initially, thoracic aortic aneurysmal disease is asymptomatic and is often identified incidentally after imaging for unrelated conditions. As an aneurysm progressively enlarges, compression or elongation of adjacent structures can lead to the development of symptoms. The most common presenting symptom is dull pain, but hoarseness secondary to stretching of the recurrent laryngeal nerve, stridor from tracheal compression, dyspnea from compression of the lung, and plethora and edema due to SVC compression are also presenting symptoms. Some patients may develop congestive heart failure due to associated aortic valve regurgitation. Not infrequently, the aneurysm wall weakens to the point of dissection or disrupture giving rise to an entirely different and more dramatic presentation: acute severe chest or back pain, neurologic impairment indicative of stroke or spinal cord ischemia, plethora or cardiovascular collapse.[12] Tearing retrosternal pain radiating to the back often suggests proximal aortic origin and back pain localized in the interscapular region may indicate descending aortic involvement. The four predominant clinical entities can present in this acute fashion include aortic disruption, aortic dissection, intramural hematoma (IMH), and penetrating aortic ulcer (PAU).[16–19]

Prevalence and Incidence

The incidence of thoracic aortic aneurysms has increased over time; population studies from Olmsted County, Minnesota revealed an estimated incidence of 5.9 cases per 100,000 person-years from 1951 to 1980 and 10.4 cases per 100,000 person-years from 1980 to 1994. The rise in incidence is believed to be due to an aging population and better diagnostic testing (CT scan).[14,20] In a study of 58,405 autopsies performed in Malmo, Sweden from 1958 to 1985, the prevalence of uncomplicated thoracic aneurysm, aneurysmal dissection, and thoracic aortic rupture increased with age with most cases found in patients older than 60 years of age. A total of 484 thoracic aneurysms were encountered for a prevalence of 829 per 100,000 autopsies. An aortic catastrophe was the direct cause of death in 293 cases (58%), dissection was encountered in 216 cases (44.7%), and rupture in 63 cases (13%).[21]

Etiology and Pathogenesis

Risk factors associated with the development of thoracic aortic aneurysms include smoking, hypertension, atherosclerosis, bicuspid aortic valve, genetic disorders of the connective tissue like the Marfan, Ehlers–Danlos, and Loeys–Dietz syndromes, as well as a family history of the less-well-characterized familial thoracic aortic aneurysm/dissections.[15,22] The ascending aorta differs from the abdominal aorta in structure, biochemistry, and cell biology. The ascending aorta has a thinner intima, thicker media, and more medial lamellar units compared to the abdominal aorta. It also has significantly higher elastin and collagen content and a lower collagen-to-elastin ratio.[23] Most of the elasticity and tensile strength of the aorta is derived from its medial layer composed of elastin, collagen, smooth muscle cells, and ground substance.[24] A small degree of elastic fiber fragmentation with subsequent increase in ascending aorta diameter is normally associated with aging.[25] However in patients with ascending aortic aneurysms, the aortic wall shows extensive structural remodeling of the extracellular matrix including fragmentation of elastic fibers, loss of vascular smooth muscle cells, loss of myocyte function, and accumulation of a basophilic amorphous material, characteristic of cystic medial degeneration.[26] Weakening of the aortic wall and loss of elasticity result in aortic dilation. The law of Laplace dictates greater wall tension with increasing aortic diameter, and, as a result, larger aneurysms tend to have a higher rate of growth. As aortic diameter increases, the risk for aortic catastrophe also increases.

The Marfan syndrome is an autosomal-dominant connective tissue disorder associated with mutations in the *Fibrillin-1* (*FBN1*) gene located in chromosome 15q21.1.[27,28] Abnormalities in fibrillin, one of the major structural components

of the elastic fiber, result in fiber disruption and histologic findings consistent with cystic medial degeneration at an early age.[29] Patients with the Marfan syndrome frequently have cardiovascular involvement. Seventy-five to eighty-five percent of patients have annuloaortic ectasia (dilation of the aortic sinuses, annulus, and proximal ascending aorta). Aortic valve incompetence is frequently seen, and its severity is directly related to the degree of aortic root dilation.[30,31] Mitral valve prolapse with mitral regurgitation is seen in 41% of patients with the syndrome but only 14% of patients progress to severe MR.[32] Patients with the Marfan syndrome have an abbreviated life expectancy with 60–80% of deaths caused by aortic rupture, acute congestive heart failure from valvular incompetence, or acute aortic dissection.[33]

Ehlers–Danlos syndrome is attributed to various defects in the synthesis of type III collagen. Type IV Ehlers–Danlos accounts for 15% of cases and is characterized by vascular rupture with or without dissection. The abdominal aorta is frequently affected, the thoracic aorta and its branches are less frequently involved.[34] Loeys–Dietz syndrome also involves the thoracic aorta; affected patients have mutations in the transforming factor B receptors and present with craniosynostosis, cleft palate, congenital heart disease, arterial aneurysms, and mental retardation.[35] Patients affected with nonsyndromic familial thoracic aortic aneurysm/dissection (TAAD) have an 11–19% chance of having a first-degree relative affected with thoracic aortic aneurysm. TAAD is inherited in an autosomal dominant fashion, and there have been four different genes identified so far in affected families. The underlying genetic heterogeneity of TAAD is reflected in the phenotypic variability with respect to age of onset, progression, penetrance, and association with additional cardiac and vascular features.[22]

Bicuspid aortic valve (BAV), the most common congenital cardiac abnormality, is present in 0.5–1.5% of the population. It is inherited in an autosomal dominant fashion with variable penetrance, with a 3:1 male preponderance.[36] BAV is a heterogeneous disease with respect to mode of valve failure and thoracic aortic involvement. BAV patients have an increased prevalence of thoracic aortic aneurysm that ranges from 35% to 80%; this wide variability depends on the type and age of the population studied, the size criteria, and the aortic location sampled.[37] BAV patients have a ninefold increase in risk of aortic dissection when compared to tricuspid aortic valve patients.[38] The exact mechanism that explains the high prevalence of TAA and increased dissection risk is still unclear. Hemodynamic flow abnormalities that increase sheer and wall stress in the greater curvature of the mid ascending thoracic aorta might be partially responsible, especially in patients with higher degrees of valve dysfunction.[37] However, when compared with patients with tricuspid aortic valves with similar degrees of valve dysfunction, the relationship still persists.[39] Evenmore, the presence of aortic dilation in the absence of significant hemodynamic dysfunction of the valve has been well documented.[40] The fact that enlargement of the BAV aorta continues even after valvular replacement with subsequent development of aneurysm and dissection points to an underlying structural abnormality of the aorta.[41-43] There is ample evidence that BAV patients with aneurysmal degeneration and dissection have an aortopathy characterized by decreased fibrillin content and increased proteolytic enzyme activity with histologic findings compatible with cystic degeneration of the media.[36,44,45]

Natural History

Untreated aneurysms of the thoracic aorta are highly lethal. Larger aneurysms have a substantial risk of aortic catastrophe: rupture or dissection. In non-operated patients, the 5-year survival ranges from 13% to 39%. Rupture of the aneurysm occurs in 42–70% of patients and is the most common cause of death. The rate of rupture and death is highest in the setting of aneurysmal dilatation of a previous dissection.[20,46,47] The risk of rupture or dissection is clearly correlated with a larger aneurysm size. The risk of rupture or dissection for ascending aortic aneurysms greater than 6 cm is 36.2%, and for descending thoracic aneurysms greater than 7 cm, it is 47.1%.[48]

Dissection involving the ascending aorta carries a very high mortality. A substantial proportion of patients die before receiving medical attention. In a recently reported autopsy series, 21% of patients died prior to hospital admission.[49] The great majority (90%) of these patients not treated surgically die within 3 months, mostly from rupture of the dissection.[49,50] In a recent report from the International Registry of Aortic Dissection (IRAD) of 289 patients with type A aortic dissection, the 81 patients that received only medical management had a 30-day mortality of 58% compared to 26% for those that were managed operatively.[51] The development of pericardial tamponade is an ominous sign; the hospital mortality for patients that presented with tamponade in IRAD was 40% for surgically treated patients and 92% for nonoperative patients.[52] In the USA, the reported mortality rates of patients undergoing surgical repair of type A aortic dissection from several single-center experiences vary from 10% to 30%, this variability might be explained by differences in case mix, referral patterns, and center experience.

The risk of development of aortic catastrophe is not equal for all aneurysms. There are several factors known to influence aneurysm growth and predispose to a higher risk of complications. Patients with a strong family history of rupture or dissection, patients with a prior dissection, and patients with saccular aneurysms are an increased risk of aortic catastrophe.[15,53] Patients with the Marfan syndrome also have an accelerated aneurysm growth and tend to rupture or dissect at smaller diameters.[54] Patients with BAV and TAA have been found to have a greater rate of growth and present at an earlier age when compared to patients with thoracic aortic aneurysm and a tricuspid aortic valve, but rupture and dissection do not necessarily tend to occur at smaller aortic diameters.[55]

Indications for Operation

Rupture and dissection are clear indications for emergent operation. Rupture of an ascending aortic aneurysm will occur within the pericardial space resulting in pericardial tamponade and death if not surgically treated. Development of pain in the absence of documented rupture or dissection should also prompt surgical repair, as development of pain can be a prodrome for impending rupture or dissection.

Most patients diagnosed with a thoracic aneurysm are actually asymptomatic. It is important to understand that the goal of elective surgical intervention is to improve long-term survival by preventing the development of an aortic catastrophe. A careful risk–benefit analysis should be considered in each case. For a patient to benefit from aneurysm repair, the risk of death and disabling complications associated with surgery must be less than the cumulative risk of aortic rupture, dissection, or death associated with ongoing aneurysm growth. Operative risk is specific to each individual patient and may also change with the surgeon and institutional experience. It is important to state that not every patient with a thoracic aortic aneurysm should have an operation when the risk of surgery, given the patient's comorbidities and underlying life expectancy, exceeds the perceived benefits of it.

Aneurysm size is the most important predictor of the risk of aortic rupture or dissection. Coady and associates at Yale University established the relationship of aortic catastrophe to aneurysm size. In the Yale series, the combined yearly rate of rupture, dissection, or death in patients with ascending aortic aneurysms between 5 and 6 cm in diameter was 11.8%, and it rose to 15.6% for aneurysms greater than 6 cm in diameter.[54,56] The median size at which rupture or dissection occurred was 6 cm for ascending aorta and 7 cm for the descending aorta. The authors reported that the size at which the risk–benefit ratio favored surgery was 5.5 cm for ascending aorta and 6.5 cm for descending aorta in their series. Other authors have advocated indexing measured aneurysm size to expected aortic size according to body surface area and age as a more reliable indicator of rupture or dissection risk.[57] A simpler index, the "aortic size index," which is the maximum aortic size divided by body surface area, was recently correlated to adverse aneurysm outcomes. An index of >4.25 cm/m^2 conveyed a yearly rate of rupture, dissection, or death of 20%, an index between 2.74 and 4.25 carried an 8% yearly risk of adverse events.[58] However, size is not the only indicator of aortic complication risk; recent data released from the IRAD revealed that 59% of 591 patients that presented with a type A dissection had an aortic diameter less than 5.5 cm, and 40% presented with an aortic diameter less than 5 cm.[59]

Some subsets of patients show exaggerated aneurysm growth which sets them at a higher risk of aortic complications in a shorter time frame. The average growth rates for patients with ascending aortic aneurysms in large reported series vary from 0.10 to 0.32 cm/year and there seems to be a large variability in growth rate among patients in all studies. Some aneurysms seem to remain stable, while others tend to have a rapid growth rate.[48,60,61] It has been well demonstrated that the growth rate is higher at larger aneurysm sizes and that patients with ascending aortic aneurysms have a lower growth rate compared to patients with aneurysm of the aortic arch and the descending aorta. Other factors that have been associated with a greater rate of expansion include a history of prior dissection, tobacco use, diastolic hypertension, COPD, bicuspid aortic valve, as well as both syndromic and nonsyndromic associated thoracic aortic aneurysms.[15,48,53,55,61–63] As a result, growth rate of an aneurysm must be examined in the context of each individual patient. A rate of expansion of greater than 1 cm/year is a well-accepted indication for intervention.

There are subgroups of patients with aortopathy that leads to a severely weakened aortic wall. These patients have a higher incidence of aortic catastrophe at smaller aneurysm sizes. In patients with prior dissection, patients with the Marfan syndrome, and patients with a strong family history of aortic dissection, elective aneurysm repair at smaller sizes is justified[46,48]

Some patients present with hemodynamically significant aortic valve dysfunction and ascending aorta dilation. Approximately a third of patients with severe AR and an ascending aorta >4 cm that undergo isolated AVR go on to develop aortic dissection or subsequent aneurysmal enlargement in the following 5 years.[64,65] Aortic valve geometry and function is progressively impaired by ongoing aortic root aneurysm growth, and there is emerging evidence that the functional outcomes of aortic valve-sparing root replacement techniques may fare better when aneurysms are repaired at smaller sizes before evolving aortic cusp pathology limits their reparability.

In summary, asymptomatic thoracic aneurysms should be intervened upon an elective basis once the risk of aortic catastrophe outweighs the risk of surgery. The timing of repair is influenced by initial aortic aneurysm size, growth rate, etiology of the aneurysm, need for other cardiac surgery procedures, desire for valve-sparing procedures, patient size, age, associated comorbidities, and both surgeon and institutional experience. It is reasonable to recommend repair when the ascending aortic diameter exceeds 5 cm as the risk of aortic catastrophe starts to go up significantly beyond this point. Exceptions include patients with intrinsic weakening of the aortic wall such as prior dissection or those with syndromic and non-syndromic thoracic aortic aneurysms, and these should often be repaired earlier. In patients with aortic valvular indications for surgery, a dilated ascending aorta should usually be replaced if over 4.5 cm or even if over 4 cm when there are other substantive risk factors present given the rapid rate of continued dilatation in this subset of patients. An annual growth rate of 1 cm or greater is also an accepted indication for TAA repair. Symptomatic aneurysms should be repaired rather urgently to avoid imminent aortic catastrophe. Patients presenting with aortic dissection or rupture should be emergently repaired.

Preoperative Imaging

Contrast CT is the most common modality used to determine precise aneurysm size, extent, and location of aortic involvement. A CT angiogram of chest, abdomen, and pelvis provides excellent resolution of the entire aorta including the aortic bifurcation as well as axillary, subclavian, iliac, and femoral vessels. Cross-sectional imaging is important to delineate areas of aortic calcification, luminal thrombus, atheromatous plaques,

and dissection to help direct cannulation sites. CTA may be unsuitable for patients with dye allergies or those with tenuous renal function.[66] Magnetic resonance angiography with gadolinium enhanced (MRA) also provides excellent three-dimensional images of the entire aorta and can be used as an alternative for patients with iodinated contrast allergies.[67] In patients with poor renal function, gadolinium may not be a good alternative as it can induce nephrogenic systemic fibrosis.[68]

Transthoracic echocardiography is used to evaluate aortic root and ascending aorta anatomy, ventricular morphology, ventricular systolic and diastolic function, regional wall motion abnormalities, and valvular pathology. It is useful in predicting the dimensions of the sinotubular junction, coronary sinuses, and aortic annulus as well as the number, characteristics, and function of the aortic cusps. It is crucial to accurately understand the mechanism of valvular regurgitation and the characteristics of regurgitation jets. The severity of aortic regurgitation should be carefully documented, as even mild degrees of regurgitation will influence the conduct of these operations.

Operative Approach

Choice of Procedure

The choice of procedure performed depends on the extent of aneurysmal disease, the underlying pathology, the patient's age, the patient's comorbidities and expected long-term survival, the status of the aortic valve, the desire to avoid anticoagulation or to avoid a reoperation, and the surgeon and institutional experience. Patients with degenerative isolated ascending aortic aneurysm may only require replacement of the ascending aorta from the sinotubular junction to the proximal aortic arch. Patients with aneurysms of the ascending aorta and aortic root (annuloaortic ectasia) will usually need both ascending aortic and aortic root replacement. If the distal ascending aorta or the proximal aspect of the aortic arch are involved the repair is often best performed with an open distal (i.e., unclamped) aorta under conditions of hypothermic circulatory arrest. In this case, the lesser curvature of the aortic arch is resected, and the distal anastomosis is performed in an open fashion – the so-called hemiarch reconstruction. Patients with extensive involvement of the aortic arch warrant total aortic arch replacement under hypothermic circulatory arrest conditions.

Incisions

Most patients with pathology of the aortic valve, aortic root, ascending aorta, and aortic arch are usually approached via a median sternotomy. The sternotomy may be extended into the neck along either sternocleidomastoid if more cephalad exposure is needed. For young patients undergoing extensive reconstructions of ascending, arch, and descending aorta in a single stage, a bilateral thoracosternotomy (clamshell) incisions can be used to offer better exposure to the descending thoracic aorta from an anterior approach.

In the reoperative setting it is important to minimize the possibility of injury to the right ventricle or great vessels upon reentry. A CT scan of the chest can help delineate the anatomy to anticipate the degree of difficulty of reentry. Most patients can safely undergo reentry via resternotomy unless an aneurysm or pseudoaneurysm is stuck to the sternum, in which case exposure of peripheral vessels for cannulation prior to sternotomy is prudent. A small subset of patients at very high risk of aortic injury on reentry may require remote institution of CPB (femoral or axillary) and cooling prior to sternotomy. Institution of CPB prior to sternotomy is generally undesirable because it significantly lengthens the time on CPB and may invoke bleeding complications.

Cannulation

The cannulation strategy is dictated by the extent of repair needed, the intended strategy for cerebral protection, the quality of the aorta and peripheral vessels, as well as the urgency of the clinical presentation. Arterial cannulation can be performed centrally on the distal ascending aorta/proximal arch or peripherally via the femoral or axillary arteries. When cannulating centrally, a bolus of 300 u/kg of heparin is given before cannulation. Axillary artery cannulation is easiest when performed before sternotomy; a bolus of 5,000 units of heparin is used during instrumentation of the artery, with full heparinization given after sternotomy is performed. In cases that require establishment of peripheral CPB prior to sternotomy, full heparinization is required.

Aortic cannulation can be safely performed when the aorta is free of atheromatous disease. In most patients the anterior or anteroinferior surface of the arch is the preferred location for cannulation. In some patients an aneurysm itself can be cannulated directly if there is no atheroma or intraluminal clot; this cannulation site is usually resected along with the aneurysm specimen and the graft used for replacement is cannulated after a period of hypothermic circulatory arrest. In patients with poor aortic quality, an alternative site for cannulation is indicated. Right axillary or subclavian artery cannulation is now commonly used in these patients and in patients that are undergoing complex repairs that may require an extended period of moderate or deep hypothermic circulatory arrest to facilitate antegrade cerebral perfusion via the right carotid as a neurocerebral protection strategy. The subclavian artery can be cannulated directly, or an 8–10 mm silo graft sewn end to side to the artery allows continued distal upper extremity perfusion and has been associated with a lower vascular complication rate. Femoral artery cannulation is also used safely by many centers. Femoral cannulation may be particularly useful for hemodynamically unstable emergent cases when there is little time for axillary cannulation or in redo cases when CPB must be established in response to or for prevention of a reentrant injury.

Venous cannulation is typically performed via the right atrium with a two-stage venous cannula. If retrograde cerebral perfusion is planned, the superior vena cava is cannulated separately, and a bridge is placed between the arterial inflow tubing and the superior vena cava tubing, or alternatively the SVC cannula can be attached to the cardioplegia line. In cases with hemodynamic instability, femoral venous cannulation may be used to establish CPB after which central right atrial or bicaval cannulation can be converted if drainage is inadequate.

General Conduct of Operation

After full heparinization, arterial and venous cannulation, and placement of cardioplegia cannulas, CPB is established. For patients requiring hypothermic circulatory arrest (HCA), systemic cooling is initiated shortly after placement on CPB. The cross-clamp is then placed at the distal ascending aorta and fastidious myocardial protection ensured with antegrade and/or retrograde cardioplegia. The proximal aortic reconstruction (e.g., aortic root replacement) is begun during systemic cooling in order to minimize total CPB time. When temperature and time of cooling are adequate for neurocerebral protection and HCA, the arch portion of the repair is completed. Following arch reconstruction, arterial perfusion is reinstituted. Rewarming is initiated and attention is returned to the completion of the proximal portion of the reconstruction and reestablishment of aortic continuity. This operative sequence of events provides the most efficient use of CPB time. When the patient's core temperature has returned to 36°C, and hemostasis is adequate, the patient is weaned from CPB.

Neurocerebral Protection

Neurologic complication following proximal aortic reconstruction can manifest as either a stroke or transient neurologic dysfunction. These phenomena are secondary to either embolic events or cerebral ischemia secondary to hypoperfusion or inadequate neurocerebral protection following a period of circulatory arrest. Strategies to minimize neurologic injury focus on minimizing

embolic phenomena, maintenance of adequate neurocerebral perfusion during periods of CPB, and reduction of cerebral metabolism with systemic cooling during periods of circulatory arrest. Maneuvers aimed at reduction of embolic phenomena include careful intraoperative screening for aortic atherosclerotic debris, calcium deposits or thrombus using TEE and/or epiaortic ultrasound, appropriate selection of cannulation site, avoidance of cross-clamping these hostile aortic territories, minimal dissection of arch aneurysms prior to circulatory arrest, complete exclusion and excision of the diseased aortic arch, and removal of debris and air using retrograde cerebral perfusion.

The primary method that has been used effectively to lower cerebral oxygen and metabolic demand and reduce ischemic injury is the establishment of deep cerebral hypothermia. Additional pharmacologic adjuncts that decrease neuronal activity (barbiturates) or limit cerebral edema (mannitol and steroids) may play a role. Deep or profound hypothermia (cerebral temperature 12–18°C) allows a brief period of time (approximately 20 min) to safely complete open aortic arch repairs in the absence of any brain perfusion. The incidence of neurologic injury increases exponentially with periods of HCA exceeding 30 min. Most hemiarch reconstructions can be safely accomplished in this short time frame. However, more complex total aortic arch reconstructions require longer periods of neurocerebral protection than can be facilitated by HCA alone.

In order to improve neurocerebral protection beyond what HCA alone can achieve and to reduce the degree of systemic cooling necessary to achieve adequate neurocerebral protection, a variety of adjunctive perfusion strategies have been developed:

- Retrograde cerebral perfusion (RCP) via the SVC and internal jugular veins maintains continuous and uniform cerebral cooling during HCA while also facilitating retrograde flushing of particulate debris and air from the brachiocephalic circulation during open arch surgery.

- Antegrade cerebral perfusion (ACP) via direct catheterization of the carotid arteries provides continuous regional arterial perfusion during systemic circulatory arrest and maintains adequate oxygen and nutrient delivery to the brain. This strategy has allowed safe straight-forward arch reconstructions at moderate hypothermia 23–28°C and, in combination with deep HCA, has allowed for quite extended periods of safe systemic circulatory arrest (>60 min) with maintenance of adequate neurocerebral protection.

- Selective antegrade cerebral perfusion (SACP) has referred to unilateral brain perfusion via right axillary or subclavian artery perfusion in combination with proximal innominate arterial occlusion. This strategy relies on an assumed or demonstrated intact circle of Willis to provide contralateral hemispheric protection. SACP can be combined with direct catheterization of the left carotid artery to provide bilateral hemispheric antegrade perfusion.

Surgical Techniques

Ascending Aorta Aneurysm Repair

Determination of the proximal and distal extent of ascending aortic replacement is predicated on the surgeon's ability to completely excise the aneurysmal aorta with or without a cross-clamp in place, the quality of the aorta adjacent to the aneurysm (connective tissue abnormality, no atheromatous debris, or calcifications) to which each anastomosis will be completed, and the ability of the patient to tolerate the extent of the operation. Strict adherence to myocardial and neurocerebral protection throughout aortic reconstruction is fundamental to the conduct of these operations. Patients with moderate or severe aortic regurgitation will require cardioplegic induction via retrograde delivery to prevent cardiac ejection upon initial aortotomy. Following aortotomy, direct coronary ostial delivery of antegrade cardioplegia can then occur. Relying only on retrograde cardioplegia in these circumstances may result in inadequate protection of the right ventricle and should be avoided. Adequacy of repeated administration of cardioplegia at regular intervals to maintain an asystolic cardiac arrest

can be monitored by electrocardiogram and continuous septal myocardial temperature probe when cold cardioplegia is used. With isolated ascending aortic aneurysm, the aorta is typically transected at the sinotubular junction, and a braided or woven polyester graft is sewn to sinotubular junction of the aortic root. The aneurysm is then excised either to the aortic cross-clamp or to the proximal and/or hemiarch if circulatory arrest is planned. With excision of the aneurysm, care is taken to avoid injury to the right pulmonary artery which is adherent to the posterior wall of the aneurysm. The distal anastomosis is completed using either the same graft as used for the proximal or a separate graft that is then trimmed and sewn to the proximal graft. The decision of whether to use one or two grafts for the aortic replacement is based on establishing a normal curvature to the ascending aorta so that the graft(s) do not kink. Following completion, the neo-ascending aorta is vented to remove all air from the left side of the heart; the cross-clamp is removed, and the patient weaned from CPB. For patients in whom the aneurysm involves the distal ascending aorta and proximal aortic arch, the distal anastomosis is performed with an open technique under a brief period of hypothermic circulatory arrest with or without antegrade or retrograde cerebral perfusion (Fig. 5.1).[69] Once the distal anastomosis is completed, upper and lower body perfusion is reinitiated by cannulating the graft itself. The patient is rewarmed and the proximal portion of the reconstruction completed.

Some patients with ascending aorta aneurysm have dilation involving the sinotubular junction but otherwise normal aortic root anatomy. Central aortic regurgitation that results from a lack of central coaptation of the aortic cusps is common in these patients. Reduction of the sinotubular junction diameter with an appropriately sized graft can restore aortic root geometry allowing appropriate cusp coaptation thus eliminating aortic regurgitation in this situation.[70] Freedom from moderate to severe AR of 80%, freedom from severe AR of 98%, and freedom of reoperation of 97% at 10 years of follow-up have been reported with this technique.[71]

a

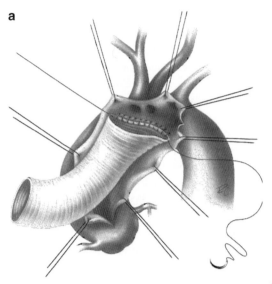

b

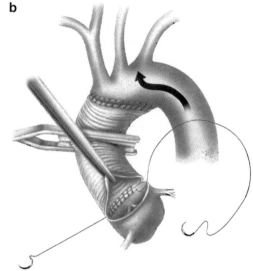

Fig. 5.1 Hemiarch reconstruction. For patients in whom the aneurysm involves the distal ascending aorta and proximal aortic arch, the distal anastomosis has to be performed with an open technique under a brief period of deep hypothermic circulatory arrest (DHCA). Once DHCA is established, the aneurysm is resected including the lesser curvature of the aortic arch; the anastomosis is then performed with a graft that is beveled to replace the portion of resected arch (Used with permission from Coselli et al. [69])

Patients with ascending aortic aneurysm, no dilatation of the aortic root but with concomitant aortic valve pathology can be treated by combining aortic valve replacement with isolated ascending aortic replacement. This approach is not generally used in patients with connective tissue disorders or those with dilation of the aortic root since progressive dilation of the unreplaced aortic root segment may result in future rupture or dissection and the need for subsequent reoperation.

Surgical Options for Aortic Root Aneurysms

Aortic root replacement strategies include the composite mechanical valved conduit, a bioprosthetic valved conduit, a stentless porcine xenograft, a homograft, the pulmonary autograft, and a valve-sparing aortic root replacement with or without aortic valve repair. The type of aortic root replacement planned may depend on the indication for the procedure, the age of the patient, the desire for avoiding anticoagulation, the hemodynamic profile, or the anticipated degree of difficulty and need of a future reoperation.

Mechanical valved conduits are extremely durable but have a higher thromboembolic risk than other choices and mandate the use of lifelong anticoagulation yielding its associated bleeding risk. Bioprosthetic valved conduits do not require long-term anticoagulation, but the valves have a limited durability often imparting the risk of reoperation. Stentless porcine xenografts, homografts, and pulmonary autografts are technically more demanding operations and also have more limited durability than mechanical valved conduits but have superb hemodynamic characteristics. Homografts are often used in cases of aortic root endocarditis when there is destruction of the aortic annulus because they can be tailored to accommodate annular reconstruction and in some cases they may have a lower risk of endocarditic recurrence than other options. Pulmonary autografting is popular in younger patients with its excellent hemodynamic profile but subjects the patient to a risk of reoperation for both the replaced pulmonic and aortic roots. Valve-sparing aortic root replacement can be the most technically difficult, but this strategy can offer the potential for long-term durability without the need for anticoagulation and is becoming increasingly popular.

Prefabricated Aortic Root Replacement

Following aortic transection, the noncoronary sinus is excised and both main coronary arteries are dissected and coronary buttons created to facilitate their orthotopic transfer. The aortic valve is excised and the annulus debrided of any calcium deposits. The annulus is then appropriately sized and a preassembled valved conduit consisting of a polyester graft with either a mechanical or bioprosthetic valve housed within the leading edge of the graft. Bioprosthetic valved conduits are not currently commercially available but can

be fabricated at the time of surgery by sewing a porcine or bovine pericardial valve into a polyester graft to create such a valved conduit. Valved conduits are typically implanted using an intraannular suture technique with everting mattress sutures placed around aortic annulus from the aortic to ventricular aspect, then through the valve sewing cuff. The valved conduit is lowered into position and the sutures are tied in place. The coronary buttons are tailored to include a small ring (3–4 mm) of aortic sinus around each coronary ostia. A circular opening is created on the graft, precisely located to allow easy, tension-free orthotopic transfer of first the left then the right coronary button onto the graft. Hemostasis is tested by delivering cardioplegia down the graft (this manuever also helps determine the site of implantation of the right coronary button.) The distal aortic anastomosis is completed last (Fig. 5.2).[72]

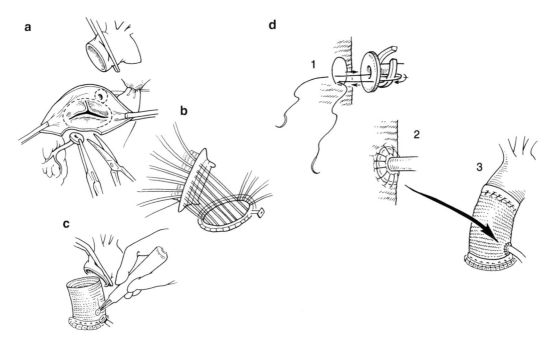

Fig. 5.2 Composite aortic root replacement. The aneurysm is transected at the ascending aorta and at the level of the sinotubular junction. The aneurysm is excised; then the aortic cusps are resected. The aortic sinuses are dissected to the level of the aortic annulus. The noncoronary sinus is excised followed by excision of the left and right sinuses with creation of coronary buttons. The aortic annulus is appropriately sized. A preassembled commercially available mechanical valved conduit is selected.

Everting 2-0 Ethibond mattress sutures are placed on the aortic annulus leaving the needles in place; the sutures are then placed through the ring of the composite valved conduit. (**a**) The valved conduit is lowered into position and the sutures are tied in place. (**b**) The left coronary button is implanted into an openings created on the graft. The distal aortic anastomosis is completed followed by implantation of the right coronary button (Used with permission from Downing and Kouchokos[72])

Implantation of stentless xenograft aortic roots follows the same guideline as for valved conduits with one exception: the coronary button transfer. The porcine xenograft aortic root have coronary sinus anatomy that differs from the human with respect to the position of the right coronary ostium such that the angle relative to the central point of valve cusp coaptation between the left and right coronary ostia is only 90–110° compared to the human which is typically 130–170°. This can be accommodated by either more extensive coronary button mobilization combined with clockwise rotation of the xenograft 15–20° or by counterclockwise rotation of the xenograft 120° with implantation of the native right coronary button to the porcine noncoronary sinus rather than the right coronary sinus.[73]

Pulmonary Autograft

Pulmonary autograft transfer for aortic valve replacement was first described by Donald Ross in 1967 as a subcoronary implantation technique and later as a full root replacement technique.[74,75] The pulmonary autograft has a number of advantages including freedom from anticoagulation, improved hemodynamics relative to prosthetic valves, and continued growth of the autograft with time in children. The primary disadvantages include the technical difficulty of the operation and the conversion of single-valve disease into two-valve disease with its associated replacement of the pulmonary valve. The Ross procedure is contraindicated in patients with known connective tissue disorders in whom the propensity for aneurysmal dilation of the autograft is inherent. The Ross operation is most commonly used in young patients with aortic stenosis in whom long-term anticoagulation is not desired.[76] Patients with large aortic root aneurysms with associated aortic regurgitation may not be ideal candidates for pulmonary autografting because dilation of the aortic annulus may create too distinct a size mismatch relative to the pulmonary autograft, and many of these patients have an underlying aortopathy that may also affect the pulmonary autograft

once transferred, for example, bicuspid aortic valve patients.

Initially the conduct of Ross procedure is similar to any root replacement. However, the first step is to ensure that the pulmonary valve is normal and appropriate for transfer. The main pulmonary artery (PA) and valve are harvested by transverse transection of the PA at its bifurcation. It is then dissected out posteriorly. Injury to the left main coronary artery, left anterior descending, and first septal perforator must be avoided. The dissection continues close to the PA until the septal musculature is encountered. While looking through the pulmonary valve into the right ventricle, the surgeon identifies a point below the pulmonary annulus to perform a transverse ventriculotomy directed by a right-angle clamp passed through the valve into the right ventricular outflow tract. The right ventricle is divided 3–4 mm below the annulus. The right ventricular musculature is divided and the harvest of the pulmonary autograft is completed from anterior to posterior. Next, a transverse aortotomy is made above the origin of the right coronary artery (RCA). The left and right coronary buttons are tailored and mobilized. The aortic root and valve are excised. The autograft is correctly positioned by placing the posterior sinus of the pulmonary valve as the new left coronary sinus. Three interrupted sutures are placed between the nadir of the pulmonary sinuses and the nadir of the aortic sinuses to secure this orientation. The proximal suture line is then completed with either running or interrupted sutures. Each coronary button is transferred as with other root replacement techniques. More recently, surgeons have also wrapped the pulmonary autograft with prosthetic graft material or created a tubularized autograft by placing the autograft within a polyester graft prior to implantation in order to prevent subsequent autograft dilatation. Following root replacement, the aortic cross-clamp is removed, and a pulmonary homograft or other bioprosthesis is sutured to the right ventricular outflow tract avoiding injury to the septal coronary arteries. The distal end of the homograft is then anastomosed to the transected pulmonary artery trunk.

Valve-Sparing Root Reconstructions

Patients with aortic root aneurysm or dissection and aortic cusps that are either normal or amenable to repair may be candidates for root replacement with valve preservation. Two distinct strategies were first described as the "remodeling" and "reimplantation" techniques by Yacoub and David, respectively.[77,78] Valve features that preclude a valve-sparing approach to root replacement include significant cusp calcification, fibrosis or sclerosis and severely elongated cusps with large stress fenestrations as are found in large root aneurysms with associated long-standing severe aortic regurgitation. Transesophageal echocardiography is the primary tool used to assess the aortic valve at the time of surgery. A detailed evaluation of the dimensions of the aortic annulus, aortic sinuses, and sinotubular junction and of the character and quality of the aortic cusps should be obtained. The number of cusps, their thickness, the quality of their free margins, the excursion of each cusp, and the line and height of their coaptation should be carefully interrogated. The direction and size of the regurgitant jets should be clarified to help direct aortic valve repair maneuvers.

Remodeling Technique

The technique of root remodeling was introduced by Sarsam and Yacoub in 1979.[77] The aorta is transected approximately above the sinotubular junction at a level. The three aortic sinuses are excised leaving behind a small rim (3–5 mm) of aortic tissue attached to the aortic annulus to allow a cuff of aorta to which a tailored graft will be attached. Right and left coronary buttons are also created for subsequent implantation in a fashion identical to any root replacement. An appropriately sized graft is chosen based on the desired diameter of the sinotubular junction and three longitudinal incisions are created in the proximal end of the graft corresponding to the anatomic location of the three aortic valve commissural attachments. These create three tongues of graft that are then rounded off to facilitate sewing the edge of each tongue to the corresponding residual sinus segment aortic cuff along the aortic annulus. The commissural posts are suspended in the graft,

the scalloped end of the graft is attached to the residual cuff of the aortic root just above the valve attachment site with a running suture. The coronary buttons are transferred to their respective neoaortic sinus. The distal end of the graft is sutured to normal ascending aorta (Fig. 5.3).[79] Advantages of this procedure include the use of a single suture line for proximal attachment, and there is creation of neoartic sinuses that may impart less stress on the aortic cusps. Disadvantages include a higher incidence of bleeding from the proximal graft attachment site, and the aortic

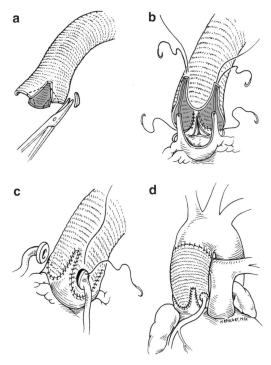

Fig. 5.3 Valve-sparing aortic root replacement-remodeling technique. The aorta is transected approximately 2 cm above sinotubular junction at a level where the ascending aorta is of normal caliber. The three aortic sinuses are excised leaving behind a small rim (5 mm) of tissue attached to the aortic annulus preserving aortic cusps attachment. *Right* and *left* coronary buttons are also created. Three longitudinal incisions are created in the proximal end of the graft corresponding to the anatomic location of the three commissural posts. The commissural posts are suspended in the graft; the scalloped end of the graft is attached to the remnants of the aortic root above the valve leaflets with a running 4-0 Prolene suture. The coronary buttons are reimplanted in their respective neoaortic sinus. The distal end of the graft is sutured to normal ascending aorta recreating aortic root anatomy (Used with permission from Patel et al.[79], p 192)

annulus is not fixed within the graft so the annulus is susceptible to subsequent dilation portending the development of aortic regurgitation. In Yacoub's series of 158 patients, the freedom from aortic valve replacement at 10 years was 89%, but 33% of patients had some degree of aortic regurgitation at latest follow-up.[80]

Reimplantation Technique

The reimplantation technique was developed by David in 1988.[78] This technique also involves excision of the aortic root, preservation of the valve, and reimplantation of the coronaries. In this case, the entire aortic valve and annulus structure is reimplanted inside a graft that is attached to and around the aortic annulus. The graft encircles the aortic annulus preventing subsequent annular dilation. The aorta is similarly transected, the aortic sinuses are excised completely, and the coronary buttons are prepared. Next, the annulus itself is circumferentially dissected away from the surrounding structures to allow placement of a graft just below the annular plane. A polyester graft is then affixed to the left ventricular outflow tract (LVOT) by placing sub-valvular horizontal mattress sutures out of the LVOT and through the graft. Care is taken to avoid passage of these needles through the conduction system. The valve commissures are then resuspended into the neo-root to the appropriate height, and a second running suture is used to distinctly secure the aortic annulus and small residual cuff of aorta to the inside of the graft. The commissural resuspension sutures are then tied down, and a neosinotubular junction is fashioned above the commissures. The coronary buttons are then orthotopically transferred (Fig. 5.4).[81] The two proximal suture lines of this technique significantly minimize bleeding at this level. Aortic annular fixation by the graft is expected to prevent future annular enlargement to allow better long-term valve function. However, this operation is technically difficult and requires longer CPB time compared to the remodeling technique. Since the aortic valve is resuspended inside the tubular graft, there has been concern about increased stress on the aortic cusps due to the lack of aortic sinuses. Consequently, some surgeons

have advocated new techniques aimed at decreasing the stress on the cusps: tailoring of the conduit by pleating the graft and creating neo-sinuses, using grafts with one premade sinus (Valsalva graft), or using a two-graft technique in which the root graft is larger than the distal graft allowing billowing sinuses at the level of the root.[81-83] Early

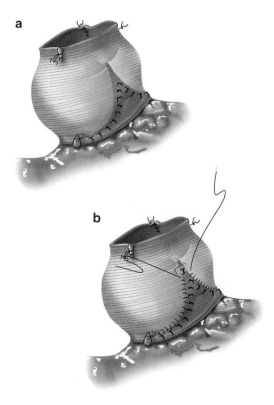

Fig. 5.4 Valve-sparing root replacement-reimplantation technique. The aorta is transected, the aortic sinuses are excised and the coronary buttons are prepared. Each commissural post is tagged with a 4-0 Prolene suture used for future fixation inside the graft. A graft is selected. A row of 3-0 Ethibond subvalvular horizontal mattress sutures are placed from the left ventricular outflow tract below the nadir of the aortic cusps exiting the outside the remnant of the aortic annulus, following the natural scallop of the valve. The subvalvular sutures are attached to the graft; the commissural post sutures are then placed inside the graft and the subvalvular sutures are then tied. The commissural post sutures are secured to the graft at the desired height to allow proper geometry of the root and valve competency. A second running 4-0 Prolene is used to secure the remnant of the aortic annulus to the inside of the graft. Then the left coronary artery is reimplanted, and the distal anastomosis to the ascending aorta is completed followed by reimplantation of the right coronary button (Used with permission from Gleason[81])

laboratory data and clinical indicate better flow dynamics with the creation of sinuses,[84,85] but long-term data is currently unavailable.

Valve-sparing aortic root replacement with aortic valve reimplantation is currently the technique favored by most thoracic aortic surgeons.[86] In David's series, the freedom from moderate or severe aortic insufficiency at 10 years was 94 ± 4%; the freedom from aortic valve replacement at 10 years was 95 ± 3%. Independent predictors of death included age >65 years, advanced functional class, and ejection fraction <40%.[87] The reimplantation technique has been used in patients with Marfan syndrome and bicuspid aortic valves with comparable mid- and long-term results.[88-91]

Aortic Arch Aneurysms

Total aortic arch replacement (TAAR) is a challenging and technically difficult operation that requires meticulous attention to end-organ protection in order to achieve good outcomes. Techniques have evolved over time with the goal of minimizing global cerebral ischemia during the period of mandatory circulatory arrest and to avoid embolic events of air or atheromatous debris associated with manipulation of the head vessels. As many TAAR will require a period of circulatory arrest that exceeds 30 min, most surgeons have adopted techniques that allow ongoing cerebral perfusion during the arrest period. Either direct cannulation of the carotids or selective antegrade cerebral perfusion using the right axillary artery as inflow supplemented with cannulation of the left carotid artery can be used for to achieve this goal.

TAAR was first reported by Griepp in 1975.[92] During a period of hypothermic circulatory arrest, the aortic arch is opened and excised leaving an island of aorta containing the three arch vessels taking care to avoid injury of the left vagus, recurrent laryngeal, and phrenic nerves. The distal anastomosis is completed with an end-to-end anastomosis between a prosthetic graft and the proximal descending aorta. An opening of adequate size is created on the greater curve of the graft to allow reimplantation of the island of aorta containing the arch vessels end to side. The graft is then recannulated and cerebral and total body perfusion is reinitiated. The proximal anastomosis is completed, and, after rewarming, the patient is weaned from CPB (Fig. 5.5).[93] As experience with the technique accrued, it was clear that cerebral ischemic times invariably exceeded 30 min and that neurologic injury was common. A direct correlation between neurologic injury and the circulatory arrest time was established.[94]

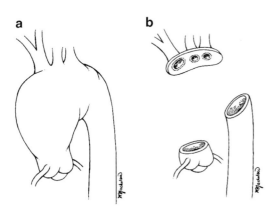
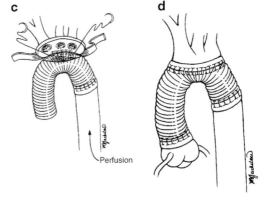
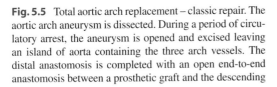

Fig. 5.5 Total aortic arch replacement – classic repair. The aortic arch aneurysm is dissected. During a period of circulatory arrest, the aneurysm is opened and excised leaving an island of aorta containing the three arch vessels. The distal anastomosis is completed with an open end-to-end anastomosis between a prosthetic graft and the descending aorta. An opening of adequate size is created on the graft to allow reimplantation of the island of aorta containing the arch vessels. The graft is then recannulated, and cerebral and total body perfusion is reinitiated. The proximal anastomosis is completed followed by rewarming and separation from CPB (Used with permission from Galla[93], p 326)

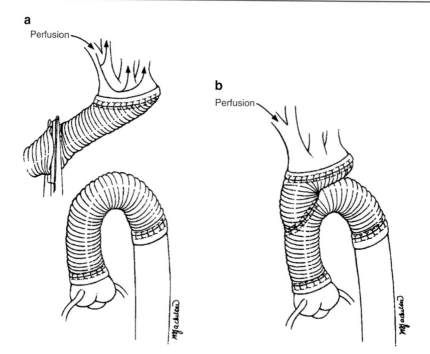

Fig. 5.6 Total aortic arch replacement – "arch first" repair. The aortic arch aneurysm is dissected. During a period of circulatory arrest, the aneurysm is opened and excised leaving an island of aorta containing the three arch vessels. The island of arch vessels is reattached "first" to an "arch" graft allowing early reinitiation of upper body perfusion at the completion of this anastomosis. While still on lower body circulatory arrest, an open distal end-to-end anastomosis to the descending aorta is then performed with a separate graft. The proximal anastomosis is then completed. The "arch" graft is then anastomosed end to side to the ascending to descending graft using either a side-biting clamp or a brief second period of DHCA. Full body perfusion is reestablished. The patient is then rewarmed and separated from CPB (Used with permission from Galla[93], p 327)

In 1994, Ergin and Griepp described the "arch first" technique.[95] With this technique the surgical approach to the arch aneurysm was similar with creation of an island of aorta housing the brachiocephalic branches, but the sequence of the anastomoses performed while under circulatory arrest was modified. First, the island of arch vessels was anastomosed end to end to a distinct "arch" graft allowing early reinitiation of upper body perfusion at the completion of this anastomosis. While still on lower body circulatory arrest an open distal end-to-end anastomosis was then performed with a separate graft to the descending aorta followed by completion of the proximal anastomosis. The arch graft was then anastomosed end to side to the ascending-to-descending graft using either a side-biting clamp or a brief second period of circulatory arrest. The patient is then rewarmed and separated from CPB (Fig. 5.6).[93]

In an effort to further reduce embolic neurologic injury, more aggressive techniques of TAAR have evolved that include transection of the arch vessels approximately 2 cm from their origin in the arch. In theory, at this point the vessels are usually more pliable with less atherosclerotic disease. The arch vessels are then separately reimplanted into specially devised branched grafts. Spielvogel has popularized the use of the trifurcation graft technique. In this approach, right axillary cannulation is used to allow selective cerebral perfusion. During circulatory arrest, the arch aneurysm is resected as previously described, a trifurcated graft is used to separately reimplant each one of the head vessels with sequential reinitiation

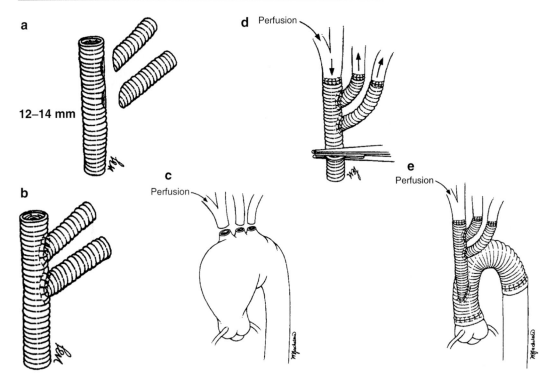

Fig. 5.7 Total aortic arch replacement – trifurcated graft repair. This technique uses right axillary arterial inflow for CPB. The aortic arch aneurysm is dissected. During a brief period of DHCA, the aneurysm is opened and excised. The arch vessels are transected approximately 2 cm from their origin in the arch and antegrade selective cerebral perfusion is initiated. Using the "arch first" concept, each arch vessel is separately reimplanted into a specially constructed trifurcated graft. Complete antegrade cerebral perfusion is reinitiated. While still on lower body circulatory arrest an open distal end-to-end anastomosis to the descending aorta is then performed with a separate graft. The proximal anastomosis is then completed. The "arch" graft is then anastomosed end to side to the ascending to descending graft using either a side-biting clamp or a brief second period of DHCA. Full body perfusion is reestablished. The patient is then rewarmed and separated from CPB (Used with permission from Galla[93], p 328)

of perfusion to each brachiocephalic artery (Fig. 5.7).[93,96,97] Kasui described replacement of the total arch using individual branch vessel grafts that each come off the primary arch graft in an anatomic fashion. Antegrade cerebral perfusion is immediately established with perfusion catheters inserted into each of the brachiocephalic branches. An open distal anastomosis is performed end to end between a special four branch graft and the descending aorta allowing establishment of lower body perfusion though the fourth branch of the graft. Next, the left subclavian is reimplanted and perfused. Finally, the left carotid and innominate are reimplanted into the remaining two branches and the remaining proximal reconstruction completed (Fig. 5.8).[79,98]

For patients with extensive involvement of the ascending, arch, and proximal descending thoracic aorta (so-called mega-aorta syndrome), there are two general approaches. The first involves a two-stage approach in which the first-stage operation addresses the aneurysmal area at greatest risk followed by repair of the area of lesser risk at a second-stage operation. Usually the ascending aorta and the arch are repaired first through a median sternotomy, followed by repair of the descending aorta through a thoracotomy incision at a later date.[99] The "elephant trunk" technique, first described by Borst in 1983, is a modification of the open distal anastomotic technique where the graft used for the anastomosis is invaginated into itself

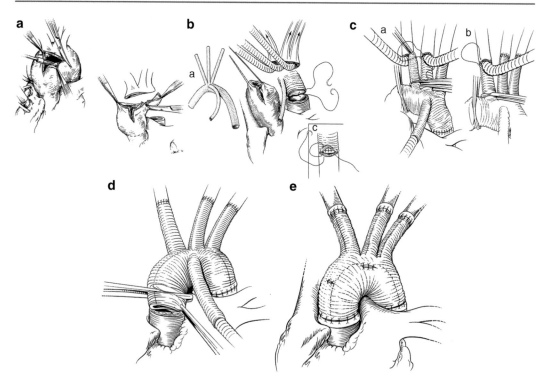

Fig. 5.8 Total aortic arch replacement – Kazui's technique. During a brief period of HCA, the arch aneurysm and origin of the arch vessels are completely resected with establishment of antegrade cerebral perfusion with perfusion catheters inserted into each one of the head vessels. An open distal anastomosis is performed end to end between a special four branch graft and the descending aorta followed by establishment of lower body perfusion though the fourth branch of the graft. Then the left subclavian is separately reimplanted and perfused followed by the left carotid and innominate arteries. After all the arch vessels are implanted, total body perfusion is resumed and the proximal anastomosis is completed during rewarming (Used with permission from Patel et al.[79], p 193)

and introduced inside the descending aorta, the distal anastomosis is performed, and then the invaginated portion of the graft is retrieved from the aorta and used for the arch and ascending aorta reconstruction. At the second stage of the repair, the elephant trunk is retrieved and utilized to perform the proximal anastomosis of the descending aortic replacement simplifying dissection and avoiding possible injury to adjacent structures (Fig. 5.9).[69,100] Unfortunately, up to one third of patients do not return for their second-stage operation, and the additive mortality for the two procedures and the interval wait approaches 20%.[99] Consequently, Kouchoukos suggested a single-stage repair for extensive aortic aneurysms using a bilateral thoracosternotomy (or "clam-shell") incision. Arterial inflow is established with right axillary artery cannulation, under DHCA and selective cerebral perfusion; the aneurysm is completely resected, and the arch vessels are reimplanted into a three-branched graft with initiation of antegrade cerebral perfusion. The distal end of the graft is passed underneath the pedicle of the left phrenic nerve. The graft is then anastomosed to the distal descending aorta followed by reinitiation of total body perfusion. The patient is then rewarmed while the proximal anastomosis is performed (Fig. 5.10).[101,102] Great care must be given to ligation of all bronchial and intercostal arteries emanating from the replaced segment of descending aorta.

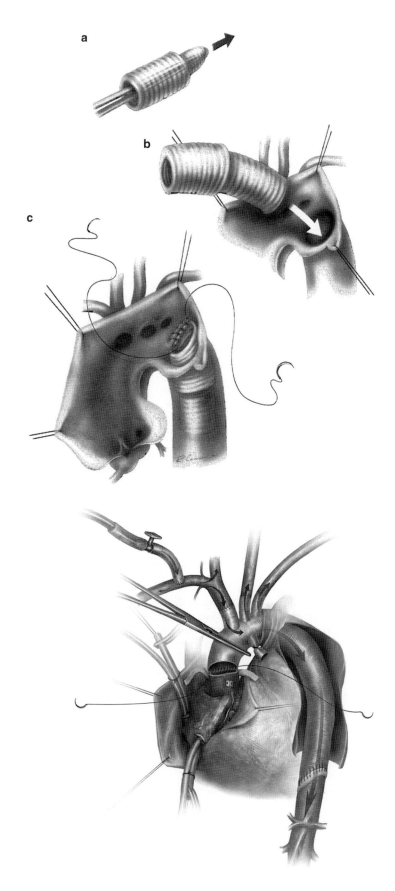

Fig. 5.9 The "elephant trunk" anastomotic technique. The graft used for the anastomosis is invaginated into itself and introduced inside the descending aorta; the distal anastomosis is performed. The invaginated portion of the graft is retrieved from the aorta and used for arch and ascending aorta reconstruction. At the second-stage repair of the descending aorta, the segment of 5–8 cm of graft left inside of the descending aorta is retrieved and utilized to perform the proximal anastomosis (Used with permission from Coselli et al.[69], p 263)

Fig. 5.10 Single-stage total aortic replacement through a bilateral thoracosternotomy incision. Arterial inflow is established with right axillary artery cannulation; under DHCA and selective cerebral perfusion, the aneurysm and origin of the arch vessels are completely resected. Using the "arch first" concept, the arch vessels are reimplanted into a three-branched graft with initiation of antegrade cerebral perfusion. The distal end of the graft is passed underneath the pedicle of the left phrenic nerve. The graft is then anastomosed to the distal descending aorta followed by reinitiation of total body perfusion. The patient is then rewarmed while the proximal portion of the operation is performed (Used with permission from Kouchoukos[103])

References

1. Stehbens WE. History of aneurysms. *Med Hist.* 1958;2(4):274–280.
2. Castiglioni A. In: Knopf AA, ed. *A History of Medicine.* New York: Knopf; 1941:370.
3. Oschner A. Discussion. Surgical considerations of intrathoracic aneurysms of the aorta and great vessels. *Ann Surg.* 1952;135(5):686.
4. Cooley DA, DeBakey ME. Surgical considerations of intrathoracic aneurysms of the aorta and great vessels. *Ann Surg.* 1952;135(5):660–680.
5. Craaford C, Nylin G. Congenital coarctation of the aorta and its surgical treatment. *J Thorac Surg.* 1945;14:347.
6. Gross R, Hurwitt E, Bill A. Preliminary observation on the use of human arterial grafts in the treatment of certain cardiovascular defects. *N Engl J Med.* 1948; 239:578.
7. Cooley DA, DeBakey ME. Successful resection of aneurysm of thoracic aorta and replacement by graft. *JAMA.* 1953;152:673.
8. De Bakey ME. Cooley DA, Crawford ES, et al. Clinical application of a new flexible knitted dacron arterial substitute. *Am Surg.* 1963;27(4):779–783.
9. Cooley DA, De Bakey ME. Resection of entire ascending aorta in fusiform aneurysm using cardiac bypass. *J Am Med Assoc.* 1956;162(12):1158–1159.
10. Starr A, Edwards ML, McCord CW, Grisworld HE. Aortic replacement: clinical experience with a semi-rigid ball-valve prosthesis. *Circulation.* 1963;27(4): 779–783.
11. Bentall H, De Bono A. A technique for complete replacement of the ascending aorta. *Thorax.* 1968; 23(4):338–339.
12. Kouchoukos NT, Dougenis D. Surgery of the thoracic aorta [see comment]. *N Engl J Med.* 1997;336(26): 1876–1888.
13. Johnston KW, Rutherford RB, Tilson MD, et al. Suggested standards for reporting on arterial aneurysms. Subcommittee on Reporting Standards for Arterial Aneurysms, Ad Hoc Committee on Reporting Standards, Society for Vascular Surgery and North American Chapter, International Society for Cardiovascular Surgery [see comment]. *J Vasc Surg* 1991;13(3):452–458.
14. Clouse WD, Hallett JW Jr, Schaff HV, et al. Improved prognosis of thoracic aortic aneurysms: a population-based study. *JAMA.* 1998;280(22):1926–1929.
15. Coady MA, Rizzo JA, Goldstein LJ, et al. Natural history, pathogenesis, and etiology of thoracic aortic aneurysms and dissections. *Cardiol Clin.* 1999;17(4): 615–635. vii.
16. Vilacosta I, Roman JA. Acute aortic syndrome. *Heart.* 2001;85(4):365–368.
17. Reece TB, Green GR, Kron IL. Cardiac surgery in the adult. In: Cohn L, ed. *Aortic Dissection.* New York: McGraw-Hill; 2008.
18. Sundt TM, Sundt TM. Intramural hematoma and penetrating aortic ulcer. *Curr Opin Cardiol.* 2007; 22(6):504–509.
19. Stanson AW, Kazmier FJ, Hollier LH, et al. Penetrating atherosclerotic ulcers of the thoracic aorta: natural history and clinicopathologic correlations. *Ann Vasc Surg.* 1986;1(1):15–23.
20. Bickerstaff LK, Pairolero PC, Hollier LH, et al. Thoracic aortic aneurysms: a population-based study. *Surgery.* 1982;92(6):1103–1108.
21. Svensjo S, Bengtsson H, Bergqvist D. Thoracic and thoracoabdominal aortic aneurysm and dissection: an investigation based on autopsy. *Br J Surg.* 1996; 83(1):68–71.
22. Pannu H, Avidan N, Tran-Fadulu V, et al. Genetic basis of thoracic aortic aneurysms and dissections: potential relevance to abdominal aortic aneurysms. *Ann NY Acad Sci.* 2006;1085:242–255.
23. Guo DC, Papke CL, He R, et al. Pathogenesis of thoracic and abdominal aortic aneurysms. *Ann NY Acad Sci.* 2006;1085:339–352.
24. Wolinsky H, Glagov S. A lamellar unit of aortic medial structure and function in mammals. *Circ Res.* 1967;20(1):99–111.
25. Pearce WH, Slaughter MS, LeMaire S, et al. Aortic diameter as a function of age, gender, and body surface area. *Surgery.* 1993;114(4):691–697.
26. Lesauskaite V, Tanganelli P, Sassi C, et al. Smooth muscle cells of the media in the dilatative pathology of ascending thoracic aorta: morphology, immunoreactivity for osteopontin, matrix metalloproteinases, and their inhibitors. *Hum Pathol.* 2001;32(9):1003–1011.
27. Dietz HC, Cutting GR, Pyeritz RE, et al. Marfan syndrome caused by a recurrent de novo missense mutation in the fibrillin gene. *Nature.* 1991;352(6333):337–339.
28. Kainulainen K, Pulkkinen L, Savolainen A, et al. Location on chromosome 15 of the gene defect causing Marfan syndrome. *N Engl J Med.* 1990;323(14):935–939.
29. Schoen F. Robbins and Cotran pathologic basis of disease. In: Kumar V, Abbas AK, Fausto N, eds. *Blood Vessels.* Philadelphia, PA: Elsevier Saunders; 2005.
30. Pyeritz RE, McKusick VA. The Marfan syndrome: diagnosis and management. *N Engl J Med.* 1979; 300(14):772–777.
31. Marsalese DL, Moodie DS, Vacante M, et al. Marfan's syndrome: natural history and long-term follow-up of cardiovascular involvement. *J Am Coll Cardiol.* 1989; 14(2):422–428.
32. Pyeritz RE, Wappel MA. Mitral valve dysfunction in the Marfan syndrome. Clinical and echocardiographic study of prevalence and natural history. *Am J Med.* 1983;74(5):797–807.
33. Murdoch JL, Walker BA, Halpern BL, et al. Life expectancy and causes of death in the Marfan syndrome. *N Engl J Med.* 1972;286(15):804–808.
34. Oderich GS, Panneton JM, Bower TC, et al. The spectrum, management and clinical outcome of Ehlers-Danlos syndrome type IV: a 30-year experience. *J Vasc Surg.* 2005;42(1):98–106.

35. Loeys BL, Schwarze U, Holm T, et al. Aneurysm syndromes caused by mutations in the TGF-beta receptor. *N Engl J Med.* 2006;355(8):788–798.

36. Tadros TM, Klein MD, Shapira OM, et al. Ascending aortic dilatation associated with bicuspid aortic valve: pathophysiology, molecular biology, and clinical implications. *Circulation.* 2009;119(6):880–890.

37. Della Corte A, Bancone C, Quarto C, et al. Predictors of ascending aortic dilatation with bicuspid aortic valve: a wide spectrum of disease expression. *Eur J Cardio-Thorac Surg.* 2007;31(3):397–404.

38. Larson EW, Edwards WD. Risk factors for aortic dissection: a necropsy study of 161 cases. *Am J Cardiol.* 1984;53(6):849–855.

39. Keane MG, Wiegers SE, Plappert T, et al. Bicuspid aortic valves are associated with aortic dilatation out of proportion to coexistent valvular lesions. *Circulation.* 2000;102(19 Suppl 3):III35–III39.

40. Pachulski RT, Weinberg AL, Chan KL. Aortic aneurysm in patients with functionally normal or minimally stenotic bicuspid aortic valve. *Am J Cardiol.* 1991;67(8):781–782.

41. Russo CF, Mazzetti S, Garatti A, et al. Aortic complications after bicuspid aortic valve replacement: long-term results. *Ann Thorac Surg.* 2002;74(5): S1773–S1776.

42. Borger MA, Preston M, Ivanov J, et al. Should the ascending aorta be replaced more frequently in patients with bicuspid aortic valve disease? *J Thorac Cardiovasc Surg.* 2004;128(5):677–683.

43. Yasuda H, Nakatani S, Stugaard M, et al. Failure to prevent progressive dilation of ascending aorta by aortic valve replacement in patients with bicuspid aortic valve: comparison with tricuspid aortic valve. *Circulation.* 2003;108(Suppl 1): II291–II294.

44. Nataatmadja M, West M, West J, et al. Abnormal extracellular matrix protein transport associated with increased apoptosis of vascular smooth muscle cells in marfan syndrome and bicuspid aortic valve thoracic aortic aneurysm. *Circulation.* 2003;108(Suppl 1): II329–II334.

45. Fedak PW, de Sa MP, Verma S, et al. Vascular matrix remodeling in patients with bicuspid aortic valve malformations: implications for aortic dilatation. *J Thorac Cardiovasc Surg.* 2003;126(3):797–806.

46. Perko MJ, Norgaard M, Herzog TM, et al. Unoperated aortic aneurysm: a survey of 170 patients. *Ann Thorac Surg.* 1995;59(5):1204–1209.

47. Pressler V, McNamara JJ. Thoracic aortic aneurysm: natural history and treatment. *J Thorac Cardiovasc Surg.* 1980;79(4):489–498.

48. Coady MA, Rizzo JA, Hammond GL, et al. What is the appropriate size criterion for resection of thoracic aortic aneurysms? *J Thorac Cardiovasc Surg.* 1997;113(3):476–491.

49. Meszaros I, Morocz J, Szlavi J, et al. Epidemiology and clinicopathology of aortic dissection. *Chest.* 2000;117(5):1271–1278.

50. Anagnostopoulos CE, Prabhakar MJ, Kittle CF. Aortic dissections and dissecting aneurysms. *Am J Cardiol.* 1972;30(3):263–273.

51. Hagan PG, Nienaber CA, Isselbacher EM, et al. The International Registry of Acute Aortic Dissection (IRAD): new insights into an old disease. *JAMA.* 2000;283(7):897–903.

52. Gilon D, Mehta RH, Oh JK, et al. Characteristics and in-hospital outcomes of patients with cardiac tamponade complicating type A acute aortic dissection. *Am J Cardiol.* 2009;103(7):1029–1031.

53. Coady MA, Davies RR, Roberts M, et al. Familial patterns of thoracic aortic aneurysms. *Arch Surg.* 1999;134(4):361–367.

54. Davies RR, Goldstein LJ, Coady MA, et al. Yearly rupture or dissection rates for thoracic aortic aneurysms: simple prediction based on size. *Ann Thorac Surg.* 2002;73(1):17–27.

55. Davies RR, Kaple RK, Mandapati D, et al. Natural history of ascending aortic aneurysms in the setting of an unreplaced bicuspid aortic valve. *Ann Thorac Surg.* 2007;83(4):1338–1344.

56. Coady MA, Rizzo JA, Hammond GL, et al. Surgical intervention criteria for thoracic aortic aneurysms: a study of growth rates and complications. *Ann Thorac Surg.* 1999;67(6):1922–1926.

57. Ergin MA, Spielvogel D, Apaydin A, et al. Surgical treatment of the dilated ascending aorta: when and how? *Ann Thorac Surg.* 1999;67(6):1834–1839.

58. Davies RR, Gallo A, Coady MA, et al. Novel measurement of relative aortic size predicts rupture of thoracic aortic aneurysms. *Ann Thorac Surg.* 2006;81(1):169–177.

59. Pape LA, Tsai TT, Isselbacher EM, et al. Aortic diameter > or = 5.5 cm is not a good predictor of type A aortic dissection: observations from the International Registry of Acute Aortic Dissection (IRAD). *Circulation.* 2007;116(10):1120–1127.

60. Hirose Y, Hamada S, Takamiya M. Predicting the growth of aortic aneurysms: a comparison of linear vs exponential models. *Angiology.* 1995;46(5):413–419.

61. Dapunt OE, Galla JD, Sadeghi AM, et al. The natural history of thoracic aortic aneurysms. *J Thorac Cardiovasc Surg.* 1994;107(5):1323–1332.

62. Masuda Y, Takanashi K, Takasu J, et al. Expansion rate of thoracic aortic aneurysms and influencing factors. *Chest.* 1992;102(2):461–466.

63. Albornoz G, Coady MA, Roberts M, et al. Familial thoracic aortic aneurysms and dissections–incidence, modes of inheritance, and phenotypic patterns. *Ann Thorac Surg.* 2006;82(4):1400–1405.

64. Michel PL, Acar J, Chomette G, et al. Degenerative aortic regurgitation. *Eur Heart J.* 1991;12(8): 875–882.

65. Prenger K, Pieters F, Cheriex E. Aortic dissection after aortic valve replacement: incidence and consequences for strategy. *J Card Surg.* 1994;9(5):495–498.

66. Yu T, Zhu X, Tang L, et al. Review of CT angiography of aorta. *Radiol Clin North Am.* 2007; 45(3):461–483.

67. Sakamoto I, Sueyoshi E, Uetani M, et al. MR imaging of the aorta. *Radiol Clin North Am.* 2007; 45(3):485–497.
68. Marckmann P, Skov L, Rossen K, et al. Nephrogenic systemic fibrosis: suspected causative role of gadodi-amide used for contrast-enhanced magnetic resonance imaging. *J Am Soc Nephrol.* 2006;17(9):2359–2362.
69. Coselli JS, LeMaire SA, Koksoy C. Thoracic aortic anastomoses. *Oper Tech Thorac Cardiovasc Surg.* 2000;5(4):261–265.
70. Olson LJ, Subramanian R, Edwards WD. Surgical pathology of pure aortic insufficiency: a study of 225 cases. *Mayo Clin Proc.* 1984;59(12):835–841.
71. David TE, Feindel CM, Armstrong S, et al. Replacement of the ascending aorta with reduction of the diameter of the sinotubular junction to treat aortic insufficiency in patients with ascending aortic aneurysm. *J Thorac Cardiovasc Surg.* 2007;133(2):414–418.
72. Downing SW, Kouchoukos NT. Ascending aotic aneurysm. In: Edmunds LHJ, ed. *Cardiac Surgery in the Adult.* New York: McGraw-Hill; 1997:1163.
73. Gleason TG, David TE, Coselli JS, et al. St. Jude Medical Toronto biologic aortic root prosthesis: early FDA phase II IDE study results. *Ann Thorac Surg.* 2004;78(3):786–793.
74. Ross DN. Replacement of aortic and mitral valves with a pulmonary autograft. *Lancet.* 1967;2(7523):956–958.
75. Somerville J, Ross DN. Pulmonary autograft for replacement of the aortic valve. *G Ital Cardiol.* 1974; 4(4):413–425.
76. Elkins RC. Pulmonary autograft. In: Franco KL, Verrier ED, eds. *Advanced Therapy in Cardiac Surgery.* Hamilton: BC Decker; 2003:156–167.
77. Sarsam MA, Yacoub M. Remodeling of the aortic valve anulus. *J Thorac Cardiovasc Surg.* 1993;105(3): 435–438.
78. David TE, Feindel CM. An aortic valve-sparing operation for patients with aortic incompetence and aneurysm of the ascending aorta. *J Thorac Cardiovasc Surg.* 1992;103(4):617–621.
79. Patel HJ, Deeb GM, Patel HJ, et al. Ascending and arch aorta: pathology, natural history, and treatment. *Circulation.* 2008;118(2):188–195.
80. Yacoub MH, Gehle P, Chandrasekaran V, et al. Late results of a valve-preserving operation in patients with aneurysms of the ascending aorta and root. *J Thorac Cardiovasc Surg.* 1998;115(5):1080–1090.
81. Gleason TG. Current perspective on aortic valve repair and valve-sparing aortic root replacement. *Semin Thorac Cardiovasc Surg.* 2006;18(2):154–164.
82. Demers P, Miller DC, Demers P, et al. Simple modification of "T. David-V" valve-sparing aortic root replacement to create graft pseudosinuses. *Ann Thorac Surg.* 2004;78(4):1479–1481.
83. Pacini D, Settepani F, De Paulis R, et al. Early results of valve-sparing reimplantation procedure using the Valsalva conduit: a multicenter study. *Ann Thorac Surg.* 2006;82(3):865–871.
84. Maselli D, De Paulis R, Scaffa R, et al. Sinotubular junction size affects aortic root geometry and aortic valve function in the aortic valve reimplantation procedure: an in vitro study using the Valsalva graft. *Ann Thorac Surg.* 2007;84(4):1214–1218.
85. Liu X, Weale P, Reiter G, et al. Breathhold time-resolved three-directional MR velocity mapping of aortic flow in patients after aortic valve-sparing surgery. *J Magn Reson Imaging.* 2009;29(3):569–575.
86. Miller DC, Miller DC. Valve-sparing aortic root replacement: current state of the art and where are we headed? *Ann Thorac Surg.* 2007; 83(2):S736–S739.
87. David TE, Feindel CM, Webb GD, et al. Long-term results of aortic valve-sparing operations for aortic root aneurysm. *J Thorac Cardiovasc Surg.* 2006; 132(2):347–354.
88. Schafers HJ, Aicher D, Langer F, et al. Preservation of the bicuspid aortic valve. *Ann Thorac Surg.* 2007;83(2):S740–S745. discussion S785–90.
89. Cameron DE, Alejo DE, Patel ND, et al. Aortic root replacement in 372 Marfan patients: evolution of operative repair over 30 years. *Ann Thorac Surg.* 2009;87(5):1344–1349.
90. Aicher D, Langer F, Kissinger A, et al. Valve-sparing aortic root replacement in bicuspid aortic valves: a reasonable option? *J Thorac Cardiovasc Surg.* 2004; 128(5):662–668.
91. Patel ND, Weiss ES, Alejo DE, et al. Aortic root operations for Marfan syndrome: a comparison of the Bentall and valve-sparing procedures. *Ann Thorac Surg.* 2008;85(6):2003–2010.
92. Griepp RB, Stinson EB, Hollingsworth JF, et al. Prosthetic replacement of the aortic arch. *J Thorac Cardiovasc Surg.* 1975;70(6):1051–1063.
93. Galla JD. Aneurysms of the aortic arch. In: Franco KL, Verrier ED, eds. *Advanced Therapy in Cardiac Surgery.* Hamilton: BC Decker; 2003:326–328.
94. Ergin MA, Galla JD, Lansman L, et al. Hypothermic circulatory arrest in operations on the thoracic aorta. Determinants of operative mortality and neurologic outcome. *J Thorac Cardiovasc Surg.* 1994;107(3):788–797.
95. Ergin MA, Griepp EB, Lansman SL, et al. Hypothermic circulatory arrest and other methods of cerebral protection during operations on the thoracic aorta. *J Card Surg.* 1994;9(5):525–537.
96. Spielvogel D, Etz CD, Silovitz D, et al. Aortic arch replacement with a trifurcated graft. *Ann Thorac Surg.* 2007;83(2):S791–S795.
97. Spielvogel D, Strauch JT, Minanov OP, et al. Aortic arch replacement using a trifurcated graft and selective cerebral antegrade perfusion. *Ann Thorac Surg.* 2002;74(5):S1810–S1814.
98. Kazui T, Washiyama N, Muhammad BA, et al. Total arch replacement using aortic arch branched grafts with the aid of antegrade selective cerebral perfusion. *Ann Thorac Surg.* 2000;70(1):3–8.

99. Safi HJ, Miller CC 3rd, Estrera AL, et al. Optimization of aortic arch replacement: two-stage approach. *Ann Thorac Surg.* 2007;83(2):S815–S818.

100. Borst HG, Walterbusch G, Schaps D. Extensive aortic replacement using "elephant trunk" prosthesis. *Thorac Cardiovasc Surg.* 1983;31(1):37–40.

101. Kouchoukos NT, Masetti P, Mauney MC, et al. One-stage repair of extensive chronic aortic dissection using the arch-first technique and bilateral anterior thoracotomy. *Ann Thorac Surg.* 2008;86(5): 1502–1509.

102. Kouchoukos NT, Mauney MC, Masetti P, et al. Optimization of aortic arch replacement with a one–stage approach. *Ann Thorac Surg.* 2007;83(2):S811–S814.

103. Kouchoukos NT. One-stage repair of extensive thoracic aortic aneurysm using the arch-first technique and bilateral anterior thoracotomy. *Oper Tech Thorac Cardiovasc Surg.* 2008;13(4):229.

Anesthesia for Surgery of the Ascending Aorta and Aortic Arch

6

Andrew W. Murray and Kathirvel Subramaniam

Introduction

Disease of the ascending aorta is always a serious development in any patient. The nature of the disease and the severity of the particular disease will typically determine whether the patient will ultimately have to proceed with immediate surgical intervention or observation and medical management.

Surgery of the ascending aorta is very complex. Anesthesia delivery for these patients requires strict attention to detail to ensure preservation of the patient's system functions while providing the ideal surgical working environment for the successful repair of the aorta. This requires a very close collaboration and meticulous communication between the surgical and the anesthesiology teams.

Common diseases of thoracic aorta requiring ascending and arch surgery include aneurysms and dissections (Fig. 6.1). Inflammatory arteritis and infectious diseases of aorta are other indications for thoracic aortic surgery. A basic knowledge of pathology of the diseases affecting ascending aorta and arch of aorta is essential for anesthesiologists practicing anesthesia for aortic surgery.

A.W. Murray (✉)
Department of Anesthesiology, University of Pittsburgh
Medical Center – Presbyterian and VA Hospital,
Pittsburgh, PA, USA
e-mail: murrayaw@anes.upmc.edu

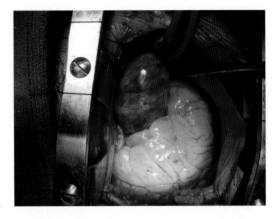

Fig. 6.1 Surgical exposure showing acute type A dissection involving ascending aorta

Aneurysmal Diseases of Thoracic Aorta

The dimensions of the aortic root and ascending aorta show considerable variability in normal populations. Nomograms have been developed for adolescents and adults that account for age and body surface area.[1] For example, 2.1 cm/m² has been considered as the upper limit of aortic sinus of Valsalva. Aortic dilatation is considered an increase in diameter above the norm for age and body surface area, and an aneurysm has been defined as a 50% increase over the normal diameter. Aortic aneurysm is also defined as a twofold increase of the transverse diameter of the aorta compared with normal aortic segment. In patients with diffuse aneurysms, aortic diameter can be compared with the size pulmonary artery. Normally, their diameters are equal.

True aneurysm has all the layers of aorta in its wall. Among the thoracic aortic aneurysms, 51% involve ascending aorta, 38% descending aorta, and the remaining 11% in aortic arch.[2] Pathologically, damage occurs in the aortic tunica media layer, which results in weakening and dilatation of the aortic wall. In addition to enlarged diameter, the aorta also increases in length causing distortion and tortuosity of distal and affected segments.

Based on the shape of the aneurysmal sac, aneurysms can be classified into saccular, fusiform, and cylindrical (Fig. 6.2). Fusiform aneurysms have symmetric dilatations of the aortic lumen and the aneurysm sac is in direct continuity with normal aorta. The enlargement can be eccentric and may involve considerable lengths to produce cylindroid aneurysms. Mural thrombus can be seen lining the aneurysmal wall. Saccular aneurysms are spherical protrusions or outpouching of aorta and connect to the true lumen of tubular aorta, traumatic and mycotic aneurysms are typical examples.

Cystic medial degeneration is the most common reason for ascending aortic aneurysms. This is characterized by depletion of smooth muscle cells and elastic tissue leading to fragmentation and weakening of aortic wall resulting in aneurysm formation. A group of hereditary connective tissue disorders result in aortopathy that can account for at least 20% of aortic aneurysms. Marfan syndrome (MFS), Ehler–Danlos syndrome (EDS), familial aortic dissecting aneurysms, adult polycystic kidney disease, and Turner syndrome are a few of the disorders associated with aortopathy.

MFS serves as prototype for the chronology of hereditary disorders. It is an autosomal dominant disorder with an incidence of 1 in 7,000 caused by more than 100 mutations involving fibrillin-1 gene. Cardiovascular manifestations are given in Table 6.1. Complications of aortopathy such as rupture and dissection are responsible for 80% of deaths in MFS with average age of death in the fourth and fifth decades. Although the risk of dissection increases as the aortic diameter increases, aortic dissection can occur with normal-sized aortas. It is difficult to predict which patients are prone for dissection, but a positive family history is a strong predictor. Other features of MFS include arachnodactyly, scoliosis, pectus excavatum, eye abnormalities, spontaneous pneumothorax, and emphysema. MFS type 2 is associated with central and peripheral aortopathy, cerebrovascular and peripheral arteriopathy, congenital heart disease, and neoplastic disorders.

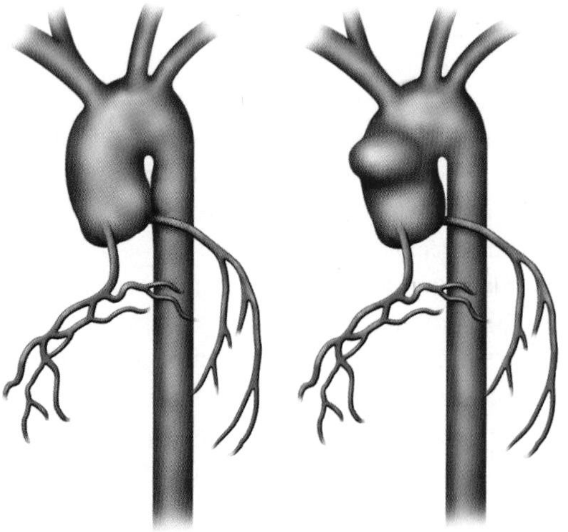

Fusiform aneurysm   Saccular aneurysm

Fig. 6.2 Classification based on the shape of the aneurysm

Table 6.1 Cardiovascular manifestations of Marfan syndrome

Aortopathy
Dilatation of aortic root due to stretch of sinus of valsalva
Dilatation of proximal aorta with abnormal elastic properties (decreased distensibility, increased stiffness, and increased pulse wave velocity)
Aortic dissection (predominantly type A)
Aortic valve
Mega valve cusps
Floppy aortic valve
Aortic valve prolapse
Bicuspid aortic valve
Aortic valvular regurgitation
Mitral and tricuspid valve
Floppy mitral and tricuspid valve
Mitral/tricuspid valve prolapse
Mitral/tricuspid regurgitation
Mitral annular calcification

Compared to non-MFS patients, valve-sparing operations are less successful because of subsequent development of degeneration and regurgitation of the valve. Composite graft replacement of the aortic root and ascending aorta remains the gold standard for MFS patients. Additional late aortic operations may be needed.

Annuloaortic ectasia refers to aortic annular and ascending aortic dilatation. The histopathologic changes seen are similar to those seen with medial necrosis. Like MFS, this disorder is associated with reduced life expectancy.

Bicuspid aortic valve (BAV) is the most common congenital cardiac malformation. BAV is associated with aortic dilatation, aortic dissection, coarctation of aorta, and interrupted aortic arch. Hence, BAV is considered as a disease of the entire aorta. Aortic dilatation occurs even without valve stenosis and regurgitation. Most patients develop stenosis or regurgitation, and they are at increased risk for infective endocarditis.

Atherosclerotic aneurysms usually affect the abdominal aorta severely, and thoracic aortic involvement is less extensive unless the patients have diabetes, previous aortitis, and hyperlipidemias. Atherosclerosis and the attendant weakening of the aortic media may eventually lead to aneurysmal dilation in some patients while others develop heavy calcification and obstructive disease. However, atherosclerosis may be superimposed on aneurysm of any etiology.

Hypertension is the most prevalent risk factor found in patients with aortic aneurysms and aortic dissections.[3] Other etiological factors for aortic aneurysms include poststenotic dilatation due to aortic stenosis, postsurgical trauma, and inflammatory and infective mycotic aneurysms.

Aortic Pseudoaneurysms

Pseudoaneurysms of the aorta involve disruption of at least one layer of the vessel wall with containment by the remaining vessel wall layers or by surrounding mediastinal structures. Pseudoaneurysms of aorta may result from aortic pathology such as dissection, penetrating atherosclerotic ulcer, intramural

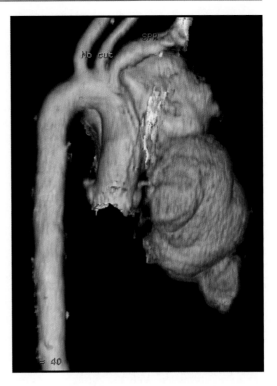

Fig. 6.3 CT reconstruction showing pseudoaneurysm arising from ascending aorta

hematoma, trauma, infections, ruptured aneurysms, and more commonly, postoperative following cardiac surgery.[4-10] Spontaneous rupture with pseudoaneurysm formation has also been reported.[11]

Common sites for postoperative pseudoaneurysms are the aortic cross-clamp, aortotomy, proximal bypass graft anastomosis, aortic cannulation, cardioplegia needle, and aortic vent sites (Fig. 6.3). After aortic surgery, pseudoaneurysms can form at implantation site of coronary arteries, proximal graft anastomotic site, and, least commonly, at distal graft anastomotic site. Pseudoaneurysms have been reported as late as 21 years after previous cardiac surgery. Pseudoaneurysms can present as cardiogenic shock after rupture.

Inflammatory Aortic Disease

Syphilis was the main cause of inflammatory aortitis until the early part of twentieth century when aortitis was linked with other diseases.

Anesthesiologists may occasionally be involved with care of patients with such diseases, and knowledge of the diseases is essential. Inflammatory aortitis can be classified into infective and noninfectious aortitis.

Infectious Aortitis

Pre-existing atherosclerotic disease, intraluminal thrombus of aneurysmal disease, and aortic trauma (iatrogenic or traumatic) all act as nidus for aortitis in the presence of bacteremia. Infectious endocarditis, vegetations, and intravenous drug abuse may be associated. Salmonella, streptococcus, and staphylococcus are frequently isolated organisms. Focal saccular aneurysm formation and wall thickening occur in atypical locations of the aorta. The aorta may be normal in adjacent areas or there may be intraaortic debris.[12] Aortic aneurysm develops mostly in ascending aorta.

Syphilis generally involves ascending aorta and arch. Lesions consist of calcifications and pseudoaneurysm formation with the thrombus. Aortic insufficiency (29%) and coronary ostial stenosis (26%) with wall motion changes/myocardial ischemia are associated features. Tuberculosis can also cause aortitis and aneurysms of the aorta.

Noninfectious Aortitis

Takayasu arteritis is a primary chronic inflammatory occlusive aortitis involving aortic arch, thoracic and abdominal aorta. Aneurysm formation has been reported. Involvement of origin of arch vessels with thrombus formation is characteristic. Multisegmental involvement with normal areas in between is typical. Fibrosis and wall thickening may be mistaken for intramural hematoma or dissection by imaging techniques. Marked global decrease in aortic distensibility and concentric wall thickening are echocardiographic characteristics. Dilatation of aortic segments was observed in 37% and 48% in two different studies, respectively.[13]

Other inflammatory disorders such as Behcet's disease, rheumatoid arthritis, ankylosing spondylitis, Reiter's syndrome, Kawasaki's syndrome, and giant cell arteritis may also be associated with aortic pathology.

Preoperative Preparation

The goals of the preoperative evaluation in patients undergoing thoracic aortic surgery are: to accurately categorize the extent of aneurysmal disease, to define the type of repair needed, to evaluate patient's characteristics that will have an impact on the execution of the surgical procedure, and, in the protection of end organs during surgery, to recognize other cardiac conditions that may require concomitant surgical intervention, and to detect and optimize the comorbid status.

A thorough history and physical must be conducted with detailed questioning regarding cardiopulmonary status, renal and liver function, bleeding diathesis, cerebrovascular and peripheral vascular disease. All information regarding prior cardiac and aortic interventions must be obtained. It is also important to determine the current functional status of the patient. The physical examination must include detailed neurological, cardiopulmonary, and peripheral vascular assessments. Laboratory studies should include a complete blood count, serum electrolytes, creatinine and estimated glomerular filtration rate, coagulation indices, and blood type and crossmatch to ensure availability of sufficient blood products for the intended procedure.

Coronary artery disease (CAD) must also be considered. Coronary angiography should be performed in patients older than 50 years of age or younger patients with risk factors for CAD. Patients who require root, ascending aorta, or arch surgery may need to undergo coronary bypass grafting at the time of surgery. For patients with descending or thoracoabdominal aortic disease, coronary revascularization may have to be undertaken prior to aneurysm resection depending on the severity of CAD. Limited CAD can be treated with angioplasty and stenting; however, the use of drug-eluting stents in this setting may be discouraged as the need for clopidrogel may complicate surgery.

Cerebrovascular and peripheral vascular diseases are also relevant. In patients with either a history of prior cerebrovascular disease or previous stroke or transient ischemic attacks, a CTA or MRA of head and neck vessels may be helpful in guiding neurocerebral protection strategies. Patients with carotid bruits, patients older than 65, and patients with severe peripheral vascular disease may benefit from Duplex examination of their carotids, as intervention on a severely stenotic carotid may be warranted prior to aortic aneurysm repair.

Renal function must be carefully assessed prior to surgical repair. The development of renal failure has a profound impact on patient's outcomes impairing early and late survival. All patients should be counseled as to the risks of developing renal failure and the potential need for hemodialysis postoperatively. In patients with moderate renal dysfunction, every effort must be taken to protect renal function before, during, and after surgery. Avoidance of nephrotoxic contrast material and nephrotoxic medications is paramount. Patients with severely decreased renal function or on hemodialysis have a significantly higher perioperative risk of morbidity and mortality after complex aortic repairs.

In patients with history of chronic pulmonary disease, classification of disease severity is important. Pulmonary function testing may help to identify patients who are at a substantially higher risk of developing postoperative pulmonary complications. These patients may benefit from preoperative pulmonary rehabilitation. More simply, the use of incentive spirometry and pulmonary toilet techniques can be taught pre-operatively. Patients who are currently using tobacco should stop its use. Patients with chronic bronchitis and significant sputum production can be treated with preoperative antibiotics with surgery delayed.

Anesthetic Management

Discussion with the Patient

The procedure for repair of the ascending aorta and arch is very complex and fraught with much risk that needs to be discussed with the patient as length. Our surgical colleagues do discuss this with the patient, but it is the author's opinion that the major risks should be discussed again with the patient. Emergency surgery of the ascending aorta and arch carries significantly higher morbidity and mortality that needs to be discussed frankly with the patient and/or their family making sure that they are aware of the risks.

Discussion should include, but need not be restricted to, the risk of death, major cardiac events, transfusion risks, the risk of respiratory failure requiring prolonged mechanical ventilation, and major neurologic complications. Studies have shown that the use of deep hypothermic circulatory arrest (DHCA) is a significant cause for postsurgical neurological defects, both transient and permanent. Fleck and colleagues showed that irrespective of the use of retrograde cerebral perfusion, the duration of DHCA was most predictive of the postoperative transient neurologic complications such as confusion, agitation, and delirium.[14] They found that patients who underwent DHCA for greater than 40 min as opposed to less than 30 min were placed at a 2.73 times greater risk.[14] A study by Hagl in 2001 suggested that antegrade cerebral perfusion, by selective cannulation of the carotid arteries, provided greater protection and increased the safe duration for DHCA to 40 min.[15] The author has found that discussing these issues with the patient and their family has been especially helpful.

Planning

The anesthetic management of patients who present for surgery of the ascending aorta and aortic arch can be exceedingly complex. The complexity needs to be addressed in the planning and preoperative work-up phase to ensure that as many modifiable factors as possible are taken care of prior to the patients arriving in the operating room for their surgery. Extensive planning is often required. Planning should include a discussion with the surgeon to clearly delineate the surgical plan. Topics that should be discussed are: the monitors needed (e.g., site of invasive arterial pressure monitoring), the potential for blood transfusion, the use of antifibrinolytics, the use of adjunct medications for cerebral protection, perfusion adjuncts for cerebral protection, depth of hypothermia, and the plan for rewarming the patient after hypothermic arrest.

Monitoring

Hemodynamic Monitoring

American Society of Anesthesiology (ASA) standard monitors are used. Electrocardiogram (leads II and V5) remains the gold standard for ischemia monitoring. Selection of the site for invasive arterial monitoring should be considerate of aortic cannulation and clamp site, surgical plan, and the disease process. Various approaches exist and are mostly guided by institutional preference. The author's opinion is that central aortic pressure in the form of a femoral arterial line gives the most accurate arterial pressure, especially during rewarming phase (when residual vasospasm of the radial artery may cause the central arterial pressure to be underestimated) and post cardiopulmonary bypass (CPB) period when it is extremely important to be able to achieve precise blood pressure control and avoid stress on the suture lines. Consideration has to be given to the surgical approach, as the surgeons may want to gain access for CPB through femoral arterial cannulation. Femoral arterial pressures reproduce central aortic pressures more reliably than brachial and radial pressures after CPB.[16] However, brachial arterial pressures are more reliable than radial arterial pressures in patients undergoing CPB and are used in some institutions with acceptable risk.[17]

If upper limb arterial lines are used, left radial or brachial is accessed because right radial arterial line may read excessively high if the surgeons have utilized right subclavian artery for cannulation. This will occur when there is inadequate snaring of the distal limb of the artery. Of note is the fact that this may also lead to edema of the right arm postoperatively that resolves spontaneously. Alternatively, it may be entirely lost if the aortic cross-clamp is placed distal to the innominate artery origin. However, right radial arterial pressure may be useful to monitor the perfusion pressures of antegrade perfusion given through right axillary or subclavian artery under DHCA. In such situations, bilateral upper extremity or right radial with a femoral access is used. Right radial pressure is maintained at around 40 mmHg during antegrade perfusion. One great risk is the inadvertent placement of the arterial line of a dissection patient into the false lumen. Invasive arterial pressure should be obtained at two different sites and correlated with noninvasive blood pressure cuff. It may be useful to remember that dissection process more often involves iliac artery on the left side. Common femoral artery is rarely involved.

All patients undergoing aortic surgery with DHCA have central venous access via a 9F catheter with a pulmonary artery catheter placed in right jugular vein. Apart from monitoring central venous pressure, pulmonary artery pressures, cardiac output, and mixed venous saturations before and after CPB, superior vena caval (SVC) pressure is monitored during retrograde cerebral perfusion (RCP). This can be done either by a catheter in external jugular vein or by connecting the transducer to the introducer side port. SVC pressures are maintained between 15 and 25 mmHg.[18] Higher pressures may be associated with cerebral edema and neurological dysfunction. Multimodal neurophysiologic monitoring should be used to ensure safe delivery of RCP with higher SVC pressures (40 mmHg).[19] Pulmonary artery catheter is pulled back 3–5 cm during the DHCA to prevent the possibility of distal migration during cardiac manipulation and avoid perforation of pulmonary vasculature by the stiffening catheter (due to hypothermia).

Echocardiography

Transesophageal echocardiography (TEE) and epiaortic ultrasound (EUS) are indicated in aortic surgery for many reasons. TEE can confirm the preoperative diagnosis, detect new or underappreciated lesions of the valves and other cardiac structures, assess the extent of aortic involvement, and give the surgical team aortic dimensions to help plan the surgery, especially if root replacement is being considered. Aortic valve involvement with regurgitation is common in patients with aneurysms and dissections (Fig. 6.4). With specific regard to aortic regurgitation, TEE allows detailed assessment of aortic root dimensions and cusp prolapse, calcification, sclerosis, perforation, fenestration, or disruption often indicating the feasibility of aortic valve repair. TEE also

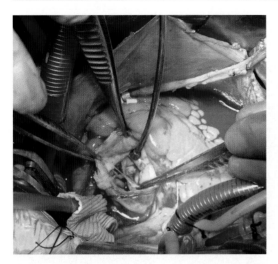

Fig. 6.4 Surgical exposure showing dissection flap involving the aortic valve

allows assessment of the quality of the aorta, and may predict embolization risk with aortic cannulation, retrograde arterial (femoral) perfusion, and intraaortic balloon pump placement. Epicardial ultrasound can also be utilized to determine the safe locations for cannulation.[20] In patients with aortic disease, it is also important to obtain baseline cardiac contractile function by TEE.

TEE is used to confirm the guidewire in the true lumen of aortic dissection and safely guide the placement of aortic cannula, as this will avoid false lumen cannulation and resulting cerebral malperfusion.[21] In re-do aortic surgery where the grafts are close to the sternum and in patients with extensive dissection or giant aneurysm, TEE is used to guide femoral arterial cannulation and inferior vena caval cannulation. TEE is used to avoid hepatic venous cannulation and help placement of cannula at SVC-right atrial junction. Right subclavian artery is exposed and a graft is sewn after full heparinization. Patient is placed on CPB and cooling is often begun immediately before sternum is opened in these patients.

In the post-bypass period, TEE is invaluable in the evaluation of the success of aortic surgery. Aortic graft is examined for laminar flow and any obvious leak around the graft. The aortic valve (native or prosthetic) is examined for gross abnormalities. Color flow Doppler is used to examine the aortic valve for paravalvular leak and residual AR (after valve repair) (Fig. 6.5). AR may be appreciated

even during full CPB by color flow Doppler though quantification of AR should be done after separation from CPB. Left ventricular distension during CPB also gives clue about developing AR.

Coronary arterial and graft flows are evaluated especially after coronary reimplantation procedures (Cabrol's and Bentall procedure). TEE can identify developing mediastinal and periaortic hematoma, which may require reexploration on CPB (Fig. 6.6). Equally important is that TEE can be utilized to investigate the overall cardiac function, regional wall motion changes, and volume status after termination of CPB.

Cerebral Monitoring

Postoperative neurological dysfunction remains the most significant cause of postoperative morbidity after otherwise successful major aortic surgery and is devastating to the patient and surgical team. This has major impact on overall costs of medical care for these patients and is an area of intense investigation recently. Advances in intraoperative neuromonitoring technology bring newer methods (near-infrared spectrometry, transcranial Doppler, and jugular venous saturation) into practice. Evidence-based guidelines are still not available though some form of neuromonitoring is used by most institutions. Currently, at our institution, standard 12-lead electroencephalogram (EEG) and somatosensory-evoked potentials (SSEP) are used in most of the patients undergoing aortic arch surgery. Neurophysiologists help with intraoperative EEG and SSEP monitoring and communicate significant changes during cooling and rewarming to the anesthesiologist and surgeon. Processed EEG using bispectral index (BIS) can be utilized as an alternative to standard EEG in emergency situations.

Temperature Monitoring

Temperature monitoring should be performed at multiple sites during aortic surgery involving DHCA. Nasopharyngeal or tympanic membrane temperature is used to monitor brain temperature. Core temperature is monitored by esophageal probe

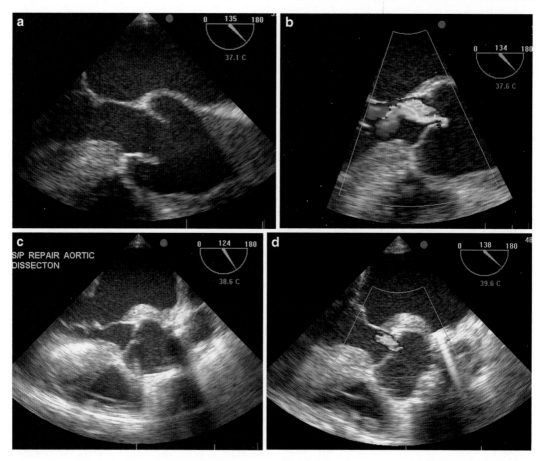

Fig. 6.5 (a–c). Pre-bypass TEE image showing dissection of the ascending aorta with morphologically normal looking aortic valve (a). Eccentric aortic regurgitation was noted (b). Valve sparing aortic replacement was performed (c). Post-bypass TEE showed trace aortic regurgitation, which was left alone (d)

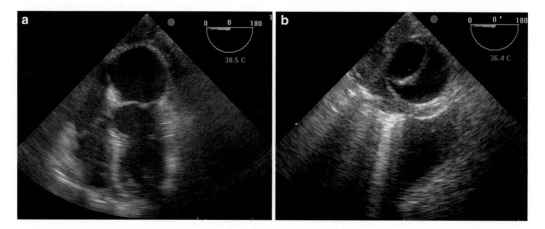

Fig. 6.6 (a and b). Post-bypass TEE showing blood collection in the oblique sinus behind left atrium (a) and periaortic hematoma (b)

or pulmonary artery catheter. Bladder or rectal temperature is monitored to make sure that no significant gradient exists during rewarming. The perfusion team closely watches arterial perfusate and venous temperature. Monitoring of temperature from each site has its advantages and drawbacks.

Arterial perfusate temperature: This is the temperature to which the brain is exposed during rewarming phase. Gradient between the actual perfusate temperature and target brain temperature (measured at different sites) during rewarming should not exceed 10°C and the absolute temperature of the perfusate should not exceed 36°C.[22]

Venous return temperature: This is a crude estimate of whole body temperature and measured in close proximity to the venous reservoir. Heat loss between the patient and reservoir in the tubings leads to underestimation of true venous temperature.[23]

Jugular bulb temperature: Temperature measured at this site closely approximates the arterial blood temperature and is always higher than that measured at other sites. This is the standard with which temperatures from other sites are compared.[24] This measurement requires an invasive procedure.

Pulmonary artery catheter temperature: Pulmonary artery catheter allows monitoring of blood temperature, which correlates most closely with brain temperature during rapid cooling and rewarming and performed better than temperature measured from other sites.[25,26] However, this can be confounded by the exposure of the heart to the room-air in open heart procedures, or by administration of cardioplegia.

Other sites: Nasopharyngeal temperature is considered a safe surrogate indicator of cooling.[24] However, this will underestimate the actual brain temperature during rewarming.[24] Rewarming to the target nasopharyngeal temperature of 36°C may avoid overheating of the brain.[22] Esophageal temperature is an alternative site for core temperature measurement and the position of the probe is important during esophageal temperature measurement so that it is not affected by myocardial topical cooling and cold cardioplegia.[23] Tympanic membrane has the risk of perforating the eardrum.

Rectal temperature is affected by the presence of feces and bladder temperature is dependent on urine flow.[23] Bladder temperature is used in all patients as the indicator of total body rewarming. Rewarming to bladder temperature of 34–36°C helps in the prevention of the afterdrop.[22]

Monitoring for aortic surgical procedures on CPB with DHCA should include assessment of coagulation status at various time periods (preoperative, during CPB, post-bypass period, and postoperative in ICU). Monitoring for blood coagulation is described in the section on coagulopathy.

Induction and Maintenance

Induction method differs between elective and emergency ascending and arch of aortic surgery. Elective patients for aneurysm repair are induced just like any other cardiac surgery with careful watch on arterial blood pressure. Invasive arterial monitoring and large bore peripheral intravenous access (14 or 16F) are typically established before induction of anesthesia for both elective and emergency aortic surgery. Adequate blood products, preprepared inotropic and vasoactive medications should be available in the room.

Induction of general anesthesia can be a stressful time especially in the patient with ascending aortic dissection and patients having symptoms of impending aneurysm rupture.[27] Preferred induction agents are thiopental (3–5 mg/kg) and etomidate (0.3 mg/kg) depending on the basal blood pressure readings noticed on arterial pressure monitoring prior to induction. Care must be taken to avoid hypertension and tachycardia during intubation and laryngoscopy, both of which can cause aneurysm rupture. Rapid-acting narcotics such as fentanyl (5–10 mcg/kg) can be used to prevent hypertensive response, but the potential for significant hypotension should be recognized when they are combined with benzodiazepines in patients with hypovolemia and poor ventricular function. Care should be taken to avoid the potential for significant blood pressure decreases that may occur with combinations of the antihypertensive medications and the anesthetic agents.

After induction of anesthesia, two large bore central venous catheters (9F & 8.5F) are inserted either through double stick of right internal jugular vein or 9F in the internal jugular (to pass PAC) and 8.5F in the femoral vein (for volume infusion). Alternatively, Advanced Venous Access (AVA) device with three large bore sidearms can be used. In patients requiring large volume infusion (ruptured aneurysm and dissection), rapid volume infusion systems and cell-saver blood-scavenging systems should be readily available.

Anesthetic maintenance can be achieved with balanced anesthetic technique using narcotics, benzodiazepines, and volatile anesthetics titrated to keep tight control of blood pressure. Requirement for anesthetics decreases after hypothermia, and overdosing of anesthetic drugs may cause vasodilatation and myocardial depression in the post-CPB period. Processed EEG monitors such as BIS and patient state index (PSI) when used to titrate anesthetic drugs have a role to improve outcomes by preventing unnecessary anesthetic administration in the early post-CPB period.[28] Large doses of narcotics are not needed since the aim is to promote rapid awakening, weaning, extubation, and neurologic assessment.[29] Fentanyl 20–25 mcg/kg and midazolam 5–10 mg are typically administered through the surgery.

Airway Management

Patients undergoing sternotomy for ascending aortic and arch surgery with CPB can be managed with standard single lumen endotracheal tube. Involvement of distal arch and proximal descending thoracic aorta will require left lung isolation by endobronchial tube for access through lateral thoracotomy. Airway compression or deviation by a large aneurysm should be suspected in patients with wheezing, dry cough, dyspnea on exertion or in supine position and stridor. Thoracic aortic lesions can lead to distortion, deviation, and compression of trachea and the mainstem bronchus.[30] Tracheomalacia and respiratory distress can be associated. Preoperative chest X-ray and computerized tomographic scans should be reviewed to rule out airway involvement (Fig. 6.7). Special

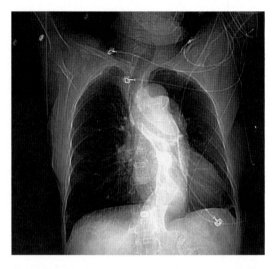

Fig. 6.7 Contrast chest CT showing tracheal deviation from huge thoracic aortic aneurysm

techniques such as fiber-optic intubation in a spontaneously breathing sedated patient in the upright position can be utilized in patients with airway compromise. The use of muscle relaxants may lead to airway obstruction and therefore are avoided if there is a significant airway compression and tracheomalacia.

Hemodynamic Management

Management of elective aortic surgery in the pre-bypass period is quite similar to any other cardiac surgery. Patients presenting for emergency surgery for aortic dissection, intramural hematoma, or impending rupture are usually hypertensive with their blood pressure and heart rate needing to be aggressively controlled with infusions of esmolol (50–300 mcg/kg/min), labetalol (0.5–2 mg/min), or nicardipine (2–15 mg/h) to the target systolic blood pressure of 100–110 mmHg. Diltiazem can be used in patients with significant bronchospastic airway disease. Antihypertensive therapy with beta-blockers is indicated to decrease the velocity of left ventricular ejection (dP/dT), which will prevent progression of dissection. If heart rate control with beta-blocker does not decrease the systolic blood pressure, vasodilators may be added. Vasodilators such as sodium nitroprusside therapy given before beta-blockers cause tachycardia leading to increased velocity of ejection (dP/dT) and extension of dissection.

Other group of patients may present to the emergency repair with already compromised hemodynamics. Hemodynamic compromise may be the result of rupture and hemopericardium (cardiac tamponade), severe aortic valve regurgitation, and coronary artery involvement (myocardial ischemia).[27] Circulation and ventilation are supported until the surgical team places the patient on CPB. Securing the airway takes priority. Consideration should be given to the possibility of full stomach. Placement of central venous access and arterial access should be achieved quickly as the surgeon prepares to initiate CPB. Heparinization should be remembered and communicated to the surgeon and perfusionist. Epinephrine, norepinephrine, milrinone, and vasopressin have all been used to good effect to support patients preoperatively. Packed red cells and fluids are administered to maintain adequate intravascular volume hematocrit. Overaggressive treatment will precipitate hypertension and should be avoided. TEE probe is inserted to perform a fast and focused examination.

Management of DHCA and CPB is described elsewhere in detail. In the post-repair phase, the hemodynamics of the patient may continue to remain deranged due to the effects of long duration of CPB and aortic cross-clamp, residual effects of preoperative myocardial compromise, and inadequate protection of the myocardium. In many instances, the stunned myocardium requires inotropic therapy. Great care should be taken to avoid a hypertensive state during post-CPB, transport, and in the immediate postoperative period. Propofol infusion can be titrated to prevent blood pressure rise and subsequent stress on the vascular suture lines during transport to intensive care unit (ICU) and early recovery period in ICU.

Coagulopathy

Patients who undergo repair of the ascending aorta and arch frequently develop a significant coagulopathy. Advanced age, renal failure, and insufficiency are risk factors for bleeding complications.[31]

The reasons for coagulopathy are multifactorial and include platelet dysfunction, disruption of the coagulation cascade, hypothermia, fibrinolysis, inflammation, and systemic anticoagulation. The use of advanced antiplatelet and antithrombotic agents worsens the situation in these patients.

The effects of the extracorporeal circuit on platelets are multiple. Mechanical destruction and hemodilution decrease the number of platelets. Functional abnormalities in platelet aggregation result from contact with artificial surfaces of the bypass circuit.[32] Von Willebrand Factor receptors, Glycoprotein IIb/IIIa receptor (fibrinogen) loss, and subsequent degranulation have been implicated, but it is also being recognized that hypothermia and heparin may play important roles in their dysfunction.[33] Attempted methods to mitigate these effects include the use of heparin-bonded bypass materials, microfilters to remove aggregates, and the use of platelet function assays to determine platelet transfusion requirements.[32]

The role of hypothermia in the impairment of the coagulation system should not be underestimated.[34,35] The mechanism is felt to be the impairment of coagulation factors, platelet dysfunction, and activation of fibrinolysis. Below 30°C, the factor activity is severely affected with 0% activity for factors VIII and IX and 5% activity for factors II and VII at 25°C. Tests of coagulation performed at the blood temperature 37°C may mask the effects of hypothermia. An *in vitro* study of rotational thromboelastography has shown temperature-dependent decrease in the function of the coagulation system.[36] The impairment in relevant measures was evident in all temperatures below 37°C.

The effects of the extracorporeal circuit on the coagulation cascade are well documented. Coagulation factors depletion occurs because of two reasons: dilution of factors in the pump prime and denaturation of coagulative proteins due to contact with artificial surfaces (e.g., cardiotomy suction). Bubble oxygenators were also a large source of this problem but have been eliminated. Reston et al. published that OPCAB had significantly lower bleeding rates versus on-pump CABG. While this does not directly apply to aortic surgery, it does illustrate the effect of the bypass system on coagulation.[37] Evidence exists that both the extrinsic and intrinsic pathways are activated. Factor XII, Factor IX, and tissue factor have all been heavily implicated as the trigger for the extrinsic pathway. Studies have shown high levels of tissue factor in blood suctioned from the pericardium. Elimination of cardiotomy suction has been shown to decrease platelet activation, thrombin generation, and even inflammation.[32]

Fibrinolysis is a homeostatic mechanism, which serves to limit clot growth. The fibrinolytic system is activated during CPB as a result of Factor XIIa in the intrinsic pathway in conjunction with tissue plasminogen activator (t-PA) and urokinase plasminogen activator (u-PA) of the extrinsic pathway.[34] Thrombin has also been implicated in releasing tissue-type plasminogen from the vascular endothelium.[35] The activation of t-PA is also enhanced with longer CPB times and intracardiac procedures. Antifibrinolytic agents have been used successfully in clinical practice to mitigate this effect.

The inflammation caused by CPB worsens coagulopathy by way of increased expression of tissue factor that occurs due to increased levels of mediators like interleukin 1, tumor necrosis factor (TNF), as well as endotoxin.[38,39] Hemodilution due to prime volume may also account for the decrease in coagulation factors and platelet count.

The final factor in coagulopathy to be discussed is the role of systemic anticoagulation. This is a topic that is still under much debate. It would seem obvious that systemic anticoagulation causes more bleeding. However, the traditional use of activated clotting time (ACT) to maintain level of anticoagulation may actually be increasing bleeding complications despite the decreased use of heparin than those patients whose heparin dosing is controlled by heparin concentration monitoring (Hep-Con). Despotis et al. showed that Hep-Con controlled patients received 32% more heparin than the ACT-controlled patients but experienced less bleeding and less need for blood products.[40,41] Patients controlled by Hep-Con had better thrombin and fibrinolysis suppression as well as better maintenance of blood levels of coagulation factors. Another study in patients undergoing aortic surgery under deep hypothermic arrest has shown better suppression of thrombin and fibrinolytic system when higher doses of

heparin are used with aprotinin as hemostatic agent.[42] The effect of the thrombin will be to potentially make the platelets dysfunctional and therefore lead to more bleeding in the postoperative period. It should be also recognized that higher doses of heparin might shield the coagulation system from excessive thrombosis and fibrinolysis and, therefore, theoretically, decrease the amount of bleeding in these patients. The assumption has to be that the heparin used intraoperatively is adequately neutralized with protamine after the termination of CPB.[31]

Apart from heparin concentration and ACT monitoring, patients during aortic surgery are monitored with point of care (POC) viscoelastic coagulation devices (thromboelastography (TEG, Haemoscope, Niles, IL) and rotational thromboelastometry (ROTEM, Pentapharm, Munich, Germany, and the Sonoclot Analyzer, and various platelet function monitors). POC tests are preferred over the traditional laboratory tests (e.g., prothrombin time, partial thromboplastin time, fibrinogen levels, and platelet counts) to monitor coagulation in the dynamic operating room environment. The advantages and limitations of POC coagulation testing are given in Table 6.2.

Among the viscoelastic POC coagulation studies, TEG is commonly used in USA while ROTEM is popular in Europe. TEG and ROTEM assess and display the viscoelastic clot formation under low shear conditions at all stages of developing and resolving clot.[43] Though TEG and ROTEM tracings look similar, the terminology and values are different (Fig. 6.8). R time (clotting time in ROTEM) indicates initial clot formation. Alpha angle and clot formation time (k time in TEG) indicate rate of fibrin polymerization. Maximum amplitude (MA in TEG) or maximum clot firmness (MCF in ROTEM) reflects number and function of platelets and their interaction with fibrin. Amplitude of the TEG/ROTEM waveforms 30 and 60 min after MA/MCF reflects fibrinolysis.

TEG and ROTEM are used in clinical cardiac surgical practice to predict the extent of post-CPB bleeding, to diagnose the cause of post-CPB bleeding and to evaluate the efficacy of hemostatic therapy.[43] The data on positive predictive value of POC tests for excessive post-CPB bleeding are

Table 6.2   Point of care coagulation testing

Advantages over traditional lab tests
Less turnover time
Provides rapid diagnostic results (10–15 min) allowing appropriate targeted therapy
Whole blood can be used, No centrifugation required
Easy to use (disposable cartridges, cups, electronic pipette, and computer display of results), can be done in the operating room by anesthesiologists and anesthesia technologists
Testing possible at patient's temperature
Sensitive in detecting fibrinogen function, fibrinolysis, platelet function, and platelet fibrin interaction
Diagnosis of hypercoagulable conditions possible
Limitations
Few studies evaluated the reliability, accuracy, validity, and reproducibility.
Age, gender, red cell mass, equipment, and activators used will alter the assay results and specificity
Lack of standardization
Inadequate quality control
Prone for errors when performed by nonlaboratory personnel, regular training required
Coagulation in the cuvette occurs in no-flow conditions so that the results have to be interpreted against the backdrop of clinical bleeding

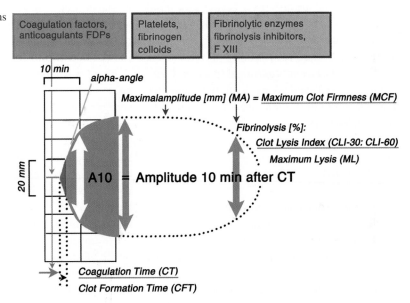

Fig. 6.8 Typical waveforms of thromboelastography (TEG) and rotational thromboelastometry (ROTEM) (Reprinted with permission from Dr Gorlinger[84])

not consistent but the negative predictive value is very high.[44–46] Hence, in the presence of a normal POC test, inadequate surgical hemostasis is more likely the cause of excessive hemorrhage.

In patients undergoing surgery for acute type A aortic dissection, ROTEM-based coagulation management decreased transfusion of blood products, postoperative adverse events, and duration of mechanical ventilation and also shortened ICU stay and reduced secondary costs.[47]

Platelet dysfunction during aortic surgery may result from impairment of platelet activation, adhesion, aggregation, and release or platelet–fibrin interaction. ROTEM and TEG does not provide specific information on platelet function related to adhesion/aggregation. Verifynow system (Accumetrics, San Diego, CA, USA), Multiplate analyzer (Dynabyte, Munich, Germany), Platelet works (Helena laboratories, Beaumont, TX, USA), and Platelet Function Analyzer-100 (PFA-100, DADE Behring, and USA) are some of the currently available monitors, which can be used to assess various platelet functions including aggregation. Monitoring of antiplatelet drugs (aspirin, clopidogrel, and glycoprotein receptor antagonists) is the main application of platelet function monitors. It is not infrequent nowadays that patients present to elective and emergency aortic surgery while taking antiplatelet therapy. A pre-bypass platelet function analysis might be able to detect residual effect of antiplatelet drugs. Their utility in cardiac surgery is evaluated in limited clinical trials. The use of POC platelet function tests in the operating room and their efficacy in reducing platelet transfusion need further investigation.

At author's institution, Platelet works study is used to measure platelet function in the pre- and post-CPB periods. Platelet works measure platelet count before and after activation with an agonist (ADP, collagen, or arachidonic acid). Nonfunctional platelets do not aggregate in the agonist tube and the difference between the basal platelet count and the count in the agonist tube indicates functional platelet number.[48] Normal patients have more than 90% of their platelets functional. TEG and functional platelet count results are analyzed along with the surgeon's assessment of clinical microvascular bleeding to guide platelet therapy.

Transfusion

Blood conservation strategies using preoperative autologous donation, intraoperative donation (acute normovolemic hemodilution), and cell savage can help avoid the use of homologous blood transfusion (HBT) in aortic surgery. Intraoperative blood salvage can also be done using automatic blood collection and washing equipment before and after CPB. During CPB, blood from cardiotomy suction can be autotransfused directly or recycled using a cell-saving device. At the end of CPB, the blood remaining in the pump prime can be processed using ultrafiltration and reinfused. In 61 patients undergoing elective thoracic aortic surgery with deep hypothermic arrest, Shibata et al.[49] using the above methods have shown avoidance of HBT in 43% of their patients during the entire hospital stay. Patients who received HBT had prolonged intubation and higher infection rate though the

direct cause–effect relationship could not be established. Svensson et al.[50] used similar blood conservation program along with reinfusion of shed blood from chest tubes in 45 elective ascending aortic and arch operations. They could avoid in hospital HBT in 69% of patients and have shown shorter hospital stay and better functional dyspnea class on discharge in those patients. Going by these reports, blood conservation and avoidance of transfusion is possible in certain patients undergoing aortic surgery. Other group of high-risk aortic surgical patients in whom anemia and coagulopathy requiring HBT cannot be completely avoided because of the reasons explained in the previous section. Measures should be taken to minimize the amount of blood products transfused in these patients as the amount of blood transfused has a profound effect on morbidity and mortality. Apaydin et al.[51] showed that transfusion of greater than four units of blood was a predictor of mortality. Published guidelines by society of thoracic surgeons and society for cardiovascular anesthesiologists should be followed for perioperative blood transfusion and conservation in these high-risk aortic surgical patients[52] (Table 6.3). Preoperative identification of patients at high risk for bleeding and application of all blood conservation measures in those patients are recommended as they account for majority of blood products consumed. Older age, preoperative anemia, preexisting coagulopathy (congenital and acquired disorders), preoperative antithrombotic and antiplatelet drug intake, small body size, complex and redo surgery with prolonged CPB duration, emergency surgery and patients with multiple comorbidities are a few of them.[52] Multimodal approach using point of care testing and institutional transfusion algorithms help minimize the use of blood products in these patients.[52]

Given the rare transmission of viral diseases with blood transfusion, fears of acquiring those diseases should not limit the administration of indicated blood products.[52] Practitioners should ensure that adequate blood products are available to be able to transfuse the patient promptly if he or she needs it. Extreme care needs to be taken to

Table 6.3 Society of thoracic surgeons and society of cardiovascular anesthesiologists recommendation summary for blood transfusion and blood conservation in cardiac surgery

Preoperative
Discontinue antiplatelet medications (e.g. aspirin and plavix) before surgery to limit blood loss (Class IIa)
Recombinant erythropoietin to prepare for autologous blood donation and predonation of two units in carefully selected routine cardiac surgical patients (Class IIa)

Intraoperative
Acute normovolemic hemodilution is not unreasonable as a part of multimodal blood conservation approach (Class IIb)
Transfusion for hemoglobin levels less than 6 g/dl, Transfusion for Hemoglobin more than 6 g/dl is indicated depending on clinical situation (e.g.,cerebrovascular disease, diabetes, poor cardiac function, myocardial ischemia, critical end organ ischemia, active blood loss) (Class IIa)
Antifibrinolytics to reduce blood loss (Class I)
Maintenance of higher or patient-specific heparin concentrations during CPB to reduce hemostatic system activation, reduce platelet and coagulation proteins consumption for procedures with longer CPB duration (2–3 h) (Class IIb)
Retrograde autologous priming of CPB circuit (Class IIb)
Modified ultrafiltration in patients with significant prime volume (Class IIb)
Routine use of red cell saving is helpful except in patients with infection and malignancy (Class I)
Use of heparin-coated bypass circuits (Class IIb)
Topical sealants to assist in the highly complex aortic repair (dissection) (Class IIb)
Post bypass
Titrate protamine or empiric low-dose protamine (50% of total heparin dose) to achieve lower protamine--heparin ratio at the end of CPB (Class IIb)
Desmopressin acetate to improve platelet function and attenuate excessive bleeding in uremia, CPB-induced platelet dysfunction, type I Von Willebrand Disease (Class IIb)
Recombinant factor VIIa concentrate for the management of intractable nonsurgical bleeding unresponsive to routine hemostatic therapy (Class IIb)

Postoperative
Therapeutic PEEP to reduce excessive postoperative bleeding (Class IIb)
Washing of shed mediastinal blood and reinfusion is not unreasonable (Class IIb)

Multimodal blood conservation approach (Class I Level A evidence)
A multimodality approach involving multiple stakeholders, institutional support, enforceable transfusion algorithms supplemented with point-of-care testing, and all of the already mentioned efficacious blood conservation interventions will limit blood transfusion and provide optimal blood conservation for cardiac operations

Reprinted with permission from (Elsevier); Casati V et al.[55]

ensure that there is no surgical source of bleeding before administration of blood products.

Antifibrinolytics

The topic of antifibrinolytics has been one of the great controversies in the anesthetic and surgical literature lately. The incidence of severe bleeding in the general cardiac surgery population is between 3.6%[53] and 4.2%.[53] Excessive chest tube output in ICU or cardiac tamponade may necessitate re-exploration in the operating room. Re-exploration for bleeding is associated with adverse outcomes after cardiac surgery.[54] An identifiable source of bleeding is found in only a minority of these patients. It is usually generalized "ooze" and this is then ascribed more to a medical cause of bleeding such as coagulopathy. CPB leads to activation of both the coagulation and fibrinolytic cascades. The consequence of this is a consumptive coagulopathy, which manifests itself as uncontrollable bleeding with no clearly identifiable surgical source. Transfusion carries the risk of immunosuppression, disease transmission (albeit low), transfusion reactions, all of which may lead to increased morbidity and possibly mortality.

Antifibrinolytics are drugs employed to decrease the transfusion rate and the number of re-explorations in cardiac surgery (Class I evidence-based recommendation). Available drugs included ε-amino caproic acid (EACA), tranexamic acid (TA), and aprotinin. EACA and TA are both lysine analogues that bind reversibly to plasminogen and plasmin and serve to interfere with the ability of plasmin to convert fibrinogen to fibrin. These agents have been shown to reduce transfusion requirements and blood loss compared to placebo in aortic surgery patients.[55–56] Aprotinin functions differently in that it is a broad-spectrum serine protease inhibitor that actively prevents the conversion of plasminogen to plasmin. It also exhibits anti-inflammatory and anti-coagulant properties. It appears to block the coagulation cascade both at the intrinsic and the tissue factor pathway. It has also been suggested that the use of aprotinin has a platelet-sparing effect for patients undergoing CPB[57]. Aprotinin's efficacy and safety profile have always been questioned in the patient population for thoracic aortic surgery with DHCA.[58-61]

There are three studies in thoracic aortic surgical population with DHCA comparing lysine analogs (EACA in 2 studies and TA in one study, 2 unpublished observations) with aprotinin. Eaton et al.[62] in a study comparing aprotinin and EACA, reported equal efficacy for both these drugs, but only EACA was associated with renal dysfunction. Fontes et al.[63] have also shown equal efficacy for aprotinin and EACA. Our own database review at the University of Pittsburgh has shown that aprotinin patients received less blood products compared to tranexamic acid and aprotinin was associated with renal dysfunction after DHCA.[64] All these studies are retrospective involving small sample size with the attendant limitations. The BART (Blood Conservation Using Antifibrinolytics in a Randomized Trial) study is a large prospective randomized study involving high-risk cardiac surgery and has shown that aprotinin produced modest reduction in massive bleeding but was associated with higher mortality.[65] Since aprotinin has been withdrawn from the market, the future clinical trials addressing the efficacy, dose response, and safety of lysine analogs should be conducted to have clear evidence-based recommendations.

The author's current practice is the use of tranexamic acid that is administered in a similar dose to the dose used in BART study. The loading dose is 30 mg/kg IV administered after heparinization for the patient and 2 mg/kg is added to the pump prime. The infusion is 15 mg/kg/h and this is continued until skin closure. TA dose should be reduced in renal insufficiency.

Implications for Cardio-Pulmonary Bypass

Cardio-pulmonary bypass is a necessity when attempting to do any open surgical repair of the ascending aorta and aortic arch. The specific aortic pathology may have important implications regarding the method that is employed to provide CPB.

Cannulation Options

Main considerations include the use of central aortic cannulation or whether it would be best for a more peripheral location for arterial access. The factors that contribute to the decision to do a peripheral cannulation relate to the extent of the aneurysmal or atherosclerotic aorta. If there is insufficient space to place an aortic cross-clamp proximal to the origin of the right subclavian artery, then this may necessitate use of alternative arterial access. Any disease involving the arch will also generate consideration of alternative access.

Femoral and axillary arteries are commonly used peripheral cannulation locations. The advantage of femoral cannulation is that it can be done percutaneously and rapidly[66] Malperfusion can occur with femoral approach in cerebral circulation and abdominal organs in patients with acute dissection. However, many believe that femoral cannulation is acceptable and yields very low complication rates as evidenced by a paper from Fusco and Colleagues.[67] This retrospective review paper suggested the ease of femoral access and the achievement of good results as well as a very low rate of malperfusion consequences (2.5%) should make the femoral approach an appropriate approach. However, the femoral artery approach does risk the retrograde showering of any descending aortic debris to the cerebral circulation.

The axillary or subclavian artery, usually the right side, is a common choice because the left subclavian is less desirable as it does not share circulation with the left common carotid. Use of axillary cannulation avoids manipulation of the atherosclerotic aorta and axillary artery, by itself, is seldom involved in severe atherosclerotic process. Axillary cannulation also allows for antegrade cerebral perfusion (Fig. 6.9a). Axillary cannulation is associated with improved neurologic outcomes.[68-70]

In patients with subclavian stenosis, the use of the axillary cannulation should be avoided as this will result in right arm overperfusion and edema. Axillary artery thrombosis and brachial plexopathy are other concerns. In addition, the use of axillary cannulation may not be useful in the emergent cases. Flow restrictions created by the use of a narrow cannula into a narrow vessel may

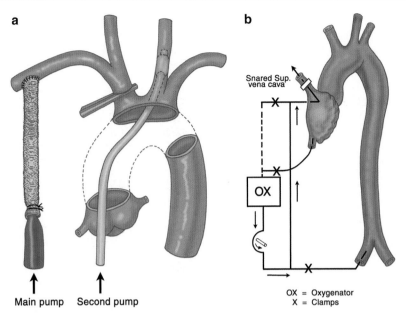

a

b

Snared Sup.
vena cava

OX

Main pump   Second pump

OX = Oxygenator
X = Clamps

Fig. 6.9 (**a**) Simplified technique for selective cerebral perfusion. Through the right axillary artery, the main pump provides a flow of 5 ml kg^{-1} min^{-1} for the right carotid artery while a second roller pump provides a flow of 5 ml kg^{-1} min^{-1} for the left carotid system (Redrawn with permission from Elsevier publishers; Mazzola[85]). (**b**) Circuit for retrograde cerebral perfusion (Modified with permission from Wiley-Blackwell Publishers; Bonser[86])

also limit the flow that can be delivered and the patient of small stature will also present difficulty for this method. Axillary artery can be cannulated directly or perfused with a side graft sewn to the artery.[71,72] The use of side graft avoids the problems of insufficient CPB flow because of the narrow vessel. Another concern regarding axillary cannulation is the risk that in the presence of axillary dissection, an antegrade carotid dissection could be caused. The involvement of axillary artery in dissections is rare.

For procedures requiring DHCA in right lateral decubitus position (for complex arch and descending thoracic aortic disease), bidirectional perfusion with femoral artery (for lower body) and another vessel (for head perfusion) is needed. Right axillary artery (cannulated with side graft in supine position before turning the patient to right lateral position)[22], left subclavian, left axillary, left common carotid, and ascending aorta are options for cerebral perfusion.[73-75] Decision is made based on the involvement of these arteries in the aneurysmal disease process.

Several authors used central aortic cannulation for type A dissection repairs successfully.[76-79]

Patients with aneurysm rupture, intramural hematoma, and false lumen thrombus are not candidates for central aortic cannulation. Aortic cannulation is achieved using Seldinger's technique.[80] A guide wire is passed into the true lumen and the position of the wire is confirmed in the true lumen with epiaortic ultrasound in the arch or with TEE in the descending aorta. Cannula is introduced over the wire and the position of the cannula is confirmed with echocardiography. After initiation of CPB, flow in the true lumen is confirmed with color Doppler ultrasound.

Another less frequently used method, although its use dates back to the 1970s, that is starting to gain attention is the cannulation of the aorta via a cardiac apical cannula. This has been promoted as a safe, rapid, and reliable technique for gaining true lumen perfusion in patients with Type A aortic dissection. The inflow cannula is positioned across the aortic valve into the proximal ascending aorta. Positioning is confirmed by the trans-esophageal echocardiography. This technique is not useful in patients who have aortic stenosis where the cannula placement may either injure the valve permanently or occlude aortic outflow entirely. The other population where the use of apical cannulation is less desirable is patients with a previous sternotomy where dissection can be very difficult.[81]

Cardiac Protection

The myocardium is always at risk during any procedure that will interrupt the normal perfusion. Repair of the ascending aorta and aortic arch is no different. In the event of a patient having significant aortic regurgitation, antegrade cardioplegia cannot be used due to the regurgitation into the left ventricle with subsequent increase in oxygen demand in the setting of no perfusion. In these instances, the initiating dose of cardioplegia will be delivered in a retrograde fashion. Subsequent dosing may be delivered in a variety of ways including direct delivery into the coronaries via hand-held probe or alternatively small cardioplegia catheters can be placed in the coronary ostia. In both these instances, the delivery is antegrade. The direct cannulation of the coronaries carries a risk of developing ostial stenosis. The risks with relying only on retrograde cardioplegia are (1) that inadequate protection of the right ventricle and posterior interventricular septum, (2) traumatic injury to the coronary sinus, (3) difficult placement of and/or (4) dislodging of the catheter. Myocardial stunning is not uncommon after prolonged CPB and DHCA. We usually start epinephrine 0.02–0.05 mcg/kg/min in these cases before separation from bypass. The dose is titrated to ventricular function on TEE and cardiac output by PAC. Ventricular pacing may be required in few patients.

Cerebral protection

Institutions reporting low incidence of stroke (3%) and neurocognitive dysfunction (2.5%) after ascending aortic and arch surgery use multimodal operative protocol involving various chemical and perfusion strategies. One such protocol used in Cleveland Clinic is given in Table 6.4.[82] The use of circulatory techniques has already been briefly mentioned in the preceding pages and detailed in the chapter on DHCA. The basic premise is to

Table 6.4 Summary of operative protocol for ascending and aortic arch operations

All patients
Electroencephalogram silence
Temperatures less than 20°C
Head packed in ice
Mannitol prime and after arrest
Alpha-stat pH control
Leukoguard filter
CO_2 flooding of field
Thiopental 5 mg/kg 5 min before arrest
Lidocaine 200 mg before arrest
Magnesium sulfate 2 g
Centrifugal pump
Membrane oxygenator
Closed circuit bag venous reservoir
Routine plasmapheresis before pump
Cell saver
Antegrade brain perfusion
Right subclavian cannulation or side graft
Innominate and carotid balloon occlusion (retrograde cardioplegia balloon occlusion catheter)
Pressure kept 40–60 mmHg
Sequential removal of catheters as arch anastomosis completed
Retrograde brain perfusion
Superior vena cava cannula
Snared below azygos vein
300–500 mL/min but less than 25–35 mmHg

Reprinted with permission from (Elsevier) Lars G Svensson.[82]

provide the brain with continuous supply of cold blood, thereby providing oxygen and nutrients in order to prolong the safe period of circulatory arrest needed to complete some of the more complex repairs. Hypothermia and perfusion of the brain are the main cerebral protective strategies. Perfusion of the brain during DHCA can be achieved either by antegrade route through the right axillary artery (to the right common carotid artery) after clamping the innominate artery close to its origin, or by retrograde route through superior vena caval cannula (Fig. 6.9b).

A number of studies have looked at medicinal or chemical methods to protect the brain from malperfusion (as is created in the DHCA patient). Many medications have been studied and ultimately there has not been any clear evidence to show that any of these work. Many have also not shown to harm and as a result their use varies. Barbiturates and steroids are probably the most widely used agents. Other agents that have been used are lidocaine, aprotinin, acadesine, nimodipine, beta-blockers, and pegorgotein.[83]

Key Notes

1. The repair of ascending aortic disease can be very complex with significant risk to the patient even in the event of a seemingly successful repair. This warrants frank discussion with the patient's family.
2. Due to the complexity of the arterial repair work combined with the complexity of the CPB arrangements, a thorough understanding of the anatomy is necessary to adequately prepare for the anesthetic planning.
3. The complexity of the perfusion system, especially if cerebral protection is being used, must be understood. Extreme vigilance is necessary to ensure that the patient is protected at all costs.
4. Management of the patient's hemodynamic status can be very tenuous and unstable. All necessary medications should be ready for use prior to starting the procedure to facilitate rapid response to instability.
5. Monitoring and protection of organ function (e.g., myocardial, cerebral, and renal) are integral aspects of successful aortic surgery.

References

1. Roman MJ, Devereux RB, Kramer-Fox R, O'Loughlin J. Two dimensional echocardiographic aortic root dimensions in normal children and adults. *Am J Cardiol.* 1989;64:507–512.
2. Bickerstaff LK, Pairolero PC, Hollier LH, et al. Thoracic aortic aneurysms: a population based study. *Surgery.* 1982;92:1103–1109.
3. Chen K, Varon J, Wenker OC, et al. Acute thoracic aortic dissection: the basics. *J Emerg Med.* 1997;15:859–867.
4. Muller JP, Reuthebuch O, Jenni R, Turina MI. Pseudoaneurysm of the left ventricle near the non-coronary sinus valsalvae after aortic valve replacement. *Eur J Cardiothorac Surg.* 2004;25:283.
5. Yasuda H, Sakagoshi N, Lim YJ, Mishima M. Pseudoaneurysm after Bentall operation diagnosed by transesophageal echocardiography. *Ann Thorac Surg.* 2004;78:1478.
6. Dhadwal AK, Abrol S, Zisbrod Z, Cunningham JN Jr. Pseudoaneurysms of the ascending aorta following coronary artery bypass surgery. *J Card Surg.* 2006;21:221–224.
7. Erkut B, Ceviz M, Becit N, Gundogdu F, Unlu Y, Kantarci M. Pseudoaneurysm of the left coronary ostial anastomoses as a complication of the modified Bentall procedure diagnosed by echocardiography and multislice computed tomography. *Heart Surg Forum.* 2007;10:E191–E192.
8. Jault F, Rama A, Cluzel P, et al. Pseudo-aneurysms of the ascending aorta in patients previously operated for acute aortic dissection. *Arch Mal Coeur Vaiss.* 2005;98:20–24.
9. Sanz O, San Román JA, Vilacosta I, et al. Clinical profile and prognosis of patients with endocarditis and periannular pseudoaneurysms. *Rev Esp Cardiol.* 2001;54:181–185.
10. Belkin RN, Kalapatapu SK, Lafaro RJ, Ramaswamy G, McClung JA, Cohen MB. Atherosclerotic pseudoaneurysm of the ascending aorta. *J Am Soc Echocardiogr.* 2003;16:367–369.
11. Staatz G, Bücker A. Spontaneous nontraumatic rupture of the descending thoracic aorta with development of a giant pseudoaneurysm. *J Vasc Interv Radiol.* 2001;12:394–395.
12. Harris KM, Malenka DJ, Plehn JF. Transesophageal echocardiographic evaluation of aortitis. *Clin Cardiol.* 1997;20:813–815.
13. Bezerra Lira-Filho E, Campos O, Lazaro Andrade J, et al. Thoracic aorta evaluation in patients with Takayasu's arteritis by transesophageal echocardiography. *J Am Soc Echocardiogr.* 2006;19:829–834.
14. Fleck TM, Czerny M, Hutschala D, et al. The incidence of transient neurologic dysfunction after ascending aortic replacement with circulatory arrest. *Ann Thorac Surg.* 2003;76:1198–1202.
15. Hagl C, Ergin MA, Galla JD, et al. Neurologic outcome after ascending aortic-aortic arch operations effect of brain protection technique in high risk patients. *J Thorac Cardiovasc Surg.* 2001;121:1107–1121.
16. Gravlee GP, Brauer SD, O'Rourke MF, Avolio AP. A comparison of brachial, femoral, and aortic intra-arterial pressures before and after cardiopulmonary bypass. *Anaesth Intensive Care.* 1989;17:305–311.
17. Bazaral MG, Welch M, Golding LA, Badhwar K. Comparison of brachial and radial arterial pressure monitoring in patients undergoing coronary artery bypass surgery. *Anesthesiology.* 1990;73:38–45.
18. Usui A, Abe T, Murase M. Early clinical results of retrograde perfusion for aortic arch operations in Japan. *Ann Thorac Surg.* 1996;62:94–104.
19. Ganzel B, Edmonds HJ Jr, Pank JR, Goldsmith LJ. Neurophysiological monitoring to assure delivery of retrograde cerebral perfusion. *J Thorac Cardiovasc Surg.* 1997;113:748–755.
20. Davila-Roman VG, Barzilai B, Wareing TH, Murphy SF, Kouchoukos NT. Intraoperative ultrasonographic evaluation of the ascending aorta in 100 consecutive patients undergoing cardiac surgery. *Circulation.* 1991;84(Supplement 5):III 47–III 53.

21. Flachskampf FA. Assessment of aortic dissection and hematoma. *Semin Cardiothorac Vasc Anesth.* 2006; 10:83–88.
22. Ergin MA. Hypothermic circulatory arrest. In: Coselli JS, Lemaire SA, eds. *Aortic Arch Surgery. Principles,Strategies and Outcomes.* 1st ed. Hoboken, NJ: Wiley-Blackwell; 2008:135–152.
23. Johnson JM, Robins S, Hyde J. Monitoring and safety in cardiopulmonary bypass. In: Kay PH, Munsch CM, eds. *Techniques in Extracorporeal Circulation.* 4th ed. London, Great Britain: Arnold; 2004:76–98.
24. Kaukuntla H, Harrington D, Bilkoo I, et al. Temperature monitoring during cardiopulmonary bypass– do we undercool or overheat the brain? *Eur J Cardiothorac Surg.* 2004;26:580–585.
25. Akata T, Yamaura K, Kandabashi T, Sadamatsu S, Takahashi S. Changes in body temperature during profound hypothermic cardiopulmonary bypass in adult patients undergoing aortic arch reconstruction. *J Anesth.* 2004;18:73–81.
26. Akata T, Setoguchi H, Shirozu K, Yoshino J. Reliability of temperatures measured at standard monitoring sites as an index of brain temperature during deep hypothermic cardiopulmonary bypass conducted for thoracic aortic reconstruction. *J Thorac Cardiovasc Surg.* 2007;133:1559–1565.
27. Bond DM, Milne B, Pym J, Sandler D. Cardiac tamponade complicating anaesthetic induction for repair of ascending aorta dissection. *Can J Anaesth.* 1987;34:291–293.
28. Edmonds HL. Advances in neuromonitoring for cardiothoracic and vascular surgery. *J Cardiothorac Vasc Anesth.* 2001;15:241–250.
29. Cooper JR. Anesthetic management. In: Coselli JS, Lemaire SA, eds. *Aortic arch Surgery. Principles, Strategies and Outcomes.* Hoboken, NJ: Wiley-Blackwell; 2007:91–97.
30. Cooper JR, Slogoff S. Thoracic aortic surgery. In: Yeager MP, Glass DD, eds. *Anesthesiology and Vascular Surgery.* Norwalk, CN: Appleton and Lange; 1990:185–210.
31. Paparella D, Brister SJ, Buchanan M. Coagulation disorders of cardiopulmonary bypass: a review. *Intensive Care Med.* 2004;30:1873–1881.
32. Hartmann M, Sucker C, Boehm O, Koch A, Loer S, Zacharowski KC. Effects of cardiac surgery on hemostasis. *Transfus Med Rev.* 2006;20:230–241.
33. Muriithi EW, Belcher PR, Menys VC, et al. Heparin-induced platelet dysfunction and cardiopulmonary bypass. *Ann Thorac Surg.* 2000;69:1827–1832.
34. Westaby S. Coagulation disturbance in profound hypothermia: the influence of anti-fibrinolytic therapy. *Semin Thorac Cardiovasc Surg.* 1997;9:246–256.
35. Wilde JT. Hematological consequences of profound hypothermic circulatory arrest and aortic dissection. *J Card Surg.* 1997;12:201–206.
36. Rundgren M, Engstrom M. A thromboelastometric evaluation of the effects of hypothermia on the coagulation system. *Anesth Analg.* 2008;107:1465–1468.
37. Reston JT, Tregear SJ, Turkelson CM. Meta-analysis of short term and mid-term outcomes following off-pump coronary artery bypass grafting. *Ann Thorac Surg.* 2003;76:1510–1515.
38. Christman JW, Lancaster LH, Blackwell TS. Nuclear factor Kappa B: a pivotal role in the systemic inflammatory response syndrome and new target for therapy. *Intensive Care Med.* 1998;24:1131–1138.
39. Baldwin AS. The NF-kappa B and I kappa B proteins: new discoveries and insights. *Annu Rev Immunol.* 1996;14:649–683.
40. Despotis GJ, Joist JH, Hogue CW Jr, et al. The impact of heparin concentration and activated clotting time monitoring on blood conservation. A prospective, randomized evaluation in patients undergoing cardiac operation. *J Thorac Cardiovasc Surg.* 1995;110:46–54.
41. Despotis GJ, Joist JH, Hogue CW Jr, et al. More effective suppression of hemostatic system in patients undergoing cardiac surgery by heparin dosing based on heparin blood concentrations rather that ACT. *Thromb Haemost.* 1996;76:902–908.
42. Okita Y, Takamoto S, Ando M, et al. Coagulation and fibrinolysis system in aortic surgery under deep hypothermic circulatory arrest with aprotinin: the importance of adequate heparinization. *Circulation.* 1997;96(Suppl 2):376–381.
43. Ganter MT, Hofer CK. Coagulation monitoring: current techniques and clinical use of viscoelastic point of care coagulation devices. *Anesth Analg.* 2008;106:1366–1375.
44. Wang JS, Lin CY, Hung WT, et al. Thromboelastogram fails to predict postoperative hemorrhage in cardiac patients. *Ann Thorac Surg.* 1992;53:435–439.
45. Mengistu AM, Wolf MW, Boldt J, et al. Evaluation of a new platelet function analyzer in cardiac surgery: a comparison of modified thromboelastography and whole blood aggregometry. *J Cardiothorac Vasc Anesth.* 2008;22:40–46.
46. Cammerer U, Dietrich W, Rampf T, et al. The predictive value of modified computerized thromboelastography and platelet function analysis for postoperative blood loss in routine cardiac surgery. *Anesth Analg.* 2003;96:51–57.
47. Gorlinger K, Herold U, Jacob H, et al. ROTEM based coagulation management in acute type A dissection: medical and economical aspects. *J Anast Intensivbeh.* 2007;14:89–90.
48. Shore-Lesserson L. Evidence based coagulation monitors: heparin monitoring, thromboelastography and platelet function. *Semin Cardiothorac Vasc Anesth.* 2005;9:41–52.
49. Shibata K, Takamoto S, Kotsuka Y, Sato H. Effectiveness of combined blood conservation measures in thoracic aortic operations with deep hypothermic circulatory arrest. *Ann Thorac Surg.* 2002;73:739–743.
50. Svensson LG, Sun J, Nadolny E, Kimmel WA. Prospective evaluation of minimal blood use for ascending aorta and aortic arch operations. *Ann Thorac Surg.* 1995;59:1501–1508.

51. Apaydin AZ, Buket S, Posacioglu H, et al. Perioperative risk factors for mortality in patients with acute Type A aortic dissection. *Ann Thorac Surg.* 2002;74:2034–2039.

52. Society of Thoracic Surgeons Blood Conservation Guideline Task Force, VA, Ferraris SP, Saha SP et al. Society of Cardiovascular Anesthesiologists Special Task Force on Blood Transfusion, Spiess BD, Shore-Lesserson L, Stafford-Smith M et al. Perioperative Blood Transfusion and blood conservation in cardiac surgery. The Society of Thoracic Surgeons and The Society of Cardiovascular Anesthesiologists clinical practice guidelines. *Ann Thorac Surg.* 2007;83(5 Suppl):S27–86.

53. Dacey LJ, Munoz JJ, Baribeau YR, et al. Reexploration for hemorrhage following coronary artery bypass grafting: incidence and risk factors. Northern New England cardiovascular disease study group. *Arch Surg.* 1998;133:442–447.

54. Moulton MJ, Creswell LL, Mackey ME, Cox JL, Rosenbloom M. Reexploration for bleeding is a risk factor for adverse outcomes after cardiac operations. *J Thorac Cardiovasc Surg.* 1996;111:1037–1046.

55. Casati V, Sandreli L, Speziali G, et al. Hemostatic effects of tranexamic acid in elective thoracic aortic surgery: A prospective, randomized, double blind, placebo-controlled study. *J Thorac Cardiovasc Surg.* 2002;123:1084–1091.

56. Shimamura Y, Nakajima M, Hirayama T, et al. The effect of intraoperative high-dose tranexamic acid on blood loss after operation for acute aortic dissection. *J Thorac Cardiovasc Surg.* 1998;46:616–621.

57. Boldt J, Schindler E, Osmer C, et al. Influence of different anticoagulation regimens on platelet function during cardiac surgery. *Br J Anaesth.* 1994;73:639–644.

58. Stundt TM, Kouchoukos NT, Saffitz JE, et al. Renal dysfunction and intravascular coagulation with aprotinin and hypothermic circulatory arrest. *Ann Thorac Surg.* 1993;55:1418–1424.

59. Westaby S, Forni A, Dunning J, et al. Aprotinin and bleeding in profoundly hypothermic perfusion. *Eur J Cardiothorac Surg.* 1994;8:82–86.

60. Parolari A, Antona C, Alamanni F, et al. Aprotinin and deep hypothermic circulatory arrest: there are no benefits even when appropriate amounts of heparin are given. *Eur J Cardiothorac Surg.* 1997;11:149–156.

61. Mora Mangano CT, Neville MJ, Hsu PH, et al. Aprotinin, blood loss, and renal dysfunction in deep hypothermic circulatory arrest. *Circulation.* 2001; 104(12 Suppl 1):I276–I281.

62. Eaton MP, Deeb GM. Aprotinin versus epsilon-aminocaproic acid for aortic surgery using deep hypothermic circulatory arrest. *J Cardiothorac Vasc Anesth.* 1998;12:548–552.

63. Fontes M, Girardi L, Koval K, et al. Post aprotinin era: Is aminocaproic acid as good in complex aortic surgery. *Anesth Analg.* 2009;108(SCA Suppl):A3.

64. Nicolau-Raducu RE, Subramaniam K, Marquez J, Hilmi IA, Sullivan EA. Safety of high dose tranexamic acid compared with aprotinin in thoracic aortic surgery. *Anesthesiology.* 2008;109:A1622.

65. Fergusson DA, Hebert PC, Mazer CD, et al. (BART study). A comparison of aprotinin and lysine analogues in high-risk cardiac surgery. *N Engl J Med.* 2008;358:2319–2331.

66. Shimazaki Y, Watanabe T, Takahashi T, et al. Minimized mortality and neurological complications in surgery for chronic arch aneurysm. *J Card Surg.* 2004;19:339–342.

67. Fusco DS, Shaw RK, Tranquilli M, et al. Femoral cannulation is safe for type A dissection repair. *Ann Thorac Surg.* 2004;78:1285–1289.

68. Reuthebuch O, Schurr U, Hellermann J, et al. Advantages of subclavian artery perfusion for repair of acute type A dissection. *Eur J Cardiothorac Surg.* 2004;26:592–598.

69. Moizumi Y, Motoyoshi N, Sakuma K, Yoshida S. Axillary artery cannulation improves operative results for acute type a aortic dissection. *Ann Thorac Surg.* 2005;80:77–83.

70. Pasic M, Schubel J, Bauer M, et al. Cannulation of the right axillary artery for surgery of acute type A aortic dissection. *Eur J Cardiothorac Surg.* 2003;24:231–235.

71. Strauch JT, Spielvogel D, et al. Axillary artery cannulation: routine use in ascending aorta and aortic arch replacement. *Ann Thorac Surg.* 2004;78:103–108.

72. Svensson LG, Blackstone EH, Rajeswaran J, et al. Does the arterial cannulation site for circulatory arrest influence stroke risk? *Ann Thorac Surg.* 2004;78:1274–1284.

73. Katoh T, Gohra H, Hamano K, Takenaka H, Zempo N, Esato K. Right axillary cannulation in the left thoracotomy for thoracic aortic aneurysm. *Ann Thorac Surg.* 2000;70:311–313.

74. Neri E, Massetti M, Barabesi L, et al. Extrathoracic cannulation of the left common carotid artery in thoracic aorta operations through a left thoracotomy: preliminary experience in 26 patients. *J Thorac Cardiovasc Surg.* 2002;123:901–910.

75. Turkoz R, Gulcan O, Demirturk OS, Turkoz A. Cannulation of the ascending aorta in left thoracotomy for thoracic aortic aneurysms. *Heart Surg Forum.* 2007;10:E81–E83.

76. Yamada T, Yamazato A. Central cannulation for type A acute aortic dissection. *Interact Cardiovasc Thorac Surg.* 2003;2:175–177.

77. Reece TB, Tribble CG, Smith RL, et al. Central cannulation is safe in acute aortic dissection repair. *J Thorac Cardiovasc Surg.* 2007;133:428–434.

78. Inoue Y, Ueda T, Taguchi S, et al. Ascending aortic cannulation in acute type A aortic dissection. *European Journal of Cardio-thoracic Surgery.* 2006;31:976–981.

79. Khaladj N, Shrestha M, Peterss S, et al. Ascending aortic cannulation in acute aortic dissection type A: the Hannover experience. *Eur J Cardiothorac Surg.* 2008;34:792–796.

80. Khoynezhad A, Plestis K. Cannulation in the diseased aorta. A safe approach using the Seldinger technique. *Tex Heart Inst J.* 2006;33:353–355.

81. Wada S, Yamamoto S, Honda J. Transapical aortic cannulation for cardiopulmonary bypass in type A aortic dissection operations. *J Thorac Cardiovasc Surg*. 2006;132:369–372.

82. Svensson LG. Progress in ascending and aortic arch surgery: minimally invasive surgery, blood conservation, and neurological deficit prevention. *Ann Thorac Surg*. 2002;74:S1786–S1788.

83. Dorotta I, Kimball-Jones P, Applegate R 2nd. Deep hypothermia and circulatory arrest in adults. *Semin Cardiothorac Vasc Anesth*. 2007;11:66–76.

84. Dr Gorlinger K. Point of care coagulation-ROTEM. 11th International Congress of Cardiothoracic and Vascular Anesthesia, Berlin, Germany, 14–18 September 2008

85. Mazzola A, Gregorini R, Villani C, Di Eusanio M. Antegrade cerebral perfusion by axillary artery and left carotid artery inflow at moderate hypothermia. *Eur J Cardiothorac Surg*. 2002;21(5):930–931.

86. Bonser RS, Harrington DK. Retrograde cerebral perfusion. In: Coselli JS, Lemaire SA, eds. *Aortic Arch Surgery. Principles, Strategies and Outcomes*. 1st ed. Hoboken: Wiley- Blackwell; 2008:167–176.

Deep Hypothermic Circulatory Arrest

7

Tomas Drabek and Joseph J. Quinlan

Cardiopulmonary bypass (CPB) and deep hypothermic circulatory arrest (DHCA) are techniques, which provide a bloodless field and enable the repair of complex congenital or acquired pathologies in cardiac surgery,[1] as well as other conditions that require complete cessation of flow, for example, clipping of giant cerebral aneurysms.[2] The protective effects of hypothermia have been known for centuries and possibly millenniums; however, the exact mechanisms that allow the temporary suspension of animation remain to be elucidated. There is extensive evidence that transient periods of no-flow can be tolerated and that the duration of this safe period is related to the level of hypothermia. The practical conduct of CPB and DHCA is dictated by the underlying pathology and has become standardized during recent decades. The compelling clinical success of routine DHCA could be one of the reasons why limited effort has been made to further facilitate the paramount protective effects of hypothermia, to extend the safe period, and to improve organ protection. Selective perfusion of the most vulnerable organs has been introduced into clinical practice only recently. Monitoring of the brain's metabolism is still limited to experimental settings. Current molecular tools also enable the investigation of the physiologic and biochemical changes that are responsible for the protection. Recently published studies in cardiac arrest showing beneficial effects of hypothermia applied even after ischemic insult have sparked a renewed interest in hypothermia research. We will review the current practice of DHCA, key mechanisms germane to hypothermic protection against ischemia-reperfusion injury, CPB perfusion strategies before and after DHCA, the role of pharmacological adjuncts, and alternative methods of neuroprotection, and discuss future directions in research.

Historical Notes

Hypothermia at the dawn of the twenty-first century represents a quite unique approach that has been tested for many clinical conditions. Although it may appear simplistic when compared to other technologies used in the current medical environment, hypothermia has proven to be one of the most powerful tools in our armamentarium to augment the outcome of some of the most severe insults. While the concept of therapeutic hypothermia has a rich history, we have yet to fully explore its potential and the mechanisms underlying its effects.

The interest in hypothermia dates back to Hippocrates who suggested topical cooling to prevent bleeding. Napoleon's surgeon later observed that wounded soldiers that were put farther from the fire died later than those closer to fire. In the 1930s, Fay used cooling for

T. Drabek (✉)
Department of Anesthesiology, University of Pittsburgh Medical Center, Presbyterian Hospital, Pittsburgh, PA, USA
e-mail: drabekt@anes.upmc.edu

K. Subramaniam et al. (eds.), *Anesthesia and Perioperative Care for Aortic Surgery*,
DOI 10.1007/978-0-387-85922-4_7, © Springer Science+Business Media, LLC 2011

extremities in patients with tumors; in 1940, he described better-than-expected results of patients with severe traumatic brain injury kept hypothermic for 4–7 days. Hypothermia has been explored during the infamous Nazi experiments on inmates of concentration camps. The breach of moral laws, along with persistent controversies over the scientific validity of the experiments, prevented the use of the acquired data in an ethical world.

The use of hypothermia in modern history dates back to the 1950s when elective moderate hypothermia (28–32°C) induced by surface cooling during general anesthesia was used for brain and heart protection. This was supported by the experimental work of Bigelow et al. who pioneered modern hypothermic research.[3] In 1950, he demonstrated protective effects of hypothermia during prolonged periods of ischemia compared to normothermic controls. Using surface cooling, he subjected dogs to total circulatory arrest for 15 min under deep hypothermia (20°C), without apparent ill effect.[4] Similar experiments using extracorporeal cooling via femoral–femoral shunt were carried out by Boerema et al.[5] In 1953, Lewis and Taufic reported a successful repair of an atrial septal defect in a 5-year-old girl, using surface cooling to induce hypothermia (28°C) that allowed protection for a short period of no-flow (5.5 min).[6] The same technique was successfully used by Swan et al. in a series of patients.[7] At the same time, CPB became clinically available and allowed complex cardiac surgery to flourish. Drew et al. used patient's own lungs as an oxygenator, along with CPB to facilitate cooling and rewarming.[8] In 1960, Dubost et al. reported the use of profound hypothermia with circulatory arrest in cardiac surgery.[9] Kirklin et al. at Mayo Clinic reported in 1961 results from 52 patients operated under DHCA, using either subject's own lungs as an oxygenator, or extracorporeal oxygenation.[10] Initially, surface cooling was used almost exclusively to induce deep hypothermia, especially in pediatric patients. CPB was used only after surface cooling was applied to further decrease the temperature and for rewarming. Since the 1970s, CPB has been used for both cooling (core cooling) and rewarming almost exclusively.

Hypothermic Cerebral Protection

Grades of Hypothermia

The level of hypothermia used in different settings varies widely and there is no generally accepted range to describe various levels of hypothermia. In clinical practice, temperatures of 32–34°C are usually referred to as mild hypothermia, 28–32°C as moderate hypothermia, and below 28°C as deep hypothermia.[11] Temperatures in the range from 15°C to 23°C are generally used in DHCA. In experimental work, even lower temperatures are explored, usually referred to as profound hypothermia (<15°C) or ultra-profound hypothermia (<10°C).

Mechanisms of Hypothermic Cerebral Protection

The initial hypothesis that hypothermia works by decreasing oxygen consumption was explored in animal models in the 1950s. During the next decades, many other protective mechanisms of hypothermia have been identified.[12] Deep hypothermia used in cardiac surgery could employ different mechanisms than mild hypothermia used to improve outcome after cardiac arrest and other events. Hypothermia significantly alters tissue energy charges in individual organs.[13] It alters gene[14] and protein[15-17] expression, protects against ischemia-induced apoptosis,[18] attenuates free oxygen radical production,[19] and mitigates reperfusion injury. Hypothermia protects against accumulation and release of excitatory neurotransmitters[20] and Ca^{++} influx.[21] The blood–brain barrier disruption is moderated by hypothermia.[22] Vascular permeability and capillary leakage are attenuated at mild to moderate levels of hypothermia; on the contrary, deep hypothermia is associated with plasma "skimming" and plasma leakage into interstitial space.[23] The overall effect is probably a result of multiple mechanisms that may vary with the level and duration of hypothermia.

Brain is metabolically very active and responsible for 20% of total body consumption. Oxygen consumption (VO_2) has been used historically as a measure of metabolic activity. Hypothermia reduces energy requirements, as reflected by decrease in VO_2. The effect of temperature on VO_2 is numerically expressed using van't Hoff's law, which relates the logarithm of a chemical reaction directly to temperature. The global effects of hypothermia on metabolism are defined by Q_{10}, which represents the reaction rate difference for a 10°C temperature difference.

Initial studies in surface-cooled dogs suggested Q_{10} of 2.7.[3,24,25] Surface cooling combined with CPB-assisted core cooling in dogs yielded similar results, with Q_{10} of 2.8.[26] The oxygen consumption at the extremes of temperatures (5°C) was similar to oxygen consumption in hibernating species.[27] Also, Q_{10} is not linear. In a canine model, brain Q_{10} was 2.23 between 37°C and 27°C, was doubled to 4.53 between 27°C and 14°C,[28] and returned to 2.19 below 14°C.[29] In a rat model, overall brain Q_{10} for temperatures 38–28°C was 5.2, with a two-component response: Q_{10} was 12.1 in 38–30°C, and 2.1 in 30–28°C.[30] In vitro studies showed that there also exist differences in cerebral metabolic rate for oxygen ($CMRO_2$) rates between white and gray matter. Young mammals usually survive deeper hypothermia than adults. This has been found to be true of many species of animals: that is, guinea pigs,[31] rats,[32] and dogs. Moreover, young animals tolerate the same degree of deep-body cooling for much longer periods than adults.

Those data suggest that Q_{10} varies between species, between age groups, and also between individual organs in one body. Hence, hypothermia may confer different level of protection for the same organ between species, resulting in different outcomes despite similar insults.

It is important to acknowledge that oxygen consumption is not reduced to zero even at very low temperatures approaching the freezing point. The continuing metabolic activity is responsible for a tendency to spontaneously rewarm. This suggests that the "safe" period of DHCA is not infinite even at ultra-profound temperatures. Ehrlich et al. showed in pigs that metabolic activity was 50% of baseline values at 28°C, 19% at 18°C, and 11% at 8°C.[33] Steen et al. showed in dogs that cerebral metabolic rate decreases to 7% at 14°C.[34] However, other studies indicate the reduction in $CMRO_2$ is modest than reported earlier. At 18°C, activity on electroencephalography (EEG) was still present, and $CMRO_2$ was 39% of baseline questioning the safety of this temperature for prolonged periods of hypothermic arrest.[35]

Greeley et al. studied cerebral metabolic suppression in neonates, infants, and children undergoing deep hypothermic arrest. Q_{10} was determined to be 3.65.[36] At 18°C, based on this coefficient, safe period of DHCA was calculated as 39–65 min. Long-term follow-up of children after a repair of a congenital heart defect using DHCA indicated that neurodevelopmental outcomes were generally not adversely affected unless the duration of DHCA exceeded a threshold of 41 min.[37]

McCullough et al., in a human study of adult patients undergoing DHCA, quantified Q_{10} for cerebrum as 2.3. $CMRO_2$ was 17% of baseline at 15°C, and they predicted a safe duration of DHCA for 29 min at this temperature. It is suggested currently that the duration of DHCA should not exceed 30 min at 12–15°C.[38] Safe duration of circulatory arrest based on the reduction in $CMRO_2$ at various hypothermic conditions is given in Table 7.1.

Profound Hypothermia and Hibernation

Animal experiments have shown that favorable outcome after even longer periods of DHCA (up to 3 h) can be achieved with profound or ultra-profound hypothermia, with or without additional interventions.[39–42] Newborn ground squirrels, natural hibernators, were able to survive up to 11.5 h of DHCA when supercooled to −4°C.[43]

Hibernation represents a naturally occurring phenomenon used by some species to overcome harsh winter conditions. It is a much more complex process than just hypothermia, which represents only one of the facets of this fascinating event. The research of hibernating species could provide some evidence that could be applied in DHCA and other conditions that utilize extreme temperature, for example, transplantation medicine. A single induction trigger that sets the cascade of actions resulting

Table 7.1 Effect of temperature on cerebral metabolic rate

Temperature (°C)	CMR (% baseline)	Duration of safe CA (min)	$CMRO_2$ (mL/100 g/min)
37	100	5	1.48
32	70(66–74)	7.5(6.5–8)	0.82
30	56(52–60)	9(8–10)	0.65
28	48(44–52)	10.5(9.5–11.5)	0.51
25	37(33–42)	14(12–15)	0.36
20	24(21–29)	21(17–24)	0.20
18	17(20–25)	25(21–30)	0.16
15	14(11–18)	31(25–38)	0.11

CMR cerebral metabolic rate, *CA* circulatory arrest, $CMRO_2$ cerebral metabolic rate for oxygen
Reprinted with permission from McGraw Hill Professional publications, Table reproduced from[174].

in hibernation remains to be characterized. Hibernation-induction triggers were used previously to induce hypothermia in natural hibernators. Plasma from hibernating woodchucks was used to induce hibernation in summer-active ground squirrels. Hibernation was also successfully induced with administration of delta-opioid agonist DADLE. Unfortunately, the same effect could not be reproduced in non-hibernators.

While profound hypothermia is tested in animal models, moderate hypothermia is also being used clinically to avoid extreme cooling, rewarming, and their associated complications.

Moderate Hypothermia and Aortic Surgery

Several studies addressed the potential of performing complex procedures under moderate hypothermia, with or without antegrade cerebral perfusion (ACP), in order to shorten the CPB duration and prevent complications ascribed to deep hypothermia.

Favorable outcomes in aortic arch surgery can be achieved with short, moderate hypothermic circulatory arrest (<10 min) at 25–28°C without additional cerebral protection.[44] In a follow-up study of 85 patients, this less-invasive approach yielded superior results when compared to "classic" DHCA technique combined with ACP in terms of postoperative mortality, neurologic complications, renal failure, pneumonia, and length of an ICU and in-hospital stay. Of note, rapid

rewarming in the moderate hypothermic circulatory arrest group was initiated with a "hot shot" of preheated CPB priming to 40°C – without apparent neurologic catastrophe. However, the no-flow time in the "classic" group was 64 ± 13 min, while in the less-invasive group only 21 ± 5 min.[45] Superior results could be explained by shorter cerebral exclusion time, CPB time, and overall surgical duration. There is also a possible role of other protective mechanisms that were not accounted for in the original studies focused on the oxygen metabolism.

In a retrospective non-randomized study, Kamiya et al. have shown no difference in neurologic outcome or complication rate in patients undergoing aortic arch repair performed at two different levels of hypothermia (23°C versus 26°C) using hypothermic ACP in both groups.[46] Minatoya et al. used moderate hypothermia (26°C) with high flow rate hypothermic ACP (20 mL/kg/min) in radical aortic arch reconstructions. Mean duration of circulatory arrest was 46 ± 13 min. No increase in neurological complications was noted compared to patients who were operated with DHCA at 16°C and ACP at 9 mL/kg/min.[47] To conclude, moderate hypothermia with or without ACP could be considered a viable option for aortic arch surgery with anticipated shorter circulatory arrest time. However, current experience with this method comes from a few single-center retrospective studies with limited postoperative follow-up and abridged neurologic assessment. Although it seems that using higher temperatures during hypothermic circulatory arrest is not inferior to "classic" DHCA, especially when augmented by hypothermic ACP, further prospective randomized studies are needed to evaluate this approach. The protection of a spinal cord and other extracerebral organs in this setting becomes a key issue that needs to be addressed.

DHCA and Postoperative Neurologic Dysfunction

Increasing clinical experience has revealed that two distinct forms of neurological injury occur after DHCA. Traditionally, evaluation of neurological outcome was limited to reporting the incidence of postoperative stroke related to ischemic infarcts due to particulate embolization. Though stroke is mainly related to embolization during aortic surgery, a higher incidence of stroke was also observed when DHCA was longer than 40 min.[48,49] More recently, the symptom complex defined as "temporary neurological dysfunction" (TND) was recognized as a functional manifestation of subtle and presumably transient brain injury, in comparison to "permanent neurologic dysfunction" (PND). Central nervous system injury is common even after cardiac surgery with CPB, but the incidence and severity of the impairment decreases over time.[50] Complex neurocognitive testing using a battery of eight tests revealed that early poor performance after DHCA was a significant predictor of delayed poor performance. DHCA of 25 min or more and advanced age were associated with memory and fine motor deficits and prolonged hospital stay.[51] Thus, TND may not be a benign self-limited condition, but rather a clinical marker for insidious but significant neurological injury associated with measurable long-term deficits in cerebral function.[52]

Brain injury after DHCA is related to ischemia and reperfusion. Cerebral ischemia is mediated by a complex biochemical process involving depletion of energy stores, anaerobic glycolysis, intracellular acidosis, accumulation of excitatory amino acids (glutamine), calcium influx, and finally structural cell damage.

Reperfusion injuries are related to the formation of oxygen free radicals, platelet aggregation, and neutrophil adhesion. Inflammatory mediators and vasoactive substances play an important role. Though the experimental studies are focused on reperfusion injury and its prevention, the clinical importance of this phenomenon is still not clearly established. Cerebral protection during vulnerable ischemic period is the main goal of various surgical, anesthetic (pharmacologic), and perfusion measures during and after DHCA in aortic surgery.

DHCA and Extracerebral Organs Dysfunction

Deep hypothermia protects spinal cord, kidneys, liver, and other lower body organs against ischemia. Low incidences of paraplegia and renal failure have been reported with DHCA for extensive thoracoabdominal and arch of aorta reconstructions.[53,54] DHCA has been successfully used to avoid clamping and other CPB-related insults in thoracic and abdominal aortic surgery to protect kidneys in patients with history of kidney transplantation.[55,56] However, with increasing use of ACP for cerebral protection during moderate hypothermic circulatory arrest, protection of other organs such as kidney, spinal cord, and liver becomes a major concern. Whole body perfusion (ACP with axillary cannulation and thoracoabdominal perfusion through femoral artery cannulation) has been successfully used for arch and thoracic aortic surgery with moderate hypothermia and is associated with lower rate of end-organ complications.[57,58] This technique requires clamping of distal aorta.

Temperature Management and Monitoring

The temperature changes associated with DHCA present a challenging situation. Brain temperature during cooling determines the safe conduct of DHCA and its duration. Rapid rewarming after arrest period with resulting higher cerebral temperature is associated with adverse neurologic sequelae. Thus, it is important to monitor temperature from a site that closely approximates brain temperature during cooling and rewarming.

Multiple temperature monitoring sites (nasopharyngeal, esophageal, pulmonary artery catheter, jugular bulb, tympanic membrane, bladder, and rectal) are used with variable success.[59] In the bypass circuit, both arterial inflow and venous return temperatures can be monitored. It is ideal to measure the temperature from more than one site since each site has its own inherent advantages and disadvantages.

Cooling

The ideal method, timing, and duration of cooling remain to be elucidated in further trials. Central cooling is typically done slowly over 30 min. During this phase of CPB, surgery on aortic root can be completed. Almond et al. showed that wide cooling gradients during rapid cooling were associated with brain damage.[60] This may be the result of uneven lowering of brain temperature. Rapid cooling may not produce uniform cooling of all organs of the body for adequate hypothermic protection. Rapid cooling also encourages the formation of gaseous microemboli within the patient's circulation. Active cooling to DHCA is continued until electrical silence on EEG is achieved or until jugular venous saturation reaches 95%.[61]

Adjuvants to central cooling are useful. Cooling blanket under the drapes, packing the head with ice, and lowering the room temperature to 18–20°C are used. DHCA caused an impairment of cerebral metabolism that was directly proportional to its duration, and recovery of metabolic function after 60 min of DHCA improved more than 50% if the head was packed in ice.[12,62] Topical cooling with ice packs around the head during DHCA is a common practice in some institutions, while others feel this does not have any additional protective value with the current practice of ACP and retrograde cold blood cerebral perfusion. Systems of continuous cooling of the head during DHCA have been developed for better efficacy and found to be useful.[63] Surface cooling usually produces smaller temperature gradients between sites, with rectal temperature being lower than nasopharyngeal.[64]

Rewarming and Reperfusion

Several reports suggest that there may be a certain benefit from a delayed rewarming. Ten minutes delay in rewarming after reperfusion following DHCA resulted in faster restoration of cerebral blood flow (CBF) to pre-bypass baseline levels.[65] The recirculation is initially started with a cold solution at low perfusion pressures (30–50 mmHg) instead of a "jump start" with a preheated oxygenator. Attempts to increase the temperature quickly result in neurological injury and may not achieve whole body rewarming resulting in higher chance of developing post-bypass afterdrop. There is a high possibility of formation of gaseous microembolism within the heat exchanger during rapid rewarming.

Maintenance of adequate oxygen delivery, perfusion pressure, and normoglycemia are important in the prevention of reperfusion injury during this critical phase of deranged autoregulation and increased cerebrovascular resistance. Vulnerable period can last 6–8 h after initiation of reperfusion.

Afterdrop

In the post-CPB period, the presence of core-periphery temperature gradients because of inadequate warming of the periphery leads to redistribution of heat and afterdrop of the core temperature.[66] Heat loss from the incisions is also partly responsible. Hypothermia inhibits coagulation, induces shivering, increases myocardial workload, and reduces resistance to surgical infections. Forced air warming of the periphery and vasodilatation with sodium nitroprusside during rewarming reduce the afterdrop.[67] Prolonged rewarming also decreases the afterdrop.

Deliberate Postoperative Hypothermia

Mild therapeutic hypothermia has been shown to be protective against cerebral ischemia in multiple animal models[68] and in cardiac arrest survivors.[69,70] Of note, hypothermia has been initiated in a delayed fashion only after the insult.

Considering the fact that DHCA represents similar ischemia-reperfusion insult, it could be speculated that postoperative mild hypothermia could also be beneficial in this setting. Current results suggest that postoperative hyperthermia in cardiac surgery[71] and DHCA[72] is detrimental. In our dog model of prolonged exsanguination circulatory arrest followed by 60 min of asanguineous DHCA at 12°C, prolonged hypothermia (36 h) was required to achieve favorable neurologic outcome. Neurologic status of dogs subjected to only 12 h postoperative mild hypothermia later deteriorated and several dogs exhibited seizure activity.[73] At this time, there is limited evidence that prolonged mild postoperative hypothermia after DHCA would be beneficial.

Cardiopulmonary Bypass Management

Pulsatile Flow

Postischemic endothelial dysfunction after DHCA tends to close the cerebral vasculature.[74] Pulsatile flow before and after DHCA may be useful in keeping the cerebral vascular bed open allowing better perfusion. Pulsatile perfusion produces less trauma to the blood, therefore, reducing blood viscoelasticity during CPB support before and after DHCA.[75] Experimental animal studies showed that cerebral vascular resistance was reduced, cerebral blood flow and cerebral metabolic recovery improved with pulsatile flow after DHCA.[76,77]

pH Management Strategies

The optimal pH strategy in CPB and DHCA continues to be widely discussed and remains unresolved issue despite many experimental and clinical studies. Alpha-stat management is targeted to maintain normal pH (7.40) and $paCO_2$ (40 mmHg) measured at 37°C and uncorrected for the actual temperature of the patient's blood. The administration of the gas via the oxygenator is kept at levels appropriate for normothermia.

Alpha-stat strategy is usually preferable on the cellular or enzyme level, including Na-K ATPase, lactate dehydrogenase, and phosphofruktokinase. This has been designated alpha-stat management because it maintains a constant buffering capacity of alpha-imidazole, resulting in a relative respiratory alkalosis during hypothermia.[78]

In contrast, pH-stat management corrects to the temperature of the patient's blood during hypothermia. pH-stat management produces a nearly constant pH of 7.4 at all temperatures. This results in a state of respiratory acidosis and hypercarbia, which translates into an increase in a CBF. This may offer some advantage to the brain oxygen metabolism in the setting of DHCA. On the contrary, pH-stat strategy may result in a "luxurious" perfusion that provides more opportunity for shedding of cerebral emboli. This may be one of the underlying mechanisms why alpha-stat strategy appears to be more beneficial in adults, while pH-stat strategy is preferred in infants undergoing CPB.

The experimental work in intact animals subjected to DHCA shows that the use of pH-stat results in higher CBF, better oxygen metabolism, energy restoration,[79,80] and neurologic outcome after DHCA.[81] Possible mechanisms for this difference are (1) improved oxygen delivery and homogeneity of brain cooling before DHCA and (2) greater CBF and reduced reperfusion injury during rewarming. To identify which of these mechanisms is dominant, Hiramatsu et al. tested pH-stat or alpha-stat strategies in both cooling and rewarming phases in a piglet model, creating four groups: alpha/alpha, alpha/pH, pH/alpha, and pH/pH. CBF was greater with pH-stat than alpha-stat during cooling (56% ± 4% vs. 33% ± 2% of normothermic baseline values). Recovery of ATP levels in the initial 45 min of reperfusion was more rapid in group pH/pH compared with the other groups. Recovery of cerebral intracellular pH in the initial 30 min was faster in group pH/pH compared with that in group alpha/alpha. This study suggests that there are mechanisms in effect during both cooling and rewarming phases before and after DHCA that could contribute to an improved cerebral outcome with pH-stat relative to more alkaline strategies.[82] In a similar fashion, Skaryak et al. tested various alpha-stat and pH-stat combinations during cooling before DHCA at 18°C or 14°C; for rewarming, alpha-stat was used in all groups. At any given temperature, pH-stat strategy provided better suppression of $CMRO_2$. The use of pH-stat strategy during initial cooling to 14°C followed by a switch to alpha-stat strategy just before arrest (for 5 min) resulted in better recovery of cerebral metabolism after DHCA compared with the recovery with either strategy used alone.[83]

Study in adult pigs showed a decrease in CBF during cooling with alpha-stat compared to no change with pH-stat. In moderate hypothermia (31°C), brain O_2 saturation was greater in alpha-stat than in pH stat. However, cerebral oxygenation was better in pH-stat during profound hypothermia at 15°C.[84]

During hypothermic (28°C) CPB for coronary artery bypass grafting (CABG), CBF was significantly greater in the pH-stat group than in the alpha-stat group.[85] Patients receiving alpha-stat management had less disruption of cerebral autoregulation during CPB, accompanied by a reduced incidence of postoperative cerebral dysfunction.[86] Several other studies indicate better neurologic outcome with alpha-stat in adult cardiac patients undergoing moderately hypothermic CPB.[87,88]

The effects of pH management in pediatric patients have been systematically investigated by the group from Children's Hospital in Boston. In a retrospective study of 16 children with transposition of the great arteries and intact ventricular septum, alpha-stat strategy during rapid cooling (15 min) before onset of DHCA was associated with worse developmental outcome.[89] These data challenged the notion that alpha-stat management is a superior strategy for organ protection during reparative operations in infants using DHCA. A follow-up randomized trial of pH-stat versus alpha-stat strategy in infants undergoing DHCA showed that pH-stat was associated with lower postoperative morbidity, shorter recovery time to first EEG activity, and in selected subgroups shorter duration of intubation and intensive care unit stay.[90]

Surprisingly, another study from the same institution evaluating developmental and neurologic effects of alpha-stat versus pH-stat strategies for

DHCA in infants did not show any advantage of one method over another, but patient characteristics were determined to be one of the important factors influencing outcome after surgery.[91] Recent advances in the molecular field allowed a more detailed insight into the mechanisms beyond the differences in pH management strategies. The data from a piglet model of DHCA showed that pH-stat strategy is associated with an increase in the phosphorylation and levels of proteins that play an important role in cell survival, without altering the level of the major pro-apoptotic protein. Based on those observations, pH-stat strategy may extend the "safe" period of DHCA by 15 min.[92]

Given the different pathologies in adult versus pediatric population, alpha-stat may be the preferable method for the adults, protecting the brain from microemboli, while pH-stat may be preferred in children to enhance the brain protection. Some experts also suggest the "crossover strategy" with initial cooling using pH-stat strategy to allow rapid onset of brain cooling with the "luxury" perfusion, switching to alpha-stat at deeper levels before stopping the circulation and using alpha-stat for rewarming.

Oxygen Transport

At least seven mechanisms could potentially affect the transport and utilization of oxygen during hypothermia: (1) changes in the metabolic rate, (2) changes in the solubility of oxygen, (3) acid–base strategy, (4) changes in the oxygen–hemoglobin dissociation curve, (5) changes in the cardiac output or CPB flow, (6) changes in the concentration of hemoglobin, and (7) changes in the "critical pO_2".[93]

With decreasing temperature, P_{50} (the oxygen tension [PO_2] at 50% hemoglobin saturation) decreases. This increase in hemoglobin affinity impairs oxygen transfer from hemoglobin to tissues. Cooling from 37°C to 25°C results in decrease in P_{50} from 27 to 13 mmHg. Infants undergoing CPB at 17°C with alpha-stat strategy have P_{50} 5 mmHg, and adults 7 mmHg. The oxygen consumption decreases, too. On the contrary, the solubility of oxygen in blood increases. At 15°C, dissolved oxygen accounts for 2–17% of arterial oxygen content, depending on PaO_2 and hemoglobin concentration. Under the condition of full-flow CPB at 18°C and $paO_2 > 180$ mmHg, the cerebral metabolic rate for oxygen obtained from dissolved oxygen represents 77%±19%. Thus, the brain uses mostly dissolved oxygen during profoundly hypothermic CPB.[94] This finding opens a potential for alternative oxygen carriers that would more readily release oxygen to tissues or other solutions that may use just the dissolved oxygen to support cerebral oxygenation, thus overcoming the limitations associated with blood transfusions. The use of such a strategy is still experimental and a variety of solutions (Kreb's solution,[95] hypothermosol,[96] and hetastarch[97]) have been tested in various animal models. For example, replacement of the blood in the CPB circuit by Hextend-based solution (hematocrit < 1%) with additional electrolytes allowed survival after 120 min DHCA at 2–4°C in dogs. However, no control group was studied in this experiment.[97] Selective perfusion of the cerebral circulation with asanguineous solutions also yielded mixed results.

The optimal strategy of oxygenation (normoxia vs. hyperoxia) during CPB before and after DHCA has been a subject of controversy. While high oxygen levels can provide an extra storage of fuel for the period of DHCA, reperfusion with high oxygen levels can trigger a massive release of free oxygen radicals that will further damage the ischemic tissue. Using a piglet model, Nollert et al. evaluated the effects of normoxia versus hyperoxia after 120 min DHCA at 15°C. Six hours after reperfusion, histologic examination revealed a significant increase in brain damage in the normoxia group, especially in the neocortex and hippocampus. Near-infrared spectroscopy suggested that the mechanism is hypoxic injury, which presumably overwhelmed any injury caused by increased oxygen free radicals.[98]

Hemodilution

Historically, the first priming solution for CPB circuit was whole blood.[99,100] Hemodilution was later advocated to reduce transfusion requirements.[101] The initial experience with 5% dextrose as priming solution also revealed a decrease in the number of clinical complications.[102] The hemodilution strategy was deemed safe and well compensated by improved viscosity, especially in the presence of hypothermia.[103,104] Clinically, it seemed that hematocrit below 30%, and sometimes as low as 15%,[105] was clinically well tolerated. The decrease in hematocrit is compensated with increased CBF. This mechanism allows to maintain normal cerebral metabolism even at extremely low hematocrit levels.[106] However, it exposes the brain to a higher microembolic load.

Those physiologic changes led to an intriguing question, "what is the optimal hematocrit during hypothermia?" This dilemma is especially pertinent to the smallest of our patients who have small blood volume. The introduction of small-volume oxygenators did not completely eliminate this problem. In light of the adverse effects linked to transfusion,[107,108] a lower hematocrit seemed the lesser of two evils.

Surprisingly, few studies have challenged the safety of hemodilution. Since the 1990s, the group at Harvard addressed this issue systematically in both laboratory and clinical settings. In a piglet model of DHCA, they showed that extreme hemodilution (hematocrit <10%) during CPB may cause inadequate oxygen delivery during early cooling. The higher hematocrit with a blood prime was associated with improved cerebral recovery after DHCA.[109]

Experimental studies showed that cerebral microcirculation is impaired with hematocrit of 10% versus 30%.[110] Both higher hematocrit (30% vs. 20%) and higher colloid oncotic pressure with pentafraction improved cerebral recovery after DHCA in piglets. The higher hematocrit improved cerebral oxygen delivery but did not reduce total body edema. Modified ultrafiltration after CPB was less effective than having a higher initial prime hematocrit or colloid oncotic pressure.[111] A complex study comparing the effects of intra-arrest temperature, hematocrit, and pH strategy in piglets showed that higher temperature, lower hematocrit level, more alkaline pH, and longer DHCA duration were predictive of more severe histological damage to the brain. The higher temperature exacerbated the disadvantage of a lower hematocrit level and longer arrest times, but not pH strategy.[112]

Jonas et al. compared the effects of two different levels of hemodilution on cognitive impairment and hemodynamic instability in infants. Patients in the lower-hematocrit group (22%) versus higher-hematocrit group (28%) showed worse cardiac performance in the early postoperative course, and worse developmental outcome scores at 1 year.[113] In a follow-up study from the same center, hemodilution to hematocrit levels of 35% compared with 25% had no major benefits or risks overall among infants undergoing two-ventricle repair using hypothermic CPB, as reflected by similar neurodevelopmental outcome at 1 year after the surgery.[114] Combining data from those two aforementioned trials suggests that a hematocrit level at the onset of low-flow CPB of approximately 24% or higher was associated with higher Psychomotor Development Index scores and reduced lactate levels. Because the effects of hemodilution may vary according to diagnosis, age at operation, bypass variables such as pH strategy and flow rate, and other perioperative factors, this study could not ascertain a universally "safe" hemodilution level.[115]

Ultrafiltration is an alternative method to achieve desirable hematocrit while avoiding unnecessary transfusion. Skaryak et al. explored the effect of hematocrit on cerebral metabolism after DHCA in a neonatal piglet model. Hematocrit in the modified ultrafiltration group and transfusion group was targeted to >40% in the post-CPB period. Cerebral oxygen delivery after DHCA increased significantly above baseline with ultrafiltration or transfusion and decreased below baseline in the control group. Cerebral metabolic oxygen consumption was impaired after DHCA in the control and transfusion groups. After ultrafiltration, however, cerebral metabolic oxygen consumption increased significantly from baseline, indicating that the decrease in cerebral metabolism immediately after DHCA is reversible and may not represent permanent cerebral injury.[116]

Although most studies used pediatric models, it seems prudent to maintain hematocrit levels at or above 25% during cooling and DHCA. Modified ultrafiltration during rewarming can help to avoid further transfusions and improve recovery. It should also be noted that the animal studies generally use fresh whole blood for transfusion, which is not the case in a clinical setting where stored blood is used. This provides an additional theoretical rationale for rapid ultrafiltration during CPB when hematocrit is marginal. The transfusion should be limited to situations when the decrease in hematocrit needs to be corrected rapidly; however, no formal studies, especially in adults, are available to set a hematocrit trigger that would require a transfusion to rapidly increase hematocrit, instead of a slower correction with ultrafiltration.

Pharmacological Adjuncts to DHCA

A recent survey among the members of the Association of Cardiothoracic Anaesthetists about the current practice in the use of pharmacological agents as cerebral protectants during DHCA revealed that 83% of respondents used some form of pharmacological agent specifically for cerebral protection. Fifty-nine percent of respondents used thiopental, 29% used propofol, and 48% also used a variety of other agents, the most common of these being a steroid. There were variations in the dose and timing of administration of drugs. Few respondents believed that there was a body of evidence to support this use of pharmacological agents. Only 35% of respondents believed there is sufficient evidence to support the use of thiopental. Similarly, only 11% of respondents believed that there was evidence supporting the use of propofol, and 16% the use of steroids.[117] These results truly reflect the fact that current practice of DHCA remains more "art" than "science."

Hypothermia by itself produces electrical silence. With the protective effects of hypothermia being paramount, there is seemingly only a limited potential for pharmacological adjuncts that would increase safety or allowable no-flow time. However, the actual temperature in which isoelectric EEG occurs could be highly variable. In a dog model, this was shown to occur at 12 ± 1 or at 17–18°C.[13,30] In pediatric patients, some studies documented EEG activity at the initiation of DHCA at temperatures at 17–23°C,[118] or even at 12°C.[119] Given the imperfections of the cooling process, there is a potential for additional protection produced by pharmacological agents. In the Boston Circulatory Arrest Study, infants that were subjected to DHCA had a greater incidence of neurologic abnormalities at 1-year follow-up compared to low-flow CPB.[120,121] The reasons are probably multifactorial but definitely indicate that better protection is needed for those patients who could not be managed without DHCA. Among the pharmacological drugs, the rich history of thiopental made it a reasonable first choice to be tested.

Thiopental

The speculations that thiopental and other barbiturates would confer additional neuroprotection benefit stemmed from studies on various brain ischemia models. The exact mechanisms are not fully understood and the postulated mechanisms include reduction in $CMRO_2$, reduction in CBF (thus carrying less emboli to the brain during cardiac surgery), reduction in cerebral edema, suppression of seizure activity, effects on free radical formation, and attenuation of release of excitatory amino acids and calcium influx during ischemia.

Rung et al. showed that after core cooling to 18°C, eight out of nine infants had persistent electrical activity that ceased in six of them after thiopental administration.[122] Thiopental would provide no cerebral protection in situations where cerebral function is abolished per se (i.e., during isoelectric EEG activity produced by hypothermia or cardiac arrest). However, in situations of hypoxia with continued cerebral function (active EEG), thiopental does afford some protection; in the absence of function (isoelectric EEG), no protection is apparent.[123] In another study exploring combined effects of hypothermia and barbiturates, $CMRO_2$ was unaffected by barbiturates at 14°C and 18°C, but there was a 55% reduction in $CMRO_2$ with thiopental at 37°C and the beneficial effect of thiopental persisted at 28°C (Fig. 7.1)[34].

The studies focused on the protective use of thiopental in cardiac surgery yielded conflicting

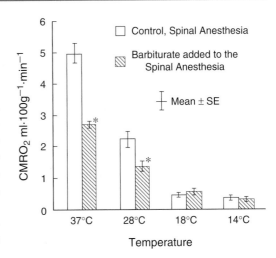

Fig. 7.1 $CMRO_2$ at different temperatures during spinal anesthesia with and without barbiturates. *Asterisk* indicates significant difference with and without barbiturate at the same temperature (Reprinted with permission; Steen et al.[34])

results. In adult patients undergoing valve replacement using mildly hypothermic CPB, thiopental was associated with a decreased incidence of neurological dysfunction on the tenth postoperative day.[124] In contrast, there were no differences in neurologic outcome in thiopental- or saline-treated low-risk patients scheduled for CABG using moderately hypothermic CPB.[125]

There is no randomized clinical trial showing the benefit or lack of benefit for barbiturates in adult aortic surgical patients undergoing DHCA. There is evidence that barbiturates may adversely impair cerebral metabolism and decrease the protection offered by HCA in a larger animal model.[126] Another important issue with large doses of barbiturates used for cerebral protection is that they can cause significant vasodilatation and hypotension, tachycardia, increased need for inotropes, prolonged time to awakening and extubation, and possibly higher complication rate.[125,127]

Barbiturates have shown mixed results in protecting against focal ischemia in animal models but failed to improve outcomes in global ischemia. Cerebral emboli are one of the "mechanistic" causes of focal neurological damage. In the adult population, atheromatous debris represents the major embolic load, while gaseous emboli are probably the most common in pediatrics. This results in a slightly different situation than DHCA, which is considered a global ischemic insult. Timing of administration of thiopental can influence its cerebral protective effects. It is advisable to administer protective agents before DHCA. Thus, the entire brain tissue could be protected against subsequent insults. If drugs are held till the initiation of reperfusion, the instant shedding of air bubbles might prevent the drugs to exert its effects when they are most needed. Thiopental has been shown to further decrease $CMRO_2$ when administered prior to DHCA, as reflected by the increase in oxygen partial pressure monitored in the jugular bulb (PjO_2). The rate of PjO_2 decrease was slower after thiopental administration, which could possibly result in better functional outcome.[128] After thiopental 10 mg/kg, continuous EEG activity was observed after 280 min after the onset of rewarming – a significant delay compared to previous studies without barbiturates, when EEG activity was detected after 15–30 min.[129,130] This prolonged electrical silence could be protective against air emboli with radii of 0.6 mm that are usually absorbed in 90 min. Some macroscopic bubbles obstructing major cerebral vessels require more than 12 h to be absorbed. Additional protection could be needed there.

In adults undergoing aortic reconstruction with DHCA, the brain is exposed to possible embolic load from atherosclerosis during various phases of surgery (e.g., cannulation, aortic cross clamping, aortic manipulations, rewarming, and decannulation). Lack of benefit of thiopental observed in few adult studies could be related to the fact that thiopental levels were not adequately maintained during these periods of embolic insults.

Other Anesthetics

Shorter-acting agents, like propofol or inhalational anesthetics, could represent reasonable alternatives to thiopental. Propofol, with its more favorable pharmacokinetic profile, successfully induced burst suppression during valve surgery in adults but failed to prevent neurologic deficits.[131] Isoflurane at two minimal alveolar concentrations (that produces similar burst-suppression pattern) is associated with more severe hypotension.[132]

Steroids

Controversies similar to those associated with thiopental also exist with steroid therapy. According to the results of a recent international survey on the use of steroids in cardiac surgery, there is high variability in the current practice. Most centers (97%) use steroids for cardiac surgery in general, yet only 40% administer steroids in every case. Of the 21 centers that selectively use steroids, 12 do so only for neonates, five administer steroids based on surgeon preference, and four administer steroids for cases anticipated to involve CPB time >2 h or DHCA. Of the 35 centers using steroids, 11 deliver a single dose in the circuit prime, 18 administer a single dose to the patient, and 6 give multiple doses.[133]

CPB alone is associated with systemic inflammatory reaction that could aggravate the neurologic injury associated with DHCA. Methylprednisolone (MP) has been used most frequently to ameliorate systemic inflammation via multiple mechanisms including antioxidant effects, inhibition of release of pro-inflammatory cytokines or excitatory amino acids. The exact mechanism of neuroprotection is yet unknown. The interest in steroids dates back to the 1960s when hydrocortisone was shown to attenuate the detrimental effects of prolonged CPB (acidosis, increase in lactate levels).[134] Hydrocortisone 50 mg/kg prevented some late motor disturbances in dogs after 60 min DHCA, and was associated with improvement of cardiac function.[135] MP then became the preferred glucocorticoid due to its apparent lack of sodium and water retention.

The groundbreaking study by Dietzman et al. showed that MP 30 mg/kg effectively reversed "low output syndrome" when combined with isoproterenol, which was not effective alone. This therapeutic combination improved survival from 22% to 65%.[136] Follow-up studies revealed some beneficial effects on pulmonary vasculature exposed to CPB, and the use of MP 30 mg/kg became a widespread practice. The pharmacodynamic studies showed that the MP levels are halved after the initiation of CPB due to dilution with the priming solution.[137] Administration of the second dose at the commencement of CPB was recommended, and at many institutions this regimen continues to be used.

Several additional studies of variable design and quality of reporting showed that patients treated with MP showed decreased vascular resistance, improved cardiac performance, and fewer postoperative complications.[138,139] However, other well-designed studies did not confirm those promising results.[140] Unlike MP, dexamethasone 6 mg/kg was no better than placebo in improving outcome after cardiac surgery.[141]

It is essential to realize that the original studies were performed in the era of bubble oxygenators that were much more prone to elicit systemic inflammatory reaction than currently used membrane oxygenators. This was elegantly shown by a study comparing three groups: bubble oxygenators, bubble oxygenators plus MP, and membrane oxygenators. The groups using bubble oxygenators plus MP and membrane oxygenators behaved similarly. The group using bubble oxygenator without MP exhibited significantly increased complement activation and leukocyte sequestration,[142] one of the main mechanisms of CPB-associated injury.

The use of steroids during CPB and DHCA is not without risk. MP increases pulmonary shunt with decrease of pulmonary compliance and hinder early extubation.[143] It has also been shown to increase glucose levels,[144] a condition that was associated with adverse outcome. Glucocorticoids were shown to potentiate ischemic injury to neurons.[145] Several well-controlled studies show no advantage of MP in the modern cardiac surgery environment using membrane oxygenators. A recently published review of the role of corticosteroids in CPB suggested that corticosteroids offer no clinical benefits to patients undergoing CPB, and in fact may be detrimental.[146]

The role of steroids in DHCA has been subjected to much less scrutiny, despite the fact that the unquestionable effect of MP on inflammatory mediators could be beneficial in prolonged exposure to CPB circuits. In contrast, to investigate the effects of MP on cerebral oxygen metabolism, Langley et al. subjected 1-week-old piglets to 60 min DHCA at 18°C. The treatment group received two intramuscular doses of MP 30 mg/kg

8 and 2 h before anesthesia. Recovery of global $CMRO_2$ was significantly better in the MP group versus controls, as well as CBF in selected brain regions. The renal blood flow was also preserved better.[147] Schubert et al. used a more challenging model of neonatal piglets subjected to 120 min DHCA at 15°C. The treatment group received MP 30 mg/kg 24 h before the experiment. Systemic pretreatment with MP resulted in persistent hyperglycemia after reperfusion. Neuronal necrosis and apoptosis was increased in selectively vulnerable brain regions in the MP group versus controls. The regional CBF was not different between groups except for the basal ganglia where CBF was higher during reperfusion in the MP group.[148]

It is quite easy to understand the high variability of the type, dosing, route, and timing of steroid administration, given the fact that the outcomes from both experimental and clinical studies yield conflicting results. A large, multiple-center clinical trial to evaluate the risks and benefits of steroid administration before DHCA will answer the question. The side effects of steroid administration, namely hyperglycemia, should be taken into account and a strict protocol should be followed.

Other Potential Pharmacologic Adjuncts to Hypothermia

There is a plethora of pharmacologic agents that proved to be beneficial in multiple cerebral ischemia models. However, very few of them have produced those benefits consistently across models and withstood the challenge of clinical trials. Hydrogen sulfide, DADLE (a delta opioid agonist), neurotensin, poloxamer 188, pentazocine, and diazoxide are few such drugs studied. The presence of deep hypothermia further complicates the assessment of potentially promising pharmacological candidates in the setting of DHCA due to profoundly altered metabolism. While newer drugs constantly emerge on the horizon, some previously promising agents are already excluded due to other reasons – aprotinin is the classic example. Many other drugs have been tested in cardiac surgery with CPB but not involving DHCA. Lidocaine has shown some potential neuroprotective effects in small study of patients undergoing valve surgery, but the same group have shown no neuroprotective benefits in a recent study involving all cardiac surgery patients.[149,150] NMDA receptor antagonists (ketamine, dextromethorphan, remacemide, and magnesium), statins, acadesine (adenosine regulating agent), alpha-2 agonists, and beta-blockers are other potential adjuncts being investigated for their neuroprotective effects in cardiac surgery.

Glucose Control and Insulin

Hyperglycemia is not uncommon during DHCA. This phenomenon could be ascribed to hypothermia, catecholamine release, inhibition of insulin secretion, insulin resistance, or administration of corticosteroids. Adverse effects of hyperglycemia are related to anaerobic conversion of glucose to lactate during periods of ischemia leading to intracellular acidosis and exacerbation of neurological injury. Experimental studies have shown adverse effects of hyperglycemia on focal and global ischemia.[151] Hyperglycemia (blood glucose >250 mg/dL) was associated with poor neurological outcome in patients undergoing aortic arch reconstruction with DHCA.[152] However, the situation in neonates could be different.[153] Glucose supplementation during or at the end of hypoxia has been shown to reduce infarct size in a neonatal model.[154] Extreme hyperglycemia offered complete neuroprotection. There may be theoretical advantages of providing the brain with more "fuel" before it is exposed to a period of limited resources. DeFerranti et al. have shown that hyperglycemia was not associated poor neurological outcome after DHCA for arterial switch operations.[155]

Recent published randomized clinical trials have shown intensive insulin therapy to reduce blood glucose levels less than 100 mg/dL was not associated with improved survival but increased mortality in medical intensive care unit.[156,157] However, a meta-analysis has shown that patients in surgical intensive care unit seemed to benefit from intensive insulin therapy.[158] Intraoperatively, maintenance of strict blood glucose control is labor-intensive. Adverse effects of "overshooting" such as

hypoglycemia and hypokalemia should be watched for.[159] Currently, maintenance of blood glucose between 100 and 150 mg/dL before and after DHCA seems to be a reasonable compromise.

Improvements in Surgical Techniques

Duration of DHCA can be shortened by modification of surgical techniques. A separate graft anastomosis to the arch island or trifurcated graft with sequential anastomosis of individual arch vessels followed by the rest of the reconstruction with SCP decreased DHCA duration (Fig. 7.2). SCP can be given through the right axillary artery and left common carotid artery in both the instances. The incidences of stroke (1%) and TND (5.4%) were significantly reduced with trifurcated graft technique.[60]

Alternative and Supplemental Methods to Improve Outcome After DHCA

While DHCA is capable of producing a bloodless field, the protection of vital organs remains time-limited. One logical solution to that limitation is

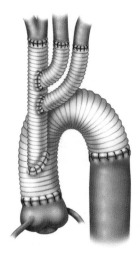

Fig. 7.2 Trifurcated aortic arch graft. Selective antegrade perfusion via right axillary artery and sequential anastomosis of head vessels to the trifurcated graft limit the circulatory arrest times

to maintain at least some circulation in situations when it would not interfere with the surgical procedure. Techniques employed included low-flow CPB (virtually replacing DHCA with deep hypothermic low-flow CPB), intermittent perfusion during DHCA, or selective brain perfusion.

Low-Flow CPB

Cerebral protection is the most important time-limiting factor during surgical procedures necessitating DHCA and low-flow CPB. Swain et al. used magnetic resonance spectroscopy to assess the degree of cerebral protection during deep hypothermic low-flow CPB and DHCA. Both DHCA and a flow rate of 5 mL/kg/min resulted in severe intracellular acidosis and depletion of high-energy phosphates. In contrast, deep hypothermia with CPB flows as low as 10 mL/kg/min maintained brain high-energy phosphate concentrations and intracellular pH for 2 h in sheep.[160]

Both DHCA and low-flow CPB are used to support vital organs during heart surgery in infants. The developmental and neurologic sequelae of these two strategies were compared in 155 patients 1 year after surgery. The infants assigned to DHCA, as compared with those assigned to low-flow CPB, had a higher risk of delayed motor development and neurologic abnormalities. The risk and severity of neurologic abnormalities increased with the duration of DHCA.[120]

Intermittent Perfusion

Langley et al. investigated the effects of intermittent perfusion during DHCA on the recovery of $CMRO_2$ after CPB and correlated these findings with electron microscopy of the cerebral microcirculatory bed. The intermittent perfusion was maintained for 1 min every 15 min during 60 min DHCA. Uninterrupted DHCA resulted in significant impairment to recovery of $CMRO_2$, and electron microscopy revealed extensive damage characterized by perivascular intracellular and organelle edema, and vascular collapse. Intermittent perfusion during DHCA, on the other hand, produced a pattern of normal $CMRO_2$ recovery

identical to controls, and the electron microscopy was normal. The damage to the vasculature was independent of the pH management used during cooling.[161] These results were supported by previous evidence from another work focused on the effects of asanguineous perfusate. The control group using intermittent perfusion with blood in CPB (5 min every 25 min) showed better neurobehavioral and histological outcome than control group subjected to uninterrupted DHCA.[162]

The timing of the intermittent perfusion may also play an important role. Kimura et al. studied the effects of intermittent perfusion carried out for 10 min every 20 min or 30 min during 120 min DHCA. Cerebral oxygen extraction rate increased significantly during the arrest periods and returned to normal after each 10-min period of systemic reperfusion in both groups. Cerebral energy metabolism became predominantly anaerobic within the first 20 min of DHCA. This suggests that intermittent perfusion should be carried out every 20 min to prevent cerebral anaerobic metabolism during long periods of DHCA that are required to complete complicated surgical repairs.[163]

The rate of flow during intermittent perfusion during 80 min DHCA was predictive of the recovery of cerebral metabolism. High flow (80 mL/kg/min) during 5-min perfusion every 20 min restored cortical oxygen pressures better than low flow (20 mL/kg/min), and improved extracellular dopamine release. The oxygen pressure decreased during subsequent DHCA periods to values not significantly different from those of DHCA without intermittent perfusion.[164] This suggests that oxygen stores might be depleted quickly, and even earlier replenishing more frequently than every 20 min may be required to achieve better outcome.

It is conceivable that intermittent perfusion during DHCA, when clinically practical, results in better recovery of brain metabolism and short-term outcome.

Antegrade and Retrograde Cerebral Perfusion

The initial experience revealed that DHCA is not capable of preventing neurologic impairment after prolonged period of no-flow. The brain remains the culprit of postoperative morbidity. The incidence of postoperative neurologic dysfunction, either temporary or permanent, varies from 2.4% to 33.3%.[165] The promising concept of maintaining low-flow CPB or at least intermittent perfusion may not be feasible in all clinical scenarios when complete circulatory arrest is required. Thus, the research focused on selective protection of the brain. The distinct circulatory system of the brain enables separate perfusion of the brain via the circle of Willis. This allows to employ the most powerful protective strategy, that is, hypothermia, and enhance it with the delivery of nutrients to the brain cells. Both techniques of selective cerebral perfusion, antegrade and retrograde cerebral perfusion, were introduced into clinical practice in the 1990s. Antegrade cerebral perfusion (ACP) closely approximates physiologic perfusion but lacks its pulsatility. Retrograde cerebral perfusion (RCP) reverses flow in brain vasculature and is also nonpulsatile. There are fundamental physiologic differences that stem from those opposing perfusion techniques (Table 7.2).

Clinical benefits and limitations of ACP and RCP are summarized in Tables 7.3 and 7.4. RCP uses uniformly cold perfusion at 10–12°C. The main operating mechanism here is probably deeper hypothermia since vascular flow studies suggested that only limited amount of infused perfusate (<3%) actually reaches brain capillaries to deliver nutrients. Most of the infused volume (80–90%) is derived to the circulation via collaterals to the inferior vena cava (IVC). Only 10–13% returns to aortic arch vessels. Most centers use perfusate of lower temperature than body core temperature. Others suggest to use perfusate just 2–3°C colder than systemic temperature.[166] Lower temperatures (10–15°C) seem to be more neuroprotective than higher temperatures (20–25°C) despite prolonged recovery of brain functions.[167] In contrast, an experimental study using a similar setting showed that ACP with 20°C yielded better results than 10°C or 30°C.[168] ACP provided superior CBF compared with total body perfusion with CPB at 20°C. In none of the brain regions studied CBF decreased below 20% of baseline with ACP.[169] The cerebral

autoregulation is maintained during ACP. On the contrary, autoregulatory mechanisms are disrupted with RCP even at postoperative period up to 1 week.[170] In a retrospective evaluation of data from 717 patients operated on at the Mount Sinai Hospital, TND was significantly attenuated with ACP.[171] Existing data summarized in recent reviews suggest that ACP provides more physiologic CBF than RCP and yields better results.[166,167] A recently introduced novel method of intermittent pressure augmentation (to 45 mmHg) during RCP yielded results similar to ACP.[172,173]

Key Notes

1. DHCA represents a clinically unique scenario that enables complex cardiac procedures with complete cessation of flow. The powerful protective effects of hypothermia allow performing most procedures without additional protective measures.

2. The duration of a "safe" period is limited and corresponds with the level of intra-arrest hypothermia. Both temporary and permanent neurologic impairment can result from incomplete protection. Thus, there is a need for additional techniques or pharmacologic adjuncts that would augment hypothermia. The role of the currently used drugs is limited, but selective cerebral perfusion is a valuable tool in ameliorating neurological damage.

3. Advanced monitoring techniques need to be developed to allow real-time assessment of the brain. This should allow us to optimize the use of protective techniques.

4. Advances in molecular biology should provide us with specific targets in the cell-death cascades that could be addressed by novel therapies.

Practical Tips and Tricks for DHCA

Cooling Phase

Forty minutes of CPB cooling are usually needed to achieve a uniform cooling. Temperatures from the PA catheter show the best correlation with the brain temperature. Arterial vasodilatation

Table 7.2 Results of comparative experimental studies between ACP and RCP (Adapted from[165] with permission of Expert Reviews Ltd)

Parameter of interest	Methodology	ACP	RCP
Blood distribution	MRI-perfusion	Uniform distribution	Little or no detectable distribution
	Microembolization	Massive embolization	Trivial embolization
	India ink	Uniform allocation in 100% of capillaries	Trivial, in 10% of capillaries Sequestration in brain venous sinuses Deviation to IVC via azygos vein
	CBF in medulla	Complete distribution	Complete distribution
	CBF in cortex	100% distribution	16% distribution
	Tchn99-albumine	Dominant fixation in brain capillaries	No fixation in brain capillaries
Cerebral blood flow	Fluorescence microscopy	No significant change (from baseline)	Trivial capillary flow
Brain edema	Brain water content	Minimal water content	Excessive water content
	Fluid sequestration	−200 mL	+760 mL
Histopathologic changes	Histopathologic scoring	No morphologic changes	Neuronal injury varying severity
		Minimal infarctions	Excessive infarctions
		Minimal edema	Excessive edema
Influence on SEPs	SEP abolition recovery	Complete abolition and automatic recovery by interruption	Complete abolition after application and no recovery
Acid–base changes	Neural cells pH	Unchanged pH levels	Decrease to 6.4 Recovery by reperfusion
Brain metabolism	ATP levels	Light decrease (baseline)	2–3% of baseline
	Phosp-31 MRI	Unchanged ATP-levels	High decrease in ATP levels Recovery by perfusion
	Cerebral oxygen consumption	6.66 mL/min	1.37 mL/min
Postoperative neurological status	Behavioral scoring	Gradually improved	No improvement
	Behavioral recovery	Complete	Complete

ACP Antegrade cerebral perfusion, *CBF* Central blood flow, *IVC* Inferior vena cava, *RCP* Retrograde cerebral perfusion, *SEPS* Somatosensory evoked potentials

Table 7.3 Antegrade cerebral perfusion (ACP)

Aim
To supply oxygenated blood to the brain during DHCA, prevents ischemic injury to brain
To meet the metabolic demands of the brain
To wash away the metabolic wastes
To achieve selected temperature of the brain

Temperature of the perfusate
10–15°C
Kazui's school adapted higher temperature 20–22°C

Flow rate
10 mL/kg/min (600–1,000 mL/min), flow rates increased 20–30% for patients at high risk for postoperative neurologic dysfunction

(continued)

Table 7.3 (continued)

Perfusion pressure
Sites: Right radial, bilateral perfusion catheter tip pressure, bilateral temporal artery pressure
Target: Right radial pressure 40 mmHg. In patients at high risk for stroke the flow rates are increased to achieve higher target pressure of 50–70 mmHg
Hemispheric versus bihemispheric perfusion
Selective or bihemispheric cerebral perfusion through direct cannulation of two out of three arch vessels, namely, innominate and left common carotid arteries. Left subclavian is occluded
Nonselective perfusion uses right axillary artery as a route for ACP and rely on intact circle of Willis for perfusion of left side brain
No clear data exists for the superiority of one versus other method
Indications for left subclavian perfusion: Occlusion of right vertebral artery, lack of intracranial communications, dominant left vertebral artery
Monitoring
Transcranial Doppler (TCD) monitoring of bilateral middle cerebral artery (MCA) flows
Near-infrared spectroscopy
Jugular bulb venous oxygen saturation (target above 90%)
Low flow velocity on the left MCA on TCD or low saturation on the left side (20% discrepancy between two sides) during nonselective perfusion is an indication for converting to bihemispheric perfusion
Advantages
Extend the safe period of circulatory arrest up to 90 min allowing meticulous repair of complex aortic pathology (total arch)
Obviates the need for deep hypothermia? Moderate hypothermia with ACP is an option for less-complex aortic procedures (hemiarch), lessens CPB time, rewarming and cooling time, coagulopathy, and other deep hypothermia related complications
Maintains autoregulation
Drawbacks
Malperfusion because of improper cannulation in the false lumen
Cerebral embolism this could be lessened by cannulation away from the orifice of the arch vessels, where atherosclerosis is marked, or by cannulation of axillary artery since this is part is rarely atherosclerotic)
Cluttered operative field with cannulae obstructing the surgical view and prolongation of DHCA time
Cumbersome procedure
Dissection of common carotid arteries by cannulation
Obstruction to the flow in the artery by improper position of cannulae in the lumen

Table 7.4 Retrograde cerebral perfusion (RCP)

Benefits
Provides hypothermic blood and produces uniform cooling of the brain
Flushes the air and particulate emboli out of arch vessels
Provide some oxygen and substrates to the brain and remove metabolic wastes
Temperature of the perfusate
10–12°C
Flow rate for RCP
Most surgeons flow 300–500 mL/min to SVC pressure 15–25 mmHg
SVC pressures up to 40 mmHg and flow rates up to 1,600 mL/min with multimodal neurophysiological monitoring
Monitoring during RCP
SVC pressure (monitored from the side port of internal jugular vein 9F introducer)
Transcranial Doppler (TCD): Bilateral middle cerebral artery flow monitoring can help alter cannulation and guide perfusion pressure and flows required to achieve cerebral perfusion. TCD can also diagnose reactive hyperemia after DHCA
Near-infrared spectroscopy can also be used to adjust flows and temperature

(continued)

Table 7.4 (continued)

Clinical outcome
Incidence of stroke and mortality low in RCP patients in few retrospective studies
Studies comparing ACP and RCP have shown reduction in transient neurological dysfunction only for ACP
Neuropsychological outcome
No benefit, few studies noted negative outcome
Drawbacks
Flow through SVC is directed into extracranial veins and inferior vena cava through azygos system
Amount of RCP reaching cerebral circulation to provide nutrition is only 5–10% of total perfusate with the pressures commonly used (15–25 mmHg)
Excessive flows and pressure can cause cerebral edema
Valves in the venous system prevent effective delivery of RCP
Veins prone for torsion, collapse, and kinking preventing effective delivery of RCP

with short-acting agents like nitroprusside or phentolamine may facilitate the rate and uniformity of cooling. Complete neuromuscular blockade further decreases oxygen consumption. pH-stat blood gas management is recommended especially in the pediatric population; 100% oxygen should be used before stopping the circulation. Hematocrit should be maintained at 25% or higher. Topical cooling of the head with ice is beneficial. Thiopental may be used in moderate doses (5 mg/kg) especially if there is persistent EEG activity. Large doses could be detrimental for cardiac recovery. Administration of MP does not have a strong support in the current literature. Pretreatment would be required to elicit its extracerebral effects.

DHCA Phase
Any flow is better than no flow. Low-flow CPB is superior to DHCA when clinically feasible. Alternatively, intermittent perfusion at high flow could be considered at least every 20 min. Cerebral perfusion during DHCA is beneficial and could extend the "safe" period of DHCA. ACP seems to be superior to RCP.

Rewarming Phase
Rewarming should be initiated with 100% oxygen. A brief period of cold reperfusion before rewarming should be considered. High CPB flows may be initiated even at low temperatures. Prevention of "overshooting" to hyperthermia is of paramount importance even if the duration of CPB is prolonged. The temperature of the arterial line of the

CPB machine reflects the maximum temperature of the brain. Alpha-stat blood gas management should be used especially in adults to limit microembolism. Post-reperfusion ultrafiltration may be beneficial. Glucose control should be employed to maintain normoglycemia.

Post-CPB Phase
Prolonged mild hypothermia after the procedure is not currently substantiated but should be considered if neurologic complications occur.

References

1. Kirklin J, Barratt-Boyes B et al. *Hypothermia, Circulatory Arrest, and Cardiopulmonary Bypass. Cardiac Surgery.* New York: Churchill Livingstone; 1993:61–127.
2. Solomon RA, Smith CR, Raps EC, Young WL, Stone JG, Fink ME et al. Deep hypothermic circulatory arrest for the management of complex anterior and posterior circulation aneurysms. *Neurosurgery.* 1991;29: 732–737. discussion 737–8.
3. Bigelow WG, Lindsay WK et al. Oxygen transport and utilization in dogs at low body temperatures. *Am J Physiol.* 1950;160:125–137.
4. Bigelow WG, Callaghan JC, Hopps JA. General hypothermia for experimental intracardiac surgery; the use of electrophrenic respirations, an artificial pacemaker for cardiac standstill and radio-frequency rewarming in general hypothermia. *Ann Surg.* 1950;132:531–539.
5. Boerema I, Wildschut A, Schmidt WJ, Broekhuysen L. Experimental researches into hypothermia as an aid in the surgery of the heart. *Arch Chir Neerl.* 1951;3:25–34.
6. Lewis FJ, Taufic M. Closure of atrial septal defects with the aid of hypothermia; experimental accomplishments and the report of one successful case. *Surgery.* 1953;33:52–59.

7. Swan H, Zeavin I, Blount SG Jr, Virtue RW. Surgery by direct vision in the open heart during hypothermia. *J Am Med Assoc.* 1953;153:1081–1085.
8. Drew CE, Keen G, Benazon DB. Profound hypothermia. *Lancet.* 1959;1:745–747.
9. Weiss M, Piwnica A, Lenfant C, et al. Deep hypothermia with total circulatory arrest. *Trans Am Soc Artif Intern Organs.* 1960;6:227–239.
10. Kirklin JW, Dawson B, Devloo RA, Theye RA. Open intracardiac operations: use of circulatory arrest during hypothermia induced by blood cooling. *Ann Surg.* 1961;154:769–776.
11. Safar PJ, Kochanek PM. Therapeutic hypothermia after cardiac arrest. *N Engl J Med.* 2002;346:612–613.
12. Mault JR, Ohtake S, Klingensmith ME, Heinle JS, Greeley WJ, Ungerleider RM. Cerebral metabolism and circulatory arrest: effects of duration and strategies for protection. *Ann Thorac Surg.* 1993;55:57–63.
13. Swain JA, McDonald TJ Jr, Balaban RS, Robbins RC. Metabolism of the heart and brain during hypothermic cardiopulmonary bypass. *Ann Thorac Surg.* 1991;51:105–109.
14. Qin HP, Mei GH, Wei L, Jiang JY. Effect of profound hypothermia on genomics of hippocampus following complete cerebral ischemia in rats. *Neurol Res.* 2008;30:536–541.
15. Sheikh AM, Barrett C, Villamizar N, et al. Proteomics of cerebral injury in a neonatal model of cardiopulmonary bypass with deep hypothermic circulatory arrest. *J Thorac Cardiovasc Surg.* 2006;132:820–828.
16. Zaitseva T, Schultz S, Schears G, et al. Regulation of brain cell death and survival after cardiopulmonary bypass. *Ann Thorac Surg.* 2006;82:2247–2253.
17. Pastuszko P, Liu H, Mendoza-Paredes A, et al. Brain oxygen and metabolism is dependent on the rate of low-flow cardiopulmonary bypass following circulatory arrest in newborn piglets. *Eur J Cardiothorac Surg.* 2007;31:899–905.
18. Ditsworth D, Priestley MA, Loepke AW, et al. Apoptotic neuronal death following deep hypothermic circulatory arrest in piglets. *Anesthesiology.* 2003;98:1119–1127.
19. Globus MY, Busto R, Lin B, Schnippering H, Ginsberg MD. Detection of free radical activity during transient global ischemia and recirculation: effects of intraischemic brain temperature modulation. *J Neurochem.* 1995;65:1250–1256.
20. Baker CJ, Fiore AJ, Frazzini VI, Choudhri TF, Zubay GP, Solomon RA. Intraischemic hypothermia decreases the release of glutamate in the cores of permanent focal cerebral infarcts. *Neurosurgery.* 1995;36:994–1001.
21. Mitani A, Kadoya F, Kataoka K. Temperature dependence of hypoxia-induced calcium accumulation in gerbil hippocampal slices. *Brain Res.* 1991;562:159–163.
22. Dietrich WD, Busto R, Halley M, Valdes I. The importance of brain temperature in alterations of the blood-brain barrier following cerebral ischemia. *J Neuropathol Exp Neurol.* 1990;49:486–497.
23. Chen RY, Wicks AE, Chien S. Hemoconcentration induced by surface hypothermia in infants. *J Thorac Cardiovasc Surg.* 1980;80:236–241.
24. Ross DN. Hypothermia. 2. Physiological observations during hypothermia. *Guys Hosp Rep.* 1954;103:116–138.
25. Penrod KE. Oxygen consumption and cooling rates in immersion hypothermia in the dog. *Am J Physiol.* 1949;157:436–444.
26. Kent B, Peirce EC 2nd. Oxygen consumption during cardiopulmonary bypass in the uniformly cooled dog. *J Appl Physiol.* 1974;37:917–922.
27. Kent KM, Peirce EC 2nd. Acid-base characteristics of hibernating animals. *J Appl Physiol.* 1967;23:336–340.
28. Michenfelder JD, Milde JH. The relationship among canine brain temperature, metabolism, and function during hypothermia. *Anesthesiology.* 1991;75:130–136.
29. Michenfelder JD, Milde JH. The effect of profound levels of hypothermia (below 14 degrees C) on canine cerebral metabolism. *J Cereb Blood Flow Metab.* 1992;12:877–880.
30. Klementavicius R, Nemoto EM, Yonas H. Basal Q10 for cerebral metabolic rate for oxygen (CMRO2) in rats. *Adv Exp Med Biol.* 1996;388:191–195.
31. Miller JA Jr. Effects of variations in body temperature upon resistance to asphyxia in the neonatal guinea pig. *Cold Spring Harb Symp Quant Biol.* 1954;19:152–154.
32. Adolph EF. Responses to hypothermia in several species of infant mammals. *Am J Physiol.* 1951;166:75–91.
33. Ehrlich MP, McCullough JN, Zhang N, et al. Effect of hypothermia on cerebral blood flow and metabolism in the pig. *Ann Thorac Surg.* 2002;73:191–197.
34. Steen PA, Newberg L, Milde JH, Michenfelder JD. Hypothermia and barbiturates: individual and combined effects on canine cerebral oxygen consumption. *Anesthesiology.* 1983;58:527–532.
35. Mezrow CK, Midulla PS, Sadeghi AM, et al. Evaluation of cerebral metabolism and quantitative electroencephalography after hypothermic circulatory arrest and low flow cardiopulmonary bypass at different temperatures. *J Thorac Cardiovasc Surg.* 1994;107:1006–1019.
36. Greeley WJ, Kern FH, Ungerleider RM, et al. The effect of hypothermic cardiopulmonary bypass and total circulatory arrest on cerebral metabolism in neonates, infants, and children. *J Thorac Cardiovasc Surg.* 1991;101:783–794.
37. Wypij D, Newburger JW, Rappaport LA, et al. The effect of duration of deep hypothermic circulatory arrest in infant heart surgery on late neurodevelopment: the Boston circulatory arrest trial. *J Thorac Cardiovasc Surg.* 2003;126:1397–1403.
38. McCullough JN, Zhang N, Reich DL, et al. Cerebral metabolic suppression during hypothermic circulatory arrest in humans. *Ann Thorac Surg.* 1999;67:1895–1899.

39. Bailes JE, Leavitt ML, Teeple E Jr, et al. Ultraprofound hypothermia with complete blood substitution in a canine model. *J Neurosurg*. 1991;74:781–788.
40. Popovic V, Popovic P. Survival of hypothermic dogs after 2-h circulatory arrest. *Am J Physiol*. 1985;248: R308–R311.
41. Behringer W, Safar P, Wu X, et al. Survival without brain damage after clinical death of 60–120 mins in dogs using suspended animation by profound hypothermia. *Crit Care Med*. 2003;31:1523–1531.
42. Tisherman SA, Safar P, Radovsky A, et al. Profound hypothermia (less than 10 degrees C) compared with deep hypothermia (15 degrees C) improves neurologic outcome in dogs after two hours' circulatory arrest induced to enable resuscitative surgery. *J Trauma*. 1991;31:1051–1061.
43. Popovic P, Popovic V. Survival of newborn ground squirrels after supercooling or freezing. *Am J Physiol*. 1963;204:949–952.
44. Kamiya H, Hagl C, Kropivnitskaya I, et al. Quick proximal arch replacement with moderate hypothermic circulatory arrest. *Ann Thorac Surg*. 2007;83: 1055–1058.
45. Hata M, Suzuki M, Sezai A, et al. Outcome of less invasive proximal arch replacement with moderate hypothermic circulatory arrest followed by aggressive rapid re-warming in emergency surgery for type A acute aortic dissection. *Circ J*. 2008;73:69–72.
46. Kamiya H, Hagl C, Kropivnitskaya I, et al. The safety of moderate hypothermic lower body circulatory arrest with selective cerebral perfusion: a propensity score analysis. *J Thorac Cardiovasc Surg*. 2007;133:501–509.
47. Minatoya K, Ogino H, Matsuda H, et al. Evolving selective cerebral perfusion for aortic arch replacement: high flow rate with moderate hypothermic circulatory arrest. *Ann Thorac Surg*. 2008;86:1827–1831.
48. Svensson LG, Crawford ES, Hess KR, et al. Deep hypothermia with circulatory arrest. Determinants of stroke and early mortality in 656 patients. *J Thorac Cardiovasc Surg*. 1993;106:19–28.
49. Ergin MA, Galla JD, Lansman L, Quintana C, Bodian C, Griepp RB. Hypothermic circulatory arrest in operations on the thoracic aorta. Determinants of operative mortality and neurologic outcome. *J Thorac Cardiovasc Surg*. 1994;107:788–797.
50. Newman MF, Mathew JP, Grocott HP, et al. Central nervous system injury associated with cardiac surgery. *Lancet*. 2006;368:694–703.
51. Reich DL, Uysal S, Sliwinski M, et al. Neuropsychologic outcome after deep hypothermic circulatory arrest in adults. *J Thorac Cardiovasc Surg*. 1999;117:156–163.
52. Ergin MA, Uysal S, Reich DL, et al. Temporary neurological dysfunction after deep hypothermic circulatory arrest: a clinical marker of long-term functional deficit. *Ann Thorac Surg*. 1999;67:1887–1890.
53. Fehrenbacher JW, Hart DW, Huddleston E, Siderys H, Rice C. Optimal end organ protection for thoracic and thoracoabdominal aortic aneurysm repair using deep hypothermic circulatory arrest. *Ann Thorac Surg*. 2007;83:1041–1046.
54. Kouchoukos NT, Masetti P, Rokkas CK, Murphy SF. Hypothermic cardiopulmonary bypass and circulatory arrest for operations on the descending thoracic and thoracoabdominal aorta. *Ann Thorac Surg*. 2002; 74:S1885–S1887.
55. Takahashi T, Ohshima K, Hasegawa Y, Nameki T, Morishita Y. Surgical treatment with deep hypothermia for thoracic aortic aneurysm in a patient with renal transplantation. *Jpn J Thorac Cardiovasc Surg*. 2006;54:27–30.
56. Yagdi T, Buket S, Tokat Y, et al. Circulatory arrest to protect transplant kidney in a patient with chronic type II dissection. *Ann Vasc Surg*. 2001;15:575–577.
57. Emrecan B, Yilik L, Tulukoglu E, et al. Whole body perfusion under moderate degree hypothermia during aortic arch repair. *Heart Surg Forum*. 2006;9: E686–E689.
58. Della Corte A, Scardone M, Romano G, et al. Aortic arch surgery: thoracoabdominal perfusion during antegrade cerebral perfusion may reduce postoperative morbidity. *Ann Thorac Surg*. 2006;81:1358–1364.
59. Stone JG, Young WL, Smith CR, et al. Do standard monitoring sites reflect true brain temperature when profound hypothermia is rapidly induced and reversed? *Anesthesiology*. 1995;82:344–351.
60. Almond CH, Jones JC, Snyder HM, Grant SM, Meyer BW. Cooling gradients and brain damage with deep hypothermia. *J Thorac Cardiovasc Surg*. 1964;48: 890–897.
61. Van der Starre PJA. Deep hypothermic circulatory arrest. In: Rousseau H, Verhoye JP, Heautot JF, eds. *Thoracic aortic diseases*. 1st ed. Berlin: Springer; 2006:101–108.
62. Griepp RB, Ergin MA, McCullough JN, et al. Use of hypothermic circulatory arrest for cerebral protection during aortic surgery. *J Card Surg*. 1997;12:312–321.
63. Lighthall GK, Cartwright CR, Haddow GR. An improved method for topical cerebral cooling during deep hypothermic circulatory arrest. *J Thorac Cardiovasc Surg*. 2000;120:403–404.
64. Civalero LA, Moreno JR, Senning A. Temperature conditions and oxygen consumption during deep hypothermia. *Acta Chir Scand*. 1962;123: 179–188.
65. Rodriguez RA, Austin EH 3rd, Audenaert SM. Postbypass effects of delayed rewarming on cerebral blood flow velocities in infants after total circulatory arrest. *J Thorac Cardiovasc Surg*. 1995;110: 1686–1690.
66. Pujol A, Fusciardi J, Ingrand P, et al. After drop after hypothermic cardiopulmonary bypass: the value of tympanic membrane temperature monitoring. *J Cardiothorac Vasc Anesth*. 1996;10: 336–341.
67. Rajek A, Lenhardt R, Sessler DI, et al. Efficacy of two methods for reducing postbypass afterdrop. *Anesthesiology*. 2000;92:447–456.

68. Colbourne F, Corbett D. Delayed and prolonged post-ischemic hypothermia is neuroprotective in the gerbil. *Brain Res*. 1994;654:265–272.

69. Bernard SA, Gray TW, Buist MD, et al. Treatment of comatose survivors of out-of-hospital cardiac arrest with induced hypothermia. *N Engl J Med*. 2002;346: 557–563.

70. Hypothermia after Cardiac Arrest Study Group. Mild therapeutic hypothermia to improve the neurologic outcome after cardiac arrest. *N Engl J Med*. 2002;346: 549–556.

71. Nussmeier NA. Management of temperature during and after cardiac surgery. *Tex Heart Inst J*. 2005;32: 472–476.

72. Shum-Tim D, Nagashima M, Shinoka T, et al. Postischemic hyperthermia exacerbates neurologic injury after deep hypothermic circulatory arrest. *J Thorac Cardiovasc Surg*. 1998;116:780–792.

73. Wu X, Drabek T, Kochanek PM, et al. Induction of profound hypothermia for emergency preservation and resuscitation allows intact survival after cardiac arrest resulting from prolonged lethal hemorrhage and trauma in dogs. *Circulation*. 2006;113:1974–1982.

74. Cooper WA, Duarte IG, Thourani VH, et al. Hypothermic circulatory arrest causes multisystem vascular endothelial dysfunction and apoptosis. *Ann Thorac Surg*. 2000;69:696–702.

75. Vinten-Johansen J, Guyton RA, Undar A, et al. The effects of pulsatile versus nonpulsatile perfusion on blood viscoelasticity before and after deep hypothermic circulatory arrest in a neonatal piglet model. *Artif Organs*. 1999;23:717–721.

76. Onoe M, Mori A, Watarida S, et al. The effect of pulsatile perfusion on cerebral blood flow during profound hypothermia with total circulatory arrest. *J Thorac Cardiovasc Surg*. 1994;108:119–125.

77. Watanabe T, Washio M. Pulsatile low-flow perfusion for enhanced cerebral protection. *Ann Thorac Surg*. 1993;56:1478–1481.

78. Swan H. The importance of acid-base management for cardiac and cerebral preservation during open heart operations. *Surg Gynecol Obstet*. 1984;158: 391–414.

79. Kurth CD, O'Rourke MM, O'Hara IB. Comparison of pH-stat and alpha-stat cardiopulmonary bypass on cerebral oxygenation and blood flow in relation to hypothermic circulatory arrest in piglets. *Anesthesiology*. 1998;89:110–118.

80. Aoki M, Nomura F, Stromski ME, et al. Effects of pH on brain energetics after hypothermic circulatory arrest. *Ann Thorac Surg*. 1993;55:1093–1103.

81. Priestley MA, Golden JA, O'Hara IB, McCann J, Kurth CD. Comparison of neurologic outcome after deep hypothermic circulatory arrest with alpha-stat and pH-stat cardiopulmonary bypass in newborn pigs. *J Thorac Cardiovasc Surg*. 2001;121:336–343.

82. Hiramatsu T, Miura T, Forbess JM, et al. pH strategies and cerebral energetics before and after circulatory arrest. *J Thorac Cardiovasc Surg*. 1995;109:948–957.

83. Skaryak LA, Chai PJ, Kern FH, Greeley WJ, Ungerleider RM. Blood gas management and degree of cooling: effects on cerebral metabolism before and after circulatory arrest. *J Thorac Cardiovasc Surg*. 1995;110:1649–1657.

84. Li ZJ, Yin XM, Ye J. Effects of pH management during deep hypothermic bypass on cerebral oxygenation: alpha-stat versus pH-stat. *J Zhejiang Univ Sci*. 2004;5:1290–1297.

85. Patel RL, Turtle MR, Chambers DJ, Newman S, Venn GE. Hyperperfusion and cerebral dysfunction. Effect of differing acid-base management during cardiopulmonary bypass. *Eur J Cardiothorac Surg*. 1993;7: 457–463.

86. Patel RL, Turtle MR, Chambers DJ, James DN, Newman S, Venn GE. Alpha-stat acid-base regulation during cardiopulmonary bypass improves neuropsychologic outcome in patients undergoing coronary artery bypass grafting. *J Thorac Cardiovasc Surg*. 1996;111:1267–1279.

87. Murkin JM, Martzke JS, Buchan AM, Bentley C, Wong CJ. A randomized study of the influence of perfusion technique and pH management strategy in 316 patients undergoing coronary artery bypass surgery. II. Neurologic and cognitive outcomes. *J Thorac Cardiovasc Surg*. 1995;110:349–362.

88. Stephan H, Weyland A, Kazmaier S, Henze T, Menck S, Sonntag H. Acid-base management during hypothermic cardiopulmonary bypass does not affect cerebral metabolism but does affect blood flow and neurological outcome. *Br J Anaesth*. 1992;69:51–57.

89. Jonas RA, Bellinger DC, Rappaport LA, et al. Relation of pH strategy and developmental outcome after hypothermic circulatory arrest. *J Thorac Cardiovasc Surg*. 1993;106:362–368.

90. du Plessis AJ, Jonas RA, Wypij D, et al. Perioperative effects of alpha-stat versus pH-stat strategies for deep hypothermic cardiopulmonary bypass in infants. *J Thorac Cardiovasc Surg*. 1997;114:991–1000.

91. Bellinger DC, Wypij D, du Plessis AJ, et al. Developmental and neurologic effects of alpha-stat versus pH-stat strategies for deep hypothermic cardiopulmonary bypass in infants. *J Thorac Cardiovasc Surg*. 2001;121:374–383.

92. Markowitz SD, Mendoza-Paredes A, Liu H, et al. Response of brain oxygenation and metabolism to deep hypothermic circulatory arrest in newborn piglets: comparison of pH-stat and alpha-stat strategies. *Ann Thorac Surg*. 2007;84:170–176.

93. Willford DC, Hill EP, Moores WY. Theoretical analysis of oxygen transport during hypothermia. *J Clin Monit*. 1986;2:30–43.

94. Dexter F, Kern FH, Hindman BJ, Greeley WJ. The brain uses mostly dissolved oxygen during profoundly hypothermic cardiopulmonary bypass. *Ann Thorac Surg*. 1997;63:1725–1729.

95. Copeland JG, Reitz BA, Roberts AJ, Michaelis LL. Hypothermic asanguineous circulatory arrest in adult dogs. *Ann Surg*. 1974;180:728–733.

96. Taylor MJ, Bailes JE, Elrifai AM, et al. A new solution for life without blood. Asanguineous low-flow perfusion of a whole-body perfusate during 3 hours of cardiac arrest and profound hypothermia. *Circulation.* 1995;91:431–444.

97. Letsou GV, Breznock EM, Whitehair J, et al. Resuscitating hypothermic dogs after 2 hours of circulatory arrest below 6 degrees C. *J Trauma.* 2003;54:S177–S182.

98. Nollert G, Nagashima M, Bucerius J, et al. Oxygenation strategy and neurologic damage after deep hypothermic circulatory arrest. II. Hypoxic versus free radical injury. *J Thorac Cardiovasc Surg.* 1999;117:1172–1179.

99. Gibbon JH Jr. Application of a mechanical heart and lung apparatus to cardiac surgery. *Minn Med.* 1954;37:171–185.

100. Kirklin JW, Donald DE, Harshbarger HG, et al. Studies in extracorporeal circulation. I. Applicability of Gibbon-type pump-oxygenator to human intracardiac surgery: 40 cases. *Ann Surg.* 1956;144:2–8.

101. Neptune WB, Bougas JA, Panico FG. Open-heart surgery without the need for donor-blood priming in the pump oxygenator. *N Engl J Med.* 1960;263:111–115.

102. Cooley DA, Beall AC Jr, Grondin P. Open-heart operations with disposable oxygenators, 5 per cent dextrose prime, and normothermia. *Surgery.* 1962;52:713–719.

103. Gordon RJ, Ravin M, Rawitscher RE, Daicoff GR. Changes in arterial pressure, viscosity and resistance during cardiopulmonary bypass. *J Thorac Cardiovasc Surg.* 1975;69:552–561.

104. Greer AE, Carey JM, Zuhdi N. Hemodilution principle of hypothermic perfusion. A concept obviating blood priming. *J Thorac Cardiovasc Surg.* 1962;43:640–648.

105. Laver MB, Buckley MJ, Austen WG. Extreme hemodilution with profound hypothermia and circulatory arrest. *Bibl Haematol.* 1975;41:225–238.

106. Sungurtekin H, Cook DJ, Orszulak TA, Daly RC, Mullany CJ. Cerebral response to hemodilution during hypothermic cardiopulmonary bypass in adults. *Anesth Analg.* 1999;89:1078–1083.

107. Engoren MC, Habib RH, Zacharias A, Schwann TA, Riordan CJ, Durham SJ. Effect of blood transfusion on long-term survival after cardiac operation. *Ann Thorac Surg.* 2002;74:1180–1186.

108. Koch CG, Khandwala F, Li L, Estafanous FG, Loop FD, Blackstone EH. Persistent effect of red cell transfusion on health-related quality of life after cardiac surgery. *Ann Thorac Surg.* 2006;82:13–20.

109. Shin'oka T, Shum-Tim D, Jonas RA, et al. Higher hematocrit improves cerebral outcome after deep hypothermic circulatory arrest. *J Thorac Cardiovasc Surg.* 1996;112:1610–1620.

110. Duebener LF, Sakamoto T, Hatsuoka S, et al. Effects of hematocrit on cerebral microcirculation and tissue oxygenation during deep hypothermic bypass. *Circulation.* 2001;104:I260–I264.

111. Shin'oka T, Shum-Tim D, Laussen PC, et al. Effects of oncotic pressure and hematocrit on outcome after hypothermic circulatory arrest. *Ann Thorac Surg.* 1998;65:155–164.

112. Sakamoto T, Zurakowski D, Duebener LF, et al. Interaction of temperature with hematocrit level and pH determines safe duration of hypothermic circulatory arrest. *J Thorac Cardiovasc Surg.* 2004;128: 220–232.

113. Jonas RA, Wypij D, Roth SJ, et al. The influence of hemodilution on outcome after hypothermic cardiopulmonary bypass: results of a randomized trial in infants. *J Thorac Cardiovasc Surg.* 2003; 126:1765–1774.

114. Newburger JW, Jonas RA, Soul J, et al. Randomized trial of hematocrit 25% versus 35% during hypothermic cardiopulmonary bypass in infant heart surgery. *J Thorac Cardiovasc Surg.* 2008;135:347–354. 354 e1–4.

115. Wypij D, Jonas RA, Bellinger DC, et al. The effect of hematocrit during hypothermic cardiopulmonary bypass in infant heart surgery: results from the combined Boston hematocrit trials. *J Thorac Cardiovasc Surg.* 2008;135:355–360.

116. Skaryak LA, Kirshbom PM, DiBernardo LR, et al. Modified ultrafiltration improves cerebral metabolic recovery after circulatory arrest. *J Thorac Cardiovasc Surg.* 1995;109:744–751. discussion 751–2.

117. Dewhurst AT, Moore SJ, Liban JB. Pharmacological agents as cerebral protectants during deep hypothermic circulatory arrest in adult thoracic aortic surgery. A survey of current practice. *Anaesthesia.* 2002;57: 1016–1021.

118. Reilly EL, Brunberg JA, Doty DB. The effect of deep hypothermia and total circulatory arrest on the electroencephalogram in children. *Electroencephalogr Clin Neurophysiol.* 1974;36:661–667.

119. Pagni CA, Courjon J. Electroencephalographic Modifications Induced by Moderate and Deep Hypothermia in Man. *Acta Neurochir Suppl.* 1964;14(Suppl 13):35–49.

120. Bellinger DC, Jonas RA, Rappaport LA, et al. Developmental and neurologic status of children after heart surgery with hypothermic circulatory arrest or low-flow cardiopulmonary bypass. *N Engl J Med.* 1995;332:549–555.

121. Newburger JW, Jonas RA, Wernovsky G, et al. A comparison of the perioperative neurologic effects of hypothermic circulatory arrest versus low-flow cardiopulmonary bypass in infant heart surgery. *N Engl J Med.* 1993;329:1057–1064.

122. Rung GW, Wickey GS, Myers JL, Salus JE, Hensley FA Jr, Martin DE. Thiopental as an adjunct to hypothermia for EEG suppression in infants prior to circulatory arrest. *J Cardiothorac Vasc Anesth.* 1991;5: 337–342.

123. Michenfelder JD, Theye RA. Cerebral protection by thiopental during hypoxia. *Anesthesiology.* 1973;39: 510–517.

124. Nussmeier NA, Arlund C, Slogoff S. Neuropsychiatric complications after cardiopulmonary bypass: cerebral protection by a barbiturate. *Anesthesiology*. 1986;64:165–170.

125. Zaidan JR, Klochany A, Martin WM, Ziegler JS, Harless DM, Andrews RB. Effect of thiopental on neurologic outcome following coronary artery bypass grafting. *Anesthesiology*. 1991;74: 406–411.

126. Siegman MG, Anderson RV, Balaban RS, Ceckler TL, Clark RE, Swain JA. Barbiturates impair cerebral metabolism during hypothermic circulatory arrest. *Ann Thorac Surg*. 1992;54:1131–1136.

127. Todd MM, Drummond JC, HS U. The hemodynamic consequences of high-dose thiopental anesthesia. *Anesth Analg*. 1985;64:681–687.

128. Hirotani T, Kameda T, Kumamoto T, Shirota S, Yamano M. Protective effect of thiopental against cerebral ischemia during circulatory arrest. *Thorac Cardiovasc Surg*. 1999;47:223–228.

129. Weiss M, Weiss J, Cotton J, Nicolas F, Binet JP. A study of the electroencephalogram during surgery with deep hypothermia and circulatory arrest in infants. *J Thorac Cardiovasc Surg*. 1975;70:316–329.

130. Fisk GC, Wright JS, Hicks RG, et al. The influence of duration of circulatory arrest at 20 degrees C on cerebral changes. *Anaesth Intensive Care*. 1976;4: 126–134.

131. Roach GW, Newman MF, Murkin JM, et al. Ineffectiveness of burst suppression therapy in mitigating perioperative cerebrovascular dysfunction. Multicenter Study of Perioperative Ischemia (McSPI) Research Group. *Anesthesiology*. 1999;90:1255–1264.

132. Stevens WC, Cromwell TH, Halsey MJ, Eger EI 2nd, Shakespeare TF, Bahlman SH. The cardiovascular effects of a new inhalation anesthetic, Forane, in human volunteers at constant arterial carbon dioxide tension. *Anesthesiology*. 1971;35:8–16.

133. Checchia PA, Bronicki RA, Costello JM, Nelson DP. Steroid use before pediatric cardiac operations using cardiopulmonary bypass: an international survey of 36 centers. *Pediatr Crit Care Med*. 2005;6:441–444.

134. Moses ML, Camishion RC, Tokunaga K, Pierucci L Jr, Davies AL, Nealon TF Jr. Effect of corticosteroid on the acidosis of prolonged cardiopulmonary bypass. *J Surg Res*. 1966;6:354–360.

135. Mohri H, Barnes RW, Winterscheid LC, Dillard DH, Merendino KA. Challenge of prolonged suspended animation: a method of surface-induced deep hypothermia. *Ann Surg*. 1968;168:779–787.

136. Dietzman RH, Casteda AR, Lillehei CW, Ersera, Motsay GJ, Lillehei RC. Corticosteroids as effective vasodilators in the treatment of low output syndrome. *Chest*. 1970;57:440–453.

137. Thompson MA, Broadbent MP, English J. Plasma levels of methylprednisolone following administration during cardiac surgery. *Anaesthesia*. 1982;37: 405–407.

138. Dietzman RH, Lunseth JB, Goott B, Berger EC. The use of methylprednisolone during cardiopulmonary bypass. A review of 427 cases. *J Thorac Cardiovasc Surg*. 1975;69:870–873.

139. Fecht DC, Magovern GJ, Park SB, et al. Beneficial effects of methylprednisolone in patients on cardiopulmonary bypass. *Circ Shock*. 1978;5:415–422.

140. Morton JR, Hiebert CA, Lutes CA, White RL. Effect of methylprednisolone on myocardial preservation during coronary artery surgery. *Am J Surg*. 1976; 131:419–422.

141. Niazi Z, Flodin P, Joyce L, Smith J, Mauer H, Lillehei RC. Effects of glucocorticosteroids in patients undergoing coronary artery bypass surgery. *Chest*. 1979;76:262–268.

142. Cavarocchi NC, Pluth JR, Schaff HV, et al. Complement activation during cardiopulmonary bypass. Comparison of bubble and membrane oxygenators. *J Thorac Cardiovasc Surg*. 1986;91: 252–258.

143. Chaney MA, Nikolov MP, Blakeman B, Bakhos M, Slogoff S. Pulmonary effects of methylprednisolone in patients undergoing coronary artery bypass grafting and early tracheal extubation. *Anesth Analg*. 1998;87:27–33.

144. Chaney MA, Durazo-Arvizu RA, Nikolov MP, Blakeman BP, Bakhos M. Methylprednisolone does not benefit patients undergoing coronary artery bypass grafting and early tracheal extubation. *J Thorac Cardiovasc Surg*. 2001;121:561–569.

145. Sapolsky RM, Pulsinelli WA. Glucocorticoids potentiate ischemic injury to neurons: therapeutic implications. *Science*. 1985;229:1397–1400.

146. Chaney MA. Corticosteroids and cardiopulmonary bypass: a review of clinical investigations. *Chest*. 2002;121:921–931.

147. Langley SM, Chai PJ, Jaggers JJ, Ungerleider RM. Preoperative high dose methylprednisolone attenuates the cerebral response to deep hypothermic circulatory arrest. *Eur J Cardio-Thorac Surg*. 2000;17: 279–286.

148. Schubert S, Stoltenburg-Didinger G, Wehsack A, et al. Large-dose pretreatment with methylprednisolone fails to attenuate neuronal injury after deep hypothermic circulatory arrest in a neonatal piglet model. *Anesth Analg*. 2005;101:1311–1318.

149. Mitchell SJ, Pellett O, Gorman DF. Cerebral protection by lidocaine during cardiac operations. *Ann Thorac Surg*. April 1999;67(4):1117–1124.

150. Mitchell SJ, Merry AF, Frampton C, et al. Cerebral protection by lidocaine during cardiac operations: a follow-up study. *Ann Thorac Surg*. 2009;87:820–825.

151. Vannucci RC, Mujsce DJ. Effect of glucose on perinatal hypoxic-ischemic brain damage. *Biol Neonate*. 1992;62:215–224.

152. Ceriana P, Barzaghi N, Locatelli A, Veronesi R, De Amici D. Aortic arch surgery: retrospective analysis of

outcome and neuroprotective strategies. *J Cardiovasc Surg (Torino)*. 1998;39:337–342.

153. Hattori H, Wasterlain CG. Posthypoxic glucose supplement reduces hypoxic-ischemic brain damage in the neonatal rat. *Ann Neurol*. 1990;28:122–128.

154. Vannucci RC, Rossini A, Towfighi J. Effect of hyperglycemia on ischemic brain damage during hypothermic circulatory arrest in newborn dogs. *Pediatr Res*. 1996;40:177–184.

155. de Ferranti S, Gauvreau K, Hickey PR, et al. Intraoperative hyperglycemia during infant cardiac surgery is not associated with adverse neurodevelopmental outcomes at 1, 4, and 8 years. *Anesthesiology*. 2004;100:1345–1352.

156. NICE-SUGAR Study Investigators, Finfer S, Chittock DR, Su SY, et al. Intensive versus conventional glucose control in critically ill patients. *N Engl J Med*. 2009;360:1283–1297.

157. Arabi YM, Dabbagh OC, Tamim HM, et al. Intensive versus conventional insulin therapy: a randomized controlled trial in medical and surgical critically ill patients. *Crit Care Med*. 2008;36:3190–3197.

158. Griesdale DE, de Souza RJ, van Dam RM, et al. Intensive insulin therapy and mortality among critically ill patients: a meta-analysis including NICE-SUGAR study data. *CMAJ*. 2009;180:821–827.

159. Chaney MA, Nikolov MP, Blakeman BP, Bakhos M. Attempting to maintain normoglycemia during cardiopulmonary bypass with insulin may initiate postoperative hypoglycemia. *Anesth Analg*. 1999; 89:1091–1095.

160. Swain JA, McDonald TJ Jr, Griffith PK, Balaban RS, Clark RE, Ceckler T. Low-flow hypothermic cardiopulmonary bypass protects the brain. *J Thorac Cardiovasc Surg*. 1991;102:76–83.

161. Langley SM, Chai PJ, Miller SE, et al. Intermittent perfusion protects the brain during deep hypothermic circulatory arrest. *Ann Thorac Surg*. 1999;68:4–12.

162. Miura T, Laussen P, Lidov HG, DuPlessis A, Shin'oka T, Jonas RA. Intermittent whole-body perfusion with "somatoplegia" versus blood perfusate to extend duration of circulatory arrest. *Circulation*. 1996;94:II56–II62.

163. Kimura T, Muraoka R, Chiba Y, Ihaya A, Morioka K. Effect of intermittent deep hypothermic circulatory arrest on brain metabolism. *J Thorac Cardiovasc Surg*. 1994;108:658–663.

164. Schultz S, Antoni D, Shears G, et al. Brain oxygen and metabolism during circulatory arrest with intermittent brief periods of low-flow cardiopulmonary bypass in newborn piglets. *J Thorac Cardiovasc Surg*. 2006;132:839–844.

165. Apostolakis E, Shuhaiber JH. Antegrade or retrograde cerebral perfusion as an adjunct during hypothermic circulatory arrest for aortic arch surgery. *Expert Rev Cardiovasc Ther*. 2007;5:1147–1161.

166. Apostolakis E, Akinosoglou K. The methodologies of hypothermic circulatory arrest and of antegrade and retrograde cerebral perfusion for aortic arch surgery. *Ann Thorac Cardiovasc Surg*. 2008;14:138–148.

167. Strauch JT, Spielvogel D, Lauten A, et al. Optimal temperature for selective cerebral perfusion. *J Thorac Cardiovasc Surg*. 2005;130:74–82.

168. Khaladj N, Peterss S, Oetjen P, et al. Hypothermic circulatory arrest with moderate, deep or profound hypothermic selective antegrade cerebral perfusion: which temperature provides best brain protection? *Eur J Cardiothorac Surg*. 2006;30:492–498.

169. Strauch JT, Spielvogel D, Haldenwang PL, et al. Changes in regional cerebral blood flow under hypothermic selective cerebral perfusion. *Thorac Cardiovasc Surg*. 2004;52:82–89.

170. Neri E, Sassi C, Barabesi L, et al. Cerebral autoregulation after hypothermic circulatory arrest in operations on the aortic arch. *Ann Thorac Surg*. 2004;77: 72–79.

171. Hagl C, Ergin MA, Galla JD, et al. Neurologic outcome after ascending aorta-aortic arch operations: effect of brain protection technique in high-risk patients. *J Thorac Cardiovasc Surg*. 2001;121: 1107–1121.

172. Kitahori K, Takamoto S, Takayama H, et al. A novel protocol of retrograde cerebral perfusion with intermittent pressure augmentation for brain protection. *J Thorac Cardiovasc Surg*. 2005;130:363–370.

173. Kawata M, Takamoto S, Kitahori K, et al. Intermittent pressure augmentation during retrograde cerebral perfusion under moderate hypothermia provides adequate neuroprotection: an experimental study. *J Thorac Cardiovasc Surg*. 2006;132:80–88.

174. Pretre R, Turina MI. Deep hypothermic circulatory arrest. In: Cohn LH, Edmunds LH, eds. *Cardiac surgery in the adult*. 3rd ed. New York: McGraw Hill; 2008:431–442.

Cerebral Monitoring During Aortic Surgery

8

Parthasarathy D. Thirumala, John M. Murkin, Donald J. Crammond, Miguel Habeych, Jeffery Balzer, and Kathirvel Subramaniam

Introduction

Neurological complications occur frequently after aortic surgery and are associated with increased hospital mortality, and length of hospital and intensive care unit stay.[1] The incidence of stroke varies from 2% to 33% and transient neurologic dysfunction (TND) has been reported to occur up to 35% of patients after aortic surgery.[2–6] Neurological complications are also associated with poor long-term outcome and impaired quality of life.[7,8] Various surgical strategies and intraoperative neuromonitoring (IONM) techniques have been developed in recent years in an effort to reduce the neurological dysfunction after aortic surgery. Intraoperative neuromonitoring (IONM) techniques include somatosensory evoked potentials (SSEP), electroencephalography (EEG), transcranial Doppler (TCD), near-infrared spectroscopy (NIRS), and jugular venous oxygen saturation ($SJVO_2$). Neuromonitoring has become an integral part of neuroprotection and many centers use a single method or multimodal monitoring during aortic surgery. According to a nationwide survey conducted by German Society of Anesthesiology, the methods used for IONM are SSEP (40%), EEG (60%), TCD (17.5%), and NIRS (40%) with some using a combination of methods.[9] Although there are no outcome studies published with regard to the benefits of neuromonitoring in aortic surgery, these monitoring techniques can identify the intraoperative events responsible for the development of cerebral ischemia/infarction such as cerebral hypoperfusion, malperfusion, and embolism.[10] This chapter will describe the equipment needed to perform IONM, parameters used to acquire data with the equipment, and safety of the equipment in the operating room (OR). The effects of pharmacologic (anesthesia drugs) and physiologic variables (e.g., hypothermia, arterial blood gas) on different monitoring methods along with advantages and limitations of each monitoring modality will be discussed. Existing literature on the use of IONM in aortic surgery and deep hypothermic circulatory arrest (DHCA) will also be reviewed. Information presented in the chapter is based on literature review and our vast experience at University of Pittsburgh medical center in monitoring several hundred aortic repairs.

Intraoperative Neurophysiological Monitoring

Instrumentation

Intraoperative Neurophysiological Monitoring (NIOM) machines are connected to the patients using disposable subdermal needle electrodes.

P.D. Thirumala (✉)
Department of Neurosurgery,
University of Pittsburgh Medical Center,
Pittsburgh, PA, USA
e-mail: thirumalapd@upmc.edu

K. Subramaniam et al. (eds.), *Anesthesia and Perioperative Care for Aortic Surgery*,
DOI 10.1007/978-0-387-85922-4_8, © Springer Science+Business Media, LLC 2011

b

a

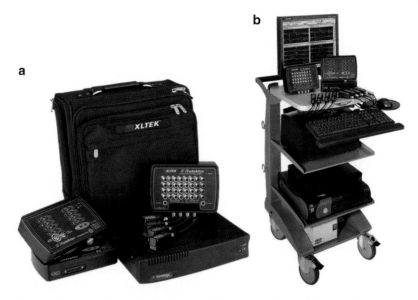

Fig. 8.1 (**a** and **b**) IOM machines shown above the portable format, which can fit in a travel bag, and desktop format to fit the needs of our practice (Published with permission from Natus Medical incorporated)

We use Rhythmlink® (Rhythmlink, SC) electrodes, which are color coded for both stimulating and collecting data from a patient (Fig. 8.1a and b). These are made from high tensile strength stainless steel with varying wire and needle lengths. The advantage of the subdermal needle electrodes is quicker setup, lower impedances, and their disposability. They however can increase the risk of needle stick injury.

placed on the scalp and in the periphery using the standard 10–20 system.[11] SSEP are generated via stimulation of the median or ulnar nerves and tibial or popliteal nerves, respectively. TcMEPs are generated using electrodes placed at C1 and C2 or C3 and C4 with responses recorded from the muscles in the upper and lower limbs, typically abductor pollicis brevis and tibialis anterior, respectively.

Stimulation and Acquisition Parameters for SSEP, EEG, MEP

Multimodality neurophysiological monitoring requires optimal parameters to be set for each modality collected and displayed. During ascending aortic or arch surgeries, upper and lower limb SSEP and EEG are continuously and concomitantly acquired during the procedure. Thoracoabdominal aneurysm repairs require the addition of transcranial motor evoked potentials (tcMEP) with SSEP and EEG. Some of the common stimulation and acquisition parameters are displayed in Table 8.1. Recording electrodes are

Electrical Safety

Generally the bioengineering department in the hospitals will check and monitor any equipment used to deliver current to the patient. The equipment should be checked for adequate grounding, and leakage currents. Electrical burns in the arms or legs secondary to excessive stimulation with needle electrodes are rare. If they occur these are generally minor and heal quickly. During transcranial electrical stimulation, the current output and intensity has to be monitored as this can induce seizures, tongue lacerations, and scalp burns.

Table 8.1 Common stimulation and acquisition parameters

Modalities	Stimulation sites	Recoding channels	Stimulation rate	Stimulation intensity	Latency range[21]		Amplitude range		Bandwidth
					Mean	3SD	Mean	3SD	
SSEP	MS, MD	P3/Fz, P4/Fz	2.35 Hz	20–40 mA	19.8	23.0	2.2	0.6	Cortical: 10–250 Hz
	US, UD	Cv2-Fz			13.3	14.5	2.3	0.5	Sub cortical: 30–1 KHz
	TS, TD	P3-P4, Pz-Fz	2.35 Hz	20–65 mA	38.0	43.9	13.4		
	PS, PD	Cv2-FZ			29.2	34.7	7.4	10.2	
MEP	Tc	Upper and lower limb muscles	Variable	200–800 V	Variable		Variable		3–1,000 Hz
EEG	None	Cortical	None	None	None		2–100		1–70 Hz

MS Left median nerve, *MD* Right median nerve, *US* Left ulnar nerve, *UD* Right ulnar nerve, *Tc* Transcranial, *PD* Left peroneal nerve, *PS* Left peroneal nerve, P3, P4, Fz, CV2 are placed in accordance to the international 10–20 system

Somatosensory Evoked Potentials (SSEP)

Recording SSEP

SSEP are generated in the spinal cord, the brain stem, and the cerebral cortex, following peripheral nerve stimulation. Following median or ulnar nerve stimulation at the wrist and tibial or peroneal nerve stimulation in the leg, electrical signals travel along the sensory nerve, dorsal columns of the spinal cord, the brain stem, and the contralateral thalamus and terminate in the primary somatosensory cortex. The integrity of these structures, which play a role in generation of SSEP responses, can be monitored during surgery. Specifically, the peripheral sensory nerve generates an action potential in response to an electrical current delivered by pad or subdermal needle electrodes. This action potential travels along the sensory nerve to the spinal dorsal columns. Potentials are recorded along the peripheral nerve (Fig. 8.2) at the erbs point (N9), or the popliteal fossa in the upper and lower extremities, respectively.[12] The spinal dorsal columns are white matter tracts containing no synapses until reaching the lower medullary nuclei. The responses recorded in the cervical region (Fig. 8.2) appear to be generated from the upper cervical cord and lower brain stem.[12] Postsynaptic fibers from the nuclei cross to the contralateral side of the brain stem and ascend as the medial lemniscus to the ventroposterior nucleus of the thalamus and then eventually terminating in the primary somatosensory cortex. Cortical responses are recorded on the scalp (Fig. 8.2a) from the contralateral somatosensory cortex.[12]

Factors Affecting SSEP

Anesthetic drugs, mean arterial pressure, blood gas tensions, hematocrit, and temperature can have profound effect on the cortical SSEP amplitude and latencies.[13] Both hypercarbia and hypocarbia can affect SSEP signals. Hemodilution and low hematocrit also increase latency. Hemodilution and hypotension are synergistic to depress SSEP waveforms.[13]

Anesthesia Drugs

General anesthetics act primarily on the synaptic chemical transmission process itself and do not affect the conduction of impulses in nerve axons or change the electrical excitability of neurons. Hence, optimal management of anesthesia is required for recording cortical evoked potentials.[14] A balanced anesthetic technique is used for aortic surgery, which includes an induction agent (thiopental, etomidate, or propofol), amnestic (midazolam), analgesic (fentanyl), and maintenance inhalational anesthetics (IA) (isoflurane, sevoflurane, or desflurane) or maintenance intravenous agent (propofol).

Primary effects of inhalational anesthetics (IA) are observed as an increase in the latency and a decrease in the amplitude of the cortical SSEP response.[14–17] Subcortical latencies and amplitudes are not altered significantly though monitoring subcortical potentials are not always possible and desirable.[17,18] Maintenance dose of IA should not only allow interpretation of cortical SSEP but also prevent the awareness from occurring. Addition of nitrous oxide to IA compounds this observed decrease in amplitude of cortical SSEP response.[19] Since nitrous oxide is not used in aortic surgery, this is not a concern here unlike spine surgery. There is considerable debate on the differential effects of each IA at equivalent minimum alveolar concentration (MAC) on the amplitude and latency of cortical SSEP responses. Most of the evidence comes from spine and neurosurgery literature and is applicable to cardiac and aortic surgery.

Isoflurane is the most commonly used IA in cardiac surgery followed by sevoflurane and desflurane. The use of sevoflurane and isoflurane up to 1 MAC is compatible with intraoperative SSEP monitoring.[20] Zhang et al. compared the effects of isoflurane and desflurane on cortical SSEPs. Both decreased N20 amplitude and latency significantly. Cortical waveforms disappeared with both the agents at 1.5 MAC. Isoflurane maintained bispectral index (BIS) less than 60 compared to

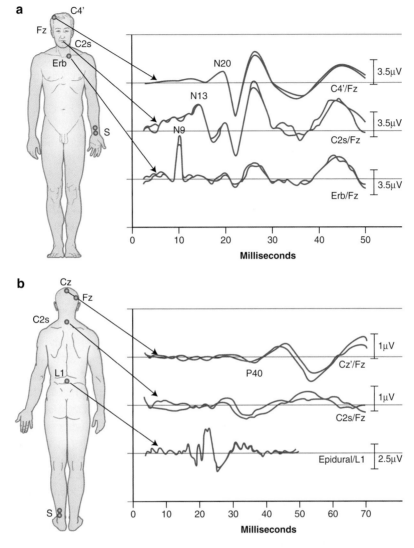

Fig. 8.2 (**a**) Somatosensory evoked potentials after stimulation to the left median nerve, recorded transcutaneously from points along the somatosensory pathway: from Erb's point (Erb/Fz) over the second cervical spinous process (C2s/Fz) and over the somatosensory cortex (C4'/Fz). The difference between N13 and N20 waveform peaks represents the central conduction time.

(**b**) Somatosensory evoked potentials after stimulation to the left tibial nerve, recorded from points along the somatosensory pathway: from the first lumbar epidural space (epidural/L1) from the skin overlying the second cervical spinous process (C2s/Fz) and from the scalp overlying the somatosensory cortex (CZ'/Fz) (Redrawn with permission from Lake[84])

desflurane at 0.75 MAC.[21] Rehberg et al. have shown that sevoflurane and desflurane are better suited for NIOM because SSEP amplitudes are better preserved compared to isoflurane.[22] Schindler et al. studied various concentrations of desflurane on cortical SSEP and concluded that the use of desflurane up to 1 MAC is compatible with intraoperative SSEP monitoring.[23]

Induction dose of thiopental (5 mg/kg) followed by 2 mg/kg/h had little effect on amplitude but prolonged latency of cortical SSEP responses.[24] Thiopental bolus 4 mg/kg also produced similar results in another study.[25] Higher doses produced a significant decrease in the amplitude and an increase in the latency but still compatible with recording of cortically recorded

SSEP responses.[26] Etomidate and ketamine increase the signal amplitude of SSEPs.[13]

The effects of propofol on SSEP were similar to thiopental. Propofol used as a continuous infusion to maintain anesthesia preserves SSEP waveforms better than isoflurane and sevoflurane.[27,28] In adolescents undergoing spinal fusion, both isoflurane 0.6% in air and propofol infusion (120 ug/kg/min) preserved SSEP signals though propofol performed better. Average BIS values were lower for propofol than for isoflurane.[29] However, few studies described advantages of propofol over sevoflurane anesthesia. Fung et al. compared propofol-remifentanil with sevoflurane-remifentanil anesthesia in providing optimal conditions for SSEP monitoring. Propofol administered patients had less within patient variability in cortical amplitude and latency. However, sevoflurane patients had faster suppression with increasing concentration and faster recovery after stopping the drug.[30] The implication is that if there is light anesthesia and hypertensive response during maintenance, deepening anesthesia with sevoflurane may be preferable to giving intravenous bolus of propofol because recovery of SSEP to baseline will be faster with sevoflurane. Ku et al. reported similar findings in patients undergoing scoliosis surgery. In addition, patients who received sevoflurane were more cooperative and more lucid during recovery from anesthesia in their study.[31]

High-dose narcotics produce modest alterations in cortical SSEP but are suitable for intraoperative monitoring.[24,32,33] Benzodiazepines also can produce modest changes similar to narcotics. Midazolam 0.2 mg/kg followed by 5 mg/h produced depression of cortical amplitude without altering latency.[34] Another study used a similar dose and found that midazolam prolonged latency without any change in amplitude.[25]

Neuromuscular blocking drugs do not directly influence SSEP, but they increase the signal to noise ratio by eliminating the electromyography artifact thereby improving SSEP recordings.[35]

In summary, different classes of anesthetic drugs can affect SSEP to a varying degree. Drugs and doses that will minimally affect the waveform amplitude and latency should be used. In general, intravenous anesthetics affect SSEP less than inhalational anesthetics. IA can be used, provided the concentrations can be limited to 1 MAC. A baseline SSEP should be obtained after induction when a steady state anesthetic state is reached. Intravenous boluses of anesthetic drugs or sudden increases in IA concentration should be communicated to the neurophysiologist so that false-positive interpretation of cerebral ischemia can be avoided.

Cerebral Blood Flow (CBF), Mean Arterial Blood Pressure (MAP), and SSEP

Adequate cerebral blood flow is necessary for viable neuronal cell function in the cerebral cortex to generate SSEP responses. Normal CBF in an awake adult is approximately 50 mL/100 g/min, with cortical regions (gray matter) requiring higher levels as compared to subcortical regions (white matter tracts).[36] Cerebral autoregulation maintains a constant CBF with MAP between 60 and 150 mmHg.[36,37] Decreases in MAP below 60 mmHg results in oligemia and consequent decrease in the CBF. It is important to note that outside the cerebral autoregulation window there is nonlinear correlation between the CBF and MAP, which results in significant drop in CBF with insignificant decreases in MAP. When CBF decreases below the functional threshold, electrophysiological changes begin to appear.[38] Mild hypoperfusion (22 mL/100 g/min) is well tolerated and typically does not induce neuronal dysfunction. CBF in the range of 14–16 mL/100 g/min results in a sharp decline in the evoked response, with a 50% reduction of the response observed at 16 mL/100 g/min.[39] Primate models indicate complete absence of evoked responses at levels below 12 mL/100 g/min. This has been termed as "electrical failure." The CBF threshold for failure of energy metabolism or "energy failure" or for the maintenance of the ionic pumping mechanisms of cell membranes is lower than that for electrical failure.[39] Animal studies indicate that CBF levels of approximately 10 mL/100 g/min results in significant increase in the extracellular potassium, which indicates an ionic or energy failure. However, normal concentrations of extracellular potassium were present in the face of a complete loss of evoked potentials. This finding indicates a clear difference in CBF threshold levels for neuronal and electrical function.[39] Time-dependent reversible changes in the CBF can return the SSEP changes back to control levels.[40–42] These studies emphasize optimizing MAP in the operating room and the need to quickly reverse changes in MAP to maintain adequate CBF.

Hypothermia and SSEP

At the normal body temperature of 37°C, the brain can tolerate approximately 4–5 min of circulatory arrest (Fig. 8.3a, b). At lower temperatures, the circulatory arrest can be extended 20–40 min with minimal neurological complications.[43,44] Arrest extending for 1–2 h was associated with 15% risk of significant neurological injury.[44] The "safe period" can be extended with antegrade[3] or retrograde cerebral perfusion (RCP) with deep hypothermic circulatory arrest

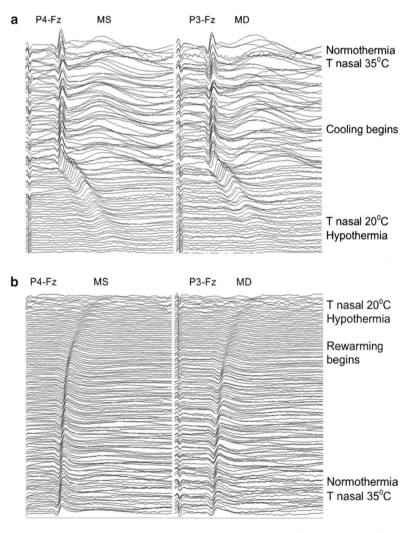

Fig. 8.3 This shows the effect of bilateral cortical median nerve SSEP responses in response to cooling (**a**) and warming (**b**) during an aortic surgery repair. The *left column* shows the cortical responses N20-P30 complex (P4-Fz channel) from the left median nerve SSEPs, and the *right column* shows the cortical responses (P3-Fz channel) from the right median nerve

(DHCA).[45] Optimal hypothermic temperature for DHCA during cardiac surgeries has been a matter of debate. Temperatures in the range of 10–25°C have been used to reduce postoperative neurological deficits.[2,46,47] Nasopharyngeal or rectal temperatures do not accurately predict brain temperatures; therefore, targeting of optimal temperature may be difficult. SSEP and EEG recordings can be an electrophysiological marker to evaluate adequate hypothermia during DHCA. This notion is summarized in a large study performed by Stecker MM et al.[48,49] who examined neurophysiological monitoring changes during DHCA. They found that the cortical SSEP N20-P30 complex disappeared at a nasopharyngeal temperature of 21.4°C ± 4°C, and subcortical (N13) responses disappeared at temperatures of 17.3°C ± 4°C. Cortical SSEP responses reappeared at nasopharyngeal temperature 18.6°C ± 3°C, and subcortical N13 responses reappeared at 17.2°C ± 3°C. The time frame observed for recovery of the SSEP cortical N20-P30 complex correlated to the length of circulatory arrest. The nasopharyngeal temperature was higher for reappearance of cortical N20-P30 in patients presenting with postoperative stroke.[48–51] The subcortical N13 potentials disappeared at a lower temperature and its reappearance did not depend on the length of circulatory arrest.[48,49,52] Hence, SSEP recorded under optimal anesthetic conditions can be helpful in improving prognosis after DHCA.[52]

Role of Intraoperative SSEP in Aortic Surgery

SSEP monitoring has several important roles in ascending and aortic arch surgery. In the pre-bypass period, several patients presenting for emergency surgery (aortic dissection and ruptured aneurysms) are already intubated and full neurological examination is not possible. Baseline SSEP abnormalities may indicate great vessel involvement and alert the surgical and anesthesia team to prepare for immediate initiation of CPB, rapid cooling, and appropriate blood pressure management for protecting cerebral circulation.[52] Disappearance of SSEP at higher temperature in the pre-bypass cooling period also indicates

neurological compromise and should also be addressed immediately.[53]

Target temperature for initiation of DHCA varies between patients. Cooling titrated to fixed nasopharyngeal temperature may not reflect brain temperature required for adequate cerebral protection. Too deep cooling may increase the rewarming period, total CPB time, inflammatory response, and coagulopathy. Disappearance of both cortical and subcortical SSEP has been used as the end point for cooling and initiation of DHCA. Ghariani et al. reported successful neurological outcome in their patients using this criterion.[54]

As described in the previous section, time to reappearance of SSEP signals during rewarming was correlated with postoperative neurological dysfunction. New asymmetry of SSEP signals in the post-reperfusion period should alert the team to look for graft patency and embolism. SSEP cannot differentiate embolism from hypoperfusion.[55]

Delayed onset of neurological abnormalities in the postoperative period with no SSEP abnormalities in the intraoperative period may occur. Strategy of extending the neuromonitoring into the intensive care unit in intubated, paralyzed, and sedated patients may be helpful.

Electroencephalography

EEG is spontaneous brain activity recorded from the scalp using subdermal needle electrodes. Ideally, 8 or 16 channel recordings are obtained covering both the hemispheres equally. Electrodes are placed in accordance to the standard international 10–20 system.[11] Compressed and digital spectral assays that display quantitative EEG can be used in addition to the traditional raw EEG display to identify focal and hemispheric changes. EEG activity is classified based on frequency. Frequencies include alpha (8–13 Hz), beta (>14 Hz), theta (5–7 Hz), and delta (0.5–4 Hz). Interpretation of EEG recorded and intraoperatively poses significant challenges due to general anesthesia, artifacts secondary to use of electrical equipment, and the patient's neurological and hemodynamic status.

EEG and Anesthetic Drugs

Most anesthetic agents produce an initial excitatory stage characterized by desynchronization (possibly loss of inhibitory synaptic function). Amplitude is observed to increase as the EEG becomes synchronized, with a predominance of activity in the alpha range. Increasing IA levels cause progressive slowing until the EEG achieves burst suppression and, finally, electrical silence.[56] (Fig. 8.4).

The choice of the anesthetic agent depends on the procedure and specific goal of neurophysiological monitoring. In general, IA shifts the dominant alpha rhythm to the frontal lobes similar to sleep spindles. Intravenous agents (opioids and ketamine) have minimal effects as compared to IA on the EEG. However at high doses these can produce similar effects to inhalational agents and nitrous oxide. Neuromuscular blocking agents do not affect the EEG directly however can increase the signal-to-noise ratio by decreasing muscle artifacts.[56] During aortic surgeries halogenated agents at less than 0.5 MAC with IV medications is desirable to effectively interpret the cortical SSEPs and EEG.[52]

EEG and Cerebral Blood Flow

EEG changes in response to decreased cerebral perfusion are similar to cortical SSEP amplitude changes. Changes in frequency and amplitude of EEG are dependent on the degree of hypoperfusion. Initial changes include decrease of alpha and beta activity followed by an increase in the theta and delta activity ultimately reaching electrocerebral silence. These changes have been correlated to changes in cerebral blood flow. The initial or minor changes in EEG characterized as a loss of fast activity seem to appear at or below 20–22 mL/100 g/min. Severe changes in EEG characterized by complete attenuation of faster activity and/or a significant increase in the delta activity less than 1 Hz is observed with CBF below 15 mL/100 mg/min. Appearance of delta activity and attenuation of faster activity appears in between the above-mentioned CBF values.[57–61] Complete loss of EEG activity is observed at perfusion levels of 7–15 mL/100 g/min.[62] Animal studies have indicated that changes in EEG occur well before there is a cellular ionic change.[39] As with changes in cortical SSEPs, the EEG changes can be reversed if CBF is restored early. During

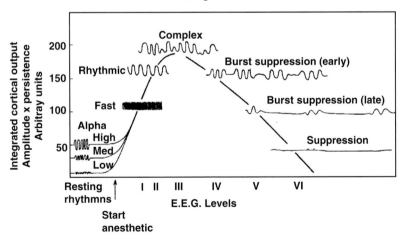

Fig. 8.4 Typical anesthesia induced changes in the EEG at different levels of anesthesia with inhalational agents and several intravenous agents. Mean frequency gradually decreases with increasing depth of anesthesia. Mean EEG amplitude increases initially and then decreases (Reprinted with permission from Stockard and Bickford[120])

aortic surgery, this principle can be used for monitoring the recovery of EEG after DHCA to evaluate the adequacy of cerebral perfusion.

Hypothermia and EEG

Isoelectric EEG recording can be used a physiological marker for hypothermia as there are no criteria to select the optimal temperature or a reliable means to measure it.[49,63] EEG was tested as a means of measuring the adequacy of cerebral protection and prognosis after DHCA in adult and pediatric

patients.[48,49,64–66] The findings are summarized in a large study conducted by Stecker MM et al.,[48,49] who reviewed neurophysiological changes during DHCA (Fig. 8.5). Bilateral or unilateral periodic complexes are the first changes to appear in the baseline EEG under anesthetic influence at a nasopharyngeal temperature of 30°C (±5°C). As cooling continues at the rate of 0.7°C/min, the periodic complexes give way to a burst suppression pattern at a nasopharyngeal temperature of 24.4°C (±4°C). With progressive cooling, isoelectric EEG appears at a nasopharyngeal temperature at 17.8°C (±4°C). The importance of using temperature as an

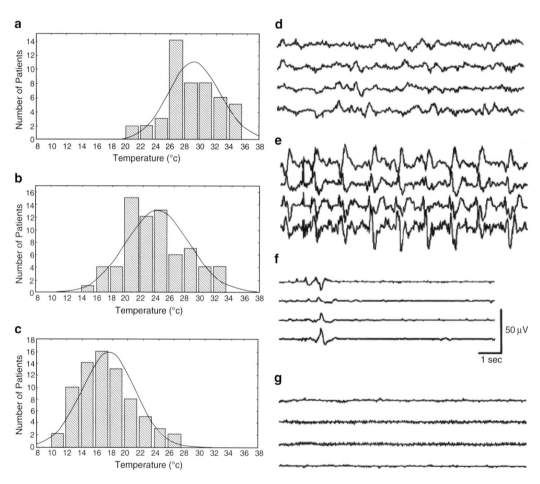

Fig. 8.5 Distribution of nasopharyngeal temperatures at which various electroencephalogram (EEG) landmarks occur: (**a**) appearance of periodic complexes, (**b**) appearance of burst suppression, and (**c**) electrocerebral silence. Examples of typical EEG patterns during cooling are also shown: (**d**) precooling, (**e**) appearance of periodic complexes, (**f**) appearance of burst suppression, and (**g**) electrocerebral silence. Each of the EEG samples represents the following four channels recorded from the left hemisphere (Fp1–F7, F7–T3, T3–T5, and T5–O1) (Reprinted with permission from Stecker et al.[49])

important physiological indicator is enhanced with findings from studies in pediatric population. Isoelectric EEG or electrocerebral silence was defined as absence of electrocerebral activity of more than 2 µV for more than 3 min duration.

EEG and Aortic Surgery

Both EEG and SSEP are used in aortic surgery with DHCA. Whether to use SSEP loss of potentials or EEG isoelectricity for initiation of DHCA has not been addressed by randomized trials. Cortical sensory evoked potentials disappear before electrocerebral silence on EEG and subcortical potentials may be demonstrated at lower temperature even after EEG isoelectricity. So, some institutions use disappearance of both cortical and subcortical SSEP waveforms as the end point for cooling.

Continuous EEG activity is seen after the onset of antegrade circulation at a nasopharyngeal temperature of 30°C (±5°C). There appears to be a correlation between poor postoperative neurological outcomes and the return of EEG activity at higher temperatures. EEG is a very useful monitoring modality to assess the adequacy of cerebral perfusion, guide to cerebral protection with hypothermia, and provide prognostic information after DHCA.

Transcranial Doppler (TCD)

TCD is based on the principle of ultrasonic echoes from a piezoelectric crystal penetrating adult human skull in the thinnest temporal regions.[67] These ultrasonic echoes from crystals are reflected by the erythrocytes and the direction and velocity of the red cell movement through the largest intracranial arteries can be determined by the Doppler principle. Typically, middle cerebral artery (MCA) flow velocities are monitored during cardiac and aortic surgery since the artery carries 75–80% of ipsilateral carotid blood flow. Pulse wave spectral Doppler method measures the peak systolic, end-diastolic, and mean flow velocities at a predetermined distance or at multiple distances from the probe. In contrast to pulse

wave Doppler, M-mode records time series display of signal amplitude at each depth gate.[68]

There is no data regarding the extent of maximum velocity suppression associated with postoperative neurologic dysfunction in cardiac surgery. Data in carotid endarterectomy patients showed that neurologic damage is unlikely if V max was maintained at 40% or greater than its preclamp value.[69] Flow velocity reduction to 70% of its basal value has been used as intervention threshold in cardiac surgery.

Also, flow velocity is not directly related to absolute cerebral blood flow. However, the changes in cerebral blood flow can be indirectly detected with changes in flow velocity. Two important factors affect the relation of flow velocity and blood flow. First, changes in middle cerebral artery diameter (nitroglycerine vasodilatation) affect the flow velocity with no change in CBF. Second, the orientation of pulse wave Doppler relative to the direction of MCA blood flow affects the measurement of flow velocity. Significant underestimation of flow velocity will result if the angle of insonation is more than 30°.

Malperfusion

TCD during aortic surgeries can detect malperfusion syndromes at the initiation of cardiopulmonary bypass.[68] Flow through the false lumen may force a portion of torn intimae across the opening of arch vessels. Since the obstruction may not involve upper limb arterial pressure monitoring sites, early detection and correction by TCD is essential to avoid catastrophic brain injury.

Rewarming from DHCA

During rewarming, the brain is prone for ischemia for two reasons. CBF does not increase in response to increased metabolism as there is flow metabolism uncoupling during DHCA. CBF becomes pressure dependent because of loss of autoregulation in deep hypothermia. TCD during reperfusion shows immediate hyperemia followed by lower than basal flow velocities during

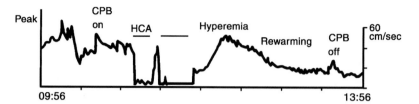

Fig. 8.6 The trend plot of changes in middle cerebral artery peak flow velocity during pediatric aortic arch reconstruction. *CPB* cardiopulmonary bypass, *HCA* hypothermic circulatory arrest. With the resumption of systemic perfusion at the end of HCA, peak flow velocities increased above pre-CPB baseline indicating flow-metabolism uncoupling. Later, this translates into cerebral ischemia as the falling velocity signifies a flow insufficient to meet the hypermetabolic demand of the rewarming brain (Reprinted with permission (Wiley-Blackwell) from reference 70)

most of the rewarming (Fig. 8.6). Adjustment of systemic perfusion and mean blood pressure according to TCD velocities may aid in preventing ischemia of rewarming.[70,71]

Retrograde Cerebral Perfusion (RCP) and Antegrade Cerebral Perfusion (ACP)

Evaluation of RCP and antegrade cerebral perfusion (ACP) during DHCA is an important application of TCD during aortic surgery.[72–74] Effectiveness of RCP may be limited by several anatomical factors such as valves in venous system, thin-walled veins with their tendency for collapse and kinking, and the drainage of perfusion through the azygos system. TCD flow velocity can be used to evaluate the efficacy of RCP and detect inadequate perfusion. Estrera et al.[75] studied patients undergoing acute type A resection with retrograde perfusion and DHCA. TCD altered cannulation and guided retrograde perfusion in 28.5% and 78.6% of the patients, respectively. TND was significantly reduced (14.8%) in TCD monitored patients compared to unmonitored patients (51.8%). Retrograde superior vena caval pressures necessary to achieve effective RCP can be titrated using TCD. Tanoue et al. were able to detect TCD signals in 3 of 15 patients with SVC pressures of 15–25 mmHg.[73] With higher SVC pressures (40 mmHg), Ganzel et al. demonstrated TCD signals in 16 of 18 of their patients.[76] Inadequate RCP also causes reactive hyperemia after systemic reperfusion, which will result in neurological damage unless detected and treated by lowering blood pressure and thereby lowering flow velocity.[73] TCD can diagnose reactive hyperemia after RCP and aid in the management.

Anterograde cerebral perfusion (ACP) methods have similar anatomical limitations. Functionally inadequate cerebral collateral blood flow from a single carotid, or axillary arterial cannula may be expected because of incomplete circle of Willis. Bilateral TCD monitoring provides the only means to directly document the initiation and maintenance of bihemisphericante grade cerebral perfusion through large arteries.[77] TCD can also be used to limit the excessive pump flow and prevent hyperperfusion syndrome.[78]

Detection of Emboli

Transcranial Doppler can detect embolization, which are important sources of brain injury and long-term cognitive dysfunction during cardiac and aortic surgery.[79,80] Microembolism is not uncommon during open cardiac and aortic surgery. However, there is a correlation between the number of microemboli detected by TCD and postoperative neurologic dysfunction.[81] TCD can also evaluate technical aspects designed to reduce these emboli during aortic manipulation[82] or trap atheromatous emboli.[83] Audible feedback to the surgeon helps in modification of techniques resulting in reduction of microemboli.[81] Modification of techniques include avoidance of reinfusing unwashed cardiotomy suction blood, elimination of partially occluding clamps, carbon dioxide purging of nitrogen in the surgical field, and transesophageal echo and TCD guided deairing maneuvers. Use of well-designed venous reservoirs that minimize air entrapment and replacement of bubble oxygenators by membrane oxygenators also decreased emboli counts.

Limitations

TCD is not without its limitations.[70,84] The technique is very user dependent. Temporal windows are difficult to obtain in patients with thick skull because of poor transmission of ultrasound signals. TCD used for intraoperative monitoring requires a fixation device to the head. Minor probe movements can cause loss of signals, which should be differentiated from flow cessation during aortic surgery. TCD flow velocity is not indicative of absolute CBF as described above.

Jugular Bulb Venous Oxygen Saturation (SJVO2)

Jugular bulb venous oxygen saturation ($SJVO_2$) monitoring measures the cerebral oxygenation on an intermittent or continuous basis via a catheter placed in the jugular bulb.[85] Normal $SJVO_2$ values range from 55% to 75%, or up to 85%. This value reflects the normal degree of coupling between the oxygen supply to the brain and oxygen demand.

Because of the linear relation and strong correlation between $SJVO_2$ and $CMRO_2$, $SJVO_2$ can be used as a surrogate of residual cerebral metabolic activity during cooling phase of DHCA for aortic arch surgery (Fig. 8.7). $SJVO_2$ is specifically useful in determining the duration and thus the end point of cooling to DHCA. After $SJVO_2$ reaches 95%, DHCA can be initiated safely.[86] Lower $SJVO_2$ values before DHCA were associated with neurological dysfunction postoperatively.[87] Cooling to a fixed temperature or to isoelectric EEG can leave significant residual metabolic activity.[88]

$SJVO_2$ has also been used to monitor ACP during DHCA and values maintained above 90%.

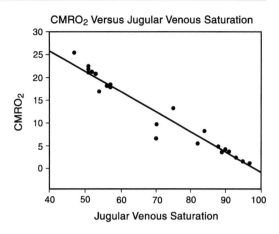

Fig. 8.7 Graph showing close linear relationship between $SJVO_2$ and $CMRO_2$ during cooling phase of profound hypothermia in human brain (Reprinted with permission from (Elsevier); McCullough et al.[121])

Lower values suggest an insufficient oxygen supply to the brain to meet the demands and ACP flows and perfusion pressure are adjusted accordingly to achieve a higher $SJVO_2$.[89] $SJVO_2$ is also a useful measure of cerebral metabolism if aortic arch surgery is performed with moderate hypothermia and ACP.[90]

$SJVO_2$ monitoring requires additional invasive procedure. Contamination of extracranial facial veins should be avoided by slow aspiration of the blood sample. $SJVO_2$ values indicate global oxygen supply–demand balance and the major limitation is its inability to detect regional cerebral ischemia. No correlation could be demonstrated between regional oxygen saturation measured by NIRS and $SJVO_2$.[91] $SJVO_2$ is subject to "wall-artifact," or interference with oximeter signal due to catheter impingement against the vessel wall.

Near-Infrared Regional Spectroscopy

Near-infrared regional spectroscopy (NIRS)[92] and $SJVO_2$ both can provide information about cerebral oxygenation. This information is not available using SSEP, EEG, and TCD. Transcranial cerebral oximetry, based on the principle of NIRS, has been successfully used in the OR during cardiac surgical procedures. The ability of continuous cerebral NIRS monitoring of cerebral tissue oxygenation to detect and optimize cerebral hypoperfusion in the setting of aortic surgery and DHCA will be discussed.

Basic Principle of NIRS: Lambert Law

The ability to measure the concentration of various substances, specifically tissue hemoglobin content as well as cerebral tissue oxygen saturation, is predicated on the concept that the concentration of a substance in a solution can be determined by measuring the difference in intensity between transmitted and received light when delivered at specific wavelengths. This is what is described by the Beer–Lambert law, wherein a change in light intensity is equivalent to the quantity (depth) of the substance and the amount of light absorbed by a known quantity of that substance.

In the 700–1,300 nm range, near-infrared light effectively penetrates tissue several centimeters.[93] Within the NIR range, the primary light absorbing molecules in mammalian tissue are metal complex chromophores: hemoglobin, bilirubin, and cytochrome. The absorption spectrum of oxyhemoglobin (HbO_2) shows a broad peak between 700 and 1,150, deoxyhemoglobin ranges from 650 to 1,000 nm, and cytochromeoxidase aa3 has a broad low peak at 820–840 nm.[94] The frequency of NIR light in commercial devices utilizes wavelengths selected to be sensitive to these biologically important chromophores and generally ranges between 700 and 850 nm where the absorption spectra of Hb and HbO_2 are maximally separated and there is minimal overlap with H_2O.

Correction for Extracerebral Tissue

In order for noninvasive NIRS interrogation of cerebral tissue, photons must penetrate several tissue layers including scalp, skull, and dura. These tissues contain various concentrations of blood and tissue derived chromophores, which potentially confound the signal derived from cortical brain tissue. Using various models employing both computer simulation and experimental tissue preparations, it has been demonstrated that with percutaneous transillumination photons follow an elliptical pathway centered around the transmitter. The mean depth of tissue penetration is proportional to approximately one third the separation distance of the transmitting to receiving optodes.[95] Increasing transmitter/receptor distance increases depth of penetration, but within the safe power limits to prevent direct thermal tissue damage, and since signal intensity decreases exponentially with increasing distance, 5 cm separation appears to be the functional maximal spacing providing a mean depth of NIRS penetration approximating 1.7 cm and enabling interrogation of outer layers of cerebral cortex.[95] However, even with increased transmitter/receiver separation, there is still significant attenuation from extracerebral tissue necessitating further corrections.

Spatial Resolution

Since mean depth of photon penetration approximates one third the transmitter/receiver separation, by utilizing two differentially spaced receiving optodes – one spaced more closely and the other spaced farther from the transmitter – a degree of spatial resolution can be achieved. Accordingly, the closer receiver (e.g., 3 cm separation) detects primarily superficial tissue, while the farther optode (e.g., 4 cm separation) reflects deeper tissue. Incorporation of a subtraction algorithm enables calculation of the difference between the two signals and thus a measure of deeper, cortical tissue saturation. Thus, differential spacing of receiving optodes can provide spatial resolution to distinguish signals from cerebral versus extracerebral tissues.[96]

Temporal Resolution

With time domain NIRS techniques, those photons detected as arriving at a receiver later relative to those detected sooner following a pulsed optical signal have a longer tissue pathlength. This longer pathlength may be assumed to correspond to greater depth of tissue penetration and thus reflective of cerebral tissue. An important assumption in this analysis is the homogeneity of interrogated tissue – a condition that is not necessarily consistent with biological reality.

Partitioning of Cerebral Arterial and Venous Blood

All cerebral NIRS devices measure mean tissue oxygen saturation and, as such, reflect hemoglobin saturation in venous, capillary, and arterial blood comprising the sampling volume. For cerebral cortex, it can be demonstrated that on average tissue hemoglobin is distributed in a proportion of 70% venous and 30% arterial, based on correlations between position emission tomography (PET) and NIRS.[97] However, clinical studies have demonstrated that there may be considerable biologic variation in individual cerebral arterial/venous ratios between patients, further underscoring that use of a fixed ratio may produce significant divergence from actual in vivo tissue oxygen saturation thus confounding even "absolute" measures of cerebral oxygenation, such as frequency domain NIRS and time domain NIRS.[98]

In clinical practice, therefore, the use of cerebral NIRS as a trend monitor with interventions designed to preserve an individual patient's cerebral saturation values close to their individual baseline values (e.g., equating each patient's unique baseline saturation value to 100%, and treating deviations from that 100% baseline) has produced a significantly lower incidence of adverse clinical events in patients undergoing coronary artery bypass (CAB) surgery.[99] A trend monitoring approach thus minimizes confounds introduced by biologic variation in individual cerebral arterial/venous ratios and outer layer tissue composition since these can produce an "offset" in measured saturation values and result in inaccurate therapy if based on the assumption that a device is measuring "absolute" in vivo cerebral oxygenation. Indications for interventions based on NIRS are summarized in Table 8.2.

An important clinical factor is that measurement of cortical oxygen saturation is uninfluenced by perfusion characteristics, enabling measurements to be made continuously during non-pulsatile cardiopulmonary bypass and circulatory arrest states. The advantages and limitations of NIRS are summarized in Table 8.3.

Table 8.2 Indications for intervention

Absolute values less than 55% especially if the drop was sustained for more than 5 min
Difference between left and right hemispheres exceeding 30%
Current to baseline values ratio less than 0.8

Table 8.3 Advantages and limitations of cerebral oximeter as neuromonitor during aortic surgery

Advantages
Noninvasive
Easy application and interpretation
Continuous monitor
Useful even in non-pulsatile circulation (CPB, circulatory arrest with ACP)
Portable
No significant hazard from photons
Bilateral
Limitations
Cannot diagnose the etiology of low values (emboli vs. hypoperfusion)
Regional saturation limited to frontal lobe, ischemia of other regions may go unnoticed
Electrocautery may interfere with readings
Ratio of arterial to venous blood may vary during anesthesia causing inaccuracies, so trends rather than single value should be followed, baseline value should be obtained
External carotid blood flow interruption or ischemia in external carotid artery territory can cause low saturations
Normal rSO$_2$ has been recorded in brain with no flow such as in brain-dead patients

NIRS and Retrograde Cerebral Perfusion

There have been a variety of case reports of the ability of cerebral NIRS to detect onset of cerebral ischemia during aortic arch surgeries and there is growing interest in the role of cerebral NIRS as a measure of adequacy of RCP and ACP in this setting.[92,100–102] While RCP may provide additional cooling and may act to minimize cerebral embolization during circulatory arrest[103] factors that likely explain the success seen by some groups using this technique – there is recognition that RCP provides less than 10% of anterograde cerebral blood flow as determined in both a swine model and a study in nonhuman primates.[104,105] This has been reflected in lower regional cerebral tissue oxygen saturation (rSO_2) values seen during clinical NIRS monitoring in RCP versus ACP.[106,107] While clinical outcomes are variable, several large experiential reviews have concluded that for an extended interval, ACP appears to result in lower risk of CNS injury.[108,109]

NIRS and Anterograde Cerebral Perfusion (ACP)

In assessing the role of NIRS monitoring during ACP, a study was undertaken in 46 consecutive aortic arch surgery patients in whom ACP was established by perfusion of the right subclavian artery (with or without left carotid artery perfusion) or by separate concomitant perfusion of the innominate and the left carotid arteries. In this study, bilateral regional cerebral tissue oxygen saturation index was monitored using INVOS 4100 NIRS and the study utilized stroke as the primary clinical end point.[110] Six patients died in hospital, and six patients (13%) experienced a perioperative stroke. In patients with stroke, rSO_2 values were significantly lower during ACP, and rSO_2 also tended to be lower in the affected hemisphere. Their analysis indicated that during ACP, rSO_2 decreasing to between 76% and 86% of baseline had a sensitivity of up to 83% and a specificity of up to 94% in identifying individuals with stroke. In their assessment, it was concluded

that monitoring of rSO_2 by using NIRS during ACP allows detection of clinically important cerebral desaturations and that it could help predict perioperative neurologic sequelae thus supporting its use as a noninvasive trend monitor of cerebral oxygenation.[110] In another study of 59 DHCA patients managed with ACP, it was reported that a sustained drop in cerebral rSO_2 below 55% correlated with transient neurological events, with the important caveat that cerebral NIRS was limited for detection of embolic events or hypoperfusion in the basilar region.[102]

NIRS and Cerebral Malperfusion

In adult patients during aortic arch and minimal access surgery, cerebral malperfusion can occur either as a consequence of ascending aortic dissection with occlusion of carotid lumen,[111,112] perfusion cannula malfunction, or due to migration of aortic endoclamp cannula during minimal access cardiac surgery all producing compromise of cerebral perfusion.[113] During DHCA with ACP cerebral ischemia can occur due to kinking or obstruction of the perfusion cannula during selective cerebral perfusion for circulatory arrest procedures – an event which has been documented during slightly more than 10% of such procedures.[114] Coincident with the onset of profound NIRS desaturation, in some cases it is possible to directly visualize the cause – migration of the perfusion catheter with obstruction of the common carotid artery by the catheter balloon – as seen on transesophageal echocardiography (TEE) and shown in Fig. 8.8. Figure 8.9 shows a schematic illustration of such cannula malposition during ACP. It is important to appreciate that in the absence of NIRS or other continuous monitoring, this is an event that would otherwise be clinically silent, as even line pressure of the perfusion cannula would not increase due to persistence of flow down the subclavian artery.

There are also an increasing number of reports indicating that bilateral rSO_2 monitoring can detect contralateral desaturation during unilateral selective antegrade cerebral perfusion (SACP).

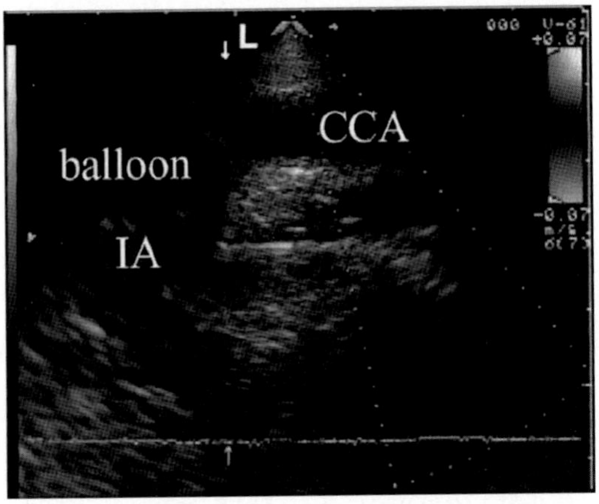

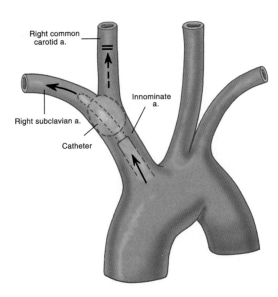

Fig. 8.8 Transesophageal echocardiogram showing the long-axis view of right common carotid artery (CCA) and the balloon at the bifurcation, obstructing the orifice of CCA during selective cerebral perfusion. *IA* innominate artery (Reprinted with permission: Orihashi et al.[114])

Fig. 8.9 Schematic illustration showing obstruction of right common carotid artery (CCA) by the balloon of catheter (CATH) for selective cerebral perfusion. The catheter tip is in the right subclavian artery (SCA). *IA* innominate artery (Redrawn with permission from Orihashi et al.[114])

This can result from an incomplete circle of Willis, which in some series has a prevalence of up to 50% and has been estimated to be a factor in cerebral malperfusion in approximately 15% of patients.[115,116] Early recognition of contralateral desaturation by NIRS during SACP in aortic

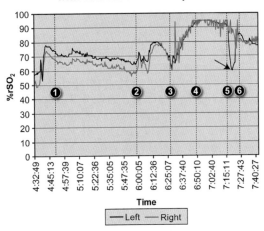

Fig. 8.10 Aortic dissection with unilateral cerebral perfusion via innominate artery. Immediate profound decrease in left rSO_2 followed by perfusion via left carotid artery cannula with restoration of left regional brain saturation (rSO_2). 1, induction of anesthesia; 2, onset of CPB; 3, cooling on CPB; 4, 18°C onset selective cerebral perfusion (SCP) via innominate artery; 5, profound left desaturation; (*arrow*) 6, perfusion via left carotid cannula. This unilateral desaturation is most probably because of incomplete circle of Willis (Reprinted with permission from the reference; André Denault et al.[122] by SAGE Publications, Inc. All rights reserved. ©)

dissection cases lead to cannulation and perfusion of the left carotid artery separately (Fig. 8.10). In a more recent case report, cerebral rSO_2 monitoring was utilized during selective cerebral perfusion in the absence of systemic CPB during repair of traumatic aortic arch rupture and detected both episodes of cerebral malperfusion and, most critically, acute thrombosis of carotid artery graft leading to thrombectomy and restoration of flow.[117] Therefore, the ability of cerebral oximetry to detect onset of critical levels of cerebral hypoperfusion is well attested and may be expected to play a critical role in up to 10–15% of such patients.

NIRS Versus $SJVO_2$ Monitoring

Since the electroencephalogram (EEG) becomes progressively attenuated below 25°C, $SJVO_2$ and cerebral NIRS have been advocated to monitor cerebral well-being during aortic surgery with

DHCA. Since NIRS is noninvasive, bilateral and more acceptable for clinical use, several authors tried to correlate $SJVO_2$ and rSO_2 measured by NIRS so that NIRS can be used as the alternative to invasive $SJVO_2$ monitoring of metabolic suppression in patients undergoing DHCA. No clear correlation has been shown between rSO_2 and $SJVO_2$ values during cardiac surgery and DHCA.[91,118,119] This discrepancy could be explained by several factors. NIRS is a highly regional measure of frontal cortical oxygen saturation, whereas $SJVO_2$ reflects global cerebral mixed venous oxygen saturation and is thus reflective of global changes in oxygenation. NIRS reflects the combined oxygen saturation in the arterial, venous, and capillary blood in the brain and can be affected by extracerebral tissue oxygenation unlike $SJVO_2$, which measures mixed venous cerebral oxygen saturation. The ratio of venous to arterial blood content changes with hypothermia and could explain the wide interindividual variation of rSO_2 and lack of correlation with $SJVO_2$. In addition to hypothermia, hemodilution during cardiac surgery may have different effects on rSO_2 and $SJVO_2$. Mild to moderate hemodilution caused decreased rSO_2 but had no effect on $SJVO_2$ values.[119] Several other perioperative factors affect rSO_2 measurements and anesthesiologists should be aware of these conditions (Table 8.4).

Table 8.4 Causes of low cerebral oximeter rSO_2 readings

Hypotension
Hypoxemia
Arterial cannula malposition on CPB
Malposition of ACP cannula
Head position and SVC cannula obstruction (may cause hyperemia and hyperperfusion)
Hemodilution
Anemia
Hypocapnia and respiratory alkalosis
Hypothermia with Alpha-stat management
Hyperthermia
Faster rate of rewarming
Convulsions
Inadequate depth of anesthesia
Cerebral embolism/hypoperfusion
Intracranial hemorrhage/increased intracranial pressure/cerebral edema
Jaundice and abnormal hemoglobins

Key Points

1. Multimodal monitoring using NIRS, EEG and TCD decreased hospital length of stay and neurologic complications after coronary bypass surgery.

2. Postoperative neurological dysfunction is more common after aortic surgery than any other cardiac surgical procedure. Neurological dysfunction leads to increased mortality and poor quality of life.

3. Multimodal neuromonitoring is useful in the early detection of events during open and endovascular aortic surgical procedures leading to postoperative neurological dysfunction. Early detection and immediate interventions (such as increasing blood pressure) may improve outcome of these patients.

4. SSEPs have several applications during aortic surgery. Baseline SSEP abnormalities, early disappearance of SSEP during cooling period, late reappearance during rewarming and appearance of new asymmetric signals in the post bypass period are indications for immediate intervention and are predictors of postoperative neurological dysfunction.

5. EEG isoelectricity and disappearance of both cortical and subcortical SSEP signals are used as end points for cooling before the initiation of DHCA.

6. TCD measured middle cerebral artery blood flow velocities can be used to diagnose malperfusion during bypass, evaluate the adequacy of antegrade and retrograde cerebral perfusion and detect microembolism during surgical manipulations of the aorta. However, TCD is user dependent and prone for artifacts.

7. Jugular venous oxygen saturation is used to assess the residual metabolic activity of the brain during cooling to DHCA. SJVO2 is also used to evaluate selective antegrade cerebral perfusion during DHCA. SJVO2 cannot reliably detect regional or focal ischemia.

8. Like SJVO2, near infrared spectroscopy also provides information about cerebral oxygenation. However, NIRS measures regional cerebral oxygen saturation. Poor correlation is expected between these two modalities.

NIRS provides useful information about cerebral perfusion and malperfusion during antegrade and retrograde perfusion.

9. NIRS is non-invasive, portable and can be interpreted easily. Lower saturation values can occur because of multiple reasons and an algorithmic approach is necessary.

10. Anesthesiologists need to have an understanding of the basic principles, applications, advantages and more importantly limitations of each and every neuromonitoring technique.

References

1. Poli de Figueiredo LF. Prevention and amelioration of neurologic dysfunction after complex aortic surgery: a task for critical care practitioners. *Crit Care Med.* 2004;32:1426–1427.
2. Di Eusanio M, Schepens MA, Morshuis WJ, et al. Brain protection using antegrade selective cerebral perfusion: a multicenter study. *Ann Thorac Surg.* 2003;76:1181–1188.
3. Ehrlich MP, Ergin MA, McCullough JN, et al. Predictors of adverse outcome and transient neurological dysfunction after ascending aorta/hemiarch replacement. *Ann Thorac Surg.* 2000;69:1755–1763.
4. Fleck TM, Czerny M, Hutschala D, Koinig H, Wolner E, Grabenwoger M. The incidence of transient neurologic dysfunction after ascending aortic replacement with circulatory arrest. *Ann Thorac Surg.* 2003;76:1198–1202.
5. Tan ME, Morshuis WJ, Dossche KM, Kelder JC, Waanders FG, Schepens MA. Long-term results after 27 years of surgical treatment of acute type A aortic dissection. *Ann Thorac Surg.* 2005;80:523–529.
6. Ueda T, Shimizu H, Ito T, et al. Cerebral complications associated with selective perfusion of the arch vessels. *Ann Thorac Surg.* 2000;70:1472–1477.
7. Ergin MA, Uysal S, Reich DL, et al. Temporary neurological dysfunction after deep hypothermic circulatory arrest: a clinical marker of long-term functional deficit. *Ann Thorac Surg.* 1999;67:1887–1890.
8. Krahenbuhl ES, Immer FF, Stalder M, Englberger L, Eckstein FS, Carrel TP. Temporary neurological dysfunction after surgery of the thoracic aorta: a predictor of poor outcome and impaired quality of life. *Eur J Cardiothorac Surg.* 2008;33:1025–1029.
9. Erdos G, Tzanova I, Schirmer U, Ender J. Neuromonitoring and neuroprotection in cardiac anaesthesia. Nationwide survey conducted by the Cardiac Anaesthesia Working Group of the German Society of Anaesthesiology and Intensive Care Medicine. *Anaesthesist.* 2009;58:247–258.
10. Daily PO, Trueblood HW, Stinson EB, Wuerflein RD, Shumway NE. Management of acute aortic dissections. *Ann Thorac Surg.* 1970;10:237–247.
11. Klem GH, Luders HO, Jasper HH, Elger C. The ten-twenty electrode system of the International Federation. The International Federation of Clinical Neurophysiology. *Electroencephalogr Clin Neurophysiol Suppl.* 1999;52:3–6.
12. American Clinical Neurophysiology Society. Guideline 9D: guidelines on short-latency somatosensory evoked potentials. *J Clin Neurophysiol.* 2006;23:168–179.
13. Banoub M, Tetzlaff JE, Schubert A. Pharmacologic and physiologic influences affecting sensory evoked potentials: implications for perioperative monitoring. *Anesthesiology.* 2003;99:716–737.
14. Richards CD. Actions of general anaesthetics on synaptic transmission in the CNS. *Br J Anaesth.* 1983;55:201–207.
15. Pathak KS, Ammadio M, Kalamchi A, Scoles PV, Shaffer JW, Mackay W. Effects of halothane, enflurane, and isoflurane on somatosensory evoked potentials during nitrous oxide anesthesia. *Anesthesiology.* 1987;66:753–757.
16. Peterson DO, Drummond JC, Todd MM. Effects of halothane, enflurane, isoflurane, and nitrous oxide on somatosensory evoked potentials in humans. *Anesthesiology.* 1986;65:35–40.
17. Samra SK, Vanderzant CW, Domer PA, Sackellares JC. Differential effects of isoflurane on human median nerve somatosensory evoked potentials. *Anesthesiology.* 1987;66:29–35.
18. Porkkala T, Kaukinen S, Hakkinen V, Jantti V. Median nerve somatosensory evoked potentials during isoflurane anaesthesia. *Can J Anaesth.* 1997;44:963–968.
19. Wolfe DE, Drummond JC. Differential effects of isoflurane/nitrous oxide on posterior tibial somatosensory evoked responses of cortical and subcortical origin. *Anesth Analg.* 1988;67:852–859.
20. Schindler E, Thiel A, Muller M, Milosevic M, Langer C, Hempelmann G. Changes in somatosensory evoked potentials after sevoflurane and isoflurane. A randomized phase III study. *Anaesthesist.* 1996;45(Suppl 1):S52–S56.
21. Zhang J, Liang WM. Effects of volatile anesthetics on cortical somatosensory evoked potential and Bispectral index. *Zhonghua Yi Xue Za Zhi.* 2005;85:2700–2703.
22. Rehberg B, Ruschner R, Fischer M, Ebeling BJ, Hoeft A. Concentration-dependent changes in the latency and amplitude of somatosensory-evoked potentials by desflurane, isoflurane and sevoflurane. *Anästhesiol Intensivmed Notfallmed Schmerzther.* 1998;33:425–429.
23. Schindler E, Muller M, Zickmann B, Osmer C, Wozniak G, Hempelmann G. Modulation of somatosensory evoked potentials under various concentrations of desflurane with and without nitrous oxide. *J Neurosurg Anesthesiol.* 1998;10:218–223.
24. McPherson RW, Sell B, Traystman RJ. Effects of thiopental, fentanyl, and etomidate on upper extremity somatosensory evoked potentials in humans. *Anesthesiology.* 1986;65:584–589.
25. Koht A, Schutz W, Schmidt G, Schramm J, Watanabe E. Effects of etomidate, midazolam, and thiopental on

median nerve somatosensory evoked potentials and the additive effects of fentanyl and nitrous oxide. *Anesth Analg.* 1988;67:435–441.

26. Drummond JC, Todd MM, Hoi Sang U. The effect of high dose sodium thiopental on brain stem auditory and median nerve somatosensory evoked responses in humans. *Anesthesiology.* 1985;63:249–254.

27. Boisseau N, Madany M, Staccini P, et al. Comparison of the effects of sevoflurane and propofol on cortical somatosensory evoked potentials. *Br J Anaesth.* 2002;88:785–789.

28. Liu EH, Wong HK, Chia CP, Lim HJ, Chen ZY, Lee TL. Effects of isoflurane and propofol on cortical somatosensory evoked potentials during comparable depth of anaesthesia as guided by bispectral index. *Br J Anaesth.* 2005;94:193–197.

29. Clapcich AJ, Emerson RG, Roye DP Jr, et al. The effects of propofol, small-dose isoflurane, and nitrous oxide on cortical somatosensory evoked potential and bispectral index monitoring in adolescents undergoing spinal fusion. *Anesth Analg.* 2004;99: 1334–1340.

30. Fung NY, Hu Y, Irwin MG, Chow BE, Yuen MY. Comparison between sevoflurane/remifentanil and propofol/remifentanil anaesthesia in providing conditions for somatosensory evoked potential monitoring during scoliosis corrective surgery. *Anaesth Intensive Care.* 2008;36:779–785.

31. Ku AS, Hu Y, Irwin MG, et al. Effect of sevoflurane/nitrous oxide versus propofol anaesthesia on somatosensory evoked potential monitoring of the spinal cord during surgery to correct scoliosis. *Br J Anaesth.* 2002;88:502–507.

32. Kalkman CJ, Leyssius AT, Bovill JG. Influence of high-dose opioid anesthesia on posterior tibial nerve somatosensory cortical evoked potentials: effects of fentanyl, sufentanil, and alfentanil. *J Cardiothorac Anaesth.* 1988;2:758–764.

33. Schubert A, Drummond JC, Peterson DO, Saidman LJ. The effect of high-dose fentanyl on human median nerve somatosensory-evoked responses. *Can J Anaesth.* 1987;34:35–40.

34. Sloan TB, Fugina ML, Toleikis JR. Effects of midazolam on median nerve somatosensory evoked potentials. *Br J Anaesth.* 1990;64:590–593.

35. Sloan TB. Nondepolarizing neuromuscular blockade does not alter sensory evoked potentials. *J Clin Monit.* 1994;10:4–10.

36. Lassen NA. Cerebral blood flow and oxygen consumption in man. *Physiol Rev.* 1959;39:183–238.

37. Paulson OB, Strandgaard S, Edvinsson L. Cerebral autoregulation. *Cerebrovasc Brain Metab Rev.* 1990;2:161–192.

38. Florence G, Guerit JM, Gueguen B. Electroencephalography (EEG) and somatosensory evoked potentials (SEP) to prevent cerebral ischaemia in the operating room. *Neurophysiol Clin.* 2004;34:17–32.

39. Symon L. The relationship between CBF, evoked potentials and the clinical features in cerebral ischaemia. *Acta Neurol Scand Suppl.* 1980;78:175–190.

40. Branston NM, Symon L, Crockard HA. Recovery of the cortical evoked response following temporary middle cerebral artery occlusion in baboons: relation to local blood flow and PO2. *Stroke.* 1976;7:151–157.

41. Matsumiya N, Koehler RC, Traystman RJ. Consistency of cerebral blood flow and evoked potential alterations with reversible focal ischemia in cats. *Stroke.* 1990;21:908–916.

42. Wilson GJ, Rebeyka IM, Coles JG, et al. Loss of the somatosensory evoked response as an indicator of reversible cerebral ischemia during hypothermic, low-flow cardiopulmonary bypass. *Ann Thorac Surg.* 1988;45:206–209.

43. Griepp RB, Ergin MA, Lansman SL, Galla JD, Pogo G. The physiology of hypothermic circulatory arrest. *Semin Thorac Cardiovasc Surg.* 1991 July;3:188–193.

44. Svensson LG, Crawford ES, Hess KR, et al. Deep hypothermia with circulatory arrest. Determinants of stroke and early mortality in 656 patients. *J Thorac Cardiovasc Surg.* 1993;106:19–28.

45. Ueda Y, Miki S, Kusuhara K, Okita Y, Tahata T, Yamanaka K. Surgical treatment of aneurysm or dissection involving the ascending aorta and aortic arch, utilizing circulatory arrest and retrograde cerebral perfusion. *J Cardiovasc Surg (Torino).* 1990;31: 553–558.

46. Borst HG, Schaudig A, Rudolph W. Arteriovenous fistula of the aortic arch: repair during deep hypothermia and circulatory arrest. *J Thorac Cardiovasc Surg.* 1964;48:443–447.

47. Griepp RB, Stinson EB, Hollingsworth JF, Buehler D. Prosthetic replacement of the aortic arch. *J Thorac Cardiovasc Surg.* 1975;70:1051–1063.

48. Stecker MM, Cheung AT, Pochettino A, et al. Deep hypothermic circulatory arrest: II. Changes in electroencephalogram and evoked potentials during rewarming. *Ann Thorac Surg.* 2001;71:22–28.

49. Stecker MM, Cheung AT, Pochettino A, et al. Deep hypothermic circulatory arrest: I. Effects of cooling on electroencephalogram and evoked potentials. *Ann Thorac Surg.* 2001;71:14–21.

50. Coles JG, Taylor MJ, Pearce JM, et al. Cerebral monitoring of somatosensory evoked potentials during profoundly hypothermic circulatory arrest. *Circulation.* 1984;70(3 Pt 2):I96–I102.

51. Guerit JM, Verhelst R, Rubay J, et al. The use of somatosensory evoked potentials to determine the optimal degree of hypothermia during circulatory arrest. *J Card Surg.* 1994;9:596–603.

52. Stecker MM. Neurophysiology of surgical procedures for repair of the aortic arch. *J Clin Neurophysiol.* 2007;24:310–315.

53. Guerit JM, Baele P, de Tourtchaninoff M, Soveges L, Dion R. Somatosensory evoked potentials in patients undergoing circulatory arrest under profound hypothermia. *Neurophysiol Clin.* 1993;23:193–208.

54. Ghariani S, Matta A, Dion R, Guerit JM. Intra- and postoperative factors determining neurological complications after surgery under deep hypothermic circulatory

arrest: a retrospective somatosensory evoked potential study. *Clin Neurophysiol.* 2000;111:1082–1094.

55. Ghariani S, Liard L, Spaey J, et al. Retrospective study of somatosensory evoked potential monitoring in deep hypothermic circulatory arrest. *Ann Thorac Surg.* 1999;67:1915–1918.

56. Sloan TB. Anesthetic effects on electrophysiologic recordings. *J Clin Neurophysiol.* 1998;15:217–226.

57. Sharbrough FW, Messick JM Jr, Sundt TM Jr. Correlation of continuous electroencephalograms with cerebral blood flow measurements during carotid endarterectomy. *Stroke.* 1973;4:674–683.

58. Blume WT, Ferguson GG, McNeill DK. Significance of EEG changes at carotid endarterectomy. *Stroke.* 1986;17:891–897.

59. Grady RE, Weglinski MR, Sharbrough FW, Perkins WJ. Correlation of regional cerebral blood flow with ischemic electroencephalographic changes during sevoflurane-nitrous oxide anesthesia for carotid endarterectomy. *Anesthesiology.* 1998;88:892–897.

60. Sundt TM Jr, Sharbrough FW, Piepgras DG, Kearns TP, Messick JM Jr, O'Fallon WM. Correlation of cerebral blood flow and electroencephalographic changes during carotid endarterectomy: with results of surgery and hemodynamics of cerebral ischemia. *Mayo Clin Proc.* 1981;56:533–543.

61. Trojaborg W, Boysen G. Relation between EEG, regional cerebral blood flow and internal carotid artery pressure during carotid endarterectomy. *Electroencephalogr Clin Neurophysiol.* 1973;34:61–69.

62. Boysen G, Engell HC, Pistolese GR, Fiorani P, Agnoli A, Lassen NA. Editorial: on the critical lower level of cerebral blood flow in man with particular reference to carotid surgery. *Circulation.* 1974;49: 1023–1025.

63. Safi HJ, Brien HW, Winter JN, et al. Brain protection via cerebral retrograde perfusion during aortic arch aneurysm repair. *Ann Thorac Surg.* 1993;56: 270–276.

64. Hicks RG, Poole JL. Electroencephalographic changes with hypothermia and cardiopulmonary bypass in children. *J Thorac Cardiovasc Surg.* 1981;81:781–786.

65. Miller G, Rodichok LD, Baylen BG, Myers JL. EEG changes during open heart surgery on infants aged 6 months or less: relationship to early neurologic morbidity. *Pediatr Neurol.* 1994;10:124–130.

66. Mizrahi EM, Patel VM, Crawford ES, Coselli JS, Hess KR. Hypothermic-induced electrocerebral silence, prolonged circulatory arrest, and cerebral protection during cardiovascular surgery. *Electroencephalogr Clin Neurophysiol.* 1989;72:81–85.

67. Aaslid R, Markwalder TM, Nornes H. Noninvasive transcranial Doppler ultrasound recording of flow velocity in basal cerebral arteries. *J Neurosurg.* 1982;57:769–774.

68. ***Edmonds HL, Jr. Monitoring of cerebral perfusion with transcranial doppler ultrasound. In: Nuwer MR, ed. *Intraoperative Monitoring of Neural Function: Handbook of neurophysiology.Vol 8,* 1st ed. Elsevier, New York; 2008:909–923.

69. Halsey JH Jr. Risks and benefits of shunting in carotid endarterectomy. The International Transcranial Doppler Collaborators. *Stroke.* 1992;23:1583–1587.

70. Edmonds HL Jr, Thomas MH, Ganzel BL, Austin EH. Monitoring brain: transcranial Doppler. In: Coselli JS, Lemaire SA, eds. *Aortic Arch Surgery, Principles, Strategies and Outcomes.* 1st ed. Hoboken, NJ: Wiley-Blackwell; 2008:128–134.

71. Greeley WJ, Ungerleider RM, Kern FH, Brusino FG, Smith LR, Reves JG. Effects of cardiopulmonary bypass on cerebral blood flow in neonates, infants, and children. *Circulation.* 1989;80(3 Pt 1):I209–I215.

72. Neri E, Sassi C, Barabesi L, et al. Cerebral autoregulation after hypothermic circulatory arrest in operations on the aortic arch. *Ann Thorac Surg.* 2004;77:72–79.

73. Tanoue Y, Tominaga R, Ochiai Y, et al. Comparative study of retrograde and selective cerebral perfusion with transcranial Doppler. *Ann Thorac Surg.* 1999;67:672–675.

74. Appoo JJ, Augoustides JG, Pochettino A, et al. Perioperative outcome in adults undergoing elective deep hypothermic circulatory arrest with retrograde cerebral perfusion in proximal aortic arch repair: evaluation of protocol-based care. *J Cardiothorac Vasc Anesth.* 2006;20:3–7.

75. Estrera AL, Garami Z, Miller CC 3rd, et al. Cerebral monitoring with transcranial Doppler ultrasonography improves neurologic outcome during repairs of acute type A aortic dissection. *J Thorac Cardiovasc Surg.* 2005;129:277–285.

76. Ganzel BL, Edmonds HL Jr, Pank JR, Goldsmith LJ. Neurophysiologic monitoring to assure delivery of retrograde cerebral perfusion. *J Thorac Cardiovasc Surg.* 1997;113:748–755.

77. Doblar DD. Intraoperative transcranial ultrasonic monitoring for cardiac and vascular surgery. *Semin Cardiothorac Vasc Anesth.* 2004;8:127–145.

78. Fraser CD Jr, Andropoulos DB. Principles of antegrade cerebral perfusion during arch reconstruction in newborns/infants. *Semin Thorac Cardiovasc Surg Pediatr Card Surg Annu.* 2008;11:61–68.

79. Pugsley W, Klinger L, Paschalis C, Treasure T, Harrison M, Newman S. The impact of microemboli during cardiopulmonary bypass on neuropsychological functioning. *Stroke.* 1994;25:1393–1399.

80. Kimatian SJ, Saliba KJ, Soler X, et al. The influence of neurophysiologic monitoring on the management of pediatric cardiopulmonary bypass. *ASAIO J.* 2008;54:467–469.

81. Spencer MP. Transcranial Doppler monitoring and causes of stroke from carotid endarterectomy. *Stroke.* 1997;28:685–691.

82. Calafiore AM, Bar-El Y, Vitolla G, et al. Early clinical experience with a new sutureless anastomotic device for proximal anastomosis of the saphenous vein to the aorta. *J Thorac Cardiovasc Surg.* 2001; 121:854–858.

83. Eifert S, Reichenspurner H, Pfefferkorn T, et al. Neurological and neuropsychological examination and

outcome after use of an intra-aortic filter device during cardiac surgery. *Perfusion*. 2003;18(Suppl 1):55–60.

84. McCullough TLA. Specialized neurophysiologic monitoring. In: Lake CL, Hines RL, Blitt CD, eds. *Clinical Neuromonitoring. Practical Applications for Anesthesia and Critical Care*. Philadelphia, PA: WB Saunders company; 2001:132–145.

85. Shaaban Ali M, Harmer M, Latto I. Jugular bulb oximetry during cardiac surgery. *Anaesthesia*. 2001;56: 24–37.

86. McCullough JN, Zhang N, Reich DL, et al. Cerebral metabolic suppression during hypothermic circulatory arrest in humans. *Ann Thorac Surg*. 1999;67: 1895–1899.

87. Greeley WJ, Kern FH, Ungerleider RM, et al. The effect of hypothermic cardiopulmonary bypass and total circulatory arrest on cerebral metabolism in neonates, infants, and children. *J Thorac Cardiovasc Surg*. 1991;101:783–794.

88. Mezrow CK, Midulla PS, Sadeghi AM, et al. Evaluation of cerebral metabolism and quantitative electroencephalography after hypothermic circulatory arrest and low-flow cardiopulmonary bypass at different temperatures. *J Thorac Cardiovasc Surg*. 1994;107:1006–1019.

89. Okada M, Sakakibara Y, Suehiro K, et al. Cerebral protection during aortic arch replacement: usefulness of continuous O2 saturation monitoring of internal jugular bulb to optimize cerebral perfusion. *Kyobu Geka*. 1993;46:668–671.

90. Kuwabara M, Nakajima N, Yamamoto F, et al. Continuous monitoring of blood oxygen saturation of internal jugular vein as a useful indicator for selective cerebral perfusion during aortic arch replacement. *J Thorac Cardiovasc Surg*. 1992;103:355–362.

91. Ali MS, Harmer M, Vaughan RS, Dunne JA, Latto IP. Spatially resolved spectroscopy (NIRO-300) does not agree with jugular bulb oxygen saturation in patients undergoing warm bypass surgery. *Can J Anaesth*. 2001;48:497–501.

92. Ogino H, Ueda Y, Sugita T, et al. Monitoring of regional cerebral oxygenation by near-infrared spectroscopy during continuous retrograde cerebral perfusion for aortic arch surgery. *Eur J Cardiothorac Surg*. 1998;14:415–418.

93. McCormick PW, Stewart M, Goetting MG, Dujovny M, Lewis G, Ausman JI. Noninvasive cerebral optical spectroscopy for monitoring cerebral oxygen delivery and hemodynamics. *Crit Care Med*. 1991;19: 89–97.

94. Jobsis FF. Noninvasive, infrared monitoring of cerebral and myocardial oxygen sufficiency and circulatory parameters. *Science*. 1977;198:1264–1267.

95. Matcher SJ, Cope M, Delpy DT. Use of the water absorption spectrum to quantify tissue chromophore concentration changes in near-infrared spectroscopy. *Phys Med Biol*. 1994;39:177–196.

96. Germon TJ, Evans PD, Barnett NJ, Wall P, Manara AR, Nelson RJ. Cerebral near infrared spectroscopy: emitter-detector separation must be increased. *Br J Anaesth*. 1999;82:831–837.

97. Ohmae E, Ouchi Y, Oda M, et al. Cerebral hemodynamics evaluation by near-infrared time-resolved spectroscopy: correlation with simultaneous positron emission tomography measurements. *Neuroimage*. 2006;29:697–705.

98. Watzman HM, Kurth CD, Montenegro LM, Rome J, Steven JM, Nicolson SC. Arterial and venous contributions to near-infrared cerebral oximetry. *Anesthesiology*. 2000;93:947–953.

99. Murkin JM, Adams SJ, Novick RJ, et al. Monitoring brain oxygen saturation during coronary bypass surgery: a randomized, prospective study. *Anesth Analg*. 2007;104:51–58.

100. Higami T, Kozawa S, Asada T, et al. A comparison of changes of cerebrovascular oxygen saturation in retrograde and selective cerebral perfusion during aortic arch surgery. *Nippon Kyobu Geka Gakkai Zasshi*. 1995;43:1919–1923.

101. Hofer A, Haizinger B, Geiselseder G, Mair R, Rehak P, Gombotz H. Monitoring of selective antegrade cerebral perfusion using near infrared spectroscopy in neonatal aortic arch surgery. *Eur J Anaesthesiol*. 2005;22:293–298.

102. Orihashi K, Sueda T, Okada K, Imai K. Near-infrared spectroscopy for monitoring cerebral ischemia during selective cerebral perfusion. *Eur J Cardiothorac Surg*. 2004;26:907–911.

103. Juvonen T, Weisz DJ, Wolfe D, et al. Can retrograde perfusion mitigate cerebral injury after particulate embolization? A study in a chronic porcine model. *J Thorac Cardiovasc Surg*. 1998;115:1142–1159.

104. Boeckxstaens CJ, Flameng WJ. Retrograde cerebral perfusion does not perfuse the brain in nonhuman primates. *Ann Thorac Surg*. 1995;60:319–327. discussion 327–318.

105. Ehrlich MP, Hagl C, McCullough JN, et al. Retrograde cerebral perfusion provides negligible flow through brain capillaries in the pig. *J Thorac Cardiovasc Surg*. 2001;122:331–338.

106. Higami T, Kozawa S, Asada T, et al. Retrograde cerebral perfusion versus selective cerebral perfusion as evaluated by cerebral oxygen saturation during aortic arch reconstruction. *Ann Thorac Surg*. 1999;67:1091–1096.

107. Okita Y, Minatoya K, Tagusari O, Ando M, Nagatsuka K, Kitamura S. Prospective comparative study of brain protection in total aortic arch replacement: deep hypothermic circulatory arrest with retrograde cerebral perfusion or selective antegrade cerebral perfusion. *Ann Thorac Surg*. 2001;72:72–79.

108. Di Eusanio M, Schepens MA, Morshuis WJ, Di Bartolomeo R, Pierangeli A, Dossche KM. Antegrade selective cerebral perfusion during operations on the thoracic aorta: factors influencing survival and neurologic outcome in 413 patients. *J Thorac Cardiovasc Surg*. 2002;124:1080–1086.

109. Matalanis G, Hata M, Buxton BF. A retrospective comparative study of deep hypothermic circulatory arrest, retrograde, and antegrade cerebral perfusion in aortic arch surgery. *Ann Thorac Cardiovasc Surg*. 2003;9:174–179.

110. Olsson C, Thelin S. Regional cerebral saturation monitoring with near-infrared spectroscopy during selective antegrade cerebral perfusion: diagnostic performance and relationship to postoperative stroke. *J Thorac Cardiovasc Surg*. 2006;131:371–379.

111. Sakaguchi G, Komiya T, Tamura N, et al. Cerebral malperfusion in acute type A dissection: direct innominate artery cannulation. *J Thorac Cardiovasc Surg*. 2005;129:1190–1191.

112. Janelle GM, Mnookin S, Gravenstein N, Martin TD, Urdaneta F. Unilateral cerebral oxygen desaturation during emergent repair of a DeBakey type 1 aortic dissection: potential aversion of a major catastrophe. *Anesthesiology*. 2002;96:1263–1265.

113. Schneider F, Falk V, Walther T, Mohr FW. Control of endoaortic clamp position during Port-Access mitral valve operations using transcranial Doppler echography. *Ann Thorac Surg*. 1998;65:1481–1482.

114. Orihashi K, Sueda T, Okada K, Imai K. Malposition of selective cerebral perfusion catheter is not a rare event. *Eur J Cardiothorac Surg*. 2005;27:644–648.

115. Hoksbergen AW, Legemate DA, Csiba L, Csati G, Siro P, Fulesdi B. Absent collateral function of the circle of Willis as risk factor for ischemic stroke. *Cerebrovasc Dis*. 2003;16:191–198.

116. Merkkola P, Tulla H, Ronkainen A, et al. Incomplete circle of Willis and right axillary artery perfusion. *Ann Thorac Surg*. 2006;82:74–79.

117. Santo KC, Barrios A, Dandekar U, Riley P, Guest P, Bonser RS. Near-infrared spectroscopy: an important monitoring tool during hybrid aortic arch replacement. *Anesth Analg*. 2008;107: 793–796.

118. Leyvi G, Bello R, Wasnick JD, Plestis K. Assessment of cerebral oxygen balance during deep hypothermic circulatory arrest by continuous jugular bulb venous saturation and near-infrared spectroscopy. *J Cardiothorac Vasc Anesth*. 2006;20:826–833.

119. Yoshitani K, Kawaguchi M, Iwata M, et al. Comparison of changes in jugular venous bulb oxygen saturation and cerebral oxygen saturation during variations of haemoglobin concentration under propofol and sevoflurane anaesthesia. *Br J Anaesth*. 2005;94:341–346.

120. Stockard J, Bickford R. The neurophysiology of anesthesia. In: Gordon E, ed. *A Basis and Practice of Neuroanesthesia*. Amsterdam: Excerpta Medica; 1975:3–46.

121. McCullough JN, Galla JD, Ergin MA, Griepp RB. Central nervous system monitoring during operations on the thoracic aorta. *Op Tech Thorac Cardiovasc Surg*. 1999;1:87–96.

122. Denault A, Deschamps A, Murkin JM, et al. A proposed algorithm for the intraoperative use of cerebral near-infrared spectroscopy. *Semin Cardiothorac Vasc Anesth*. 2007;11:274–281.

Understanding Open Repair of the Descending Thoracic and Thoracoabdominal Aorta

9

Jay K. Bhama, Scott A. LeMaire, John R. Cooper, and Joseph S. Coselli

Introduction

Although substantial innovation has characterized the field of aortic surgery during the last 50 years, successful repair remains a formidable challenge. Aortic repair has grown to encompass adjuncts designed to ameliorate specific surgical morbidities, such as spinal cord and renal ischemia, while the strategy of repair remains largely dictated by the extent of repair. Repair of the distal aorta, namely the descending thoracic and thoracoabdominal aorta, poses different risks than proximal aortic repair; thus, operative strategy and expected outcomes vary tremendously with the extent of aorta that requires replacement. An accurate understanding of the extent of aortic involvement is critical to planning appropriate management.

Distal aortic disease may be limited to the descending thoracic aorta within the chest or may extend beyond the level of the diaphragmatic hiatus to involve varying segments of the abdominal aorta, necessitating a thoracoabdominal aortic repair. Descending thoracic aortic aneurysms (DTAAs) usually begin just distal to the left subclavian artery and extend toward, but not past, the crura of the diaphragm. In contrast, repair of thoracoabdominal aortic aneurysms (TAAAs)

necessitates exposing the aorta above and below the diaphragm and generally involves replacing the segment from which the visceral arteries arise (Fig. 9.1). Thus, repairing TAAAs is generally more complicated than repairing DTAAs.

The Crawford classification schema is used to convey additional information about TAAA repairs, dividing them into four "extents" according to the amount of aorta replaced (Fig. 9.1). Crawford extent I repairs involve the aorta from just distal to the left subclavian artery to the origins of the celiac axis and superior mesenteric arteries and may also involve the renal arteries, but these repairs do not extend into the infrarenal aorta. Extent II repairs involve nearly the entire distal aorta, from near the left subclavian artery to the infrarenal abdominal aorta, often extending to the iliac bifurcation. Extent III repairs involve the mid-descending thoracic aorta (below the sixth rib) and a variable amount of the abdominal aorta. Extent IV repairs begin within the diaphragmatic hiatus and extend through the abdominal aorta. Of the four extents of TAAA repair, extent II involves the greatest risk because it requires replacing the largest amount of aorta.

Although endovascular approaches have become increasingly popular for repairing DTAA, their use remains largely experimental for TAAA repair because of the difficulty of incorporating the visceral arteries into a purely endovascular repair. Furthermore, endovascular approaches do not yet have the well-established long-term durability of open graft replacement, which has allowed

J.K. Bhama (✉)
Division of Cardiac Surgery, Department of Cardiothoracic Surgery, University of Pittsburgh Medical Center, Pittsburgh, PA, USA
e-mail: bhamajk@upmc.edu

K. Subramaniam et al. (eds.), *Anesthesia and Perioperative Care for Aortic Surgery*,
DOI 10.1007/978-0-387-85922-4_9, © Springer Science+Business Media, LLC 2011

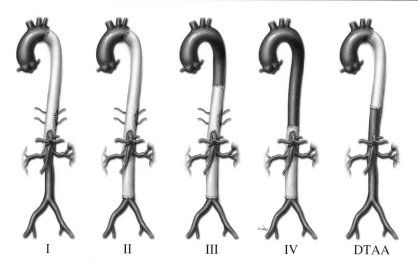

I	II	III	IV	DTAA

Fig. 9.1 The Crawford classification system for describing the extent of thoracoabdominal aortic repair. A descending thoracic aortic aneurysm (DTAA) repair is shown for comparison. Note that DTAA repair does not extend beyond the diaphragmatic hiatus to involve the visceral arteries and thus is generally a less complex repair (Reproduced with permission from Baylor College of Medicine)

that approach to remain the "gold-standard" for the management of both DTAAs and TAAAs.

Early Development of Surgical Approach

Surgical repair of the distal aorta began in the early 1950s with several successful aortic repairs in which a portion of the abdominal aorta (which did not involve any of the visceral arteries) was replaced with an aortic homograft. As aortic repair moved toward the descending thoracic aorta, it was not clear whether the ischemia caused by aortic clamping would be tolerated without complication, especially after the failed attempt at descending thoracic aortic resection and homograft replacement by Lam and Aram. In 1953, DeBakey and Cooley were able to successfully "clamp-and-sew" a homograft replacement of the descending thoracic aorta. And in 1955, Etheredge and colleagues reported a successful homograft replacement of a TAAA, and they used a small temporary shunt to deliver blood to the downstream aorta. That same year, Rob reported several TAAA repairs performed by using a "clamp-and-sew" approach. At that time, it was believed that the spinal cord and visceral organs could tolerate brief periods of ischemia, although individual patients' tolerance to ischemia varied for reasons that were not well understood.

During the next several years, the availability of Dacron grafts facilitated the use of an extra-anatomic approach in which the graft would be placed around the aneurysm and also used as a bypass shunt. For TAAAs, these repairs would be done in a bottom-to-top fashion to quickly restore blood flow to the visceral organs. However, these repairs were associated with high rates of death, paraplegia, and kidney failure.

In 1973, Crawford detailed his experience with 23 TAAA patients, revolutionizing the technique for TAAA repair by drawing on other surgical applications—Javid's anatomic graft inclusion technique, Spencer's experimental reimplantation of lumbar or intercostal arteries, and Carrel and Guthrie's experimental use of direct suture of vessel orifices to reattach the visceral arteries. By achieving a survival rate of 96%, Crawford's approach became the foundation for current surgical approaches to TAAA repair.

Symptomatology and Diagnosis

Thoracic aortic disease often remains asymptomatic until dissection or rupture occurs. When specific symptoms are present, they are usually related to aneurysmal expansion and compression of surrounding structures or to malperfusion related to dissection. Pain is the most common symptom and may be located in the chest, back, abdomen, or flank. Compression of the esophagus may lead to dysphagia, whereas impingement on the trachea or proximal bronchi may result in coughing, wheezing, or pneumonitis. Vocal cord paralysis or hoarseness may occur if the recurrent laryngeal nerve is involved. Bleeding from the airway (hemoptysis) or gastrointestinal tract (hematemesis) may occur if aneurysms erode into these structures. Spontaneous paraplegia, incontinence or abnormal urination, cold or painful extremities, nausea, vomiting, and abdominal pain may all be signs of malperfusion caused by aortic dissection. The onset of symp-

toms is generally considered an indication of impending rupture or significant perfusion failure and should prompt careful and immediate evaluation.

However, most thoracic aortic disease is discovered incidentally by imaging studies ordered for the evaluation of other, unrelated problems. Thus, the diagnosis of thoracic aortic disease is primarily dependent on radiologic imaging. A plain chest radiograph may show widening of the descending thoracic aortic shadow, which is often enhanced by calcification. More sophisticated imaging, such as computed tomography or magnetic resonance imaging, is required for a more precise understanding of the aortic disease process, as well as the disease's location and extent (Fig. 9.2). Contrast aortography is

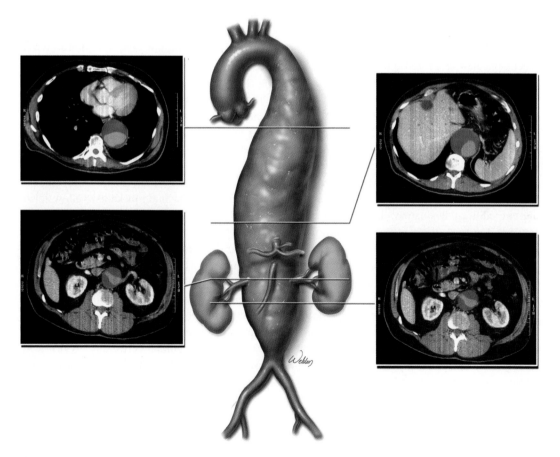

Fig. 9.2 Contrast-enhanced computed tomography (CT) images of the aorta. Such images provide important information about the severity of aortic disease, as well as identifying its anatomic location and extent. An extensive thoracoabdominal aortic aneurysm is depicted here with CT images at the level of the mid-descending thoracic aorta and the supraceliac, juxtarenal, and infrarenal abdominal aorta (Reproduced with permission from Cohn[14] Copyright © McGraw-Hill, 2008, Fig. 54.7)

generally not required, although it is often useful for evaluating other vascular problems, such as visceral or iliac artery stenosis.

Indications for Repair

Replacing the aorta can be life-saving in patients with distal aortic disease. However, surgical intervention carries significant risks for both morbidity and mortality. Surgical intervention is therefore indicated primarily when the risk of rupture or other catastrophic complications exceeds the risks associated with surgical intervention. In asymptomatic patients, elective surgical repair of distal aortic aneurysms is indicated when aneurysm diameter exceeds 6.5 cm or when the rate of expansion exceeds 1 cm per year. However, this threshold is often lowered for patients with aneurysm-causing genetic conditions, particularly connective tissue disorders. Uncomplicated distal aortic dissection is generally managed medically because the risks associated with surgical repair have traditionally exceeded those associated with medical treatment. However, in patients with a preexisting distal aortic aneurysm, acute dissection creates a particularly unstable situation that often warrants urgent surgical intervention to prevent rupture. Symptomatic patients should undergo careful and expeditious evaluation, including suitable imaging, to assess the severity and extent of aortic involvement. Acute pain and hypotension are generally considered clear indications for immediate surgical intervention in suitable candidates.

In the modern era, it is not uncommon for endovascular repair of the descending thoracic aorta to eventually fail in such a manner as to necessitate subsequent open repair in which the endovascular device is removed and replaced with a Dacron graft. A variety of factors may cause the stent-graft to fail, including continued dilatation of the aorta at the landing zones; ongoing expansion of the aneurysm because of an inadequate seal between the stent-graft and aorta (Type 1 endoleak); bleeding into the aneurysmal sac from any covered branch artery, such as an intercostal or lumbar artery (Type 2 endoleak); infection of the device; collapse, narrowing, or "bird-beaking" of the stent-graft related to placement of a straight stent-graft in a curved section of the aorta (such as that near the left subclavian artery); and device malfunctions such as fracture of the scaffolding struts.

Anesthesia

The importance of adequate intraoperative monitoring and venous access cannot be overemphasized. All patients typically undergo placement of a right radial or brachial arterial line, a pulmonary artery catheter, and a large-bore central venous catheter capable of allowing rapid fluid administration. Agents recommended for anesthesia induction are chosen according to the patient's hemodynamics and cardiac contractile state. Muscle relaxation is usually achieved with pancuronium bromide unless motor-evoked potential monitoring is to be used, in which case shorter-acting agents are administered during initial intubation and monitoring-electrode placement and then are reversed. Presence of muscle relaxants will not allow a proper motor-evoked potential response to be generated, even in intact spinal tracts. All patients are orotracheally intubated with a double-lumen endobronchial tube or left mainstem bronchial blockade to allow selective deflation of the left lung, ensuring adequate exposure of the descending thoracic aorta and reducing the chance of damage to the lung from manipulation while the patient is heparinized. Occasionally, distortion of tracheobronchial anatomy by a large aneurysm will make the use of a standard left-sided double-lumen tube impossible. In this situation, a right-sided tube, placed with fiber-optic guidance, usually works well. Placement of a lumbar spinal drain for measuring spinal fluid pressures and removing fluid is done in extent I and II TAAA repairs and occasionally in extent III and IV repairs, depending on clinical circumstances. Frequent arterial blood gas analysis and close monitoring of serum electrolytes and the hematocrit are necessary. Broad-spectrum antibiotics are given before skin incision to minimize surgical site infection.

During aortic replacement, attention to volume status by the surgeon and anesthesiologist is important to avoid wide fluctuation in blood pressure and perhaps organ dysfunction. Hydration with crystalloid solutions is initiated at the start of the operation to maintain filling pressures. Mannitol may also be administered at the induction of anesthesia to help maintain diuresis. It is important to try to keep the systemic blood pressure within a normal range during aortic cross-clamping. Hypertension is often encountered after aortic cross-clamp placement causes a large increase in afterload. Vasodilating agents such as nitroglycerin, nicardipine, or nitroprusside may be used as needed. In situations where left heart bypass (LHB) is employed as an adjunct, increasing flow through the left heart circuit can be an effective means of blood pressure control in the vessels above the proximal cross-clamp. Blood loss is closely monitored, and lost blood is replaced. The hypotension that typically occurs with removal of the aortic cross-clamp is avoided or attenuated by discontinuing vasodilating agents before declamping and especially infusing fluids to account for volume lost during the repair. It is often desirable to achieve hypervolemia with rapid fluid administration just before clamp release. Reinfusion of shed blood recycled from a cell-saving device is particularly important in decreasing the amount of transfusion and even avoiding it in some cases. In many cases, fresh frozen plasma and platelet transfusion are necessary to restore adequate clotting function. Acidosis encountered during aortic cross-clamping is treated aggressively with sodium bicarbonate infusion. At the conclusion of the procedure, changing the double-lumen tube to a single-lumen one is desirable but may not be possible because upper airway edema is common, so the exchange may need to be delayed for some hours.

Strategy for Repair

We use a multimodal repair strategy that is based on the extent of aortic replacement (Table 9.1). Less extensive disease is repaired expeditiously with a standard "clamp-and-sew" technique. For more extensive repairs, such as extent I and II TAAA repairs, we use additional perfusion strategies and techniques to manage spinal cord and other end-organ ischemia.[1-3] Additional adjuncts may be used in patients with certain comorbidities or other risk factors, such as acute presentation.

Patients undergo repair with mild permissive hypothermia (32–34°C) and moderate heparinization (1 mg/kg) to preserve the microcirculation. Aggressive reattachment of patent intercostal and lumbar arteries, particularly those between T8 and L2, and sequential aortic clamping are used whenever possible.[4]

Table 9.1   Current strategy for surgical repair of descending thoracic and thoracoabdominal aortic aneurysms

All descending thoracic and thoracoabdominal aortic repairs
- Moderate heparinization (1 mg/kg)
- Permissive mild hypothermia (32–34°C, nasopharyngeal)
- Aggressive reattachment of segmental arteries, especially between T8 and L1
- Sequential aortic clamping when possible

All thoracoabdominal aortic repairs
- Perfusion of renal arteries with 4°C crystalloid solution when possible

Crawford extent I and II thoracoabdominal aortic repairs
- Cerebrospinal fluid drainage
- Left heart bypass during proximal anastomosis
- Selective perfusion of celiac axis and superior mesenteric artery during intercostal and visceral anastomoses

Certain extensive or highly complex aortic repairs
- Hypothermic circulatory arrest
- Elephant trunk or reversed elephant trunk technique

Surgical Technique

Positioning

Operative techniques for repair of DTAAs and
TAAAs vary according to the severity and extent
of the disease being treated. Adequate exposure
is of paramount importance and remains a fundamental principle of DTAA and TAAA repair.
Ideally, the patient is positioned in a modified
right lateral decubitus position with the shoulders
at 60–80° and the hips flexed to 30–40° from
horizontal (Fig. 9.3). A beanbag is used to secure
the patient in this position. Draping should allow
access to the entire left chest, abdomen, and both
groins.

Exposure

Descending thoracic aortic aneurysms are
repaired through a left thoracotomy (Fig. 9.3a)
and are usually reached by entering through the
sixth intercostal space (although the fifth intercostal space may be used to optimize exposure of
the distal aortic arch, if necessary). For extent I
and II TAAA repairs, the incision is extended
across the costal margin and into the abdomen,
terminating at the level of the umbilicus unless
further exposure is necessary to address iliac
artery disease (Fig. 9.3b). For the less extensive
extent III repair, the seventh or eighth intercostal
space is entered, and the incision is curved into
the abdomen. Acute angulations near the costal
margin should be avoided to prevent tissue

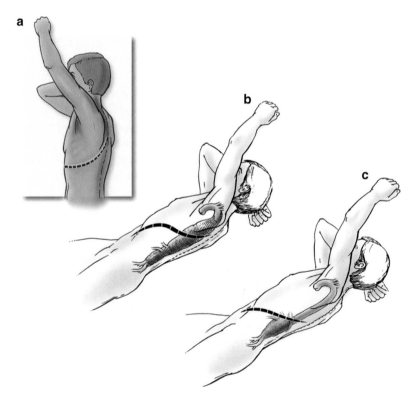

Fig. 9.3 Approaches to exposure used in descending thoracic and thoracoabdominal aortic repairs of different
extents. The patient is positioned in a modified right lateral decubitus position that optimizes exposure of the
descending thoracic and thoracoabdominal aorta while
also exposing the femoral vessels. (**a**). A lateral thoracotomy is used for descending thoracic aortic repairs.
(**b**). For Crawford extent I–III thoracoabdominal aortic
repairs, a curvilinear incision is made. (**c**). For Crawford
extent IV thoracoabdominal aortic repairs, a more linear
incision suffices (Reproduced with permission from
Baylor College of Medicine)

necrosis. For extent IV repair, a straight oblique incision is made through the ninth or tenth interspace (Fig. 9.3c). This facilitates control of the thoracic aorta while the predominantly abdominal repair is performed.

Cerebrospinal Fluid Drainage

During aortic replacement, a varying number of intercostal and lumbar arteries are sacrificed; coupled with significant fluctuations in blood pressure that are related to aortic clamping, this devascularization enhances the risk of spinal cord ischemia and resultant paraplegia or paraparesis. Therefore, in patients with the most extensive aneurysms (i.e., those necessitating extent I and II TAAA repairs), we use cerebrospinal fluid (CSF) drainage.[5,6] Other centers expand the use of CSF drainage to extent III thoracoabdominal repair, as well as to extensive endovascular thoracic repair. After induction, an 18-gauge intrathecal catheter is placed through the second or third lumbar space. The catheter permits passive drainage of CSF and allows the CSF pressure to be carefully monitored during the operation to achieve a target pressure between 8 and 10 mmHg. The CSF drain is left in place for approximately 48 h after the aortic repair because spinal cord ischemia may occur intraoperatively or in a delayed fashion postoperatively; thus, attentive monitoring is suggested. Risks associated with CSF drainage include intracranial bleeding, perispinal hematoma, and meningitis.

Motor- or somatosensory-evoked potentials may be monitored to estimate spinal cord motor neuron function during aortic replacement and to guide the use of spinal perfusion-enhancing measures, such as selecting specific intercostal arteries for reattachment, increasing perfusion pressure, or enhancing CSF drainage. Monitoring motor-evoked potentials requires preserving basal motor function. Additional strategies used by others to protect against spinal cord ischemia include inducing regional spinal hypothermia by means of direct epidural infusion of cold perfusate or the use of naloxone with barbiturate-based anesthesia to reduce spinal metabolism.[7]

Left Heart Bypass

For patients undergoing extent I and II TAAA repairs, as well as select patients with poor cardiac function, LHB is used to provide distal perfusion and effectively unload the left ventricle. A closed-circuit in-line centrifugal pump without a cardiotomy reservoir, oxygenator, or warming device is used to deliver oxygenated blood distal to the aortic segment being replaced (Fig. 9.4). After heparin (1 mg/kg) is administered, cannulas are placed in the left inferior pulmonary vein and the distal descending thoracic aorta or the left femoral artery. Cannulating the distal descending thoracic aorta has become our preferred approach because it eliminates the need for femoral artery exposure, as well as the potential complications related to femoral artery repair. Typically, LHB is instituted with flows of 1.5–2.5 L/min. Additionally, using LHB allows quick adjustment of the proximal arterial pressure and reduces the need for pharmacologic intervention.

Selective Visceral Perfusion

For patients with extent I and II TAAA repairs, the LHB circuit can be used to provide visceral perfusion (Fig. 9.4). Individual 9-F balloon perfusion catheters are placed within the origins of the celiac and superior mesenteric arteries and are perfused with oxygenated blood from a Y-branch off the arterial return tubing of the LHB circuit. This reduces the total mesenteric and hepatic ischemic times to just a few minutes, even during these complex aortic reconstructions. Potential benefits include reduced risk of postoperative coagulopathy and bacterial translocation from the bowels.

Cold Crystalloid Renal Perfusion

Whenever possible, we protect the kidneys by intermittently perfusing them with cold (4°C) crystalloid to establish renal hypothermia (Fig. 9.4). This practice is supported by our clinical trial comparing cold crystalloid to

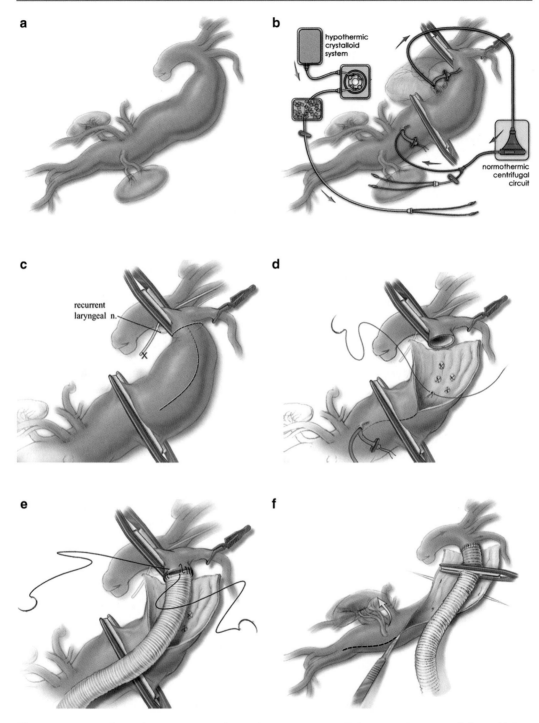

Fig. 9.4 Drawings illustrating an extent II thoracoab-dominal repair. (**a**). The diseased aortic segment extends from the left subclavian artery to the aortoiliac bifurcation. (**b**). Left heart bypass (LHB) is used to provide distal perfusion during this complex repair. Perfusion catheters branch off the LHB circuit to provide selective visceral perfusion to the celiac axis and mesenteric arteries. A separate perfusion system is set up to deliver cold crystalloid to the kidneys. (**c**). Whenever possible, the phrenic, vagus, and recurrent laryngeal nerves are preserved during the repair. The isolated segment of aorta is opened longitudinally and divided circumferentially a few centimeters beyond the proximal clamp. (**d**). Patent upper intercostal arteries are oversewn.

g

h

i

j

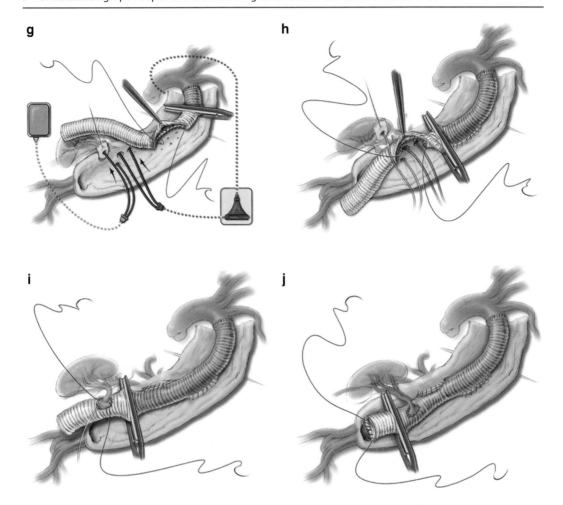

Fig. 9.4 (continued) (**e**). The proximal anastomosis is performed with continuous suture. (**f**). LHB is then stopped, and the proximal clamp is repositioned distally and onto the graft. Flow is restored to the left subclavian artery, and the remainder of the aneurysm is opened longitudinally to expose the entire extent of repair. (**g**). Balloon perfusion catheters are placed in the celiac axis and superior mesenteric artery to deliver isothermic blood and in the renal arteries to provide cold crystalloid perfusion. Patent lower intercostal arteries are reattached to an opening in the graft. (**h**). The aortic clamp is repositioned further down the graft to restore circulation to the spinal cord. An island of visceral arteries is anastomosed to a hole cut into the graft. (**i**). The left renal artery is mobilized on a button of aortic tissue and separately anastomosed to a small hole in the graft. (**j**). The clamp is again moved distally, and the final anastomosis is completed in an "open-distal" manner at the level of the aortic bifurcation in this extensive repair (Reproduced with permission from Cohn[14] Copyright © McGraw-Hill, 2008, Fig. 54.7.)

isothermic blood, which established that cold crystalloid renal perfusion protects against acute renal dysfunction.[8,9] The cold crystalloid (lactated Ringer's solution prepared with 12.5 g/L mannitol and 125 mg/L methylprednisolone) is administered as a 200–400-mL bolus every 15–20 min, with careful monitoring to ensure that the patient is not overcooled or overloaded with fluid. Our recent clinical trial comparing cold blood perfusion to cold crystalloid perfusion did not establish the superiority of one technique over the other for preventing acute renal dysfunction. However, we prefer cold crystalloid perfusion because it is easier to implement.

Use of Hypothermic Circulatory Arrest in Distal Aortic Repair

Kouchoukos and other authors routinely use HCA during repair of extensive aneurysms involving the thoracoabdominal aorta, and these investigators cite the protective effect of hypothermia against spinal cord ischemia.[10] However, we use HCA on an as-needed basis for high-risk patients, such as those with a proximal descending thoracic aorta that cannot be clamped because of rupture, severe atherosclerosis or calcification (i.e., porcelain aorta), large thrombus, or extensive aneurysm in which the aortic arch is also grossly aneurysmal (i.e., mega-aorta) (Fig. 9.5). The risks associated with HCA use in distal aortic repair include coagulopathy, cold injury to the lung, retraction injury to a heparinized lung, and adult respiratory distress syndrome.

In cases necessitating the use of HCA, cardiopulmonary bypass is initiated by establishing venous drainage through a 28–32-F, long, multiholed cannula inserted into the left femoral vein and positioned in the right atrium, as verified by transesophageal echocardiography. Vacuum-assisted venous drainage is used, and flows of 1.8–2.4 L/min/m² or 50 mL/min/kg are achieved. To prevent left ventricular distention, an angled cannula (20- or 22-F) connected to a Y-branch of the venous line is placed through the inferior pulmonary vein into the left atrium; alternatively, a cannula may be placed in the left atrial appendage or the pulmonary artery.

In younger patients with minimal atherosclerosis, the arterial return cannula is a 20- or 22-F straight cannula placed in the left femoral artery; in older patients with severe atherosclerosis or thrombus, a 22-F angled cannula is placed in the

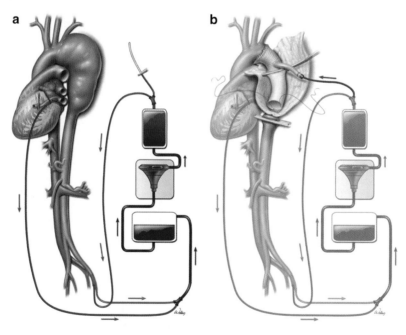

Fig. 9.5 Drawing illustrating the use of hypothermic circulatory arrest in descending thoracic aortic replacement. (**a**). Cardiopulmonary bypass is performed via a venous drainage cannula inserted into the left femoral vein and an arterial return cannula in the left femoral artery. Additional drainage and cardiac decompression are provided by a cannula placed in the left atrium via the inferior pulmonary vein. Circulatory arrest is initiated when electrocerebral silence is achieved, and the proximal anastomosis is then performed. (**b**). The branch in the replacement graft is used to restore coronary and brachiocephalic perfusion via the arterial return line while the distal aspect of the repair is performed (Reproduced with permission from Gravlee et al.[16] Copyright © Lippincott, Williams, and Wilkins, 2008, Fig. 32.5.)

lower descending thoracic aorta. Alternatively, the return cannula may be placed in the left common carotid artery or the left axillary artery, either directly or through a conduit graft. Systemic cooling is initiated, and for added protection we administer methylprednisolone (5–10 mg/kg), sodium thiopental (10–15 mg/kg), lidocaine (100 mg), and a short-acting β (beta) blocker. After the patient has been cooled to electrocerebral silence (which typically occurs at a nasopharyngeal temperature of 15–18°C), circulatory arrest is initiated. The aneurysm is opened, and the proximal anastomosis is constructed. On completion, a Y-limb from the arterial line is connected to a side branch of the graft. The graft is deaired and clamped, pump flow is restored to the upper body, and the rest of the aortic repair is performed. The traditional perfusion techniques used with HCA in aortic arch repair (such as cardioplegia or selective cerebral perfusion) are generally not employed.

Elephant Trunk Approach for Extensive Aortic Repair

Surgical repairs of extensive aortic aneurysms (i.e., repairs that involve replacing almost the entire aorta, which are often called "mega-aorta" repairs) require a specialized approach to enable sufficient exposure of all diseased segments. Such repairs are usually done in two stages. The traditional sequence involves replacing the proximal aorta during the first operation and replacing the distal aorta during the second operation.

The first stage involves a full arch replacement that leaves a 10-cm "trunk" of Dacron graft hanging beyond the distal anastomosis, into the proximal descending thoracic aorta. During the second-stage completion repair—which is usually performed several weeks later—the elephant trunk is used to facilitate the proximal anastomosis when the distal aorta is replaced. This technique allows clamping of the elephant trunk, rather than the replaced arch or proximal descending thoracic aorta. If the distal aorta is determined to be at greater risk of rupture than the proximal aorta, this procedure can be reversed; in this

reverse elephant trunk procedure, the distal aorta is replaced first, and the elephant trunk is inverted inside the most proximal section of the distal aortic replacement graft to facilitate subsequent arch repair.

Management of the Descending Thoracic Aorta

The proximal portion of the aneurysm is isolated by placing a clamp on an adjacent, healthy aortic segment (Fig. 9.6). Often, the clamp is placed distal to the left subclavian artery, but should more proximal access be required, the aorta may be clamped between the left subclavian and left common carotid arteries while a separate bulldog clamp is applied to the left subclavian artery. The vagus and recurrent laryngeal nerves are identified and protected. Then, with the electrocautery, the aorta is opened and cleared of any thrombus or debris. Upper intercostal arteries are oversewn to prevent backbleeding. The aorta is then transected 2–3 cm from the proximal clamp so as not to injure the esophagus and surrounding structures. The proximal aortic cuff is then prepared for anastomosis by separating it completely from the underlying esophagus. The graft is then anastomosed with meticulous suturing to ensure hemostasis. If the proximal aortic clamp has been placed between the left subclavian and left common carotid arteries, it should be repositioned onto the graft after the proximal anastomosis is complete to allow perfusion of the left subclavian artery.

For extensive DTAAs that approach the diaphragmatic hiatus, patent lower intercostal arteries may be reattached as buttons or islands of tissue to a small hole cut into the graft. A distal clamp is generally not used during DTAA repair, allowing an open distal anastomosis to satisfactory aortic tissue. If acute dissection is present, the false lumen is obliterated in the distal suture line whenever possible; if chronic dissection is present, a fenestration is created between the true and false lumens to minimize malperfusion.

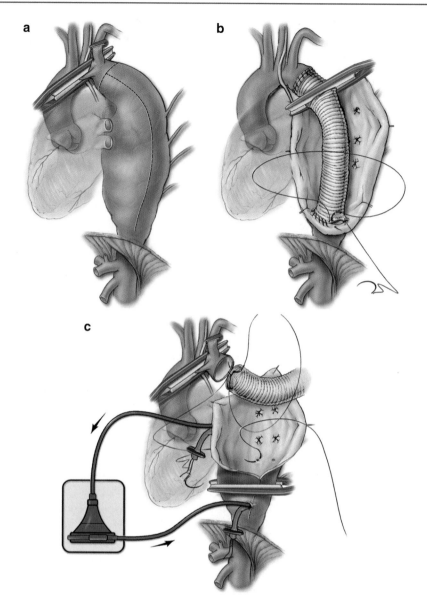

Fig. 9.6 Drawings illustrating graft repair of a descending thoracic aortic aneurysm. (**a**). The aorta has been clamped proximal to the left subclavian artery, which has also been occluded with a bulldog clamp. The descending thoracic aorta may be replaced (**b**) by using the "clamp-and-sew" technique or, (**c**) more rarely, by using left heart bypass for distal aortic perfusion (Reproduced with permission from Cohn[14] Copyright © McGraw-Hill, 2008, Fig. 54.7.)

Management of Thoracoabdominal Aorta

In patients undergoing extent I, II, or III TAAA repair (Fig. 9.4), the proximal anastomosis is completed as described above; this anastomosis is made more distally in extent III repairs than in extent I or II repairs. For extent IV TAAA repairs, the proximal clamp is placed just superior to the diaphragm, and the proximal anastomosis is usually performed end-to-end at the level of the diaphragm but may also be performed as a bevel that lies behind the origins of the visceral arteries. If the extent of repair necessitates it, the longitudinal aortotomy is extended posterior to the left renal artery origin to the distal end of the aneurysm. One or more pairs of intercostal or lumbar arteries are reattached to the replacement graft; the other pairs are oversewn to prevent back-bleeding. As needed, extent-specific protective adjuncts are adopted as described in previous sections, with the goal of enhancing survival and reducing complications in the most extensive forms of distal aortic repair, namely extent I and II TAAA repairs.

The visceral arteries are then incorporated into the repair in accordance with the extent of repair. Disease involving the visceral arteries may necessitate endarterectomy or renal artery stenting to improve circulation. In extent I TAAA repairs, the visceral arteries are incorporated by surrounding them with a beveled distal anastomosis. In extent II, III, or IV TAAA repairs, the specific needs of the patient determine whether an "island" or individual branch technique is used to incorporate the visceral arteries. The island technique is the simpler approach and involves attaching a patch of native aorta that includes the origins of all four visceral vessels to an oval opening in the graft. In this approach, the anastomosis closely follows the ostia of the vessels to reduce the amount of native aortic tissue that is incorporated into the repair. When the left renal artery has been displaced from the other visceral branches because of dissection or aneurysm expansion, it is separately reattached (Fig. 9.4).

Some patients, such as those with connective tissue disorders, are at high risk for the development of patch aneurysms involving the residual aortic tissue adjacent to reattached branch arteries.[11] In these patients, as well as in those in whom the visceral vessels themselves are compromised (i.e., severely atherosclerotic or otherwise diseased), one or more of the visceral arteries can be individually attached by using either separate small-diameter Dacron grafts sewn to the aortic graft or a prefabricated branched aortic graft.

In preparation for the distal anastomosis, the aortic clamp is often relocated distal to the visceral anastomosis to facilitate visceral-organ reperfusion. The final end-to-end anastomosis is then carried out by using an open-distal technique, usually at the level of aortic bifurcation. In cases of chronic aortic dissection, complete mobilization of the aorta with circumferential division may be required to determine the location of the true and false lumens. Additionally, in these cases, the dissecting membrane is fenestrated to ensure perfusion of both lumens. For patients with acute dissections, the false lumen is obliterated by inclusion within the suture line, effectively directing the blood flow entirely to the true lumen.

Closure

After the repair is completed, heparin is reversed with protamine sulfate. Careful attention to hemostasis cannot be overemphasized for all suture lines and cannulation sites. Before closure, the adequacy of renal, visceral, and peripheral perfusion should be assessed. The remaining aneurysm wall is then wrapped around the aortic reconstruction and secured with a running suture. Thoracic drainage tubes are placed within the posterior thorax, and a closed suction drain is placed within the retroperitoneum. After the diaphragm is reapproximated, the ribs are closed with heavy braided suture and stainless steel wire. Pericostal catheters are placed to allow delivery of local anesthetic postoperatively, and the fascia is then closed with heavy monofilament suture.

Postoperative Management

Because of the fragility of the aortic anastomosis in the early postoperative period, blood pressure is kept within a narrow range—between 80 and 90 mmHg—for the first 24–48 h. This is generally achieved with nitroprusside and intravenous β (beta)-antagonists. The target range may be reduced to 70–80 mmHg for patients with particularly fragile aortic tissue, such as those with acute dissection or Marfan syndrome. Although even short periods of hypertension can disrupt suture lines, leading to severe bleeding or pseudoaneurysm formation, periods of hypotension are of equal concern because they may lead to paraplegia or paraparesis.

In patients with a CSF drain, intrathecal pressure is kept between 10 and 12 mmHg during the early postoperative period by passively draining CSF as necessary. Once motor function of the legs is confirmed, the pressure may be increased to 12–15 mmHg. Delayed paraplegia or paraparesis is not uncommon, so patients are carefully monitored. If the patient remains neurologically intact, then the CSF drain is typically removed within 48 h. If paraplegia or paraparesis does arise, it is treated emergently and aggressively. If a CSF drain is not in place, one is inserted immediately, and the intrathecal pressure is reduced to below 10 mmHg. Other treatment modalities that may be helpful include optimizing hemodynamics, raising the mean arterial blood pressure to a higher range (85–95 mmHg), correcting anemia, administering steroids and osmotic diuretics, and preventing fever.

Emerging complications, such as pulmonary and renal complications, are carefully monitored, and corrective measures are taken (such as resuming ventilator support or increasing the patient's blood pressure to better perfuse the kidneys, respectively). Preventing graft infection is extremely important after aortic replacement, given the high mortality risk such infection carries. Meticulous surgical technique and close attention to sterility during surgery cannot be overemphasized. Broad-spectrum antibiotics are administered during the postoperative course until drains and central venous catheters have been removed. The retroperitoneal closed suction drain may be removed after 24 h, and the thoracic drainage tubes are removed when drainage is less than 300 mL/d (typically within 72 h). Aggressive physical therapy and ambulation are emphasized early in the recovery process.

A long-term surveillance protocol is initiated when patients are discharged. Even patients without connective tissue disorders remain at risk for subsequent aneurysm formation in their remaining native aortic segments, including reattachment sites. Additionally, suture lines can progressively weaken over time, especially in patients with poorly controlled hypertension, leading to the development of pseudoaneurysms.

Late infection of aortic replacement grafts may also lead to suture-line disruption and pseudoaneurysm formation. We recommend that all patients undergo at least yearly computed tomographic imaging of the chest and abdomen. This is especially important in patients with connective tissue disorders.

Outcomes

The most common complications in DTAA and TAAA repair are pulmonary complications, affecting approximately 40% of patients. The lack of standardization in defining complications makes it difficult to compare their frequency between surgical centers or between endovascular and open surgical patients. It is also difficult to assess complication risk when large series that span decades are compared to more contemporary series in which modern adjuncts are used. This being said, the most serious complications of DTAA and TAAA repair continue to be death, paraplegia, and renal failure, and emergent or urgent repairs generally involve twice the risk that elective repairs do.

We have previously published results on large series of DTAA and TAAA repairs (387 and 2,286 cases, respectively) spanning a 20-year period.[12,23] In Table 9.2, we present our contemporary experience with 406 patients who underwent various extents of DTAA and TAAA repair over a recent 3-year interval. The 30-day mortality rate was 5.4% ($n=22$) overall and ranged from 3.4% in extent I TAAA repair patients to 7.0% in extent IV TAAA repair patients. We believe that the use of a multimodal approach to spinal cord protection has dramatically reduced rates of permanent paraplegia in recent years because our overall rate is now 1.5% ($n=6$).[13] Renal failure remains a significant complication with an overall rate of 4.6% ($n=24$); rates range from 2.3% in extent I repairs to 9.3% in extent IV repairs. Patients who experience these devastating complications tend to have decreased long-term survival, as well as a diminished quality of life.

Table 9.2 Contemporary outcomes of 406 descending thoracic and thoracoabdominal aortic repairs

Extent/Type of Repair	No. of Patients	30-Day Deaths	Permanent Paraplegia	Permanent Renal Failure
DTAA	57	3 (5%)	0	4 (7%)
TAAA I	88	3 (3%)	0	2 (2%)
TAAA II	101	6 (6%)	2 (2%)	5 (5%)
TAAA III	74	4 (5%)	3 (4%)	2 (3%)
TAAA IV	86	6 (7%)	1 (1%)	8 (9%)
Total	406	22 (5.4%)	6 (1.5%)	21 (5.2%)

DTAA, descending thoracic aortic aneurysm; *TAAA*, thoracoabdominal aortic aneurysm.

Key Notes

1. Careful assessment of symptoms and thorough imaging establishes the urgency of repair, preventing inappropriate delay or hastening of surgical treatment.
2. Thorough preoperative assessment is conducted so that a patient-specific plan for optimizing physiologic reserve and a strategy for operative repair can be developed to enhance the patient's chances of survival and to reduce surgical complications.
3. Cerebrospinal fluid drainage is used in extensive TAAA repair to reduce the likelihood of postoperative paraplegia.
4. Uncomplicated chronic distal dissection is managed with medical treatment until the risk of rupture exceeds the risks associated with repair.
5. After aortic repair, patients are followed with an annual imaging surveillance protocol to enable early detection of new aortic aneurysms or pseudoaneurysms.

Acknowledgments The authors express gratitude to Stephen N. Palmer, PhD, ELS, and Angela T. Odensky, MA, of the Texas Heart Institute, as well as Susan Y. Green, MPH, for editorial assistance, and Scott A. Weldon, MA, CMI, and Carol P. Larson, CMI, for creating the illustrations and assisting with image selection.

References

1. Coselli JS. The use of left heart bypass in the repair of thoracoabdominal aortic aneurysms: current techniques and results. *Semin Thorac Cardiovasc Surg.* 2003;15:326–332.

2. Coselli JS, Bozinovski J, Cheung C. Hypothermic circulatory arrest: safety and efficacy in the operative treatment of descending and thoracoabdominal aortic aneurysms. *Ann Thorac Surg.* 2008;85:956–963. discussion 964.

3. Huh J, LeMaire SA, Bozinovski J, Coselli JS. Perfusion for thoracic aortic surgery. In: Gravlee GP, Davis RE, Stammers AH, Ungerleider RM, eds. *Cardiopulmonary Bypass: Principles and Practice.* 3rd ed. Philadelphia: Lippincott Williams & Wilkins; 2008:647–661.

4. Cambria R. Commentary: Thoracic and thoracoabdominal aneurysm repair: is reimplantation of spinal cord arteries a waste of time? *Perspect Vasc Surg Endovasc Ther.* 2008;20:221–223.

5. Coselli JS, LeMaire SA, Köksoy C, Schmittling ZC, Curling PE. Cerebrospinal fluid drainage reduces paraplegia after thoracoabdominal aortic aneurysm repair: results of a randomized clinical trial. *J Vasc Surg.* 2002;35:631–639.

6. Coselli JS, LeMaire SA, Schmittling ZC, Köksoy C. Cerebrospinal fluid drainage in thoracoabdominal aortic surgery. *Semin Vasc Surg.* 2000;13:308–314.

7. Black JH, Davison JK, Cambria RP. Regional hypothermia with epidural cooling for prevention of spinal cord ischemic complications after thoracoabdominal aortic surgery. *Semin Thorac Cardiovasc Surg.* 2003;15:345–352.

8. Köksoy C, LeMaire SA, Curling PE, et al. Renal perfusion during thoracoabdominal aortic operations: cold crystalloid is superior to normothermic blood. *Ann Thorac Surg.* 2002;73:730–738.

9. LeMaire SA, Jones MM, Conklin LD, et al. Randomized comparison of cold blood and cold crystalloid renal perfusion for renal protection during thoracoabdominal aortic aneurysm repair. *J Vasc Surg.* 2009;49:11–19. discussion 19.

10. Rokkas CK, Kouchoukos NT. Hypothermic circulatory arrest in the treatment of descending thoracic and thoracoabdominal aortic disease. *Ann Thorac Surg.* 2008;86:1399–1400.

11. Dias RR, Coselli JS, Stolf NAG, Dias AR, Mady C, Oliveira SA. Aneurysmal dilation of the reimplant segment of the visceral vessels after thoracoabdominal

aneurysm correction. *Arq Bras Cardiol*. 2003;81: 273–278.

12. Coselli JS, Bozinovski J, LeMaire SA. Open surgical repair of 2286 thoracoabdominal aortic aneurysms. *Ann Thorac Surg*. 2007;83:S862–864.

13. MacArthur RG, Carter SA, Coselli JS, LeMaire SA. Organ protection during thoracoabdominal aortic surgery: rationale for a multimodality approach. *Semin Cardiothorac Vasc Anesth*. 2005;9:143–149.

14. Cohn LH. (ed): *Cardiac Surgery in the Adult*. 3rd ed. New York: McGraw-Hill; 2008.

15. Gardner TJ, Spray TL, eds. *Operative Cardiac Surgery*. 5th ed. New York: Arnold Ltd; 2004.

16. Gravlee GP, Davis RF, Stammers AH, Ungerleider RM, eds. *Cardiopulmonary Bypass: Principles and Practice*. 3rd ed. Philadelphia: Lippincott, Williams, and Wilkins, Wolters Kluwer; 2008.

Further Reading

17. Acher CW, Wynn M. A modern theory of paraplegia in the treatment of aneurysms of the thoracoabdominal aorta: an analysis of technique specific observed/expected ratios for paralysis. *J Vasc Surg*. 2009;49: 1117–1124. discussion 1124.

18. Black JH III, Cambria RP. Contemporary results of open surgical repair of descending thoracic aortic aneurysms. *Semin Vasc Surg*. 2006;19:11–17.

19. Conrad MF, Crawford RS, Davison JK, Cambria RP. Thoracoabdominal aneurysm repair: a 20-year perspective. *Ann Thorac Surg*. 2007;83:S856–861.

20. Coselli JS, LeMaire SA. Tips for successful outcomes for descending thoracic and thoracoabdominal aortic aneurysm procedures. *Semin Vasc Surg*. 2008;21: 13–20.

21. Coselli JS, LeMaire SA, Bhama JK. Thoracoabdominal aortic aneurysm. In: Gardner TJ, Spray TL, eds. *Operative Cardiac Surgery*. 5th ed. New York: Oxford University Press; 2004:483–494.

22. Coselli JS, LeMaire SA, Carter SA, Conklin LD. The reversed elephant trunk technique used for treatment of complex aneurysms of the entire thoracic aorta. *Ann Thorac Surg*. 2005;80:2166–2172. discussion 2172.

23. Coselli JS, LeMaire SA, Conklin LD, Adams GJ. Left heart bypass during descending thoracic aortic aneurysm repair does not reduce the incidence of paraplegia. *Ann Thorac Surg*. 2004;77:1298–1303.

24. Coselli JS, LeMaire SA, Conklin LD, Koksoy C, Schmittling ZC. Morbidity and mortality after extent II thoracoabdominal aortic aneurysm repair. *Ann Thorac Surg*. 2002;73:1107–1115. discussion 1115–1106.

25. Coselli JS, LeMaire SA, Miller CC III, et al. Mortality and paraplegia after thoracoabdominal aortic aneurysm repair: a risk factor analysis. *Ann Thorac Surg*. 2000;69:409–414.

26. LeMaire SA, Carter SA, Coselli JS. The elephant trunk technique for staged repair of complex aneurysms of the entire thoracic aorta. *Ann Thorac Surg*. 2006;81:1561–1569. discussion 1569.

27. LeMaire SA, Miller CC III, Conklin LD, Schmittling ZC, Coselli JS. Estimating group mortality and paraplegia rates after thoracoabdominal aortic aneurysm repair. *Ann Thorac Surg*. 2003;75:508–513.

28. LeMaire SA, Miller CC III, Conklin LD, Schmittling ZC, Köksoy C, Coselli JS. A new predictive model for adverse outcomes after elective thoracoabdominal aortic aneurysm repair. *Ann Thorac Surg*. 2001;71:1233–1238.

29. LeMaire SA, Pannu H, Tran-Fadulu V, Carter SA, Coselli JS, Milewicz DM. Severe aortic and arterial aneurysms associated with a TGFBR2 mutation. *Nat Clin Pract Cardiovasc Med*. 2007;4:167–171.

30. Svensson LG, Crawford ES, Hess KR, Coselli JS, Safi HJ. Experience with 1509 patients undergoing thoracoabdominal aortic operations. *J Vasc Surg*. 1993;17: 357–368.

31. Wong DR, Lemaire SA, Coselli JS. Managing dissections of the thoracic aorta. *Am Surg*. 2008;74:364–380.

Anesthesia for Descending Aortic Surgery

10

Kathirvel Subramaniam and John C. Caldwell

Introduction

Anesthetic management of patients undergoing descending aortic surgery is complex and challenging. Clear understanding of patient's preoperative aortic disease and other comorbidities is important in planning intraoperative management. A preoperative visit is essential to evaluate the perioperative risk and explain the patient of possible complications. Rational planning for the anesthetic care is likely to also warrant review of relevant imaging studies, and often, face-to-face discussion with the surgeon regarding plans for surgical technique, with special attention paid to intended surgical exposure and cardiopulmonary bypass cannulation. Special anesthetic considerations include one-lung ventilation, airway, and hemodynamic and transfusion management. End-organ dysfunction such as stroke, spinal cord injury, myocardial ischemia, and renal failure accounts for morbidity and mortality in these patients. Intensive perioperative monitoring and measures should be undertaken to prevent the occurrence of such complications.

Pathology of Distal Aortic Disease

Patients presenting for descending thoracic and thoracoabdominal aortic surgery have cystic medial degeneration of the aortic media, leading to aortic aneurysm formation or to aortic dissection. Each of these entities is a known risk factor for the development of the other, and thus they often coexist. Other disease processes that may involve the distal aorta include connective tissue disorders such as Marfan syndrome, Loeys–Dietz syndrome, and Ehlers–Danlos syndrome; aortitis, infection, or thoracic trauma. Ultimately, in each of these conditions, the aortic wall may become dilated, leading to rupture and catastrophic exsanguination.

Preoperative Evaluation

Two central questions must be answered during preoperative evaluation of patients with disease of the descending thoracic and thoracoabdominal aorta: First and most important, does the patient need surgery? Second, what is the choice of the surgical technique, that is, is an open or endovascular approach most appropriate? Studies of natural history of descending thoracic aortic aneurysms (DTAA) have shown that repair-free survival is only 24% at 2 years, and survival without surgery drops to 17% (83% mortality) at 5 years. On the other hand, 5-year mortality was

K. Subramaniam (✉)
Department of Anesthesiology, University of Pittsburgh Medical Center – Presbyterian Hospital,
Pittsburgh, PA, USA
e-mail: subramaniamk@upmc.edu

K. Subramaniam et al. (eds.), *Anesthesia and Perioperative Care for Aortic Surgery*,
DOI 10.1007/978-0-387-85922-4_10, © Springer Science+Business Media, LLC 2011

shown to be 39% in matched patients who underwent thoracoabdominal aortic surgical repair.[3] While no randomized studies examining rates of survival for patients who undergo emergent surgery at the time of aortic rupture, most centers report anecdotes of poor outcomes when surgery is forced after aortic rupture. What is known is that few, if any, patients survive aortic rupture with surgery. The average rate of expansion in aortic diameter is 0.2–0.4 cm/year. Factors associated with more rapid expansion, and therefore increased risk of aneurysm disruption, are advanced patient age, aneurysm diameter greater than 60 mm, presence of pain, history of smoking, chronic obstructive lung disease, diastolic hypertension, and renal failure.[4]

Most surgeons elect to operate on symptomatic (unruptured) patients; or upon asymptomatic patients whose aortic diameters exceed 5.5 cm, or whose rates of expansion exceed 1 cm/year. Open surgical repair is ideally planned when the risk of aortic rupture, with medical management alone, exceeds operative risk. Aortic repair via endograft technique has, as of this writing, begun to supplant traditional open repair because of relative ease of surgical technique, and because of a perception of reduced surgical morbidity and mortality.[5,6] The US FDA approved three endograft stent devices for the treatment of descending thoracic aneurysms (GORE TAG thoracic endoprosthesis (approval in March 2005), Talent™ Thoracic Stent Graft System (June 2008), and Zenith® TX2® Thoracic TAA Endovascular Graft (May 2008)).

When open and endovascular techniques are carefully compared, differences in primary outcomes (mortality, stroke rate, and paraplegia) are not entirely clear, and the long-term durability of endovascular repairs is not yet known. While the endograft's indication in treating aneurysms of the descending thoracic and abdominal aorta is comparatively established, the use of endovascular stent repair remains investigational for the treatment of thoracoabdominal aortic aneurysms (TAAA). 'Hybrid' aortic debranching with endovascular repair and the use of fenestrated and branched stent grafts are two alternate therapies undergoing active clinical trials for the treatment of TAAA.

A surgical candidate's life expectancy, independent of their aortic disease, should be considered when selecting the surgical option of endovascular versus open aortic repair. Special dilemmas are posed by patients with chronic obstructive pulmonary disease (COPD) and advanced age, for example, as these factors not only increase risk of spontaneous aortic rupture, but also increase likelihood of perioperative morbidity in relation to the thoracotomy mandated by an open surgical repair. While long-term outcome after endograft repair is not yet clear, it may not be relevant if a patient's expectant survival is less than 5 years because of end-stage lung disease. Unique considerations also appear to apply to saccular aneurysms, pseudoaneurysms, and post-traumatic aneurysms, which can be better dealt with endograft coverage and exclusion of a solitary portion of the aortic wall. Endografts are also used increasingly in patients with ruptured thoracic aneurysms. Meta-analysis of open versus endovascular stenting for ruptured descending thoracic aneurysms has shown 19% 30-day mortality for endovascular repair compared to 33% mortality with open repair.[7] So long as comorbidities are limited; however, patients with Marfan syndrome should probably undergo open repair. This is because the impact of radial forces imposed by an endograft, and which persist in the Marfanoid aortic wall, are not well understood.

Once patient and technical factors dictate the need for open and elective surgical repair, preoperative evaluation, with attention to physiologic reserve, is crucial to assuring the best possible patient outcome. Given that high-risk aortic surgical procedures in high-risk patient population increase perioperative risk,[8] preoperative estimation of risk to individual organ systems, with priority given to cardiac, pulmonary, renal, and nervous systems, are essential for cogent anesthetic planning and proper informed patient consent.

Patients need substantial cardiac reserve to tolerate thoracic aortic clamping and unclamping. Transthoracic echocardiography is routinely used for preoperative assessment of ventricular and valvular function. When compromised ventricular function is observed, or when myocardial ischemia is suspected, additional testing, namely coronary angiography, may be necessary. Though preoperative coronary revascularization may not prevent all perioperative infarctions, revascularization is recommended before elective aortic replacement in those patients for whom revascularization is seen as a long-term outcome benefit.[9] In patients who have previously undergone coronary artery revascularization with the left internal thoracic artery, left carotid to subclavian artery bypass can be considered before aortic replacement, with the goal of avoiding myocardial ischemia when aortic clamp is proximal to the origin of the left subclavian artery (as is commonly done in DTAA and extent I and II TAAA repairs). When preoperative revascularization is not an option, medical optimization with beta-blockers and other cardiac medications is advised before and up to the time of surgery.

Postoperative respiratory failure is the most common complication after descending aortic surgery. Lung function is assessed preoperatively in patients at risk with pulmonary function studies, including forced expiratory volume in 1 s (FEV1), forced vital capacity (FVC), and arterial blood gas analysis. When severe derangement of lung function exists, patients should undergo the less invasive endograft repair so long as the aortic pathology is suitable. Especially when open repair is planned, preoperative respiratory optimization with cessation of smoking (4 weeks), bronchodilators, antibiotics, and incentive spirometry may lessen postoperative pulmonary complications.

Preoperative renal insufficiency is seen in substantial number of patients (13–25%) and is a strong predictor of mortality, early postoperative renal failure, visceral and neurological complications after aortic replacement.[10] A baseline creatinine >2.5 mg/dL is a relative contraindication for surgery, unless the renal artery is involved in the aneurysm process. When a compromise in renal blood supply is related to the aortic pathology, and when reconstruction may result in improved renal perfusion, surgery in fact may be more logical. If nephrotoxic contrast agents are required in patients with borderline renal function, prophylaxis with 5% dextrose and Ringer's lactate solution with 25 g/L mannitol and 1 amp/L sodium bicarbonate may be protective. Once dye loads have been given, it is prudent to examine post-dyeload renal function so that timing of surgery may be delayed until stabilization of renal function is assured.

Postoperative neurological complications (spinal cord ischemia and stroke) occur frequently after DTAA and TAAA repairs. Neurologic deficits increase mortality and disability with aortic reconstruction, irrespective of whether those deficits arose before or during surgery. Presence of cerebrovascular disease (history of stroke, transient ischemic attack, and carotid artery disease) not only increases the incidence of neurologic complications but also affects long-term survival.[10] Patients should be preoperatively screened for cerebrovascular disease, and appropriate intervention should be considered as indicated before elective aortic reconstruction is undertaken.

Review of preoperative imaging will provide useful guidance in formulating rational surgical and anesthetic management plans. Anatomic imaging features of great interest are proximal and distal extent of aortic disease, ascending aortic and arch involvement, presence of mural thrombus, atheroma, and calcification, and branch vessel involvement. Of particular interest to the anesthesiologist is presence of airway compression or distortion, whether it is tracheal or carinal. Pleural effusions may be a harbinger of contained aortic leakage, heart failure, or pulmonary vascular involvement. When possible spinal cord arterial supply, including locations of the arteria radicularis magna (ARM) (also known as Artery of Adamkiewicz), should be sought when reviewing contrast studies (Fig. 10.1). A discussion with the surgeon is required regarding the surgical strategy since it will direct anesthetic management. If the surgical repair involves arch of aorta requiring deep hypothermic circulatory arrest, all considerations of arch surgery (such as temperature management, and cerebral monitoring) will apply. A discussion with the surgeon is essential regarding the need for cerebrospinal fluid (CSF) drainage. If the surgery involves only proximal DTA or in type IV aneurysms, spinal catheter insertion may not be required.

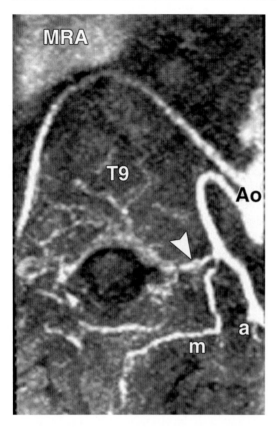

Fig. 10.1 Magnetic resonance Angiography (MRA) showing greater radicular artery of Adamkiewick (*arrowhead*) originating from posterior intercostal artery (a branch of aorta [Ao]) at T_9 level. Anterior (a) and muscular (m) branches are shown (Reprinted with permission obtained from reference[81])

Anesthetic Management

Studies revealing cardiac, pulmonary, renal, and neurologic reserve should be tailored, as earlier described, to a given patient's needs. In addition to airway evaluation, physical exam should incorporate assessment of peripheral pulses and neurologic foci. Recent routine laboratory results should be examined for coagulopathy and metabolic problems. Insertion of spinal and epidural catheters requires screening for coagulopathy. Availability of blood products should be verified, as multiple packed red blood cell units will likely be needed. Fresh frozen plasma, platelets, and cryoprecipitate are arranged in patients with preexisting coagulopathy, emergency repairs, and

redo-surgical procedures. Preoperative informed consent should stress, in relation to risk, complications including renal failure, paraplegia, stroke, ventilatory and cardiac failure, and prolonged intensive care unit stay.

Epidural and Spinal Catheter Placement

Several options exist for catheter placement and reasonable practices vary. So as to take advantage of patient cooperation and reporting of discomfort, we prefer to insert both epidural and cerebrospinal catheters before the anesthetic induction. Insertion of a thoracic epidural catheter insertion in an anesthetized patient may not be advised because of the risk of unrecognized neurological damage. Some anesthesiologists prefer to insert the epidural catheter the day prior to surgery, with the advantage that surgery need not be postponed if a bloody tap is encountered during catheter placement. Other practitioners prefer epidural catheter placement in the postoperative period, once the patient is awake and assessed neurologically. The postoperative insertion approach may be made less practical by the difficulty positioning an awake and ventilated patient with surgical drains and a painful incision. Some elderly patients do well with minimal IV narcotics alone, and epidural analgesia may not be required. Epidural analgesia is a near-must in patients with preoperative narcotic dependence, and in patients with sufficient lung disease that a difficult ventilator wean can be anticipated. The T_5–T_6 interspace is generally used for epidural insertion in DTA surgery, while a T_{10}–T_{11} interspace is accessed in TAAA surgery. Verifying epidural catheter function with local anesthetics is a good practice. Appropriateness of catheter test dosing with epinephrine, to rule out intravascular communication, can be debated. Some anesthesiologists prefer not to employ epidural regional anesthesia during surgery, citing concerns of sympathectomy and hypotension. Still other practitioners use epidural anesthesia to blunt stress response and hypertensive reactions to aortic cross clamping.

Spinal drainage catheters are ideally inserted preoperatively, although insertion after induction of anesthesia is safe in our opinion. In unstable and emergent situations such as leaking aneurysms, subarachnoid drainage may need to be deferred until surgery is complete. After identifying the subarachnoid space with a large spinal needle (14 G) at the L3–L4 interspace, free CSF flow is confirmed. Excessive loss of CSF during catheter insertion is to be avoided. The spinal needle bevel is generally turned cephalad, and the CSF drainage catheter is advanced slowly and carefully so as to leave 5 cm of catheter in the subarachnoid space. A guidewire may be used to stiffen the catheter for insertion if necessary (Fig. 10.2). A catheter should not be inserted against resistance, and if resistance is encountered great care should be used to avoid catheter shear. In the event of catheter non-threading, the needle and catheter are withdrawn as a unit and the procedure is repeated. The decision to postpone or proceed with surgery after encountering a bloody tap is debated, and should be made after discussion with the patient and the surgeon.[11,12] If there is a decision to proceed, the spinal catheter should be inserted in a different interspace. Given that drainage catheters may be maintained for several days following surgery, care is taken to secure

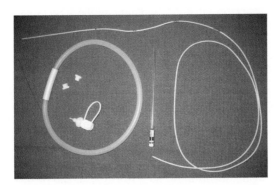

Fig. 10.2 Cerebrospinal fluid (CSF) drainage catheter insertion kit. The kit contains 80 cm closed tip and radiopaque lumbar catheter, which has multiple holes located within 17 mm of the tip and markings at 11, 16, 21, and 24 cm from the tip. It also has 14 G Tuohy needle, guidewire to facilitate insertion of the catheter, luer connector with cap and fixation collars

the catheter and to assure its patency. Catheters are generally sutured to the skin after making a loop and fixed with adhesive tape/op-site/mastasol, and finally secured on the patient's back to the right of the spine. Aspiration through the catheter is confirmed and the drain capped for patient positioning. After positioning, the subarachnoid drainage catheter is connected to a CSF drainage system, and to a manometer/transducer for CSF pressure monitoring (Fig. 10.3a and b). Absolute sterility is maintained in handling the catheter and drainage system, given concerns of meningitis.

Induction

Patients are taken to the operating room and standard ASA monitors applied. A right radial arterial line is inserted under local anesthesia and monitored during induction. If the radial artery is unavailable, brachial or axillary artery cannulation is used. A right-sided pressure monitor is preferred because aortic cross clamp may have to be placed proximal to the left subclavian artery to perform proximal anastomosis (type I and type II aneurysms). In surgery for type III and IV aneurysms, noninvasive blood pressure is first measured in both arms, and radial artery is cannulated in the arm with the higher blood pressure. Blood samples for basal arterial blood gas, activated clotting time (ACT), and thromboelastogram (TEG) are obtained after the arterial line is placed. Blood products should be available in the room before surgery is begun.

Choice of anesthetic drug is less important than titration of drug to the hemodynamic parameters. Hypertensive response and tachycardia should be avoided during anesthesia induction because of attendant increases in aortic wall tension. Fentanyl bolus (5–10 mcg/kg), esmolol (0.5–1 mg/kg), lidocaine (1–2 mg/kg), and deep anesthesia with inhalational anesthetics (1.5 MAC end-tidal concentrations) are useful in blunting hemodynamic response to intubation. Adequate muscle relaxation is required for the insertion of double lumen endotracheal tubes.

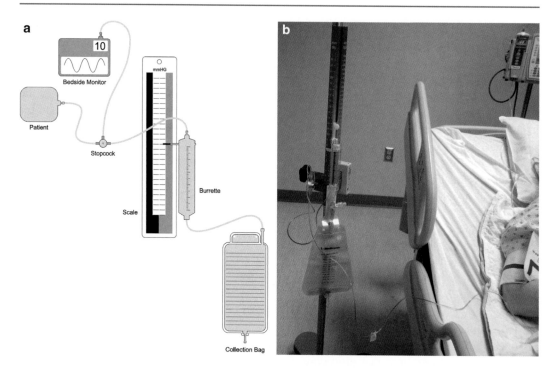

Fig. 10.3 (**a**, **b**) Cerebrospinal fluid drainage and CSF pressure monitoring system

Airway Management

A left-sided endobronchial double lumen tube is the first choice of airway instrument, provided there is no serious carinal compression or distortion created by the aortic aneurysm. The double lumen tube (DLT) is inserted within the proximal trachea, and the bronchoscope inserted through the bronchial lumen in order to guide the DLT into position. This will give an opportunity for endoscopic examination of the carina and left bronchus, and to avoid dangerous and blind insertion of the tube. One should fear catastrophe when blindly advancing an endobronchial tube in the setting of a giant aneurysm which may be compressing the left bronchus or carina. Right-sided DLT may be selected if there is significant distortion of the left bronchus. Positioning the right-sided tube to reliably avoid obstruction of the right upper lobe bronchus may be challenging. Position of the DLT should be recertified after lateral decubitus positioning, and during surgery as concerns over tube migration arise. When airway distortion is extreme, bronchial blocking

catheters may substitute for endobronchial tubes, and as a last resort, right bronchial intubation with a single lumen endotracheal tube can be considered. Hemodynamics and oxygenation should be monitored vigilantly, and should not be ignored during airway manipulations. As a general rule, airway management strategies should be sorted out at the beginning of the surgery and before positioning. Major manipulation of the airway under the surgical drapes after lateral positioning is famously difficult and may be harmful. Even when surgery must be performed with single lumen tracheal intubation, and under full cardiopulmonary bypass (CPB), as may be the case in emergencies and difficult airways, the surgeon may request lung isolation for viewing the surgical field during the post-CPB period. Again, the need for lung isolation should be discussed while the patient is on CPB and appropriate action should be taken during the CPB interval. Bronchial blockers are useful in this situation also, but gentle manipulation of the airway is advised because of bleeding risk while under full heparinization. Once the airway has been bloodied, visualization of structures and device positioning becomes even more difficult. Conversely, attempts to position blockers after cardiopulmonary bypass may result in interruption of effective ventilation, leading to dangerous episodes of hypoxia or hypertensive episodes risking hemorrhage.

Monitoring

Apart from ASA standard monitors, a pulmonary artery catheter (PAC) is inserted through right or left internal jugular vein. Subclavian access may result in catheter kinking once the patient positioned laterally. A PAC with continuous mixed venous oxygen saturation and cardiac output monitoring capabilities is useful in these complex surgical procedures. Optical PACs may be especially useful in the management of multiorgan failure in the postoperative period. A right femoral arterial catheter monitors distal perfusion pressure during partial cardiopulmonary bypass. Involvement of femoral artery in the aneurysmal process should be determined in advance and discussed with the surgeon. Right femoral wide bore central venous access (e.g., 8.5 F) is also established for rapid infusion ability. Since PAC measured pressures and derived values may not truly reflect intravascular volume status and cardiac and valvular function during cross clamping and unclamping, transesophageal echocardiography (TEE) may provide more encompassing hemodynamic monitoring during aortic reconstruction. A comprehensive examination for ventricular function, valve morphology and function, and aortic pathology is best done before positioning the patient. TEE is the modality of choice to evaluate the aortic valve, and the presence of aortic regurgitation which complicates aortic cross clamping. TEE also provides for the earliest possible diagnosis of myocardial ischemia by way of regional wall motion abnormalities (RWMA). Further, TEE assists in the surgery itself: during cannulation of the pulmonary veins, left atrium, right atrium, and descending aorta. TEE is used to confirm the presence of the guidewire in the descending aorta true lumen prior to femoral arterial cannulation.

Body core temperature should be monitored and various sites (pulmonary artery, bladder, esophageal, and nasopharyngeal) are monitored if hypothermic arrest is planned. Esophageal temperature may be misleadingly low while the chest is open and fluctuate with the temperature of the irrigation solution. ACT is used to monitor heparin effect during partial bypass and to check adequate neutralization with protamine after weaning from bypass. Points of care coagulation (POC) tests, such as thromboelastography (TEG), are useful to monitor for coagulopathy and to direct blood product administration before and after chest closure. Pulse oximeter readings, aside from accurately reflecting impaired oxygenation, may be artifactually low or unobtainable by virtue of patient position, hypovolemia, hypotension, hypothermia, and the use of vasoconstrictors. Ear, nose, and lips are few preferred locations for pulse ox transducers. Preexisting lung disease and intraoperative pathophysiology may conspire to produce large gradients between expired CO_2 values and true arterial CO_2 levels. To this end, frequent blood gas evaluation is appropriate.

The relatively high incidence of the much dreaded complication of paraplegia after TAAA repair has prompted investigation of a role for neurophysiologic monitoring modalities such as somatosensory evoked potentials (SSEP) and transcranial motor evoked potentials (tcMEP). Cunningham and Laschinger[13] described four patterns of SSEP changes during TAAA repair (Fig. 10.4). A type I pattern indicates inadequate distal perfusion, in which case they observed a loss of SSEP signals within 8–9 min of cross clamping. In some subjects, this response was reversed by institution of distal perfusion or by increasing distal perfusion pressure to more than 60 mmHg. In a subsequent observation, the same investigators showed increased incidence of paraplegia when type I SSEP responses were allowed to persist uncorrected for more than 30 min.[13] A type II pattern was indicative of adequate distal perfusion. A type III SSEP pattern was observed when spinal cord blood supply from a critical intercostal artery was interrupted. Here, SSEP were maintained after cross clamping, but declined once critical intercostal arteries were

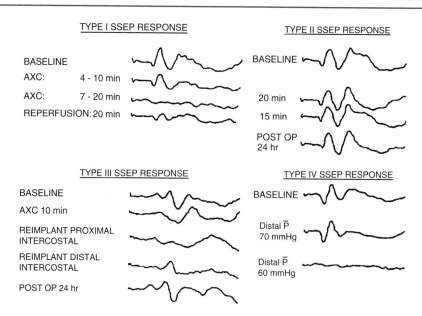

Fig. 10.4 Types of SSEP responses after aortic cross clamping during thoracoabdominal aortic repair (Reprinted with permission from[13])

ligated or clamped. Subsequent normalization of SSEP signals was observed once the intercostal artery was reimplanted. A type IV pattern was characterized by a gradual reduction in SSEP amplitude over 30 min, and is characteristic of lower extremity ischemia because of arterial dissection or embolization, or more commonly, femoral arterial cannulation. Brain stroke can also produce cortical SSEP changes but affect both lower and upper extremities. SSEPs can reliably predict paraplegia, however, only when spinal cord ischemia is extensive enough to affect global spinal cord function. Bearing in mind that SSEP monitors only the posterior sensory white matter of the spinal cord, it is appreciated that SSEP signals cannot reliably disclose ischemia involving only anterior motor neurons and corticospinal tracts. SSEP monitoring has, on the other hand, been shown to have high false-positive (67%) and false-negative (13%) rates.[14]

Transcranial motor evoked potentials (tcMEP) can detect ischemia along anterolateral white matter tracts and spinal gray matter, and reliably predict ischemia involving motor areas of spinal cord. MEP monitoring changes may trigger the surgeon and anesthesiologist to employ hemodynamic and surgical manipulations. Those include

a deliberate increase in mean arterial blood pressure (MAP), active CSF drainage, or intercostal artery reimplantation. When instituted in a timely manner, these manipulations should result in normalization of the MEP changes. Failure of the changes to normalize may indicate injury to the spinal cord and predict paraplegia after TAAA repair. To this end, clinical studies have shown improved neurologic outcomes with MEP monitoring for TAAA repair.[15,16] While a balanced anesthetic with adequate muscle paralysis and 0.5 MAC of inhalational agent permits uninhibited SSEP monitoring, MEPs are more sensitive to inhalational anesthetics, and a total intravenous anesthetic regimen is required. MEP monitoring also requires either complete avoidance of muscle relaxants or carefully monitored incomplete neuromuscular blockade.[17]

Studies comparing MEP and SSEP monitoring during TAAA surgery have shown MEPs to serve as an earlier indicator of spinal cord ischemia, generally within 1–2 min of ischemia onset. This is in contrast to the comparatively slow SSEP, which have more sluggish response to ischemia, on the order of 10–20 min after ischemia begins.[18,19] Since only 22% of MEP changes are seen in SSEP response changes, it may be that

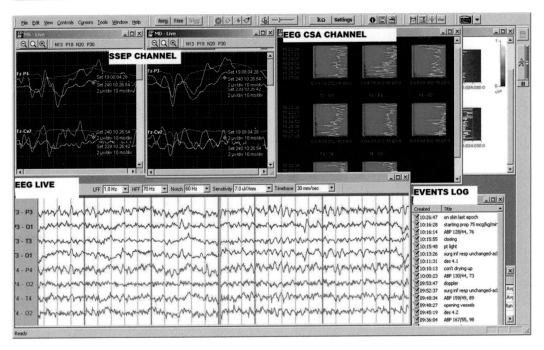

Fig. 10.5 Somatosensory evoked potential (SSEP) and electroencephalogram (EEG) monitoring module. CSA – Compressed Spectral Analysis of EEG

rapid corrections of ischemia occur even before SSEP changes appear, particularly in those instances where ischemia was not severe enough to produce clinical neurologic injury. Keyhani et al.[20] have examined this very issue and have shown good correlation between SSEPs and MEPs in the detection of those irreversible changes that led to clinical neurological injury. To this end, Keyhani et al. concluded that the addition of the more complex MEP monitoring to SSEPs did not add further meaningful information. Both MEP and SSEP had good negative predictive value, but each had poor sensitivity and positive predictive value (37% and 33% for SSEP and 22% and 45% for MEPs, respectively). In our institution, electroencephlogram (EEG) and SSEP monitoring are used in conjunction, given our preference for muscle relaxation, and the range of approaches dictated by different patients and different vascular surgeons (Fig. 10.5).

Moreover, intraoperative monitoring cannot prevent postoperative events and delayed paraplegia. In awake subjects, neurological examination can be performed to follow up spinal cord function. In sedated patients recovering from anesthesia, neuromonitoring can be continued into the postoperative period. MEPs are more painful and unacceptable in patients awakening from anesthesia.

Positioning

After placement of monitors, the patient is positioned in the right lateral decubitus position (Fig. 10.6). The thorax is positioned at 90° angle to the table but pelvis is tilted dorsad to less than 90° to facilitate cannulation of femoral vessels. As always, the anesthesiologist coordinates the move from supine to lateral position and controls airway, intravenous and monitoring lines while stabilizing the relaxed neck. It is not uncommon for the patients with aortic disease to have coexisting cerebrovascular and carotid diseases. Acute and extreme rotation of the head and neck during positioning should be avoided. Eyes, ears, and scalp should be examined frequently for excessive pressure. Stability of pelvis is obtained by flexing the

Fig. 10.6 Position for thoracoabdominal aortic repair

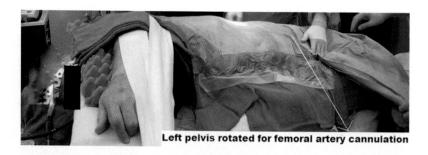

Left pelvis rotated for femoral artery cannulation

hips and knees of the lower leg while rotation of upper pelvis is done to facilitate access to femoral vessels. An inflatable bean bag is used to retain the patient position. A chest pad (known as axillary roll) is placed just caudal to axilla supporting the shoulder most portion of downside rib cage to avoid pressure on the dependent axillary neurovascular bundle. Upper extremities are positioned to avoid excessive stretch or compression of brachial plexus and peripheral nerves. Excessive lateral flexion and dorsal extension of head and neck may apply undue tension on the brachial plexus and should be avoided. After positioning, arterial lines are checked for proper waveforms and free aspiration, while venous access should be checked for free flow of fluids. Monitoring the trend of central venous pressure is recommended since the absolute numbers may not be accurate with the difficulty in defining phlebostatic axis. A pulmonary artery catheter positioned within the left pulmonary artery may lead to overestimation of left heart pressures (LVEDP) once the left lung is deflated. Positioning the catheter tip within the right pulmonary artery (RPA) can easily be done once the patient is moved into the right lateral position, since increased RPA flow will carry the catheter to the right. Position of the PAC tip is verified by TEE. Anesthesiologists should watch for sudden hemodynamic changes and ventilation perfusion mismatch which can accompany changes in position.

Aortic Cross Clamping

Aortic occlusion, a critical component of aortic surgical repair, reliably produces considerable hemodynamic effect. Three principle variables predict the nature of hemodynamic effect of cross clamping. Most important is the physical location of the clamp itself; more dramatic derangement will accompany more proximal clamping locations. Also important are the patient's baseline myocardial function, and pre-clamping intravascular blood volume. Hemodynamic changes are more pronounced upon cross clamping the thoracic aortic than those seen with infrarenal aortic clamping. Roizen et al. have observed a progression in depression of left heart function in accordance with aortic clamping site. Indices including a decrease in LVEF with regional wall motion abnormalities, and increase in end-systolic and end-diastolic ventricular cross-sectional areas were each seen on aortic clamping. Changes in these indices were mostly marked after supraceliac clamping; similar but smaller after infraceliac suprarenal clamping; and minimal when precipitated by infrarenal clamping.[21]

Kouchokous et al.[22] studied the response to cross clamping in DTAA and reported that MAP, central venous pressure, pulmonary artery pressure, and pulmonary capillary wedge pressure (PCWP) increased by 35%, 56%, 43%, and 90%, respectively, while at the same time cardiac output decreased by 29%. Each of these changes can be explained by the increases in myocardial stress, in relation to increases in preload and afterload, that are direct consequences of DTAA clamping.

Increases in afterload and proximal aortic hypertension are of multifactorial cause. In addition to the readily apparent impediment to flow created by mechanical occlusion, there are increases in systemic vascular resistance produced by release of catecholamines, renin-angiotensin, and other humoral factors. Increases in preload are explainable by redistribution of blood volume during aortic cross clamping.[23] As blood flow to organs distal to the clamp is interrupted, the venous capacitance of these organs decreases. The blood from distal organs shifts to the central venous circulation, and to those organs that are proximal to the clamp. When aortic clamping is infraceliac in location, the splanchnic vasculature acts as a reservoir and can accommodate most of the shifted blood volume. In this way, infraceliac clamping leads to modest changes in preload, filling pressures, and cardiac output. During supraceliac clamping, or when splanchnic venous tone is high, this reservoir capacity is diminished, and most of the blood with shift instead to the central circulation, and preload increases are more significant (Figs. 10.7 and 10.8).[23]

The resulting increases in preload and afterload directly trigger increases in myocardial oxygen demand which, by virtue of preload increase, may also be coupled with reductions in net coronary perfusion. While it is true that proximal hypertension increases antegrade coronary perfusion pressure, net coronary perfusion pressure may actually decline in response to rises end-diastolic pressure related to aortic cross clamping. It is this unfavorable relationship in the economy of myocardial oxygen supply and demand that serves to explain the frequent occurrence of regional wall motion abnormalities that are seen with aortic cross clamping. Presence of epicardial CAD, left ventricular hypertrophy, or diastolic and systolic dysfunction further disrupt this economy and worsen myocardial ischemia. Fayed et al. reported acute diastolic dysfunction with proximal aortic clamping during thoracoabdominal surgery, in six of nine patients, each of whom had normal E/A ratios prior to aortic clamping. Three of the patients in the Fayed series developed myocardial infarction.[24] Here again, proximity of aortic cross clamping influences the degree of diastolic dysfunction.

Although clamping of the aorta is expected to increase preload, blood loss and frank hypovolemia must not be ignored at this stage of surgery. Unexpected responses to aortic cross clamping, such as a decline or no increases in systemic pressure, may indicate severe hypovolemia or cardiac dysfunction. Such responses are investigated by measuring filling pressures and cardiac output, and by TEE evaluation. Hypovolemia exaggerates the effect of aortic cross clamping, and may precipitate cardiac ischemia through decreases in coronary perfusion pressure.

DTAA and TAAA surgeries, which necessitate very proximal aortic clamping, are accompanied not only by the reactions in preload, afterload, and myocardial oxygen balances, but are also associated with decreases in perfusion to the

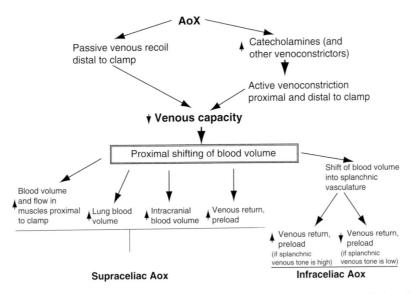

Fig. 10.7 Blood volume redistribution during aortic cross clamping (Reprinted with permission obtained from reference[23])

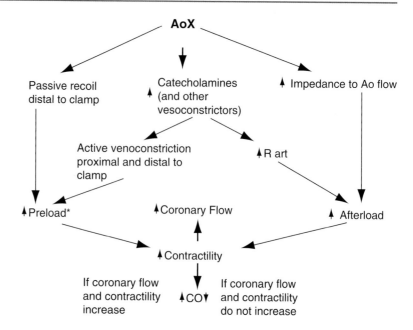

Fig. 10.8 Systemic hemodynamic responses to aortic cross clamping (Reprinted with permission obtained from reference[23])

gastrointestinal system, liver, kidneys, and spinal cord. Increases in serum lactate and metabolic acidosis indicate ischemia in those tissue beds distal to the clamp.[25] Patient management during cross clamping of the thoracic aorta therefore involves not only control of proximal hypertension and myocardial dysfunction, but also prevention of ischemia and protection of organs distal to the clamp site. Both these goals are achieved by distal arterial perfusion techniques. While distal perfusion techniques do reduce complications related to proximal clamping of the thoracic aorta, no distal perfusion technique completely eliminates the mortality and morbidity of thoracic aorta surgery.

Distal Arterial Perfusion Techniques

Passive Shunts (Gott Shunt)

Passive shunts are used to divert arterial blood from the proximal aorta, or left ventricle, to aorta sites distal to the aortic clamp. Shunts are made up of heparin-coated non-thrombogenic material, so systemic heparinization is not needed. The ascending aorta is commonly used for the shunt's origin, but the left ventricle, ascending aorta, aortic arch, or descending aorta may also be used. The left

subclavian artery is avoided as a shunting site, as this would interfere with spinal cord perfusion and cause steal phenomena. Because these shunts are passive, shunt flows cannot be controlled other than through manipulation of proximal shunt pressures, and through selection of shunt diameter and length. A shunt diameter of 9 mm is commonly used. Shunt flows of 2–2.5 L/min are reported by Verdant and colleagues.[26] Adequacy of shunt flows are monitored by visual inspection and palpation of the shunt by the surgeon, measurement of distal arterial pressure, and observation for signs of distal tissue ischemia. Clinical signs of adequate shunt flow include sufficient urine output, lack of metabolic acidosis, and favorable neurophysiological data. Difficulties with passive shunts include kinking, dislodgement, migration of the proximal end, interference with the surgical field, bleeding from origin and insertion sites, and distal embolization of atheromatous material.

Partial Cardiopulmonary Bypass

Partial CPB, achieved with either roller pump or centrifugal circuits, requires an in-line oxygenator and full systemic anticoagulation. Partial CPB incorporates right atrial drainage by way of a long reinforced cannula placed through the IVC via percutaneous femoral vein access. TEE guidance assists in placing the drainage cannula tip high in the right atrium. Arterial return is performed through cannulation of the femoral artery or distal descending aorta. A circuit heat exchanger provides active rewarming following the use of deliberate hypothermia for spinal cord protection during the repair. A venous reservoir allows addition of blood or fluids to the circulation. Pump suction, or sump sucker, may be used to return shed blood directly to the reservoir, so that a cell saver is not needed. The rate of venous drainage can be controlled by an adjustable clamp on the venous line. Arterial return rates are adjusted by roller head speed. In this way, partial CPB flow rates are deliberately manipulated to control patient hemodynamics, including moderation of proximal aortic hypertension during clamping and repair. During partial CPB, the lungs are ventilated and a beating heart perfuses the upper body, proximal to the clamp site, by way of native left heart circulation. In addition to providing a means for distal arterial perfusion, partial CPB provides the advantage of rapid conversion to full CPB should such need arise.

Left Heart Partial Bypass

Partial bypass of the left heart is the most commonly used topology for distal arterial perfusion. Partial bypass relies on a centrifugal pump, and no oxygenator or venous reservoir are incorporated. The partial bypass drainage cannula is normally placed in the left atrium (LA) by way of the left pulmonary vein, and the circuit returns to either the femoral artery or distal aorta. Absence of an oxygenator permits modest or no systemic anticoagulation. A heat exchanger may be optionally added to the circuit, and a separate cell saver device is used for field scavenge. By comparison to passive shunts, partial bypass circuit flows are moderately controllable. Flows offered by centrifugal pumps, such as the Biomedicus brand, are dependent upon circuit preload and afterload. A decrease in LA pressure, malposition of the LA cannula, or resistance to arterial return, each will precipitate decrease in partial bypass flow rates. Air embolization, particulate microembolization, platelet damage, and hemolysis are less likely with centrifugal pump when compared with those events with roller pumps.[27] Because high density anticoagulation is avoided, transfusion requirements may be more contained, but extensive cell saver has been associated with increased coagulopathy risk. The fact that partial left heart bypass does not mandate dense heparinization is particularly advantageous to patients who have suffered aortic transection in the context of multiple trauma, where associated injuries may preclude heparin use. Use of low-density heparinization is, however, common practice to maintain patency of spinal and intercostal arteries during the low flow states that may occur during surgery. Flows of 1.5–2.5 L/min (25–40 mL/kg/min) are commonly used and are titrated to mean aortic proximal, distal, and pulmonary artery pressures (Table 10.1). Partial left heart

Table 10.1 Hemodynamic management during left heart bypass

Proximal arterial pressure	Distal perfusion pressure	Pulmonary capillary wedge pressure	Left ventricular filling by TEE	Reason	Intervention
High	Low	High	Adequate	Inadequate pump flow	Increase pump flow/ evaluate drainage and return cannulae position
High	High	High	Adequate	High vasomotor tone	Deepen anesthesia/ vasodilator
Low	Adequate	High	Distension	Pump failure	Inodilators/Inotrope followed by vasodilator
Low	Low	Low	Empty	Hypovolemia	Volume infusion
Low	High	Low	Low	Increased pump flow or hypovolemia	Decrease pump flow, consider volume infusion

bypass has been credited by various investigators in reducing the incidence of spinal cord injury and perioperative renal failure after thoracic aortic reconstruction.[28-31] The use of adjuncts (CSF drainage and partial left heart bypass) is also associated with improved 10 years survival benefit.[10]

Antihypertensive Therapy

When a simple aortic cross clamping (clamp-and-sew method) is used, titration of antihypertensive drugs is the principal means of controlling proximal aortic hypertension. When a method of distal perfusion is used, manipulation of bypass circuit flows is required to maintain hemodynamics. Antihypertensive drugs may, however, still be needed and should be readily available. When titrating antihypertensive therapy, it is crucial to prevent *relative* hypotension of the proximal aortic circulation. Proximal aortic hypotension will compromise distal perfusion to collateral-dependent tissue beds, and hence, worsen visceral ischemia beyond the aortic cross-clamp site.

Adequate depth of anesthesia should be ensured before considering initiation of antihypertensive drug therapy. Beta-blockers are preferred agents when a hypertensive episode is associated with tachycardia. Esmolol infusion can be titrated (50–200 mcg/kg/min) to the HR and MAP and it has the advantage of short half-life (9 min). When a patient is well beta-blocked preoperatively, they may not benefit from intraoperative beta-blockade as a treatment for surgical hypertension. In those instances, a vasodilator is added. While sodium nitroprusside (SNP) is the most commonly used antihypertensive agent in anesthesia, SNP can increase intracranial and intraspinal pressure when used during aortic cross clamping. The observed increase in intracranial pressure may be explained either by vasodilatation of intracranial vasculature, recruitment of capacitance vessels, or it may reflect a disruption in autoregulation caused by the spinal cord ischemia related to aortic cross clamping.[32] Increased intraspinal pressure and decreased distal aortic blood pressure are detrimental to spinal

cord perfusion. Simpson et al. conducted several experimental studies investigating SNP during aortic cross clamping.[33-36] SNP use was consistently associated with poor neurological outcome. SNP further increases shunt fraction during one-lung ventilation, and causes reflex tachycardia and coronary steal, both of which are detrimental for patients with CAD. For these reasons, SNP should be used with extreme caution in aortic surgical patients. Large SNP doses or prolonged infusions should be avoided. Nitroglycerine decreases the preload associated with cross clamping, and dilates coronary vessels, both of which may be useful in patients with myocardial ischemia or CAD. Nitroglycerin is a weak antihypertensive agent and can also decrease spinal cord perfusion pressure similar to SNP.[35]

Calcium channel antagonists, such as IV nicardipine given as an infusion at 5–15 mg/h, are used as an alternate vasodilator to SNP in aortic surgery. Although the time to reach the baseline blood pressure after stopping the infusion is longer with nicardipine in comparison to SNP, nicardipine is effective and well tolerated in the perioperative setting. In addition, nicardipine is linked with increases in coronary blood flow and stroke volume, while preload and heart rate are not altered. Nicardipine was seen to increase cerebral blood flow with no clinically significant increase in CSF pressure, in subjects who did not have intracranial pathology.[37] There are no human clinical studies as of this date which compares SNP and nicardipine in patients undergoing DTAA repair. Clevidipine, an ultra-short-acting IV calcium channel blocker with a half-life of only 2 min, is an attractive antihypertensive option, but has only begun to be available in the USA for routine clinical use. The ECLIPSE trial compared clevidipine, nicardipine, SNP, and NTG in cardiac surgical patients and concluded that clevidipine is safe and as effective as other drugs.[38] In patients suffering from ventricular dysfunction and ventricular dilation, afterload reductions may be achieved with the administration of an inodilating agent, such as milrinone. Epinephrine and dopamine may be necessary in patients with severe ventricular dysfunction.

Aortic Unclamping

Hemodynamic effects of aortic unclamping can be made less dramatic during DTAA and TAAA surgery with the use of distal perfusion, and by sequential advancement cross clamp techniques. The anesthesiologist must keep abreast of surgical progress in aortic clamping and unclamping and organ reperfusion at all levels (Fig. 10.9). Knowledge of ischemic times of

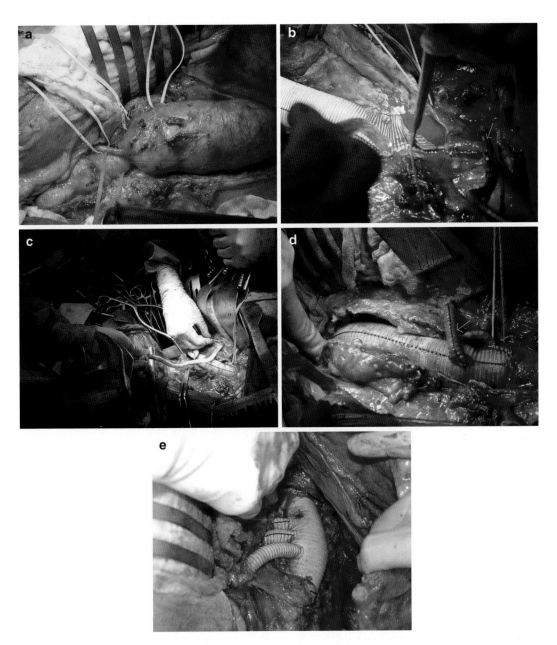

Fig. 10.9 Surgery for type IV TAAA repair, with patient's head to the image right, and feet to image left: (**a**) Surgical dissection showing celiac (*single arrow*), superior mesenteric (*double arrows*), and renal arteries (*triple arrows*). (**b**) Proximal clamp placement (*arrows*) and aorta opened for proximal anastomosis. (**c**) Clamp moved distal to the renal artery. Cold renal perfusion is given through the graft to the kidneys. (**d**) Completion of anastomosis and release of clamp for reperfusion of the graft. (**e**) Separate grafts to celiac, superior mesenteric, and renal arteries are required in some cases

organ systems such as intestines, kidneys, and lower limbs should be incorporated into the anesthetic care, and should be documented in the anesthetic record. Hypotension seen with unclamping can be moderated by a gradual release of the cross clamp, by fluid loading to pulmonary capillary wedge pressures higher than basal value, by treatment of acidosis with sodium bicarbonate, and by judicious administration of vasopressors.[39] Cardiovascular collapse may occur after unclamping even when precautions are taken and anesthesiologists should be ready for resuscitation in such situations. Temporary reclamping of the aorta may be necessary to temporize extreme circumstances. Blood pressure may overcorrect when vasopressors and inotropes have been aggressively used during unclamping, and this may complicate anastomosis bleeding.

Blood Loss and Transfusion

Blood loss from surgical dissection and back bleeding from intercostal vessels can be significant enough to require massive transfusion. Coagulopathy complicates surgical blood loss and results from heparinization, hypothermia, supravisceral aortic cross clamping, and hypoperfusion. Thoracoabdominal aneurysm repair is associated with a reduction in clotting factor activity and an increase in fibrinolysis, which occurs in supraceliac aortic clamping.[40] Profound ischemic tissue burden and visceral ischemia are the most likely precipitants of coagulation alterations.[40] Disseminated intravascular coagulation may accompany visceral ischemia and may require platelet and cryoprecipitate administration. When possible, coagulation factor replacement should be guided by POC tests. Cell saving for intraoperative blood salvage is routinely used, and a system for rapid volume transfusion should be readily available in the operating room. Antifibrinolytics have not been found to be useful in reducing transfusion or bleeding.[41]

Spinal Cord Protection

Spinal cord vascular anatomy varies between patients. The contribution of proximal collateral circulation, intercostals arteries, and distal collateral circulation to the spinal cord arterial network is unique to each patient.[42] Some patients depend heavily on proximal collateral circulation and benefit from maintaining higher perfusion pressure proximal to the aortic cross clamp. In such a patient, maintaining proximal aortic pressure is critical, and this is true irrespective of the method used for distal arterial perfusion. In other patients, proximal collateral circulation is less important for spinal cord blood supply. In this patient group, the key to prevention of paraplegia lies in maintaining distal collateral pelvic circulation, both during and after surgical repair. Assuring sufficient distal MAP during aortic occlusion, and sufficient global MAP after repair, are the most reliable means of assuring distal collateral circulation. Still other patients' spinal cord supply is critically dependent on the intercostals circulation, and such patients benefit from reimplantation of intercostal arteries. In addition, a variety of mechanisms may contribute to paraplegia such as spinal cord ischemia during cross clamping (decreased spinal cord perfusion pressure), reperfusion injury, and intraoperative embolization of the plaque or thrombi. Until techniques are available to prospectively identify the anatomy and physiology of spinal cord blood supply, and to therefore predict the mechanisms which risk neurological injury in each patient, a multimodal therapeutic approach using anatomic, surgical, physiologic, and monitoring strategies should be utilized.

Anatomic and Surgical Strategies

Cross Clamp Time

Patients vary in their abilities to tolerate spinal ischemia produced in aortic cross clamping. As a general rule, unprotected cross clamp times greater than 30 min are associated with increased incidence of spinal cord dysfunction. It is not

uncommon, however, for complex TAAA reconstruction to require cross clamp times in excess
of 30 min. Fortunately, the correlation between
extended cross clamping times and the incidence
of spinal paraplegia is much improved when
distal arterial perfusion is used[43] (Figs. 10.10
and 10.11).

Sequential Cross Clamping

Proximal and distal cross clamps are moved down
sequentially along the aorta when distal perfusion methods are used. The aim is to have the
shortest possible segment of aorta unperfused at
any point of time, so that spinal cord and visceral
ischemic times are decreased.

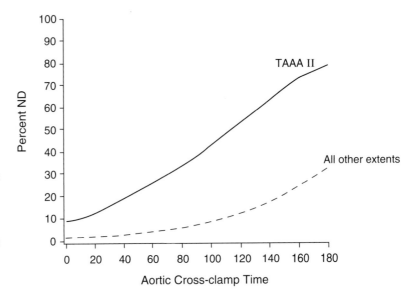

Fig. 10.10 Effect of cross
clamp duration on the
incidence of neurologic
dysfunction (ND) when
adjuncts (distal perfusion
with CSF drainage) are not
utilized (Reprinted with
permission from
reference[43])

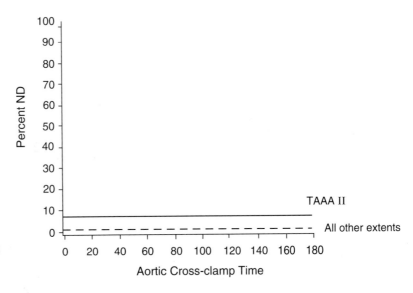

Fig. 10.11 Favorable
impact of distal arterial
perfusion and CSF
drainage in reducing
neurologic dysfunction
(ND), as a function of
aortic cross clamping
duration. Note that TAAA
type II is associated with a
higher incidence of ND
when compared to other
aneurysm types (Reprinted
with permission from
reference[43])

Preoperative Imaging of Spinal Cord Blood Supply

Preoperative description of spinal cord blood supply by computerized tomographic angiography (CTA) or magnetic resonance angiography (MRA) is potentially beneficial in reducing the incidence of paraplegia. Selective angiography of intercostal and lumbar vessels is too risky and is not employed routinely. Preoperative localization of intercostal arteries including ARM with MRA allows selective reimplantation, as opposed to mass reimplantation, of intercostal arteries. Selective reimplantation avoids the increase in clamp time and bleeding from additional anastomoses required by bulk intercostal implantation. In a review of 1,196 patients from 43 studies, MRA and CTA were able to detect the location of ARM in 67–100% (mean 80%) and 18–100% (mean 72%), respectively.[44] Patients in whom ARM could not be localized may not benefit from intercostal reimplantation. Preoperative imaging that reveals a continuous and well-developed anterior spinal artery, with good spinal cord arterial collateralization, is associated with stable spinal cord function and resistance to paraplegia with surgery. Conversely, an absence of spinal cord collateral supply increases the chance of paraplegia.[45]

Intercostal Vessel Management

Segmental reimplantation of intercostal vessels is one of the most controversial topics surrounding spinal cord protection. Some surgeons aggressively and systematically reimplant all intercostal vessels between T7 and L2 to contribute to the spinal cord collateral network. Those advocating such an approach cite lower incidence of paraplegia with segmental reimplantation as a part of their multimodal approach.[46–48] In patients with diseased intercostal vessels, acute dissections, and rupture of the aneurysms and in patients undergoing very complex aortic reconstructions, however, reimplantation may not be feasible. Other surgeons prefer to sacrifice intercostal vessels through sequential ligation, using motor evoked potentials (MEP) as a guide to the safety of ligation. Reimplantation is then only selectively performed when ligation of that artery caused

decline in evoked potentials.[49,50] In using this approach, collateral flow contribution from lumbar, cervical, and hypogastric arteries gains added importance, and therefore, the maintenance of adequate spinal cord perfusion pressure becomes critical. Alternately, surgeons may use preoperative imaging or intraoperative findings to guide selective reimplantation of intercostal arteries. With this method, larger intercostal vessels and vessels with visible back bleeding are reimplanted. Reliance on the size and back bleeding is probably a flawed methodology, however. Back bleeding from intercostals may well indicate the presence of an adequate collateral network, and lack of back bleeding may, in contrast, signify inadequate collaterals. With this in mind, it may actually be those vessels that fail to backbleed that may most benefit from reimplantation.

Physiologic Strategies

Spinal Cord Perfusion Pressure

Maintaining a spinal cord perfusion pressure (>40 mmHg) is the most important element of spinal cord protection. Blood pressure distal to the clamp should be maintained above 60 mmHg by using distal perfusion techniques. MAP proximal to the aortic clamp is maintained at preoperative levels or above 70 mmHg. CSF is drained (typically 50 cc before and 50 cc after cross clamping) with its pressure continuously maintained between 8 and 10 mmHg.

Hypothermia

Systemic Hypothermia

A patient's temperature is generally permitted to drift to 33–35° prior to application of the aortic cross clamp, with the knowledge that mild to moderate hypothermia is neuroprotective. Active cooling to low target temperatures with blankets or through the CPB circuit is rarely necessary. Coagulopathy, cardiac arrhythmias, and prolonged duration of anesthetic drugs and muscle relaxants are risks associated with hypothermia. Once the distal aortic anastomosis is complete, it is appropriate to begin active rewarming of the patient using the bypass circuit, warming blankets, warmed fluids, and by warming the operating room. Deep hypothermic circulatory arrest (DHCA) is used in complicated cases such as giant aneurysms, ruptured aneurysms, and severe calcific atherosclerotic aneurysms, when cross clamping is not possible, or in patients with aortic arch involvement. Rewarming from deep hypothermia plays an even more important role.

Regional Hypothermia

Cooling techniques that are regionally applied to thoracolumbar spinal segments put at risk by aortic clamping is used in selected hospital centers. Regional cooling is associated with low incidence of paraplegia.[51] Regional cooling is accomplished by infusing iced saline into an epidural catheter placed at T11–T12 region. A subarachnoid catheter, inserted at L3–L4 interspace, serves three purposes: Spinal temperature measurement by the attached thermister, CSF drainage, and CSF pressure measurement. A target spinal temperature of 25° is achieved through active cooling. CSF hypertension is avoided by decreasing the rate of infusion of epidural saline once the target temperature is reached and the aorta is cross clamped. Spinal cord hypothermia may confound the interpretation of evoked potential changes.

Pharmacologic Agents

There is no solid clinical evidence to support the use of any pharmacological agent to protect the spinal cord in TAAA surgery. Steroids, thiopental sodium, lidocaine, magnesium, calcium channel blockers, iloprost, sildenafil, levosimendin, and free radical scavengers have all been studied in experimental models. Though some of these drugs are used according to institutional preference, none of them has achieved widespread use.

IV naloxone (1 mcg/kg/h) has been used as an adjunct to CSF drainage in a series of reports from the University of Wisconsin. Lower rates of paraplegia (3.4%) have been reported in

their series of clamp-and-sew aortic repairs, even without the use of assisted circulation.[52,53] Kunihara et al. have shown that IV naloxone lowered CSF levels of excitatory aminoacids, which are known to be strong predictors of spinal cord injury when they are present in high concentrations.[54] Svensson et al. from Cleveland Clinic used intrathecal papaverine (30 mg) in their multimodal regimen, which also included CSF drainage, moderate hypothermia, intercostals reimplantation, and reported significant reductions in the spinal cord dysfunction to less than 5%.[55] Although interesting, it is difficult to demonstrate the effect of an individual drug when it is used as part of multimodal regimen.

Glucose Control

Data from spinal cord ischemia models suggests a deleterious effect of hyperglycemia. The likely mediator of neural injury relates to enhanced rates of lactic acidosis, which are associated with larger quantities of glucose available for metabolism.[56] Resistance to endogenous insulin has been noted in patients with spinal cord injury.[57] Since circulating insulin is also known to be protective against ischemic spinal cord injury, it is logical to conclude that avoidance of hyperglycemia prior to the onset of spinal cord ischemia lessens the risk of perioperative spinal cord injury.[58] Given that hypoglycemia is also dangerous to the nervous system, blood glucose control is in order. Serum glucose is monitored hourly during surgery, and insulin infusion is to be adjusted accordingly. Insulin infusions are continued postoperatively in the critical care unit, where glucose control remains important.

Renal Protection

Renal failure occurs with high frequency after DTA (7%) and TAAA (22.8%) repairs, and one third of those patients will require hemodialysis.[59] Renal failure increases the length of hospital stay and mortality (30% vs. 10% without renal failure) and is associated with poor long-term survival and quality of life.[59] Several papers have addressed predictors for acute renal failure after TAAA/DTA repairs.[60–63] The most predictive of postoperative renal failure was the presence of preoperative renal dysfunction. Risk factors also include advanced patient age, use of clamp-and-sew surgical technique, long cross clamp times, left renal arterial attachment, hemodynamic instability, and intraoperative transfusion in excess of five units of packed red cells or cell saver blood. Use of distal aortic perfusion, deliberate hypothermia, and selective renal perfusion with cold crystalloid (with mannitol and steroid) are adjuncts useful in preventing renal failure. Surgeries where long duration aortic cross clamping is required, and in surgical repairs involving renal arteries, make renal protection especially important.

The role of distal aortic perfusion and selective cold renal perfusion is debated in the literature. Safi et al. have shown increased renal risk with visceral perfusion.[60] Svensson et al. also have shown increased risk with the use of bypass and visceral perfusion.[61] Others described the usefulness of distal aortic perfusion and regional cold perfusion in reducing renal failure.[62,63] Jacobs et al. used volume and pressure-controlled selective renal and visceral perfusion and have shown beneficial effects in reducing renal and visceral ischemia, even in patients with preexisting renal impairment.[64,65] Cold blood perfusion appears to not be superior to cold crystalloid infusion, when used for selective visceral perfusion.[66]

Anesthesiologists commonly administer mannitol, an osmotic diuretic before cross clamping for renal protection. Mannitol produces renal vasodilatation that shifts the blood flow to the renal cortex and acts as free radical scavenger. There is little scientific evidence, however, to recommend furosemide, mannitol, steroids, dopamine, and fenoldopam for renal protection in TAAA repairs.[67]

Interestingly, Miller et al. have shown a relationship between renal failure and the SSEP changes associated with leg ischemia from femoral cannulation. Patients with SSEP changes had 41/108 (38%) postoperative renal failure compared to 49/191 (26%) without (odds ratio 1.8, $p < 0.03$).[68] This could be explained by rhabdomyolysis and free myoglobin damage to the kidneys, developing as a consequence of leg ischemia. Certainly, presence of leg ischemia may also be an indicator of generally poor arterial collaterization, and this too may be at the heart of renal ischemia. In a follow-up study, use of side-arm femoral cannulation, rather than straight cannulation, was associated with a clinically important and highly statistically significant reduction in postoperative renal complications in patients who had preoperative low GFR.[69] In another comparison, femoral cannulation was associated with more frequent renal dysfunction than distal aortic cannulation for DTA/TAAA repairs.[66]

Meseteric Ischemia

Visceral ischemia as a consequence of long duration aortic cross clamping (>40 min) in TAAA repairs was associated with multiorgan dysfunction, coagulopathy, increased morbidity and mortality, and very high health-care costs.[70] The frequency and magnitude of postoperative organ dysfunction after TAAA repair is linked to increased circulating levels of the cytokines TNF-alpha and IL-6. Of note is that increased plasma levels of these cytokines appear to require extended visceral ischemia times.[71] When cross clamping is less than 30 min, on the other hand, similar patient survival was reported for both infrarenal and visceral aortic repairs.[72] Safi et al. reported gastrointestinal complications after TAAA surgery with a perioperative incidence of 7% and mortality of 38%.[73] Hepatic dysfunction, biliary disease, and intestinal ischemia are associated with increased mortality. Peptic ulcer disease, acute pancreatitis, and GI bleeding are other perioperative complications. Coronary artery disease, renal insufficiency, and visceral artery lesions predict gastrointestinal complications, as they are indicative of widespread atherosclerotic disease.[74] Distal aortic perfusion, selective cold blood perfusion to the celiac and mesenteric arteries, and mesenteric shunting (perfusion of mesenteric and celiac artery through a perfusion catheter attached to the sidearm of the proximal aortic graft) are techniques used with the goal of reducing the severity of visceral ischemia.

Completion of Surgery

Once the perfusion to the lower extremities is restored and hemodynamics is stabilized, the patient is slowly rewarmed using the bypass circuit and external warming to normothermia. The left atrial cannula is removed and protamine is administered, if necessary, to correct the ACT to baseline. The left lung is recruited and ventilated, although it may be necessary to periodically deflate the left lung to assist in obtaining surgical hemostasis. Arterial blood gasses confirm that ventilation, oxygenation, hematocrit, and metabolic parameters are acceptable. Thromboelastography (TEG) is done to rule out and investigate coagulopathy, and blood products are administered as indicated. Once the chest is closed, the patient is turned supine and the double lumen is changed to single lumen tube over a tube exchange catheter. When the procedure is prolonged, and intraoperative fluid shifts have been large, it may be essential to not change the double lumen endotracheal tube because of significant airway edema. Hemodynamics should be watched closely during repositioning and airway manipulations. Anesthetics should not be discontinued at this point to avoid hypertension and tension on aortic suture lines.

Neuromuscular blockade is reversed and the patient is allowed to wake up for neurological examination. If the patient can move the extremities, suggesting good spinal cord function, they are sedated with propofol infusion and taken to intensive care. If spinal cord function is not reassuring, consideration is given to surgical reexploration, or to manipulation of spinal cord perfusion determinants through use of transfusion, vasoactive agents, and spinal drainage. Timing of extubation depends on variety of factors and early extubation may be possible in uncomplicated cases.

Postoperative Management

Respiratory Management

The most commonly encountered complication after DTA and TAAA repair is respiratory failure with an incidence of 21% in one series.[75] Respiratory failure had been linked with high mortality (40%). Advanced age, preexisting chronic obstructive pulmonary disease, and history of smoking are known predisposing risk factors. Surgical preservation of the phrenic nerve, and confining division to only the muscular portion of the diaphragm with preservation of central tendinous portion, may reduce the incidence of respiratory failure.[76] The left lung should be ventilated as often as possible, but only when the surgery does not mandate lung isolation. It is also important to avoid mechanical trauma to the lungs which may result in air leaks, subcutaneous emphysema, bleeding, atelectasis, and excessive lung contusion. Excessive transfusion, postoperative renal failure, and cardiac events also predict respiratory failure. Preoperative respiratory optimization, good intraoperative care, and postoperative use of respiratory exercises, aggressive pulmonary toilet, and epidural analgesia are each essential in patients at risk for respiratory failure.

Neurologic Complications

Neurologic complications such as stroke and paraplegia are frequent after open DTA/TAAA surgery. In a recent review of 224 patients who underwent type I, II, and III Crawford aneurysm repairs, spinal cord ischemia occurred in 28%, stroke in 6%, and 4% had both stroke and spinal cord ischemia.[77] Manipulation of an atherosclerotic aorta, clamping of the aorta proximal to left subclavian artery, surgery involving aortic arch with prolonged circulatory arrest are obvious risk factors for postoperative neurological dysfunction. Patient age greater than 60 years, acute aortic rupture or dissection requiring emergency surgery, history of current smoking, preoperative renal dysfunction, type II extent aneurysms, and

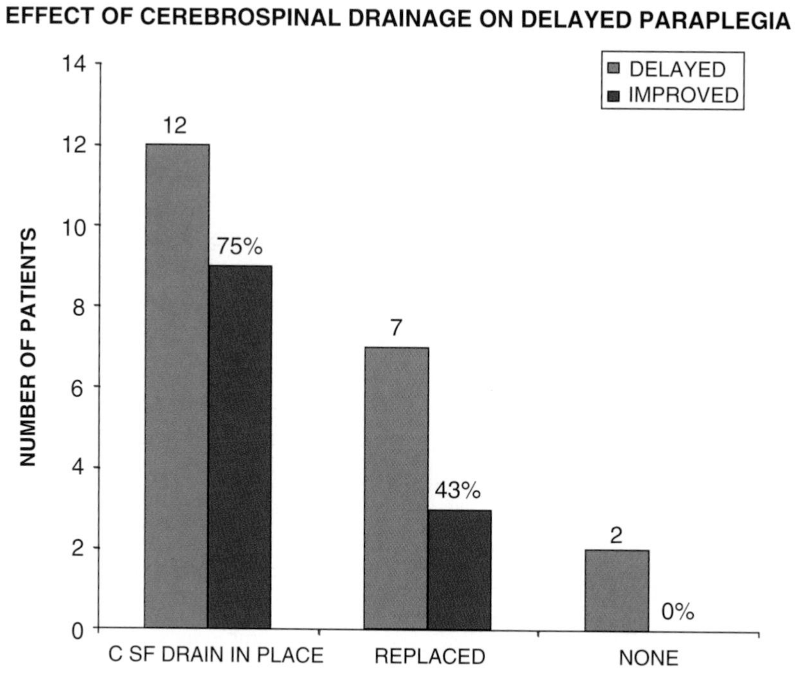

EFFECT OF CEREBROSPINAL DRAINAGE ON DELAYED PARAPLEGIA

Fig. 10.12 Percent recovery of delayed neurological deficits (Reprinted with permission from reference[79])

preexisting cerebrovascular disease are other predictors of postoperative neurological dysfunction and long-term survival.[10,43] Higher than routine cerebral perfusion pressures should be maintained in patients at special risk for stroke. Cerebral monitoring (EEG, SSEP, and cerebral oximetry) can be utilized, though their role is not yet established. Literature devoted to stroke after TAAA/DTA surgery is less plentiful than literature regarding spinal cord ischemia.

Spinal cord protection is described in detail in another chapter of this book and in the preceding sections. Alarmingly, delayed paraplegia can occur 2 h to 2 weeks after surgery (10% incidence). Postoperative hypotension, technical problems with CSF drainage, postoperative thrombosis of critical vessels, and apoptosis are proposed reasons for delayed paraplegia.[78] Aggressive management of blood pressure (MAP > 90–100 mmHg) and CSF drainage to pressure between 8 and 10 mmHg and maintenance of adequate cardiac index (>2 L) and hematocrit (>10 g) are recommended in patients who manifest delayed paraplegia. In patients without neurologic signs or

symptoms, CSF pressure is monitored for 24 h postoperatively and subarachnoid catheters removed at 48 h. Consideration should be given to the state of coagulation at the time of catheter removal, and transfusion of clotting factors should precede catheter removal in some situations. In patients who demonstrate delayed paraplegia, CSF drainage is reestablished and continued for 72 h. Paraplegia has been shown to improve in 50% of patients with this approach[79] (Fig. 10.12).

Cardiovascular Management

Cardiac complications such as myocardial ischemia, congestive heart failure, and arrhythmias are not uncommon (12–15% incidence) in this patient population following this high-risk surgery.[47,48] Beta-blockade is continued into the perioperative period, with careful monitoring to avoid hypotension and compromises in organ perfusion. Anticoagulants and antiplatelet agents are resumed when the risk for repair site bleeding is considered acceptable.

Pain Management

Epidural analgesia, while viewed as essential in some centers, is avoided in many institutions. To be sure, many patients can be managed postoperatively with intravenous narcotics alone. Epidural local anesthetics cause sympathetic block and hypotension may occur with even in dilute anesthetic concentrations. The ability to examine lower extremity neurological function at the bedside may, in some instances, be compromised with epidural local anesthesia. Epidural analgesia can, however, produce superior thoracic cage pain relief and may aid in the recovery of respiratory function. Epidural analgesia typically involves a solution of dilute local anesthetic (0.1% bupivacaine) and a narcotic (10 ug/mL of hydromorphine). It should not be difficult to differentiate spinal cord ischemia from epidural analgesia, provided that high concentration local anesthetics are avoided, and so long as a detailed neurological examination is performed. Epidural analgesia is continued as long as it is required. Coagulation should be normal before epidural catheters are removed. The use of continuous paravertebral catheter-based analgesia has been described for analgesia in thoracic aortic surgery.[80]

Reoperations

Reoperations may be required for bleeding or ischemic complications such as gut ischemia, renal artery thrombosis, or lower extremity ischemia. Supportive procedures such as percutaneous gastrostomy and tracheostomy are not uncommon after TAAA surgery in patients requiring rehabilitation for recovery.

Key Notes

1. Conventional open repair of descending thoracic and thoracoabdominal aorta still has a role in the modern era of endografts since they have proven durability. Open repair is performed in asymptomatic patients when the risk of aortic rupture with medical management exceeds operative risk.

2. High-risk aortic surgical procedure in patients with significant comorbidities increases the perioperative risk. Preoperative estimation of risk for cardiac, pulmonary, neurologic, and renal systems followed by medical optimization of the organ function is essential.

3. Age greater than 60 years, history of smoking, emergency surgery, extent two repairs, renal dysfunction, and cerebrovascular disease increase morbidity and decrease survival.

4. Discussion with the patient regarding the risks and with the surgeon regarding planned surgical procedure and anesthetic management (monitoring, cannulation, spinal drainage, and distal perfusion) are necessary.

5. Adjuncts such as cerebrospinal drainage and distal perfusion decrease postoperative complications and improve patient survival.

6. Double lumen endobronchial intubation and one-lung ventilation are needed to facilitate surgical exposure. Review of preoperative imaging should be done to rule out tracheal and carinal compression and distortion before airway intubation with double lumen tube.

7. Monitoring includes standard ASA monitoring, invasive direct arterial monitoring of proximal arterial pressure and distal perfusion pressure, pulmonary artery catheter, transesophageal echocardiography, cerebral monitors (electroencephalogram), and intraoperative neurophysiologic monitoring (somatosensory and transcranial motor evoked potentials). While SSEPs can be used with muscle paralysis and low dose inhalational agents, motor evoked potential monitoring requires avoidance of muscle relaxants and inhalational anesthetic agents.

8. Sudden and extreme hemodynamic changes may occur with aortic clamping and unclamping and anesthesiologists should be prepared to manage the crisis situations.

9. The effects of cross clamping depend on proximity of clamp site, preoperative cardiac function, and volume status. Distal perfusion methods decrease the hemodynamic changes and complications associated with cross

clamping. Manipulation of pump flow, antihypertensive therapy, volume infusion, and inotropic therapy are needed to regulate proximal and distal pressures during partial bypass.

10. Sodium nitroprusside should be used with caution and nicardipine infusion is preferred for antihypertensive management during descending and thoracoabdominal aortic surgery.

11. Spinal cord ischemia and paraplegia are devastating complications after open repair. Maintenance of spinal cord perfusion pressure is the mainstay in the prevention of immediate and delayed paraplegia.

12. Postoperative renal failure, in stark contrast to neurologic deficit, has remained resistant to every treatment that has been described in the literature. Defining the mechanism of renal injury is a priority since renal failure is associated with poor outcomes after open repair.

13. Pharmacologic protection of kidney, brain, and spinal cord are utilized according to institutional experience. Such drugs include naloxone, mannitol, steroids, and thiopental.

14. Adequate blood products should be arranged prior to open repair. Point of care coagulation tests can be used to guide transfusion management after complex open repairs. Cell savers are utilized and a rapid infuser should be readily available.

15. Respiratory failure is the most common complication after open descending aortic surgery. Postoperative pain management utilizing thoracic epidural catheters may be useful in decreasing respiratory complications.

References

1. Griepp RB, Ergin MA, Galla JD, et al. Natural history of descending thoracic and thoracoabdominal aneurysms. *Ann Thorac Surg.* 1999;67:1927–1930.
2. Elefteriades JA. Natural history of thoracic aortic aneurysms: indications for surgery, and surgical versus nonsurgical risks. *Ann Thorac Surg.* 2002;74: S1877–S1880.
3. Miller CC 3rd, Porat EE, Estrera AL, Vinnerkvist AN, Huynh TT, Safi HJ. Number needed to treat: analyzing of the effectiveness of thoracoabdominal aortic repair. *Eur J Vasc Endovasc Surg.* 2004;28:154–157.
4. Lobato AC, Puech-Leão P. Predictive factors for rupture of thoracoabdominal aortic aneurysm. *J Vasc Surg.* 1998;27:446–453.
5. Hughes GC, Daneshmand MA, Swaminathan M, et al. "Real world" thoracic endografting: results with the Gore TAG device 2 years after U.S. FDA approval. *Ann Thorac Surg.* 2008;86:1530–1537.
6. Adams JD, Angle JF, Matsumoto AH, et al. Endovascular repair of the thoracic aorta in the post-FDA approval era. *J Thorac Cardiovasc Surg.* 2009;137:117–123.
7. Jonker FH, Trimarchi S, Verhagen HJ, Moll FL, Sumpio BE, Muhs BE. Meta-analysis of open versus endovascular repair for ruptured descending thoracic aortic aneurysm. *J Vasc Surg.* 2010;51:1026–1032.
8. Coselli JS, Le Maire SA. Descending and thoracoabdominal aneurysm. In: Cohn L, ed. *Cardiac Surgery in the Adult.* 3rd ed. USA: McGraw Hill; 2008: 1277–1298.
9. Fleisher LA, Beckman JA, Brown KA, et al. ACC/AHA 2007 guidelines on perioperative cardiovascular evaluation and care for noncardiac surgery: executive summary: a report of the American College of Cardiology/American Heart Association Task Force on Practice Guidelines (Writing Committee to revise the 2002 guidelines on perioperative cardiovascular evaluation for noncardiac surgery). *Anesth Analg.* 2008;106:685–712.
10. Safi HJ, Miller CC 3rd, Huynh TT, et al. Distal aortic perfusion and cerebrospinal fluid drainage for thoracoabdominal and descending thoracic aortic repair: ten years of organ protection. *Ann Surg.* 2003;238: 372–380.
11. Sethi M, Grigore AM, Davison JK. Pro: it is safe to proceed with thoracoabdominal aortic aneurysm surgery after encountering a bloody tap during cerebrospinal fluid catheter placement. *J Cardiothorac Vasc Anesth.* 2006;20:269–272.
12. Wynn MM, Mittnacht A, Norris E. Con: surgery should not proceed when a bloody tap occurs during spinal drain placement for elective thoracoabdominal aortic surgery. *J Cardiothorac Vasc Anesth.* 2006;20:273–275.
13. Robertazzi RR, Cunningham JN Jr. Monitoring of somatosensory evoked potentials: a primer on the intraoperative detection of spinal cord ischemia during aortic reconstructive surgery. *Semin Thorac Cardiovasc Surg.* 1998;10:11–17.
14. De Haan P, Kalkman CJ. Spinal cord monitoring: somatosensory and motor-evoked potentials. *Anesthesiol Clin N A.* 2001;19:923–945.
15. De Haan P, Kalkman CJ, et al. Efficacy of transcranial motor evoked myogenic potentials to detect spinal cord ischemia during operations for thoracoabdominal aneurysms. *J Thorac Cardiovasc Surg.* 1997;113: 87–100.
16. Jacobs MJ, Meylaerts SA, et al. Assessment of spinal cord ischemia by means of evoked potential monitoring during thoracoabdominal aortic surgery. *Semin Vasc Surg.* 2000;13:299–307.

17. Sinha AC, Cheung AT. Spinal cord protection and thoracic aortic surgery. *Curr Opin Anaesthesiol.* 2010;23:95–102.

18. van Dongen EP, Schepens MA, et al. Thoracic and thoracoabdominal aortic aneurysm repair: use of evoked potential monitoring in 118 patients. *J Vasc Surg.* 2001;34:1035–1040.

19. Shine TSJ, Harrison B, De Ruyter ML, et al. Moto rand somatosensory evoked potentials: their role in predicting spinal cord ischemia in patients undergoing thoracoabdominal aortic aneurysm repair with regional lumbar epidural cooling. *Anesthesiology.* 2008;108:580–587.

20. Keyhani K, Miller CC III, Estera AL, et al. Analysis of motor and somatosensory evoked potentials during thoracic and thoracoabdominal aortic aneurysm repair. *J Vasc Surg.* 2009;41:36–41.

21. Roizen MF, Beaupre PN, Alpert RA, et al. Monitoring with two-dimensional transesophageal echocardiography. Comparison of myocardial function in patients undergoing supraceliac, suprarenal-infraceliac, or infrarenal aortic occlusion. *J Vasc Surg.* 1984;1: 300–305.

22. Kouchoukos NT, Lell WA, Karp RB, et al. Hemodynamic effects of aortic clamping and decompression with a temporary shunt for resection of the descending thoracic aorta. *Surgery.* 1979;85:25–30.

23. Gelman S. The pathophysiology of aortic cross-clamping and unclamping. *Anesthesiology.* 1995;82: 1026–1060.

24. Fayad A, Yang H, Nathan H, Bryson GL, Cina CS. Acute diastolic dysfunction in thoracoabdominal aortic aneurysm surgery. *Can J Anaesth.* 2006;53:168–173.

25. O'Connor CJ, Rothenberg DM. Anesthetic considerations for descending thoracic aortic surgery: part II. *J Cardiothorac Vasc Anesth.* 1995;9:734–747.

26. Verdant A, Page A, Cossette R, et al. Surgery of the descending thoracic aorta: spinal cord protection with the Gott shunt. *Ann Thorac Surg.* 1988;46:147–154.

27. Hyde JAJ, Delius RE. Physiology and pathophysiology of extracorporeal circulation. In: Kay PH, Munsch CM, eds. *Techniques in Extracorporeal Circulation.* 4th ed. London, Great Britain: Arnold; 2004:23–56.

28. Schepens M, Dossche K, Morshuis W, et al. Introduction of adjuncts and their influence on changing results in 402 consecutive thoracoabdominal aortic aneurysm repairs. *Eur J Cardiothorac Surg.* 2004;25:701–707.

29. Schepens MA, Vermeulen FE, Morshuis WJ, et al. Impact of left heart bypass on the results of thoracoabdominal aortic aneurysm repair. *Ann Thorac Surg.* 1999;67:1963–1967.

30. Estrera AL, Miller CC 3rd, Chen EP, et al. Descending thoracic aortic aneurysm repair: 12-year experience using distal aortic perfusion and cerebrospinal fluid drainage. *Ann Thorac Surg.* 2005;80:1290–1296.

31. Bavaria JE, Woo YJ, Hall RA, Carpenter JP, Gardner TJ. Retrograde cerebral and distal aortic perfusion during ascending and thoracoabdominal aortic operations. *Ann Thorac Surg.* 1995;60:345–352.

32. D' Ambra MN, Dewhirst W, Jacobs M, Bergus B, Borges L, Hilgenberg A. Cross-clamping the thoracic aorta. Effect of intracranial pressure. *Circulation.* 1988;78:III198–III202.

33. Simpson JI, Eide TR, Newman SB, et al. Trimethaphan versus sodium nitroprusside for the control of proximal hypertension during thoracic aortic cross-clamping: the effects on spinal cord ischemia. *Anesth Analg.* 1996;82:68–74.

34. Simpson JI, Eide TR, Schiff GA, et al. Isoflurane versus sodium nitroprusside for the control of proximal hypertension during thoracic aortic cross-clamping: effects on spinal cord ischemia. *J Cardiothorac Vasc Anesth.* 1995;9:491–496.

35. Simpson JI, Eide TR, Schiff GA, et al. Effect of nitroglycerin on spinal cord ischemia after thoracic aortic cross-clamping. *Ann Thorac Surg.* 1996;61:113–117.

36. Shine T, Nugent M. Sodium nitroprusside decreases spinal cord perfusion pressure during descending thoracic aortic cross clamping in the dog. *J Cardiothorac Anesth.* 1990;4:185–193.

37. Nishikawa T, Omote K, Namiki A, Takahashi T. The effects of nicardipine on cerebrospinal fluid pressure in humans. *Anesth Analg.* 1986;65:507–510.

38. Aronson S, Dyke CM, Stierer KA, et al. The ECLIPSE trials: comparative studies of clevidipine to nitroglycerin, sodium nitroprusside, and nicardipine for acute hypertension treatment in cardiac surgery patients. *Anesth Analg.* 2008;107:1110–1121.

39. Levine WC, Lee JJ, Black JH, Cambria RP, Davison JK. Thoracoabdominal aneurysm repair. Anesthetic management. *Int Anesthesiol Clin.* 2005;43:39–60.

40. Gertler JP, Cambria RP, Brewster DC, et al. Coagulation changes during thoracoabdominal aneurysm repair. *J Vasc Surg.* 1996;24:936–943.

41. Shore-Lesserson L, Bodian C, Vela-Cantos F, Silvay G, Reich DL. Antifibrinolytic use and bleeding during surgery on the descending thoracic aorta: a multivariate analysis. *J Cardiothorac Vasc Anesth.* 2005;19:453–458.

42. Sloan TB, James LC. Electrophysiologic monitoring during surgery to repair the thoracoabdominal aorta. *J Clin Neurophysiol.* 2007;24:316–327.

43. Safi HJ, Estrera AL, Miller CC, et al. Evolution of risk for neurologic deficit after descending and thoracoabdominal aortic repair. *Ann Thorac Surg.* 2005;80: 2173–2179.

44. Melissano G, Chiesa R. Advances in imaging of the spinal cord vascular supply and its relationship with paraplegia after aortic interventions. A review. *Eur J Vasc Endovasc Surg.* 2009;38:567–577.

45. Backes WH, Nijenhuis RJ, Mess WH, Wilmink FA, Schurink GW, Jacobs MJ. Magnetic resonance angiography of collateral blood supply to spinal cord in thoracic and thoracoabdominal aortic aneurysm patients. *J Vasc Surg.* 2008;48:261–271.

46. Kuniyoshi Y, Koja K, Miyagi K, et al. Prevention of postoperative paraplegia during thoracoabdominal surgery. *Ann Thorac Surg.* 2003;76:1477–1484.

47. Cambria RP, Clouse WD, Davison JK, et al. Thoracoabdominal aneurysm repair: results with

337 operations performed over a 15-year interval. *Ann Surg.* 2002;236:471–479.

48. Svensson LG, Crawford ES, Hess KR, et al. Experience with 1509 patients undergoing thoracoabdominal aortic operations. *J Vasc Surg.* 1993;17: 357–368.

49. Griepp RB, Ergin MA, Galla JD, Klein JJ, Spielvogel D, Griepp EB. Minimizing spinal cord injury during repair of descending thoracic and thoracoabdominal aneurysms: the Mount Sinai approach. *Semin Thorac Cardiovasc Surg.* 1998;10:25–28.

50. Galla JD, Ergin MA, Lansman SL, et al. Use of somatosensory evoked potentials for thoracic and thoracoabdominal aortic resections. *Ann Thorac Surg.* 1999;67:1947–1952.

51. Cambria RP, Davison JK. Regional hypothermia for prevention of spinal cord ischemic complications after thoracoabdominal aortic surgery: experience with epidural cooling. *Semin Thorac Cardiovasc Surg.* 1998; 10:61–65.

52. Tefera G, Acher CW, Wynn MM. Clamp and sew techniques in thoracoabdominal aortic surgery using naloxone and CSF drainage. *Semin Vasc Surg.* 2000;13:325–330.

53. Acher CW, Wynn MM, Archibald J. Naloxone and spinal fluid drainage as adjuncts in the surgical treatment of thoracoabdominal and thoracic aneurysms. *Surgery.* 1990;108:755–761.

54. Kunihara T, Matsuzaki K, Shiiya N, Saijo Y, Yasuda K. Naloxone lowers cerebrospinal fluid levels of excitatory amino acids after thoracoabdominal aortic surgery. *J Vasc Surg.* 2004;40:681–690.

55. Svensson LG. Paralysis after aortic surgery: in search of lost cord function. *Surgeon.* 2005;3:396–405.

56. Sala F, Menna G, Bricolo A, Young W. Role of glycemia in acute spinal cord injury. Data from a rat experimental model and clinical experience. *Ann NY Acad Sci.* 1999;890:133–154.

57. Duckworth WC, Jallepalli P, Solomon SS. Glucose intolerance in spinal cord injury. *Arch Phys Med Rehabil.* 1983;64:107–110.

58. Nagamizo D, Tsuruta S, Matsumoto M, Matayoshi H, Yamashita A, Sakabe T. Tight glycemic control by insulin, started in the preischemic, but not postischemic, period, protects against ischemic spinal cord injury in rabbits. *Anesth Analg.* 2007;105:1397–1403.

59. Miller CC 3rd, Estrera AL, Huynh TTT, Porat EE, Dafi HJ. Distal aortic perfusion and selective visceral perfusion. In: Rousseau H, Verhoye JP, Heautot JF, eds. *Thoracic Aortic Diseases.* 1st ed. Berlin, Heidelberg, Germany: Springer; 2006:33–53.

60. Safi HJ, Harlin SA, Miller CC, et al. Predictive factors for acute renal failure in thoracic and thoracoabdominal aortic aneurysm surgery. *J Vasc Surg.* 1996;24: 338–344.

61. Svensson LG, Coselli JS, Safi HJ, Hess KR, Crawford ES. Appraisal of adjuncts to prevent acute renal failure after surgery on the thoracic or thoracoabdominal aorta. *J Vasc Surg.* 1989;10:230–239.

62. Godet G, Fléron MH, Vicaut E, et al. Risk factors for acute postoperative renal failure in thoracic or thoracoabdominal aortic surgery: a prospective study. *Anesth Analg.* 1997;85:1227–1232.

63. Kashyap VS, Cambria RP, Davison JK, L'Italien GJ. Renal failure after thoracoabdominal aortic surgery. *J Vasc Surg.* 1997;26:949–955.

64. Jacobs MJ, Eijsman L, Meylaerts SA, et al. Reduced renal failure following thoracoabdominal aortic aneurysm repair by selective perfusion. *Eur J Cardiothorac Surg.* 1998;14:201–205.

65. Jacobs MJ, van Eps RG, de Jong DS, Schurink GW, Mochtar B. Prevention of renal failure in patients undergoing thoracoabdominal aortic aneurysm repair. *J Vasc Surg.* 2004;40:1067–1073.

66. Coselli JS, Lemaire SA, Raskin SA. Perfusion for thoracic aortic surgery. In: Gravlee GP, Davis RF, Stammers AH, Ungerleider RM, eds. *Cardiopulmonary Bypass, Principles and Practice.* 3rd ed. Philadelphia: Lippincoat Williams & Wilkins; 2008:724–736.

67. Hidatsa LF, Bakris GL, Beckman JA, et al. ACCF/ AHA/AATS/ACR/ASA/SCA/SCAI/SIR/STS/SVM guidelines for the diagnosis and management of patients with thoracic aortic disease. A Report of the American College of Cardiology Foundation/American Heart Association Task Force on Practice Guidelines, American Association for Thoracic Surgery, American College of Radiology, American Stroke Association, Society of Cardiovascular Anesthesiologists, Society for Cardiovascular Angiography and Interventions, Society of Interventional Radiology, Society of Thoracic Surgeons, and Society for Vascular Medicine. *Circulation.* 2010;121:e266-e369.

68. Miller CC 3rd, Grimm JC, Estrera AL, et al. Postoperative renal function preservation with nonischemic femoral arterial cannulation for thoracoabdominal aortic repair. *J Vasc Surg.* 2010;51:38–42.

69. Miller CC 3rd, Villa MA, Achouh P, et al. Intraoperative skeletal muscle ischemia contributes to risk of renal dysfunction following thoracoabdominal aortic repair. *Eur J Cardiothorac Surg.* 2008;33:691–694.

70. Harward TR, Welborn MB 3rd, Martin TD, et al. Visceral ischemia and organ dysfunction after thoracoabdominal aortic aneurysm repair. A clinical and cost analysis. *Ann Surg.* 1996;223:729–734.

71. Welborn MB, Oldenburg HS, Hess PJ, et al. The relationship between visceral ischemia, proinflammatory cytokines, and organ injury in patients undergoing thoracoabdominal aortic aneurysm repair. *Crit Care Med.* 2000 Sep;28(9):3191–3197.

72. Back MR, Bandyk M, Bradner M, et al. Critical analysis of outcome determinants affecting repair of intact aneurysms involving the visceral aorta. *Ann Vasc Surg.* 2005;19(5):648–656.

73. Achouh PE, Madsen K, Miller CC 3rd, et al. Gastrointestinal complications after descending thoracic and thoracoabdominal aortic repairs: a 14-year experience. *J Vasc Surg.* 2006;44:442–446.

74. Kieffer E, Chiche L, Godet G, et al. Type IV thoracoabdominal aneurysm repair: predictors of post-operative mortality, spinal cord injury, and acute intestinal ischemia. *Ann Vasc Surg.* 2008;22:822–828.

75. Svensson LG, Hess KR, Coselli JS, et al. A prospective study of respiratory failure after high risk surgery on the thoracoabdominal aorta. *J Vasc Surg.* 1991;14:271–282.

76. Engle J, Safi HJ, Miller CC 3rd, et al. The impact of diaphragm management on prolonged ventilatory support after thoracoabdominal aortic repair. *J Vasc Surg.* 1999;29:150–156.

77. Messé SR, Bavaria JE, Mullen M, et al. Neurologic outcomes from high risk descending thoracic and thoracoabdominal aortic operations in the era of endovascular repair. *Neurocrit Care.* 2008;9:344–351.

78. Huynh TT, Miller CC 3rd, Safi HJ. Delayed onset of neurologic deficit: significance and management. *Semin Vasc Surg.* 2000;13:340–344.

79. Estrera A, Miller C, Huynh T, et al. Preoperative and operative predictors of delayed neurologic deficit following repair of thoracoabdominal aortic aneurysm. *J Thorac Cardiovasc Surg.* 2003;126:1288–1294.

80. de la Linde CM, Guerrero F, Fernández R, Blanco E, Sánchez-Palencia A. Usefulness of the paravertebral block for surgery of the thoracic aorta. *Rev Esp Anestesiol Reanim.* 2004;51:466–467.

81. Yoshioka K, Niinuma H, Ohira A, et al. MR angiography and CT angiography of the artery of Adamkiewicz: noninvasive preoperative assessment of thoracoabdominal aortic aneurysm. *Radiographics.* 2003;23: 1215–1225.

Spinal Cord Protection Strategies

11

John G.T. Augoustides

Introduction

Spinal cord protection and preservation during and after reconstruction of the descending thoracic aorta (DTA) is clinically important because spinal cord injury is still common in high-risk groups and it significantly worsens perioperative mortality and morbidity.[1–3] There is a diverse set of aortic pathologies that may require reconstruction of the DTA (refer to Table 11.1 for their description and classification). Aortic repair for each of these pathologies carries a risk of spinal cord ischemia (SCI) that may present intraoperatively or postoperatively. In the contemporary era, there are three established options for reconstruction of the DTA – surgical repair (SR), thoracic endovascular aortic repair (TEVAR), and hybrid repair (involving both SR and TEVAR). The type of DTA repair is important to understand as it may significantly influence the risk for SCI. The specific details of these aortic repair techniques are covered elsewhere in this textbook.

Conventional SR of the DTA is the classic technique typically characterized by thoracotomy, aortic clamping, possible distal aortic perfusion, and aortic replacement with a Dacron interposition graft.[6] As a technique, TEVAR has recently become established, especially since government agency approval of the thoracic endovascular stent grafts and the dissemination of formal guidelines.[7,8] Hybrid repair of the thoracic aorta typically involves TEVAR with surgical translocation of aortic branches to create a safe landing zone for the endovascular stent graft, for example, the transposition of the brachiocephalic arteries to the ascending aorta for subsequent safe TEVAR in the aortic arch, and transposition of the left subclavian artery for TEVAR in the proximal DTA.[9–11]

This chapter will review the strategies for spinal cord protection during and after reconstruction of the DTA, taking into account the diverse aortic pathologies and aortic repair techniques. The typical clinical presentation of SCI associated with DTA repair will be described, followed by a discussion of its contemporary incidence, predictors, and pathogenesis, taking into consideration the current concepts of the spinal arterial collateral network. After this essential background, this chapter will discuss the spinal cord protection strategies in detail before closing with a summary of key points for the management of SCI in DTA repair.

Clinical Presentation of Spinal Cord Ischemia

The hallmark of SCI associated with DTA procedures is weakness of the lower extremities. If the weakness is severe with muscle strength weaker than gravity, it is termed paraplegia. If the weakness is present with at least movement against gravity,

J.G.T. Augoustides (✉)
Department of Anesthesiology and Critical Care,
University of Pennsylvania Medical Center,
Philadelphia, PA, USA
e-mail: yiandoc@hotmail.com

K. Subramaniam et al. (eds.), *Anesthesia and Perioperative Care for Aortic Surgery*,
DOI 10.1007/978-0-387-85922-4_11, © Springer Science+Business Media, LLC 2011

239

Table 11.1 Diseases that often require reconstruction of the descending thoracic aorta

Descending thoracic aortic aneurysm[4]	Thoracoabdominal aortic aneurysm[2]
• **Extent A**: Aneurysm originating after the left subclavian artery with distal extension to no further than the 6th thoracic vertebra (T6) • **Extent B**: Aneurysm originating after T6 with distal extension to no further than the diaphragm • **Extent C**: Aneurysm originating from the left subclavian artery with distal extension to the diaphragm	• **Extent I**: Aneurysm originating distal to the left subclavian artery but proximal to T6, with extension beyond the diaphragm to finish above the renal arteries • **Extent II**: Aneurysm originating distal to the left subclavian artery but proximal to T6, extending below the renal arteries • **Extent III**: Aneurysm originating distal to T6 but above the diaphragm, extending below the renal arteries • **Extent IV**: Aneurysm that begins distal to the diaphragm but above the renal arteries with extension below the renal arteries
Descending thoracic aortic dissection[5] Stanford classification • **Type A**: Aortic dissection originating proximal to the left subclavian artery • **Type B**: Aortic dissection distal to the left subclavian artery	Descending thoracic aortic dissection[5] DeBakey classification • **Type I**: Dissection originating in the ascending aorta with extent to the descending thoracic or abdominal aorta • **Type II**: Dissection limited to the ascending aorta and aortic arch • **Type IIIa**: Dissection distal to the left subclavian artery that ends in the descending thoracic aorta • **Type IIIb**: Dissection distal to the left subclavian artery that ends in the abdominal aorta
Thoracic aortic transection	Thoracic aortic coarctation

Table 11.2 Description of spinal ischemia after descending thoracic aortic reconstruction

Score[1,12]	Description[1,12]
Paraplegia	Paraplegia
0	No movement of lower extremity
1	Minimal movement or flicker of lower extremity
2	Movement of the lower extremity but not against resistance or gravity, for example, bend knee; move leg
Paraparesis	Paraparesis
3	Movement of the lower extremity against resistance and gravity but without ability to stand or walk
4	Ability to stand and walk with assistance

Unilateral weakness of the lower extremity is typically attributed to spinal cord ischemia unless associated with weakness of the ipsilateral upper extremity, suggestive of a stroke.

it is termed paraparesis. There is a formal scoring system that has served as a standard for grading lower extremity strength in this clinical setting: it is summarized in Table 11.2.[1,13]

The weakness of the lower extremities is typically bilateral in presentation and evolution. However, it is possible for unilateral weakness to be the presenting feature of SCI after DTA repair. In this scenario, it is important to rule out concomitant weakness of the ipsilateral upper extremity which, if present, is indicative of a stroke rather than SCI. Stroke is always possible, even in the setting of TEVAR.[14,15] If the unilateral lower extremity weakness is isolated, it is typically immediately managed as SCI to facilitate spinal recovery.[1]

The onset of SCI associated with DTA repair is classified as immediate or delayed.[1,16] Immediate onset of SCI is defined as lower extremity weakness on emergence from anesthesia within 24 h of the procedure. Delayed onset of SCI is defined as lower extremity weakness that occurs after a normal postoperative neurological examination after emergence from anesthesia. It is important to note that the delayed presentation of SCI is common and may be recurrent. In a series of 99 patients undergoing open DTA repair, Cheung et al. reported an incidence of immediate SCI of 3.0% as compared to an 8.0% incidence of delayed SCI.[17] In patients with delayed SCI, the initial episode presented at a median of 21.6 h (This is not consistent with the above definition of delayed onset. This is more like SCI of immediate onset lasting long.) after surgery (range: 6.4–110 h), with 25%

of patients having recurrent episodes that may present more than 7 days after surgery.

These findings were confirmed in a large observational study of patients ($N = 2,368$ from 1986–2006) undergoing SR of thoracoabdominal aortic aneurysm (TAAA).[6] In this single-center high-volume longitudinal experience over 20 years, the incidence of SCI was 3.9% with 63% of these cases of immediate onset SCI and 37% of delayed SCI. Delayed SCI presented clinically from 13 h (again this is not consistent with above definition) to 91 days after surgery, confirming that in certain thoracic aortic surgical patients, the risk of SCI persists for months beyond the immediate postoperative period.[6,16,17]

The incidence of delayed SCI has persisted with the advent of ER of the DTA. In a recent contemporaneous comparison of SR and TEVAR for DTA pathology ($N = 724$: 372 SR; 352 ER: 2001–2006), the incidence of SCI in the SR and ER cohorts was 7.5% (29% immediate and 71% delayed) and 4.3% (13% immediate and 87% delayed), respectively.[1] Although the lower incidence of SCI in the TEVAR cohort had borderline statistical significance (4.3% vs. 7.5%, $P = 0.08$), the proportion of immediate and delayed SCI was not significantly different between the two groups.[1]

The persistence of delayed SCI in TEVAR of the DTA is also evident in a single-center real-world case series undertaken within 2 years after US FDA approval of the Gore TAG thoracic endovascular stent (W.L. Gore and Associates, Flagstaff, AZ).[18] In this Duke ER study ($N = 91$: 2005–2007), the incidence of SCI was 5.5%. All cases were delayed in presentation, with >50% incidence of spinal cord rescue to yield a permanent SCI rate of 2.4%.

In summary, SCI associated with DTA reconstruction is possible regardless of aortic repair technique. Its clinical presentation primarily involves lower extremity weakness, whose formal grading is recommended for optimal patient care. The timing of the presentation of SCI after DTA repair is highly variable in the postoperative period. Its presentation may be unilateral as well as relapsing.

Contemporary Risk of Spinal Cord Ischemia

The risk of SCI after DTA repair has been extensively reported according to aortic pathology and aortic repair technique. In the clinical studies about SR of the DTA, further stratification of SCI has been performed according to surgical techniques such as distal aortic perfusion, and deep hypothermic circulatory arrest.[19–28] Due to the advent of TEVAR as a clinical alternative to SR of the DTA,[29] multiple recent studies have focused on the risks of SCI with either aortic repair technique. The results of these studies are summarized in Tables 11.3 and 11.4, according to repair technique.[3,8,19–47] Table 11.3 lists 14 SR studies (total $N = 5,245$) with an SCI range of 0–14%. Table 11.4 lists 23 TEVAR studies (total $N = 3,956$) with a SCI range of 0–8%.

A series of meta-analyses were subsequently completed to determine the risk of SCI specific to DTA pathology and repair technique.[48–52] These meta-analyses have been summarized in Table 11.5.[48–52] In summary, these five meta-analyses reviewed 86 studies ($N = 3,297$: SR 1798; TEVAR 1499). Regardless of DTA

Table 11.3 Risk of spinal cord ischemia with surgical repair of descending thoracic aorta

Author	Sample size	Spinal cord ischemia (%)
Greenberg[1]	372	7.5
Coselli[6]	2,286	3.9
Cheung[17]	99	11.0
Estrera[19]	300	2.3
Coselli[20]	387	2.6
Borst[21]	132	3.0
Svensson[22]	832	5.4
Verdant[23]	267	0
Kouchoukos[24]	65	3.0
Fehrenbacher[25]	63	0
Kieffer[26]	121	7.4
Misfeld[27]	56	3.6
Kieffer[28]	171	4.7
Dillavou[3]	94	14.0

Reference numbers refer to studies listed in reference list for this chapter.

pathology, TEVAR in meta-analyses is associated with a significantly lower risk of mortality ($P < 0.05$) and paraplegia ($P < 0.05$).

Table 11.4 Risk of spinal cord ischemia with endovascular descending thoracic aortic repair

Author	Sample size	Spinal cord ischemia (%)
Greenberg[1]	352	4.3
Hughes[18]	91	5.2
Kieffer[28]	52	0
Dake[30]	103	3.0
Gravereaux[31]	53	5.6
Bell[32]	67	4.5
Orend[33]	74	2.7
Bortone[34]	132	0
Hansen[35]	59	1.7
Leurs[36]	443	2.5
Makaroun[8]	142	3.0
Chiesa[37]	99	4.0
Greenberg[38]	100	6.0
Cheung[39]	75	7.0
Stone[40]	105	6.7
Iyer[41]	70	0
Khoynezhad[42]	91	8.0
Rodriguez[43]	406	2.4
Zipfel[44]	172	1.0
Hnath[45]	121	4.1
Amabile[46]	67	7.5
Dillavou[3]	140	3.0
Parker[47]	942	1.9

Reference numbers refer to studies listed in reference list for this chapter.

Predictors and Pathogenesis of Spinal Cord Ischemia

The etiology of SCI after DTA repair is a net oxygen deficit in the spinal cord where neural oxygen demand outstrips oxygen supply. This complication continues to receive major clinical attention, since it is not only a major outcome determinant but it is also eminently treatable.[53] The successful management of SCI is based on a thorough understanding of its clinical predictors and its pathogenesis, both of which are inseparably linked to the dynamics of the spinal blood supply via the spinal collateral arterial network (SCAN).

The principal clinical predictors for SCI after DTA reconstruction are summarized in Table 11.6.[1–3,6–53] The common pathway for all these predictors of SCI is often major interruption of the spinal oxygen supply via the SCAN, as is outlined in the commentary on each predictor in Table 11.6. As a consequence, the pathogenesis of SCI after DTA reconstruction is linked to a detailed understanding of the SCAN. This section will now discuss the current concepts of this arterial network which provide the framework for understanding the strategies for spinal cord protection after DTA repair.

There has been a gradual synthesis of both laboratory and clinical studies that has led to the concept of a SCAN.[54] The ground-breaking

Table 11.5 Summary of meta-analyses of descending thoracic aortic repair

Author	Sample size	Main findings
Walsh[48]	Seventeen studies with diverse aortic pathologies: $N = 1,109$ (571 SR, 538 ER)	ER significantly reduced mortality (OR 0.36, 95% CI 0.23–0.58, $P < 0.0001$) and paraplegia (OR 0.33, 95% CI 0.18–0.63, $P = 0.0007$)
Tang[49]	Thirty-three studies on traumatic thoracic aortic transection: $N = 699$ (329 SR, 370 ER)	ER significantly reduced mortality (7.6% vs. 15.2%, $P = 0.0076$) and paraplegia (0% vs. 5.6%, $P < 0.0001$)
Hoffer[50]	Nineteen studies on blunt thoracic aortic trauma: $N = 638$ (376 SR, 262 ER)	ER significantly reduced mortality (OR 0.43, 95% CI 0.26–0.70, $P = 0.001$) and paraplegia (OR 0.30, 95% CI 0.12–0.76, $P = 0.01$)
Xenos[51]	Seventeen studies on traumatic descending thoracic aortic rupture: $N = 589$ (369 SR, 220 ER)	ER significantly reduced mortality (OR 0.44, 95% CI 0.25–0.78, $P = 0.005$) and paraplegia (OR 0.32, 95% CI 0.10–0.93, $P = 0.037$)
Akowuah[52]	Ten studies on traumatic thoracic aortic rupture: $N = 262$ (153 SR, 109 ER)	ER significantly reduced mortality (7.0% vs. 19.0%, $P = 0.01$) and paraplegia (1.0% vs. 6.0%, $P < 0.01$)

SR Surgical Aortic Repair, *ER* Endovascular Aortic Repair, *OR* Odds Ratio, *CI* Confidence Interval.

Table 11.6 Predictors of spinal cord ischemia in descending thoracic aortic repair

Predictor	Comments
Extent of descending thoracic aortic repair	The risk of spinal cord ischemia increases with the extent of aortic repair due to a greater interruption of the spinal arterial supply from the intercostal and/or lumbar arterial network
Prior thoracic and/or abdominal aortic surgery, for example, open abdominal aortic aneurysm repair; thoracic aortic endovascular stent	The risk of spinal cord ischemia increases in the setting of prior aortic repair due to already sacrificed intercostal and/or lumbar arterial supply to the spinal arterial network
Surgical sacrifice of spinal segmental arterial supply, for example, intercostal arteries	The risk of spinal cord ischemia also depends on the extent of surgical preservation of the intercostal and/or lumbar arterial supply to the spinal arterial network
Aortic dissection with malperfusion	In the setting of an acute complicated type B dissection, there may already be spinal cord ischemia due to arterial malperfusion as a result of the dissection. This type of ischemic presentation is often an indication for emergency surgical intervention
Duration of aortic clamping	In the absence of distal aortic perfusion, the duration of aortic clamping to allow aortic reconstruction correlated with the risk of spinal cord ischemia. This was due to lack of arterial perfusion below the clamp and loss of spinal arterial supply in the replaced aortic segment. This pathogenesis facilitated the introduction of aortic perfusion distal to the aortic clamp with either passive flow via a Gott shunt or active flow via left heart bypass
Anemia	Acute severe anemia in this setting is most often due to severe bleeding. Acute severe anemia contributes to the risk of spinal cord ischemia from decreased oxygen-carrying capacity due to significantly decreased hemoglobin mass
Circulatory collapse, for example, aortic rupture; cardiogenic shock	Circulatory compromise interferes significantly with oxygen delivery to the spinal cord and thus is a significant risk factor for spinal cord ischemia after descending thoracic aortic reconstruction
Systemic vasodilatation and vascular steal with sodium nitroprusside	Sodium nitroprusside was utilized to control proximal hypertension associated with aortic clamping. However, due to systemic vasodilatation and consequent vascular steal, it augmented spinal cord ischemia due to lowering of arterial pressure in the spinal collateral network

Adapted from Pantin and Cheung.[12]

anatomic research of Adamkiewicz first demonstrated the vascular plexus of the anterior and posterior spinal arteries that further received cephalic, central, and caudal arterial inputs.[55] The cephalic arterial input is derived from the three brachiocephalic arteries with major supply from the vertebral arteries. The central arterial input is principally derived from multiple segmental aortic branches, namely, the intercostal and lumbar arteries. This central arterial supply typically includes a large arterial branch, most commonly at the level of the lower thoracic or upper abdominal aorta, appropriately known as the artery of Adamkiewicz or the arteria radicularis magna. The caudal arterial input that augments the arterial supply of the distal spinal cord and cauda equina is derived from the internal iliac arteries and their branches.

In the 1970s, these observations about the SCAN by Adamkiewicz were expanded by Lazorthes and colleagues who demonstrated multiple arterial plexuses outside the spinal canal, including the perivertebral and paraspinous networks.[56] Recent advances in computed tomographic angiography permit preoperative imaging of the artery of Adamkiewicz in almost all patients considered for DTA reconstruction.[57,58] These imaging studies demonstrated that this important spinal artery arises in more than 60% of cases from the left side, and in more than 90% of cases from the levels of the 8th thoracic vertebra to the 3rd lumbar vertebra (in more than 70%

of cases, from the 10th–12th thoracic vertebral levels). Magnetic resonance angiography can also image the SCAN in detail.[59] Preoperative visualization with magnetic resonance angiography of an adequate SCAN was 97% predictive for preservation of spinal cord function during DTA reconstruction. Furthermore, patients with no SCAN demonstrable on preoperative imaging were at significantly increased risk for clinical SCI in the perioperative period.[59]

Further clinical importance of the SCAN is illustrated by the significant increased risk of SCI after DTA reconstruction in patients with prior abdominal aortic replacement.[60] A recent meta-analysis ($N = 1,493$, nine studies) calculated that prior abdominal aortic replacement is a very significant risk factor for SCI after extensive DTA and TAA repair with relative risks of 11.1 (95% confidence interval 3.8–32.3, $P < 0.0001$) and 2.90 (95% confidence interval 1.26–6.65, $P = 0.008$), respectively.[60] In this meta-analysis, 12.4% of patients with DTA aneurysms and 18.7% of patients with TAAA had prior abdominal aortic replacement. Based on current concepts of the SCAN, this increased risk of SCI in this aortic repair subgroup is explained by the compromised caudal spinal arterial supply from prior abdominal aortic replacement. Although the overall risk of SCI is lower for TEVAR of the DTA, prior abdominal aortic replacement is still a significant risk factor for SCI after TEVAR due to the compromised caudal input to the SCAN.[8,29–40]

The degree of SCAN compromise and consequently increased risk of SCI has also consistently been related to the extent of DTA replacement, despite multimodal advances over the years.[6,61] Despite world-class experience and expertise in SR of TAAA ($N = 2,286$: 1986–2006), the risk of SCI was still dependent on Crawford extent as follows: extent I 3.3%, extent II 6.3%, extent III 2.6%, and extent IV 1.4% (refer to Table 11.1 for extent definitions).[6] Even at an expert center with multimodal spinal cord protection strategies sequentially introduced over 20 years, extensive compromise of the SCAN from extensive aortic repair has remained a significant risk factor for SCI.

This correlation of SCI risk and extent of aortic reconstruction also applies in DTA replacement. A recent series of DTA aneurysm repairs ($N = 300$) documented only a 2.3% incidence of SCI: all seven cases of SCI, however, occurred in patients with aneurysms of the entire DTA (160/300) or extent C aneurysms (refer to Table 11.1 for extent definitions).[19] In this series, the risk of SCI for extent C DTA aneurysm was 4.4% (7/300), as compared to 0% for extent A and extent B DTA aneurysms. Not surprisingly, multivariate analysis determined that extent C DTA aneurysm was a significant predictor for SCI with an odds ratio of 13.73 ($P = 0.02$). Furthermore, as expected, previous abdominal aortic replacement was also a significant predictor for SCI in this DTA aneurysm series with an odds ratio of 7.0 ($P = 0.005$). The clinical importance of an adequate SCAN persists regardless of aortic repair technique. Clinical markers of SCAN compromise such as extent C aneurysm and/or prior abdominal aortic replacement remain significant predictors of SCI after TEVAR of the DTA.[29,46]

Compromise of the spinal cord perfusion via the SCAN will also occur with significant perioperative hypotension during DTA reconstruction. In SR of TAAA, perioperative hypotension (defined as systolic blood pressure < 80 mmHg) was an independent predictor for SCI.[62] In particular, intraoperative hypotension after separation from cardiopulmonary bypass was the most predictive for perioperative SCI after aortic reconstruction. This clinical observation supports the concept of a critical SCAN perfusion pressure.

Relative hypotension (i.e., mean arterial pressure <80% of baseline) has also been demonstrated to have a significant association with the risk of delayed SCI after DTA reconstruction ($P = 0.03$).[63] This is an important concept since mean absolute arterial pressures may appear in the normal range, but will only be low when compared to the baseline preoperative mean arterial pressure for each patient. In this setting, each patient serves as his/her own control. This evidence suggests that the perfusion pressure in the SCAN during and after DTA repair must be managed as a function of the patient's normal baseline arterial pressure.

The concept that is inherent in the discussion of the SCAN and perioperative perfusion pressure is the principle of spinal cord perfusion pressure. Spinal cord perfusion pressure is defined as the difference between mean arterial pressure and cerebrospinal fluid (CSF) pressure. Note that if central venous pressure is consistently higher than CSF pressure, then it is substituted for CSF pressure. An elevated central venous pressure has been significantly associated with delayed SCI after DTA repair ($P = 0.03$).[63] In the setting of a significantly elevated central venous pressure, it may need to be actively managed to increase spinal cord perfusion pressure to relieve SCI.[64,65]

The spinal cord perfusion pressure can be augmented for spinal cord rescue in the setting of SCI. From the definition, it is clear that this augmentation of spinal cord perfusion may be achieved by increasing mean arterial pressure and/or decreasing CSF pressure. These two manipulations are cornerstones of perioperative management for clinical SCI in the setting of DTA repair. These perioperative interventions will be discussed in detail in the next section on clinical strategies for spinal cord protection after DTA repair.

Furthermore, it follows that aggressive systemic vasodilatation will decrease mean arterial pressure, increase vascular steal from the low-pressure SCAN, and consequently decrease spinal cord perfusion pressure to cause or aggravate SCI. These adverse spinal cord perfusion effects have been demonstrated in large animal studies with sodium nitroprusside,[66,67] encouraging perioperative teams to avoid this drug during extensive aortic reconstructions.[68]

Spinal Cord Protection Strategies: Balancing Oxygen Supply with Oxygen Demand

The five major spinal cord protection strategies are summarized in Table 11.7. All five strategies aim to preserve oxygen balance in the spinal cord. The first two strategies are to minimize ischemia due to aortic clamping and to maximize spinal

cord perfusion pressure: This pair of strategies aims to maximize oxygen supply to the spinal cord. The second two strategies are hypothermia and pharmacologic neuroprotection: This pair of strategies aims to decrease oxygen demand of the spinal cord. The last strategy is to detect spinal cord ischemia early with intensive neurological monitoring for immediate intervention: This strategy aims to limit the duration of oxygen debt and restore oxygen balance in the spinal cord. Each of these strategies will now be discussed in detail. In practice, all these strategies blend in a multimodal approach to perioperative spinal cord preservation.[69]

Minimize Interruption of Spinal Blood Supply due to Aortic Clamping

In SR of the DTA, the aorta is clamped proximally and distally to the diseased aortic segment. Aortic clamping achieves vascular isolation of the diseased aortic segment which can then be resected and replaced with a vascular graft. During the time of aortic clamping, there is interruption of normal antegrade aortic perfusion of the spinal cord, including the SCAN, and hence SCI occurs. As a result, distal aortic perfusion with left heart bypass or a Gott shunt was introduced to ameliorate the lack of arterial perfusion distal to the aortic clamps and perfuse the distal body, including the spinal cord.[21,23,54]

Replacement of the DTA, however, can be safely performed with simple aortic clamping in expert hands.[20] As an example, extensive DTA replacement in expert hands requires an average aortic clamp time of 26.9 ± 9.9 min ($N = 341$) with a paraplegia rate of 2.3%.[20] Although these results are superb, it must be remembered that they were achieved in a center of excellence with one of the longest and largest DTA experiences in the world. However, for SR of extensive TAAA (Crawford extents I and II), distal aortic perfusion with consequent perfusion of the internal iliac arteries and the caudal input to the SCAN significantly reduces the incidence of SCI.[70,71] Distal aortic perfusion with left heart bypass significantly reduced the risk of SCI, especially

Table 11.7 Spinal cord protection strategies in DTA reconstruction

Type of intervention	Clinical examples
Increase oxygen supply Maximize spinal cord perfusion during aortic clamping	• Minimize aortic clamp time • Distal aortic perfusion with passive shunt (Gott Shunt) • Distal aortic perfusion with partial cardiopulmonary bypass – Avoid aortic clamping with endovascular aortic stenting
Increase oxygen supply Maximize spinal cord perfusion pressure	• Reduction of back-bleeding from segmental arteries – Reimplantation of segmental arterial branches • Lumbar drainage of cerebrospinal fluid • Augmentation of systemic arterial pressure
Decrease oxygen demand Hypothermia	• Mild-to-moderate systemic hypothermia (32–35°C) • Deep hypothermic circulatory arrest (14–18°C) • Selective spinal cord hypothermia (epidural cooling 25°C)
Increase tissue tolerance of ischemia Pharmacologic neuroprotection of spinal cord	• Steroids • Thiopental • Magnesium sulfate • Mannitol • Naloxone • Lidocaine • Intrathecal papaverine

Early detection and intervention
Intensive clinical monitoring of spinal cord function
	• Intraoperative monitoring (patient under general anesthesia)
	  – Somatosensory evoked potentials
	  – Motor evoked potentials
	• Perioperative monitoring (patient awake)
	  – Preoperative neurologic examination to establish neurological baseline
	  – Postoperative serial neurologic examination to detect onset of spinal ischemia and spinal response to interventions
	• Aggressive intervention on detection of spinal ischemia

Adapted from Pantin and Cheung.[12]

in extent II TAAA (4.8% vs. 13.1%, $P = 0.007$[70]; 13% vs. 41%, $P < 0.003$[71]).

A survey of contemporary surgical practice reveals that distal aortic perfusion with left heart bypass (with/without an oxygenator) is utilized by most surgeons for SR of the DTA.[54] This surgical perfusion technique standardizes distal aortic perfusion and consequently augments caudal perfusion of the SCAN to minimize interruption of spinal blood supply during aortic clamping. Even in short DTA segment repairs such as in DTA traumatic transection, distal aortic perfusion with left heart bypass or the Gott shunt significantly decreases the risk of SCI (2% vs. 33%, $P = 0.007$).[72]

In TEVAR of the DTA, there is no aortic clamping. As a consequence, there is no spinal ischemia due to aortic clamping. This may be one of the reasons that the risk of SCI is significantly lower with TEVAR as compared to SR. However, there is immediate loss of spinal cord perfusion

from the segmental arterial occlusion by the endovascular stent. Hence, the extent of this coverage significantly affects SCI risk.[73]

Maximize Spinal Cord Perfusion Pressure

Management of the Segmental Arterial Supply

There is often significant retrograde bleeding from intercostal and lumbar arteries that occurs in the clamped diseased aortic segment selected for SR.[74] This bleeding from the segmental arterial supply of the SCAN directs blood flow away from the SCAN, creating vascular steal that aggravates the SCI during aortic repair (Fig. 11.1). Various interventions to minimize this segmental arterial steal have been introduced: vascular occlusion with pegs after incision of the clamped isolated aortic segment,[21] intra-aortic ligation of

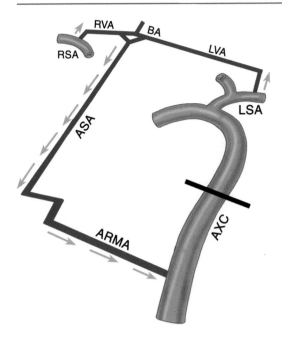

Fig. 11.1 Steal phenomenon in the excluded part of the aorta. A rerouting way through the anterior spinal artery and arteria radicularis magna steals blood from the spinal cord. *ASA* anterior spinal artery, *ARMA* anterior radicularis magna artery, *LSA* left subclavian artery, *RSA* right subclavian artery, *LVA* left vertebral artery, *RVA* right vertebral artery, *BA* basilar artery, *AXC* aortic clamping (Reprinted, with permission from Elsevier, from reference[121])

the bleeding segmental vessels,[75] segmental arterial occlusion with balloons and tourniquets,[13] clamping and division of segmental arterial vessels before aortic clamping,[68,76] and anastomosis of all segmental arteries into a vascular graft to maintain perfusion of the SCAN.[77] The principle common to all these surgical interventions is to prevent loss of perfusion pressure and consequent vascular steal from the SCAN. All these surgical adjunct techniques for segmental arterial management in DTA repair have been associated with very low rates of clinically significant SCI.

In TEVAR of the DTA, immediate occlusion of the segmental arterial system occurs with stent deployment if there is adequate apposition of the stent against the aortic wall. However, there may be retrograde flow from segmental arteries into the native diseased aorta after stent deployment: this is classified as a type II endoleak.[78] The clinical concern with type II endoleaks is that they might lead to expansion of the native diseased

aorta and ultimately lead to aortic rupture. A second concern is that retrograde flow from the segmental arteries will decrease perfusion pressure in the SCAN and aggravate SCI. Although this is theoretically possible, to the best of my knowledge (as of January 9, 2010), there has been no report of this possibility.

Endoleaks of all types occur in 29% of patients after TEVAR of the DTA: type II endoleaks account for up to 35% of all diagnosed endoleaks in this setting.[78] In this single-center series (*N* = 100), 29% of type II endoleaks spontaneously thrombosed during follow-up and there was minimal aneurysm expansion in the presence of a type II endoleak (mean of 2.9 mm).[78] No active intervention was required for type II endoleak management. In a second single-center series of SR for DTA repair (*N* = 200, 2001–2006), the endoleak II findings were similar: type II endoleaks, however, were conservatively managed in 76% of cases, and required active intervention in the remaining 26% of cases.[79] Active intervention of type II endoleaks may require additional endovascular aortic stenting or in selected cases, percutaneous transaortic needle-based embolization of segmental arteries.[80] In these reports, there were no cases of SCI that were linked to the presence of type II endoleaks.[78–80] To date, type II endoleaks in TEVAR of the DTA appear to be a risk factor for aortic rupture but not SCI.

Cerebrospinal Fluid Drainage

Lumbar drainage of CSF is an established adjunct for the management of SCI after DTA reconstruction.[12] The physiologic principle underlying its application in this setting is that reduction of CSF pressure improves spinal cord perfusion pressure via the SCAN, as explained earlier. Furthermore, it also counters perioperative increases in CSF pressure that may be due to aortic clamping, spinal cord reperfusion, increases in central venous pressure, and spinal cord edema.[81] The clinical efficacy of lumbar CSF drainage for management of SCI after SR of the DTA was first stressed in case reports.[82] Subsequently, multiple case series and randomized controlled clinical trials followed. This plethora of evidence has been

Table 11.8 Summary of meta-analyses of cerebrospinal fluid drainage in descending thoracic aortic repair

Author	Sample size	Main findings
Walsh[83]	Thirteen studies in patients with descending thoracic aortic and thoracoabdominal aortic aneurysms. (total N not listed since no data pooling was performed)	No pooling of data was performed due to the heterogeneity in study designs (two randomized trials, 11 observational case series). The conclusion was that the evidence to date was insufficient to make a clear recommendation. The authors suggested that further adequately powered randomized controlled trials were required
Tang[84]	Three randomized controlled trials in patients with Crawford extent I and extent II thoracoabdominal aortic aneurysms (total $N = 289$)	Cerebrospinal fluid drainage was associated with an 80% reduction in spinal cord ischemia (odds ratio 0.48, 95% confidence interval 0.25–0.92). The conclusion was that perioperative cerebrospinal fluid drainage reduced spinal cord ischemia in high-risk thoracoabdominal aortic aneurysm repair. The authors suggested that further experimental and clinical studies are indicated, since the current evidence was limited
Cina[85]	Three randomized controlled trials in patients with Crawford extent I and extent II thoracoabdominal aortic aneurysms (total $N = 289$) Six non-randomized studies in patients undergoing descending thoracic aortic and thoracoabdominal aortic surgery (total $N = 251$)	For the randomized studies, the odds ratio for spinal cord ischemia in the cerebrospinal fluid drainage cohort was 0.35 (95% confidence interval 0.12–0.99, $P = 0.05$) For the non-randomized studies, the odds ratio for spinal cord ischemia in the cerebrospinal fluid drainage cohort was 0.26 (95% confidence interval 0.13–0.53, $P = 0.0002$). For all studies, the odds ratio for spinal cord ischemia in the cerebrospinal fluid drainage cohort was 0.30 (95% confidence interval 0.17–0.54, $P < 0.0001$) The conclusion was that perioperative drainage of cerebrospinal fluid in expert centers is an effective adjunct for the prevention of spinal cord ischemia in extensive descending thoracic aortic and thoracoabdominal aortic reconstruction

systematically reviewed in three meta-analyses that have been summarized in Table 11.8.[83–85] In summary, the best evidence to date suggests that lumbar drainage of CSF significantly reduces the incidence of SCI after DTA repair.

Lumbar CSF drainage is performed by the percutaneous insertion of a silicon catheter via a 14-gauge Tuohy needle at the level of the L3–L4 intervertebral space, assuming that informed consent has been obtained and coagulation function is adequate. The catheter is typically advanced 10–15 cm into the subarachnoid space.[12] It is securely fastened to the skin and its open end is attached to as sterile reservoir. The lumbar CSF pressure is measured with a pressure transducer zero-referenced to the midline of the brain. The drainage of CSF is performed to maintain the lumbar CSF pressure below 10 mmHg. The catheter is typically inserted before or at the time of surgery, and CSF drainage is continued for 24 h after surgery. Subsequently, it can be capped and left in situ for the next 24 h. Thereafter, it can be removed if the patient has a normal neurologic examination and satisfactory coagulation function.[12]

The potential complications of this lumbar CSF drainage include headache, catheter fracture, epidural hematoma, meningitis, and intracranial hypotension with secondary intradural hematoma and brain herniation.[12,86,87] Despite the potential risk of neuraxial hematoma as a complication of lumbar CSF drainage in aortic surgical patients subsequently undergoing cardiopulmonary bypass with systemic heparinization, clinical practice suggests that this risk is insignificant when compared to the clinical benefits related to SCI, when CSF drainage is performed for pressures > 10 mmHg.[86] A large case series ($N = 162$, 1993–2002) of patients undergoing DTA reconstruction with cardiopulmonary bypass, systemic heparinization, and lumbar CSF drainage was reviewed for catheter-related complications.[86] The authors reported a complication rate of 3.7% (6/162): one temporary abducens nerve palsy, two fractured catheters, two cases of meningitis, and one headache. There were no catheter-related hemorrhagic complications or any permanent sequelae from all the catheter-related complications. In this series, CSF drainage was performed only when the lumbar CSF pressure was >10 mmHg and drains were removed on the second postoperative day.

Subdural hematoma due to lumbar CSF drainage for DTA repairs has been described with an incidence of 3.5% (8/230) in a single-center experience (N = 230: 1992–2001).[87] There was a 50% mortality from this complication. Furthermore, the majority of these patients underwent craniotomy or lumbar blood patch. In this series, however, CSF drainage was performed whenever CSF pressure was >5 mmHg and drains were removed on the third postoperative day. A significantly greater amount of CSF was drained from the patients who developed subdural hematomas (690 vs. 359 mL, P = 0.0013). The following interventions have been suggested for the prevention and treatment of this complication: lumbar CSF pressure drainage only when CSF pressure exceeds 10 mmHg, meticulous neurological monitoring, early neurosurgical consultation for acute subdural hematoma, and consideration of an epidural blood patch.[87,88] Meningitis is more common with prolonged CSF drainage, and often presents with fever altered mentation as well as CSF positive for bacteria and pleocytosis.[89]

An unresolved question is whether to proceed with SR of the DTA if a bloody tap occurs during placement of a lumbar CSF drain.[90,91] There is no high-quality evidence to guide decision-making on this clinical question.

Clearly, the decision must be then individualized. In emergency situations such as aortic rupture, severe malperfusion, and/or severe symptoms, it is imperative to proceed with surgical intervention since the risks from delay of aortic repair far outweigh the risks of a neuraxial hematoma. However, in the elective situation, the answer is not always so clear and collaborative discussion between all decision-makers will guide the process to a consensus-based management plan.[90,91]

The indications for CSF drainage in ER of the DTA are more stringent than in SR because the risk of SCI is significantly lower. Lumbar CSF drainage is indicated in patients at high risk for SCI in ER: those patients with prior aortic repairs and those with planned extensive endovascular repair (typically extent C DTA aneurysms; Crawford extent I and II TAAA).[3,29,39,42,45,46,73]

Augmentation of Systemic Arterial Pressure

The augmentation of systemic arterial pressure is an established intervention in the management of SCI in SR and ER of the DTA.[17,29,39,92] This intervention increases spinal cord perfusion pressure through the SCAN, as explained earlier in this chapter. The spinal cord is vulnerable to hypotensive SCI during DTA repair due to loss of significant segmental arterial input to the SCAN.[62,63] Furthermore, since SCI in DTA repair typically involves the thoracolumbar spinal cord, there is a significant sympathectomy that accompanies SCI.[17] This acute sympathectomy aggravates the severity of the SCI due to systemic vasodilatation and acute loss of spinal cord perfusion pressure. Expert opinion has recommended that the spinal cord perfusion pressure be maintained above 70 mmHg after DTA reconstruction, that is, a systemic mean arterial pressure of 80–100 mmHg.[12,54] This hemodynamic goal may require vasopressor therapy with drugs such as epinephrine, norepinephrine, phenylephrine, and/or vasopressin.[12,17,29,39,92] Although augmentation of the systemic mean arterial pressure alone may be adequate to reverse SCI, lumbar CSF drainage to maintain the CSF pressure below 10 mmHg is typically performed to further augment spinal cord perfusion pressure, especially if the patient already has a CSF drain.[12,45,54] If the patient has symptomatic SCI that does not recover with systemic hypertension, then lumbar CSF drainage is indicated. In SR of the DTA, the risks of hypotension and SCI must be balanced with the risks of hypertension and arterial bleeding especially from the new aortic suture lines. In TEVAR of the DTA, however, this is less of a concern as there are no suture lines and hence higher levels of systemic hypertension can be utilized for therapy of SCI.[45,92]

Hypothermia

Hypothermia of the spinal cord significantly lowers spinal oxygen demand and prolongs the tolerable ischemic period. A reduction in temperature of 5°C has been demonstrated in a porcine model to increase the tolerance of SCI 2.5-fold from 20 to 50 min.[93] As a result, mild systemic hypothermia has been widely adopted by experienced aortic surgeons in DTA repair as part of a multimodal approach to the management of SCI.[12,54] A greater amount of hypothermia further extends the tolerable ischemic period of the spinal cord as evidenced in deep hypothermic circulatory arrest where the spinal cord is routinely clinically normal after 2 h of ischemia at 15°C.[24]

Besides systemic hypothermia, selective spinal hypothermia with epidural cooling with cold saline has also been described.[94] With this technique, a CSF temperature of 26°C has been achieved.[94] Although this technique has typically been utilized in the clamp-and-sew aortic repair technique, it has also been described in DTA repair with cardiopulmonary bypass, including in conjunction with lumbar CSF drainage.[95,96] The clinical experience with this technique has remained limited to a few institutions.[13,94–96] An important consideration with this technique is to monitor CSF pressure carefully to avoid CSF hypertension and secondary spinal cord compression.[94,95] To obviate the possibility of CSF hypertension, self-contained spinal cooling catheter is in development for application in the subarachnoid and epidural spaces.[97,98] In large animal models, these catheters have demonstrated efficacy to cool the thoracolumbar cord significantly (25–30°C) and offer protection against SCI in DTA repair.[97,98] Although the efficacy of this technology remains to be determined in human trials, it is promising, given that hypothermia induces powerful neuroprotection and that the cooling catheter systems are self-contained.

An alternative strategy to maintain spinal hypothermia and perfusion during aortic clamping is retrograde spinal perfusion via the azygos vein.[99,100] Although this technique may offer spinal cord protection as part of a multimodal approach, it has yet to be fully tested and accepted clinically.[99,100]

Pharmacologic Neuroprotection

The search for the ideal agent for the ideal neuroprotective agent in SCI after DTA repair has been reviewed extensively.[101,102] Encouraging results from laboratory experiments have suggested possible roles for multiple agents including allopurinol, activated protein C, adenosine, barbiturates, carbamazepine, desferrioxamine, edaravone, lidocaine, magnesium, mannitol, naloxone, papaverine, prostaglandins, and steroids.[2,54,100–105] Although anesthetic agents are established preconditioners in ischemia and reperfusion, they also affect the integrity of intraoperative neuromonitoring in DTA repair. As a result, they are unlikely to be rigorously evaluated in clinical trials of SCI in DTA repair, given the central role of intraoperative neuromonitoring, a topic that will be discussed in detail in the next section. In summary, the multiplicity of agents suggests that the search for an ideal perioperative neuroprotective agent for SCI in DTA repair is ongoing.

The most widely adopted pharmacologic strategy is the administration of steroids.[54] The evidence for steroids is both based on experimental and clinical studies, but is by no means conclusive.[106,107] There is to date no randomized controlled trial that has evaluated whether steroids are protective in humans against SCI I DTA repair. Given the increasingly low incidence of SCI in contemporary series, this trial would require a large sample size. However, given the widespread adoption of ER of DTA, this study would be feasible as a multicenter trial.

An alternative strategy to limit SCI in DTA repair is ischemic preconditioning prior to aortic camping.[108] In various animal models, this powerful neuroprotective strategy has proven efficacy, whether the ischemic stimulus is delivered locally or remotely.[109–112] Ischemic preconditioning should be tested in human trials as part of a multimodal strategy to reduce the incidence of clinical SCI after DTA reconstruction.

Intensive Neurological Monitoring for Early Detection of Spinal Cord Ischemia

In the awake patient, detection of SCI is by serial neurologic assessment. The diagnosis of SCI in the awake patient after DTA repair is a clinical emergency that mandates spinal cord rescue, typically with systemic hypertension and/or lumbar CSF drainage.[17,29,39]

Intraoperative diagnosis of SCI during DTA repair is not possible with clinical neurological examination as the patient is unconscious due to general anesthesia. This is the indication for intraoperative neurophysiologic monitoring in DTA repair.[12] The detection of intraoperative SCI with somatosensory evoked potentials (SSEP) and/or motor evoked potentials (MEP) has become widely adopted as it allows modification of the intraoperative management to minimize permanent SCI after DTA repair.

Spinal cord monitoring by SSEP involves electrical stimulation of peripheral nerves followed by recording of the evoked potential at the level of the peripheral nerve, spinal cord, brain stem, thalamus, and cerebral cortex.[113] The SSEP tracings from the lower extremities diminish or disappear in the setting of SCI during DTA repair, including ER.[113–116] The SSEP tracings monitor function of the dorsal and lateral aspects of the spinal cord. Detection of intraoperative SCI by SSEP allows intraoperative spinal cord rescue with maneuvers such as deeper hypothermia, aortic clamp modification, segmental arterial implantation, augmented distal aortic perfusion, systemic hypertension, and lumbar CSF drainage.[19] Neuromonitoring with SSEP can typically be achieved with a balanced anesthetic technique consisting of narcotic, benzodiazepine, muscle relaxant, propofol, and inhaled anesthetic limited to less than 0.5 MAC.[12,112] Besides anesthetic technique, SSEP traces can be affected by hypothermia and electrical interference.

Spinal cord intraoperative monitoring with MEP involves electrical scalp stimulation followed by recording of the evoked potential in the anterior tibialis muscle.[113,117] The MEP tracings monitor function of the anterior aspects of the spinal cord. The anesthetic technique required for reliable MEP tracings is total intravenous anesthesia with partial neuromuscular blockade. As with SSEP tracings, MEP tracings are affected by anesthetic technique, hypothermia, and electrical interference. Detection of intraoperative SCI in

DTA repair is prompt and reliable, allowing spinal rescue strategies to be implemented as described for SSEP monitoring.[118,119]

A recently completed comparison of SSEP and MEP monitoring provides up-to-date insights about the perioperative applications and relevance of these monitoring modalities in contemporary DTA reconstruction ($N = 233$ SR of TAAA).[119] With irreversible SCI in DTA repair, there is 90% agreement between MEP and SSEP monitoring. Only irreversible changes in either modality correlate with immediate paraplegia in the postoperative period (odds ratio 21.9, $P < 0.00001$ for SSEP, $P < 0.0001$ for MEP). Reversible changes in SSEP and MEP racings were not associated postoperatively with spinal cord deficits. Normal intraoperative MEP and SSEP tracings essentially excluded the possibility of postoperative immediate spinal cord deficit. The authors concluded that these monitoring modalities were indicated in DTA repair, and that MEP monitoring did not add significantly to the clinical information available from SSEP monitoring alone.[119] Further studies should confirm these findings and determine the complementary roles of these intraoperative modalities for SCI in DTA repair.

Conclusion

Multiple advances have resulted in the continuously decreasing risk of spinal cord ischemia in contemporary reconstruction of the descending thoracic aorta. The future of spinal cord protection in this setting appears to be focused on endovascular aortic repair and a multimodal approach to the management of spinal cord ischemia.[120]

Key Notes

1. Spinal cord ischemia may occur with reconstruction of the descending thoracic aorta, regardless of aortic repair technique.
2. The clinical presentation primarily involves lower extremity weakness. This weakness should be formally graded to serve as an

objective measure of clinical progress and response to intervention over time.

3. Spinal cord ischemia may present at any time after repair of the descending thoracic aorta. Its presentation may be unilateral and/or relapsing.

4. The risk of spinal cord ischemia depends on aortic repair technique. Meta-analysis of the current literature has demonstrated that the risk of spinal cord ischemia is significantly lower with endovascular repair as compared to surgical repair.

5. Spinal cord ischemia in repair of the descending thoracic aorta results when neural oxygen demand exceeds its oxygen supply.

6. Spinal cord arterial perfusion depends on an extensive collateral network with arterial input from all levels of the aorta. These arterial inputs can be grouped into cephalic, central, and caudal supplies.

7. Spinal cord perfusion pressure is defined as the difference between mean arterial pressure and cerebrospinal fluid pressure.

8. The clinical predictors of spinal cord ischemia after repair of the descending thoracic aorta can all be understood in terms of their effects on the spinal collateral arterial network.

9. The clinical predictors of spinal cord ischemia after repair of the descending thoracic aorta include not only type of repair technique, but also extent of aortic replacement, prior aortic repair, duration of aortic clamping, circulatory hypotension, and anemia.

10. Perioperative spinal cord protection strategies aim to balance spinal cord oxygen supply and demand.

11. The major perioperative spinal cord protection strategies are
    - Maximization of spinal cord blood supply during aortic clamping
    - Maximization of spinal cord perfusion pressure
    - Hypothermia
    - Pharmacologic neuroprotection
    - Early detection of ischemia with intensive neuromonitoring

12. During aortic clamping, measures that increase spinal oxygen supply are minimizing the clamp time, and distal aortic perfusion with left heart bypass or a Gott shunt.

13. Spinal cord perfusion pressure and hence oxygen supply are increased by the following measures: active management of the intercostal and lumbar arteries to minimize vascular steal, lumbar drainage of cerebrospinal fluid to decrease cerebrospinal fluid pressure, and pharmacologic augmentation of systemic arterial pressure.

14. Spinal cord hypothermia decreases oxygen demand. It can be induced systemically via cardiopulmonary bypass or locally via epidural cooling. Systemic hypothermia includes deep hypothermic circulatory arrest with temperatures in the range of 14–18°C.

15. The best indicator of an intact spinal cord is a normal neurological examination in an awake and cooperative patient.

16. Intensive neurological monitoring intraoperatively while the patient is under general anesthesia is achieved with continuous monitoring of somatosensory evoked potentials and/or motor evoked potentials.

17. Detection of spinal cord ischemia in the awake or unconscious aortic surgical patient is a clinical emergency that mandates immediate spinal cord rescue with all appropriate interventions from the outlined therapeutic menu.

References

1. Greenberg RK, Lu Q, Roselli E, et al. Contemporary analysis of descending thoracic and thoracoabdominal aneurysm repair: a comparison of endovascular and open techniques. *Circulation.* 2008;118:808–817.

2. Svensson LG. Paralysis after aortic surgery: in search of lost cord function. *Surgeon.* 2005;3:396–405.

3. Dillavou ED, Makaroun MS. Predictors of morbidity and mortality with endovascular and open thoracic aneurysm repair. *J Vasc Surg.* 2008;48:1114–1120.

4. Estrera AL, Rubenstein FS, Miller CC, et al. Descending thoracic aortic aneurysm: surgical approach and treatment using the adjuncts cerebrospinal fluid drainage and distal aortic perfusion. *Ann Thorac Surg.* 2005;72:481–486.

5. Golledge J, Eagle KA. Acute aortic dissection. *Lancet.* 2008;372:55–65.
6. Coselli JS, Bozinovski J, LeMaire SA. Open surgical repair of 2286 thoracoabdominal aortic aneurysms. *Ann Thorac Surg.* 2007;83:S862–S864.
7. Svensson LG, Kouchoukos NT, Miller DC, et al. Expert consensus document on the treatment of descending thoracic aortic disease using endovascular stent grafts. *Ann Thorac Surg.* 2008;85:S1–S41.
8. Makaroun MS, Dillavou ED, Kee ST, et al. Endovascular treatment of thoracic aortic aneurysms: results of the phase II multicenter trial of the GORETAG thoracic endoprosthesis. *J Vasc Surg.* 2005;41:1–9.
9. Szeto WY, Bavaria JE, Bowen FW, et al. The hybrid aortic arch repair: brachiocephalic bypass and concomitant endovascular aortic arch stent graft placement. *J Card Surg.* 2007;22:97–102.
10. Woo EY, Bavaria JE, Pochettino A, et al. Techniques for preserving vertebral artery perfusion during thoracic aortic stent grafting requiring aortic arch landing. *Vasc Endovasc Surg.* 2006;40:367–373.
11. Drenth DJ, Verhoeven EL, Prins TR, et al. Relocation of supra-aortic vessels to facilitate endovascular treatment of a ruptured aortic arch aneurysm. *J Thorac Cardiovasc Surg.* 2003;126:1184–1185.
12. Pantin EJ, Cheung A. Thoracic aorta. In: Kaplan JA, Reich DL, Lake CL, Konstadt SN, eds. *Kaplan's Cardiac Anesthesia.* 5th ed. Philadelphia: Saunders Elsevier; 2006:723–764.
13. Cambria RP, Clouse WD, Davison JK, et al. Thoracoabdminal aneurysm repair: results with 337 operations performed over a 15-year interval. *Ann Surg.* 2002;236:471–479.
14. Gutsche JT, Cheung AT, McGarvey ML, et al. Risk factors for perioperative stroke after thoracic endovascular repair. *Ann Thorac Surg.* 2007;84:1195–2000.
15. Freezor RJ, Martin TD, Hess PJ, et al. Risk factors for perioperative stroke during thoracic endovascular aortic repairs (TEVAR). *J Endovasc Ther.* 2007;14:568–573.
16. Wong DR, Coselli JS, Amerman K, et al. Delayed spinal cord deficits after thoracoabdominal aortic aneurysm repair. *Ann Thorac Surg.* 2007;83:1345–1355.
17. Cheung AT, Weiss SJ, McGarvey ML, et al. Interventions for reversing delayed-onset postoperative paraplegia after thoracic aortic reconstruction. *Ann Thorac Surg.* 2002;74:413–419.
18. Hughes GC, Daneshmand MA, Swaminathan M, et al. 'Real world' thoracic endografting: results with the Gore TAG device 2 years after U.S. FDA approval. *Ann Thorac Surg.* 2008;86:1530–1538.
19. Estrera AL, Miller CC III, Chen EP, et al. Descending thoracic aortic aneurysm repair: 12-year experience using distal aortic perfusion and cerebrospinal fluid drainage. *Ann Thorac Surg.* 2005;80:1290–1296.
20. Coselli JS, LeMaire SA, Conklin LD, et al. Left heart bypass during descending thoracic aortic aneurysm repair does not reduce the incidence of paraplegia. *Ann Thorac Surg.* 2004;77:1298–1303.
21. Borst HG, Jurmann m, Buhner B, et al. Risk of replacement of descending aorta with a standardized left heart bypass technique. *J Thorac Cardiovasc Surg.* 1994;107:126–133.
22. Svensson LG, Crawford ES, Hess KR, et al. Variables predictive of outcome in 832 patients undergoing repairs of the descending thoracic aorta. *Chest.* 1993;104:1248–1253.
23. Verdant A. Descending thoracic aortic aneurysms: surgical treatment with the Gott shunt. *Can J Surg.* 1992;35:493–496.
24. Kouchoukos NT, Masetti P, Rokkas CK, et al. Safety and efficacy of hypothermic cardiopulmonary bypass and circulatory arrest for operations on the descending and thoracoabdominal aorta. *Ann Thorac Surg.* 2001;72:699–707.
25. Fehrenbacher JW, Hart DW, Huddleston E, et al. Optimal end-organ protection for thoracic and thoracoabdominal aortic aneurysm repair using deep hypothermic circulatory arrest. *Ann Thorac Surg.* 2007;83:1041–1046.
26. Kieffer E, Chiche L, Cluzel P, et al. Open surgical repair of descending thoracic aortic aneurysms in the endovascular era: a 9-year single-center study. *Ann Vasc Surg.* 2009;23:60–66.
27. Misfeld M, Sievers HH, Hadlak M, et al. Rate of paraplegia and mortality in elective descending and thoracoabdominal aortic repair in the modern surgical era. *Thorac Cardiovasc Surg.* 2008;56:342–347.
28. Kieffer E, Chiche L, Godet G, et al. Type IV thoracoabdominal aneurysm repair: predictors of postoperative mortality, spinal cord injury, and acute intestinal ischemia. *Ann Vasc Surg.* 2008;22:822–828.
29. Gutsche JT, Szeto W, Cheung AT. Endovascular stenting of thoracic aortic aneurysm. *Anesthesiol Clin.* 2008;26:481–499.
30. Dake MD, Miller DC, Mitchell RS, et al. The "first generation" of endovascular stent-grafts for patients with aneurysms of the descending thoracic aorta. *J Thorac Cardiovasc Surg.* 1998;116:689–703.
31. Gravereaux EC, Faries PL, Burks JA, et al. Risk of spinal cord ischemia after endograft repair of thoracic aortic aneurysms. *J Vasc Surg.* 2001;34:997–1003.
32. Bell RE, Taylor PR, Aukett M, et al. Mid-term results for second-generation thoracic stent grafts. *Br J Surg.* 2003;90:811–817.
33. Orend KH, Scharrer-Pamler R, Kapfer X, et al. Endovascular treatment in diseases of the descending thoracic aorta: 6-year results of a single center. *J Vasc Surg.* 2003;37:91–99.
34. Bortone AS, De Cillis E, D'Agostino D, et al. Endovascular treatment of thoracic aortic disease: four years of experience. *Circulation.* 2004;110:II262–II267.
35. Hansen CJ, Bui H, Donayre CE, et al. Complications of endovascular repair of high-risk and emergent descending thoracic aortic aneurysms and dissections. *J Vasc Surg.* 2004;40:228–234.
36. Leurs LJ, Bell R, Degrieck Y, et al. Endovascular treatment of thoracic aortic diseases: combined experience from the EUROSTAR and United Kingdom Thoracic Endograft registries. *J Vasc Surg.* 2004;40:670–679.

37. Chiesa R, Melissano G, Marrocco-Trischitta MM, et al. Spinal cord ischemia after elective stent-graft repair of the thoracic aorta. *J Vasc Surg.* 2005;42:11–17.

38. Greenberg RK, O'Neill S, Walker E, et al. Endovascular repair of thoracic aortic lesions with the Zenith TX1 and TX2 thoracic grafts: intermediate-term results. *J Vasc Surg.* 2005;41:589–596.

39. Cheung AT, Pochettino A, McGarvey ML, et al. Strategies to manage paraplegia risk after endovascular stent repair of descending thoracic aortic aneurysms. *Ann Thorac Surg.* 2005;80:1280–1288.

40. Stone DH, Brewster DC, Kwolek CJ, et al. Stent-graft versus open-surgical repair of the thoracic aorta: midterm results. *J Vasc Surg.* 2006;44:1188–1197.

41. Iyer VS, Mackenzie KS, Tse LW, et al. Early outcomes after elective and emergent endovascular repair of the thoracic aorta. *J Vasc Surg.* 2006;43:677–683.

42. Khoynezhad A, Donayre CE, Bui H, et al. Risk factors of neurologic deficit after thoracic aortic endografting. *Ann Thorac Surg.* 2007;83:S882–S889.

43. Rodriguez JA, Olsen DM, Shtutman A, et al. Application of endograft to treat thoracic aortic pathologies: a single center experience. *J Vasc Surg.* 2007;46:413–420.

44. Zipfel B, Hammerschmidt R, Krabatsch T, et al. Stent-grafting of the thoracic aorta by the cardiothoracic surgeon. *Ann Thorac Surg.* 2007;83:441–448.

45. Hnath JC, Mehta M, Taggert JB, et al. Strategies to improve spinal cord ischemia in endovascular thoracic aortic repair: outcomes of a prospective cerebrospinal fluid drainage protocol. *J Vasc Surg.* 2008;48:836–840.

46. Amabile P, Grisoli D, Giorgi R, et al. Incidence and determinants of spinal cord ischemia in stent-graft repair of the thoracic aorta. *Eur J Vasc Endovasc Surg.* 2008;35:455–461.

47. Parker JD, Golledge J. Outcome of endovascular treatment of acute type B dissection. *Ann Thorac Surg.* 2008;86:1707–1712.

48. Walsh SR, Tang TY, Sadat U, et al. Endovascular stenting versus open surgery for thoracic aortic disease: systematic review and meta-analysis of perioperative results. *J Vasc Surg.* 2008;47:1094–1098.

49. Tang GL, Tehrani HY, Usman A, et al. Reduced mortality, paraplegia, and stroke with stent graft repair of blunt aortic transections: a modern meta-analysis. *J Vasc Surg.* 2008;47:671–675.

50. Hoffer EK, Forauer AR, Silas AM, et al. Endovascular stent-graft or open surgical repair for blunt thoracic aortic trauma: systematic review. *J Vasc Interv Radiol.* 2008;19:1153–1164.

51. Xenos ES, Abedi NN, Davenport DL, et al. Meta-analysis of endovascular vs open repair for traumatic descending thoracic aortic rupture. *J Vasc Surg.* 2008;48:1342–1351.

52. Akowuah E, Angelini G, Bryan AJ. Open versus endovascular repair of traumatic aortic rupture: a systematic review. *J Thorac Cardiovasc Surg.* 2009;138:768–769.

53. Jacobs MJ, Mommertz G, Koeppel TA, et al. Surgical repair of thoracoabdominal aortic aneurysms. *J Cardiovas Surg (Torino).* 2007;48:49–58.

54. Griepp RB, Griepp EB. Spinal cord perfusion and protection during descending thoracic and thoracoabdominal aortic surgery: the collateral network concept. *Ann Thorac Surg.* 2007;83:S865–S869.

55. Adamkiewicz A. Die blutegefasse des menschlichen ruckenmarkes. *Sitzungsberichte Akademie der Wissen Schaften in Wein – Mathematische-Naturwissen Schaftliche Klasse – Abteilun.* 1882;84:101–130.

56. Lazorthes G, Gouaze A, Zadeh JO, et al. Arterial vascularization of the spinal cord: recent studies of the anatomic substitution pathways. *J Neurosurg.* 1971;35:253–262.

57. Nojiri J, Matsumoto K, Kato A, et al. The Adamkiewicz artery: demonstration by intra-arterial computed tomographic angiography. *Eur J Cardiothorac Surg.* 2007;31:249–255.

58. Boll DT, Bulow H, Blackham KA, et al. MDCT angiography of the spinal vasculature and the artery of Adamkiewicz. *AJR Am J Roentgenol.* 2006;187:1054–1060.

59. Backes WH, Nijenhuis RJ, Mess WH, et al. Magnetic resonance angiography of collateral blood supply to spinal cord in thoracic and thoracoabdominal aortic aneurysm patients. *J Vasc Surg.* 2008;48:261–271.

60. Felix I, Schlosser MD, Mojibian H, et al. Open thoracic or thoracoabdominal aortic aneurysm repair after previous abdominal aortic aneurysm surgery. *J Vasc Surg.* 2008;48:761–768.

61. Svensson LG, Hess KR, Coselli JS, et al. Influence of segmental arteries, extent and atriofemoral bypass on postoperative paraplegia after thoracoabdominal aortic operations. *J Vasc Surg.* 1994;20:255–262.

62. Kawanishi Y, Okada K, Matsumori M, et al. Influence of perioperative hemodynamics on spinal cord ischemia in thoracoabdominal aortic repair. *Ann Thorac Surg.* 2007;84:488–492.

63. Etz CD, Luehr M, Kari FA, et al. Paraplegia after extensive thoracic and thoracoabdominal aortic aneurysm repair: does critical spinal cord ischemia occur postoperatively? *J Thorac Cardiovasc Surg.* 2008;135:324–330.

64. Augoustides JG. Management of spinal cord perfusion pressure to minimize intermediate-delayed paraplegia: critical role of central venous pressure. *J Thorac Cardiovasc Surg.* 2008;136:796.

65. Augoustides JG. Venous function and pressure: what is their role in the management of spinal cord ischemia after thoracoabdominal aortic aneurysm repair? *Anesthesiology.* 2008;109:933.

66. Cernalanu AC, Olah A, Cilley JH Jr, et al. Effect of sodium nitroprusside on paraplegia during cross-clamping of the thoracic aorta. *Ann Thorac Surg.* 1993;56:1035–1037.

67. Simpson JI, Eide TR, Schiff GA, et al. Isoflurane versus sodium nitroprusside for the control of proximal hypertension during thoracic aortic cross-clamping:

effects on spinal cord ischemia. *J Cardiothorac Vasc Anesth*. 1995;9:491–496.

68. Griepp RB, Ergin MA, Galla JD, et al. Looking for the artery of Adamkiewicz: a quest to minimize paraplegia after operations for aneurysms of the descending thoracic and thoracoabdominal aorta. *J Thorac Cardiovasc Surg*. 1996;112:1202–1213.

69. Mac Arthur RG, Carter SA, Coselli JS, et al. Organ protection during thoracoabdominal aortic surgery: rationale for a multimodality approach. *Semin Cardiothorac Vasc Anesth*. 2005;9:143–149.

70. Coselli JS, LeMaire SA. Left heart bypass reduces paraplegia rates after thoracoabdominal aneurysm repair. *Ann Thorac Surg*. 1999;67:1931–1934.

71. Safi HJ, Campbell MP, Miller CC 3rd, et al. Cerebrospinal fluid drainage and distal aortic perfusion decrease the incidence of neurological deficit: the results of 343 descending and thoracoabdominal aortic aneurysm repairs. *Eur J Vasc Endovasc Surg*. 1997;14:118–124.

72. Crestanello JA, Zehr KJ, Mullany CJ, et al. The effect of adjuvant perfusion techniques on the incidence of paraplegia after repair of traumatic thoracic aortic transections. *Mayo Clin Proc*. 2006;81:625–630.

73. Feezor RJ, Martin TD, Hess PJ Jr, et al. Extent of aortic coverage and incidence of spinal cord ischemia after thoracic endovascular aneurysm repair. *Ann Thorac Surg*. 2008;86:1809–1814.

74. Christiansson L, Ulus AT, Heelberg A, et al. Aspects of the spinal cord circulation as assessed by intrathecal oxygen tension monitoring during various arterial interruptions in the pig. *J Thorac Cardiovasc Surg*. 2001;121:762–772.

75. Acher CW, Wynn MM. How we do it. *Cardiovasc Surg*. 1999;7:593–596.

76. Etz CD, Halstead JC, Spilvogel D, et al. Thoracic and thoracoabdominal aneurysm repair: is reimplantation of the spinal arteries a waste of time? *Ann Thorac Surg*. 2006;82:1670–1677.

77. Woo EY, McGarvey M, Jackson BM, et al. Spinal cord ischemia may be reduced via a novel technique of intercostal artery revascularization during open thoracoabdominal aneurysm repair. *J Vasc Surg*. 2007;46:421–426.

78. Parmer SS, Carpenter JP, Stavropoulos SW, et al. Endoleaks after endovascular repair of thoracic aortic aneurysms. *J Vasc Surg*. 2006;44:447–452.

79. Morales JP, Greenberg RK, Lu Q, et al. Endoleaks following endovascular repair of thoracic aortic aneurysm: etiology and outcomes. *J Endovasc Ther*. 2008;15:631–638.

80. Gorlitzer M, Mertikian G, Trnka H, et al. Translumbar treatment of type II endoleaks after endovascular repair of abdominal aortic aneurysm. *Interact Cardiovasc Thorac Surg*. 2008;7:781–784.

81. Blaisdell FW, Cooley DA. The mechanism of paraplegia and its relationship to spinal fluid pressure. *Surgery*. 1962;51:351–355.

82. Hill AB, Kalman PG, Johnston KW, et al. Reversal of delayed-onset paraplegia after thoracic aortic surgery with cerebrospinal fluid drainage. *J Vasc Surg*. 1994;20:315–317.

83. Ling E, Arellano R. Systematic overview of the evidence supporting the use of cerebrospinal fluid drainage in thoracoabdominal aneurysm surgery for prevention of paraplegia. *Anesthesiology*. 2000;93:1115–1122.

84. Khan SN, Stansby G. Cerebrospinal fluid drainage for thoracic and thoracoabdominal aortic aneurysm surgery. Cochrane Database Syst Rev. 2004;1: CD003635

85. Cina CS, Abouzahr L, Arena GO, et al. Cerebrospinal fluid drainage to prevent paraplegia during thoracic and thoracoabdominal aneurysm surgery: a systematic review and meta-analysis. *J Vasc Surg*. 2004;40:36–44.

86. Cheung AT, Pochettino A, Guvakov DV, et al. Safety of lumbar drains in thoracic aortic operations performed with extracorporeal circulation. *Ann Thorac Surg*. 2003;76:1190–1196.

87. Dardik A, Perler BA, Roseborough GS, et al. Subdural hematoma after thoracoabdominal aortic aneurysm repair: an underreported complication of spinal fluid drainage. *J Vasc Surg*. 2002;36:47–50.

88. Subramaniam B, Panzica PJ, Pawlowski JB, et al. Epidural blood patch for acute subdural hematoma after spinal catheter drainage during hybrid thoracoabdominal aneurysm repair. *J Cardiothorac Vasc Anesth*. 2007;21:704–708.

89. Coplin WM, Avelling AM, Kim DK, et al. Bacterial meningitis associated with lumbar drains: a retrospective cohort study. *J Neurol Neurosurg Psychiatry*. 1999;67:468–473.

90. Sethi M, Grigore Am, Davison JK. Pro: it is safe to proceed with thoracoabdominal aneurysm surgery after encountering a bloody tap during cerebrospinal fluid catheter placement. *J Cardiothorac Vasc Anesth*. 2006;20:269–272.

91. Wynn MM, Mittnacht A, Norris E. Con: surgery should not proceed when a bloody tap occurs during spinal drain placement for elective thoracoabdominal aortic surgery. *J Cardiothorac Vasc Anesth*. 2006;20:273–275.

92. McGarvey ML, Mullen MT, Woo EY, et al. The treatment of spinal cord ischemia following thoracic endovascular aortic repair. *Neurocrit Care*. 2007;6:35–39.

93. Strauch JT, Lauten A, Spielvogel D, et al. Mild hypothermia protects the spinal cord from ischemic injury in a chronic porcine model. *Eur J Cardiothorac Surg*. 2004;25:708–715.

94. Cambria RP, Davison JK, Carter C, et al. Epidural cooling for spinal cord protection during thoracoabdominal aneurysm repair: a five year experience. *J Vasc Surg*. 2000;31:1093–1102.

95. Motoyoshi N, Takahashi G, Sakurai M, et al. Safety and efficacy of epidural cooling for regional spinal cord hypothermia during thoracoabdominal aneurysm repair. *Eur J Cardiothorac Surg*. 2004;25:139–141.

96. Tabayashi K, Motoyoshi N, Saiki Y, et al. Efficacy of perfusion of the epidural space and cerebrospinal fluid drainage during repair of extent I and extent II thoracoabdominal aneurysm. *J Cardiovas Surg (Torino)*. 2008;49:749–755.

97. Moomiale RM, Ransden J, Stein J, et al. Cooling catheter for spinal cord preservation in thoracic aortic surgery. *J Cardiovas Surg (Torino).* 2007;48: 103–108.

98. Yoshitake A, Mori A, Shimizu H, et al. Use of an epidural cooling catheter with a closed countercurrent lumen to protect against ischemic spinal cord injury in pigs. *J Thorac Cardiovasc Surg.* 2007;134: 1220–1226.

99. Pocar M, Rossi V, Addis A, et al. Spinal cord retrograde perfusion: review of the literature and experimental observations. *J Card Surg.* 2007;22:124–128.

100. Juvonen T, Biancari F. Spinal cord protection by retrograde venous perfusion during descending thoracic and thoracoabdominal aortic surgery: fact or fiction? *Scan Cardiovasc J.* 2002;36:4–5.

101. Juvonen T, Biancari F, Rimpilainen J, et al. Strategies for spinal cord protection during descending thoracic and thoracoabdominal aortic surgery: up-to-date experimental and clinical results. *Scan Cardiovasc J.* 2002;36:136–160.

102. Tabayashi K. Spinal cord protection during thoracoabdominal aneurysm repair. *Surg Today.* 2005; 35:1–6.

103. Kohno H, Ishida A, Imamaki M, et al. Efficacy and vasodilatory benefits of magnesium prophylaxis for protection against spinal cord ischemia. *Ann Vasc Surg.* 2007;21:352–359.

104. Hamaishi M, Orihashi K, Isaka M, et al. Low-dose edaravone injection into the clamped aorta prevents ischemic spinal cord injury. *Ann Vasc Surg.* 2009; 23:128–135.

105. Sirlak M, Eryilmaz S, Inan M, et al. Effects of carbamazepine on spinal cord ischemia. *J Thorac Cardiovasc Surg.* 2008;136:1038–1043.

106. Laschinger JC, Cunningham JN, Cooper MM, et al. Prevention of ischemic spinal cord injury following aortic cross-clamping: use of corticosteroids. *Ann Thorac Surg.* 1984;38:500–507.

107. Bracken MB, Shepard MJ, Collins WF, et al. A randomized trial of methylprednisolone or naloxone in the treatment of acute spinal cord injury: results of the second national acute spinal cord injury study. *N Engl J Med.* 1990;3322:1405–1411.

108. Lee JS, Hong JM, Kim YJ. Ischaemic preconditioning to prevent lethal ischemic spinal cord injury in a swine model. *J Invest Surg.* 2008;21:209–214.

109. Benicio A, Moreira LF, Monaco BA, et al. Comparative study between ischemic preconditioning and cerebrospinal fluid drainage as methods of spinal cord protection in dogs. *Rev Bras Cir Cardiovasc.* 2007;22:15–23.

110. Monaco BA, Benicio A, Contreras IS, et al. Ischemic preconditioning and spinal cord function monitoring in the descending thoracic aorta approach. *Arq Bras Cardiol.* 2007;88(33):262–266.

111. Contreras IS, Moreira LF, Ballester G, et al. Immediate ischemic preconditioning based on somatosensory evoked potentials seems to prevent spinal cord injury following descending thoracic aorta cross-clamping. *Eur J Cardiothorac Surg.* 2005;28:274–279.

112. Selimoglu O, Ugurlucan M, Basaran M, et al. Efficacy of remote ischaemic preconditioning for spinal cord protection against ischaemic injury: association with heat shock protein expression. *Folia Neuropathol.* 2008;46:204–212.

113. Sloan TB, Jameson LC. Electrophysiologic monitoring during surgery to repair the thoracoabdominal aorta. *J Clin Neurophysiol.* 2007;24:316–327.

114. Galla JD, Ergin MA, Lansman SL, et al. Use of somatosensory evoked potentials for thoracic and thoracoabdominal aortic resections. *Ann Thorac Surg.* 1999;67:1947–1952.

115. Guerit JM, Witdoeckt C, Verhelst R, et al. Sensitivity, specificity, and surgical impact of somatosensory evoked potentials in descending aorta surgery. *Ann Thorac Surg.* 1999;67:1943–1946.

116. Weigang E, Hartert M, Siegenthaler MP, et al. Neurophysiological monitoring during thoracoabdominal aortic endovascular stent graft implantation. *Eur J Cardiothorac Surg.* 2006;29:392–396.

117. Jacobs MJ, Elenbaas TW, Schurink GW, et al. Assessment of spinal cord integrity during thoracoabdominal aneurysm repair. *Ann Thorac Surg.* 2002;74:S1864–S1866.

118. Shine TSJ, Harrison B, De Ruyter ML, et al. Motor and somatosensory evoked potentials: their role in predicting spinal cord ischemia in patients undergoing thoracoabdominal aortic aneurysm repair with regional lumbar epidural cooling. *Anesthesiology.* 2008;108:580–587.

119. Keyhani K, Miller III CC, Estrera AL, et al. Analysis of motor and somatosensory evoked potentials during thoracic and thoracoabdominal aortic aneurysm repair. *J Vasc Surg.* 2009;49:36–41.

120. Messe SR, Bavaria JE, Mullen M, et al. Neurologic outcomes from high risk descending thoracic and thoracoabdominal aortic operations in the era of endovascular repair. *Neurocrit Care.* 2008;9:344–351.

121. Biglioni P, Roberto M, Cannata, et al. Upper lower spinal cord blood supply: The continuity of the anterior spinal artery and the relevance of the lumber arteries. *J Thorac Cardiovasc Surg.* 2004;127(4): 1188–92.

Understanding Endovascular Aortic Surgery: Endovascular Repair of Aortic Aneurysmal Disease

12

Richard C. Hsu and Marc Schermerhorn

Background

In 1991, when Parodi first published his experience with placement of a balloon-expandable endograft for the treatment of abdominal aortic aneurysms in patients deemed unsuitable for open surgery,[1] interest grew in the field of endovascular approaches to the treatment of aortic aneurysms. Since that initial report, tremendous advancements have made this methodology commonplace, and more importantly, widely accepted as a viable alternative to the traditional open repair. Furthermore, refinements in the newer devices have expanded the inclusion criteria for patients previously thought to be unsuitable for endovascular repair, greatly increasing its versatility and applicability.

Open aneurysm surgery is a morbid procedure, especially considering the coexisting conditions of the patients requiring such operations. Published reports have confirmed the 3–5% perioperative mortality of open abdominal aneurysm repair.[2–5] Most patients are admitted to the intensive care unit postoperatively, and a significant number require a transitional stay in a rehabilitation facility prior to home discharge.

R.C. Hsu (✉) and M. Schermerhorn (✉)
Department of Vascular Surgery, Beth Israel
Deaconess Medical Center, 110 Francis St Suite 5B,
Boston 02215, MA, USA
e-mail: hsurc41@hotmail.com

Published Results

Two randomized trials comparing endovascular repair to open repair of abdominal aortic aneurysms have shown improved outcomes with the endovascular approach. The Dutch Randomized Endovascular Aneurysms Management (DREAM) trial[6] reported a significant decrease in perioperative morbidity and mortality in patients undergoing endovascular repair of aortic aneurysms, including lower rate of systemic complications (mainly pulmonary), decreased blood loss, and decreased length of hospital stay. These results were similar to those found in the EVAR-1 trial,[7] where a 30-day perioperative mortality of 1.7% was found in the EVAR group, compared to 4.7% in the open aneurysm repair group. Late survival was similar between the two groups in both trials. Thus, at least in patients deemed suitable for either open or endovascular repair of abdominal aortic aneurysms, the endovascular approach appears to offer a superior short-term survival advantage.

Perioperative (30-day) mortality has been described to fall between 1% and 2% on published series,[8] and is due in large part to pre-existing comorbidities. Comparison of results between endovascular and open repair of abdominal aortic aneurysms have shown an aneurysm-related survival benefit to endovascular repair,[9] and the advantage is more pronounced when only patients with significant risk factors are considered.[10] Similarly, in-hospital complication rates appear

Table 12.1 Advantages and drawbacks of endovascular aortic stent grafting treatment

Advantages

Decreased blood loss and transfusion requirements

Avoidance of major thoracic or abdominal incision, less postoperative pain, and requirement of analgesics

Avoidance of extensive dissection and surgical trauma

Avoids cross-clamping and unclamping of aorta

Avoidance of reperfusion injury

Less stress response (decreased release of plasma catecholamines, cytokines, and endotoxins)

Decreased hemodynamic stress

Decreased metabolic alterations and acid–base changes (related to bowel, leg, and visceral ischemia in open repairs)

Avoidance of general anesthesia in some patients

Decreased use of intensive care unit

Shortened hospital stay

Faster recovery to return to regular activities and normal state of health

Overall decreased perioperative mortality and morbidity

Drawbacks

Not all aortic pathology can be treated by endovascular approach

Certain anatomic limitations exist

Procedure requires contrast administration

Unique procedure-related complications (access vessel injury, distal embolization, endoleaks, postimplantation syndrome, and (others described in text))

Regular follow-up imaging required

Initial advantages of decreased perioperative mortality may not be maintained over time

Long-term advantages yet to be studied

to be lower with endovascular repair, attributable mainly to lower incidences of cardiac and pulmonary complications. The major advantages and drawbacks of this minimally invasive approach to the treatment of aortic aneurysms are given in Table 12.1.

Patient Selection

There has been no definitive study defining aneurysm size criteria justifying the endovascular treatment of aortic aneurysms. The decision to treat is based on data from open repair of aortic aneurysms, which suggest conservative management for most asymptomatic abdominal aortic aneurysms less than 5.5 cm in diameter.

Both the United Kingdom Small Aneurysm Trial (UKSAT) and the Aneurysm Detection and Management (ADAM) trial demonstrated no benefit to early surgery for small abdominal aortic aneurysms (4.0- to 5.5-cm).[11,12] Other accepted indications for repair include rapid expansion and the onset of symptoms, including pain and distal embolization. However, the ultimate decision to treat is made by consideration of a host of factors, including increased rupture risk in women, smokers, and patients with hypertension and chronic lung disease.[13] In addition, the operative risk and life expectancy of the patient must be balanced against the aneurysm rupture risk. Controversy exists regarding the treatment of mycotic aneurysms. For thoracic aortic aneurysms, treatment is not recommended for asymptomatic aneurysms less than 5 cm in diameter.[14]

Indications and Anatomic Eligibility

Endovascular stent graft therapy is typically indicated for the treatment of infrarenal abdominal aortic aneurysms. Most patients being considered for endograft treatment of aortic aneurysms require preoperative imaging. Computed tomography-angiography with 1-mm cuts and intravenous contrast enhancement is usually used. This allows for the assessment of the major branches of the aorta, as well as the characteristics of the aneurysm itself. For a patient to be deemed suitable for endograft repair of infrarenal abdominal aortic aneurysms, certain anatomic criteria have to be met.

Proximal Landing Zone

Most important of these is the proximal aortic neck, or the proximal attachment point of the endograft to the nonaneurysmal aorta.[15] A "hostile" neck, or one that has been associated with increased rate of complications, is defined as having one or more of the following properties: aortic diameter greater than 28 mm, angulation between the neck and the suprarenal aorta greater than 60°, thrombus occupying greater than 50% of the aortic circumference, distance between the start of the aneurysm sac and the most caudal renal artery of less than 10 mm, and greater than 2 mm aortic diameter expansion within 10 mm of the most proximal fixation point[16] (Fig. 12.1). Although newer devices such as those with suprarenal fixation have been successfully deployed in patients with hostile proximal aortic necks, deviation from the standard selection criteria cannot be recommended except in unusual circumstances.

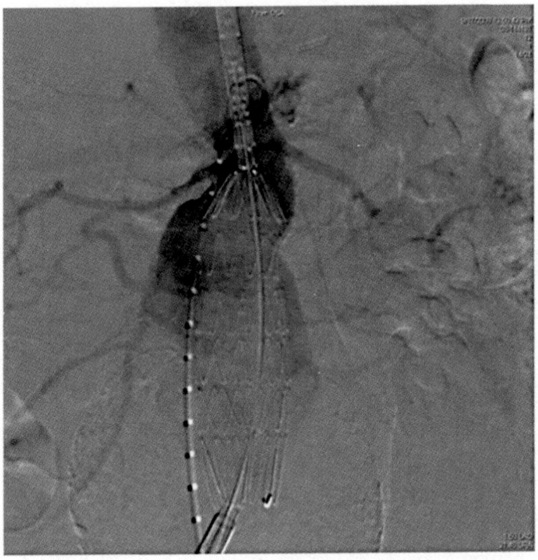

Distal Landing Zone

Other anatomic considerations include the suitability of the distal endograft landing zone.[17] Aneurysms involving the common iliac arteries can lead to inadequate sealing of the distal graft. In addition, extremely ectatic or calcified iliac arteries may lead to graft kinking or inadequate graft apposition. Techniques to address these issues include the use of flared iliac limbs, extension of the iliac limb to the external iliac arteries, typically with coil embolization of the ipsilateral hypogastric artery to prevent a type II endoleak (Fig. 12.2), and the use of branched endografts.[18,19] Exclusion of both hypogastric arteries must be performed with caution, as buttock claudication and even necrosis may occur.[20]

Fig. 12.1 An example of an infrarenal abdominal aortic aneurysm with a "hostile" neck. Note the short, wide, reverse-taper neck with severe angulation

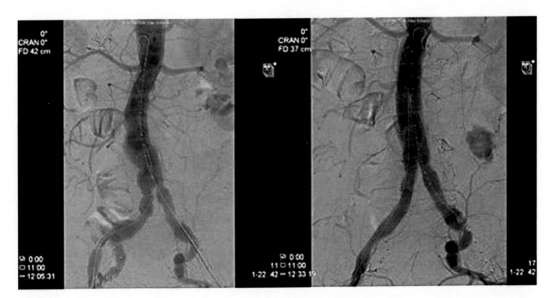

Fig. 12.2 Pre- and postprocedural arteriograms of an endovascular repair of abdominal aortic aneurysm in a patient with concomitant right common iliac artery aneurysm. Occluding coils were placed in the right internal iliac artery to treat an internal iliac artery aneurysm, and to allow extension of the right iliac limb to the external iliac artery

Access Arteries

The common femoral and external iliac arteries must be of sufficient caliber and quality to allow passage of the device. Tortuous access arteries will often straighten with the use of super stiff wires. Focal stenoses or small caliber vessels, in the absence of calcification, can be dilated with stiff dilators or balloon angioplasty. Severe calcification remains the most concerning issue. Circumferential calcification is resistant to dilation, and rupture of the calcium plaque with forceful dilation can lead to vessel rupture and severe hemorrhage. If rupture does occur, hemorrhage can be controlled with balloon occlusion followed by stent graft repair of the injured vessel[21] (Fig. 12.3). Placement of an iliac conduit to the common iliac artery via a retroperitoneal approach can bypass these issues and avoid a transabdominal incision and aortic cross-clamping.[22] Alternatively, if one iliofemoral system is suitable for access, an aorto-uni-iliac device can be used in conjunction with a femoral–femoral bypass and contralateral iliac occluder.[23]

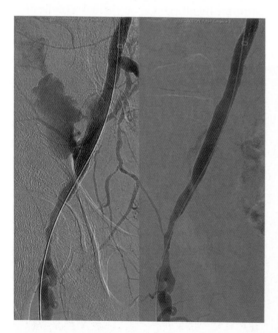

Fig. 12.3 External iliac artery rupture after balloon angioplasty and stent placement. The ruptured vessel was repaired with an additional endoluminal stent, which controlled the hemorrhage

Inferior Mesenteric Artery and Visceral Perfusion

Patients with stenosis of one or both of the celiac and superior mesenteric arteries may be dependent on the IMA for visceral perfusion. The finding of an enlarged marginal artery of Drummond or meandering mesenteric artery supports this diagnosis, and exclusion of the IMA by the endograft may lead to intestinal ischemia.[24]

Pararenal Aneurysms

Unlike infrarenal aortic aneurysms, pararenal aneurysms have inherent limitations due to insufficient neck length for secure proximal stent graft fixation. Fenestrated stent grafts overcome this difficulty while preserving renal blood flow. The device has to be patient-specific. Positioning and deployment is technically difficult. Clinical experience is limited to small series[25] and the long-term outcome is unknown.

Occlusive Disease

Lastly, endovascular therapy has also been tried in the treatment of aorto-iliac occlusive disease as an alternative to surgery. For patients with focal infrarenal aortic stenosis, it is recommended as the first-line treatment, while for chronic total aorto-iliac occlusions, it is a viable alternative to surgery.[26]

Types of Stent Grafts (Fig. 12.4)

The primary purpose of stent grafts is to exclude the aneurysm sac from arterial pressure and flow, thereby protecting the vessel from rupture, and preventing distal embolization of luminal thrombus. While a complete discussion of the different types of commercially available stent grafts is beyond the scope of this chapter, the common principles guiding the development of these

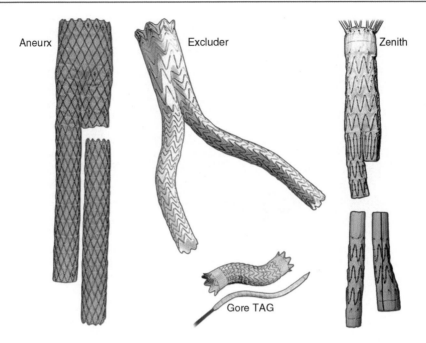

Fig. 12.4 Endograft devices in use: The AneuRx, the Excluder, the Zenith, and GORE TAG thoracic endograft

endografts are worth mentioning. Ideally, stent grafts should provide life-long protection from the dangers imposed by aortic aneurysms, be adaptable to different anatomic configurations, and be easy to deploy. Additionally, the stent graft must be flexible enough to adapt to changes in aortic anatomy as the excluded aneurysm sac shrinks, yet stiff enough to prevent collapse.[27] Most endografts today are constructed from polyester (Dacron) or polytetrafluoroethylene (PTFE) fabric firmly attached over or under full-length stents that confer columnar stiffness. The stents are manufactured from nitinol, a thermal memory alloy of nickel and titanium, or stainless steel. Radial force at the proximal and distal landing zones provides friction for fixation. Some systems embed hooks or barbs into the aortic wall for additional grip. Suprarenal fixation with bare metal stents that extend into the suprarenal aorta may provide improved proximal graft attachment in patients with less than optimal aortic necks. All endografts have radio-opaque markers that aid in accurate deployment to avoid inadvertent coverage of the renal or hypogastric arteries. The most common configuration in use today is the bifurcated endograft, which come in modular or unibody designs. The modular design allows for application in a wider range of vascular anatomy. The aorto-uni-iliac and aorto-aortic grafts are used only in specific circumstances, such as difficult access arteries[28] or in secondary procedures for treatment of endoleaks.

Radiation Safety

The technique of endovascular repair of aortic aneurysms necessitates the use of fluoroscopy. Exposure to fluoroscopic x-ray radiation has been shown to cause injuries, including skin burns, cataracts, and certain cancers,[29–31] and the radiation applied during fluoroscopically guided interventional techniques is much greater than that used in diagnostic tests. Although improvements in imaging equipment have drastically reduced the amount of radiation emitted while improving the image quality, significant injury does still occur. Radiation exerts both early and late effects, and the risks of long-term damage are additive with each exposure. Proper training of all personnel involved in performing endovascular procedures is mandatory to ensure patient and staff safety.

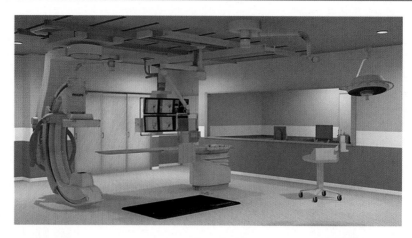

Fig. 12.5 Artist rendition of a hybrid operating room with interventional capabilities. A separate shielded booth allows for remote flurography, limiting operator radiation exposure (Courtesy of Koninklijke Philips Electronics)

Institutional protocols should be established and routinely reinforced in order to minimize radiation exposure to involved personnel. Radiation badge monitors must be worn at all times, and the dosage monitored at regular intervals by the radiation safety committee. Exposure to excessive levels mandates taking appropriate steps to reduce future exposure.

The amount of radiation exposure experienced by the patient and practitioner is determined by numerous factors, including size of the patient,[32] equipment dose rate and dose settings, beam-on time, proximity of the x-ray tube to the patient, and field collimation. Energy dissipates according to the inverse square law, where the dose rate decreases by the square of the relative increase in distance from the radiation source.[33] Maximal distance should be maintained between both the patient and the staff from the emitter at all times. Minimizing emitter on-time, using low-dose fluoroscopy, and collimating when possible are strategies to reduce the radiation exposure. Appropriate lead shielding should be used at all times. Lead aprons of at least 0.5 mm lead-equivalency is recommended, and personnel should face the emitter as much as possible, as most lead aprons provide adequate front shielding, but less protection on the sides and back. Fluorography, including digital subtraction angiography (DSA), emits a radiation dose 10–70 times that of

fluoroscopy.[34] When performing such procedures, remote control flurorography provides an ideal environment (Fig. 12.5). The operator and all assistants are positioned in a shielded booth while acquisition of images is in progress. At a minimum, additional lead shielding, such as flat panel mobile shields, should be used during fluorography. These techniques, along with consistent monitoring of radiation dose to patients and staff and improving practices as necessary, will minimize the health risks imposed by radiation.

Endovascular AAA repair can be performed in a standard operating room or preferably an operative endosuite because it allows for high-quality imaging with standard open surgical equipment. The catheterization laboratory should be avoided due to concerns for infection with groin incisions or if open conversion is required.[35] A fixed C-arm unit, compared to a portable unit, provides a larger field of view, better resolution, decreased radiation dose to patient and staff, and tableside operator controls for viewing angles and image processing.[36]

Contrast-Induced Nephropathy

Patients undergoing EVAR with pre-existing renal impairment are prone to develop contrast-induced nephropathy (CIN). Most of the recommendations for the prevention of CIN come from the studies on percutaneous coronary interventions and may be applicable to EVAR. Advanced age, diabetes mellitus, congestive heart failure, hypovolemia, and anemia are risk factors for the development of CIN.[37,38] Adequate perioperative hydration with normal saline is beneficial in preventing CIN. Forced diuresis with mannitol or furosemide was no better than hydration alone.[39] Nephrotoxic drugs such as nonsteroidal anti-inflammatory drugs and aminoglycosides should be avoided.[40] Judicious use of iso-osmolar contrast media can decrease the incidence of CIN.[41] Criado et al. used catheter-less carbon dioxide angiography conducted through the endograft delivery sheath and found this imaging modeling to be reliable for endograft deployment, safe, nontoxic, and inexpensive.[42] In patients with glomerular filtration rate (GFR) less than 60, alkalinization of urine with IV sodium bicarbonate may be performed pre- and postprocedure; and in patients with GFR less than 30, N-acetylcysteine may be added.[43]

Graft Selection and Placement

Once a patient is deemed appropriate for and elects to proceed with endovascular stent graft treatment of aortic aneurysm, the most suitable graft must be selected for the procedure. Modern endograft systems come in a wide variety of diameters and lengths, and selecting the right configuration is crucial to minimizing complications and maximizing technical success. Critical variables to consider include the diameters and lengths of the infrarenal aortic neck, aneurysm, common iliac arteries, and the diameters and quality of the access vessels, namely the external iliac and common femoral arteries. Most of this information can be obtained from the preoperative CTA. 3D image reconstructions are now widely available (Fig. 12.6), and postimage processing that allows for manipulation of view angles, centerline length, and angle measurements, and even the placement of a virtual endograft is possible from commercial software developers.

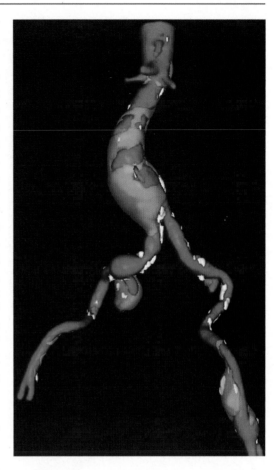

Fig. 12.6 3D reconstruction of the aorta and iliofemoral vasculature from CT-angiography performed in a patient with multiple arterial aneurysms (Courtesy of M2S)

Procedure

In an elective operation, the patient is prepped and draped similar to an open aneurysm repair. The abdominal sterile prep extends from the xiphoid to the knee and to the table laterally. Appropriate preoperative antibiotics are given, with coverage for both gram-positive and gram-negative microbes. The surgeon stands opposite the assistant, and the monitor is positioned for unobstructed viewing by both operators. The scrub nurse is positioned by the patient's feet for ease of passage of instruments and devices, as well as for distal wire monitoring and control. The anesthesiologist is positioned by the patient's

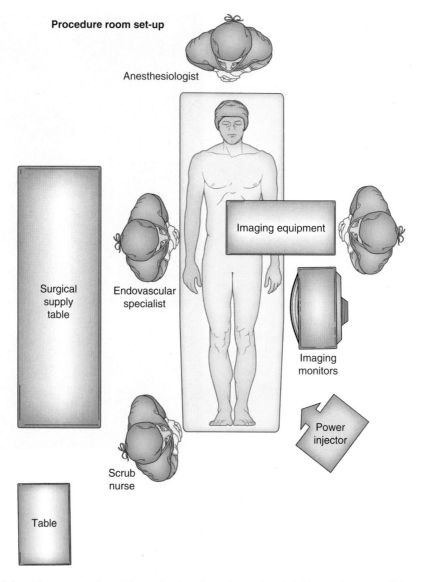

Procedure room set-up

Anesthesiologist

Imaging equipment

Surgical supply table

Endovascular specialist

Imaging monitors

Power injector

Scrub nurse

Table

Fig. 12.7 Schematic representation of the staff and equipment setup in a hybrid operating room. This configuration allows for optimal visualization by the principal operator and maximizes space efficiency within the operative field

head for airway monitoring as well as continuous vitals surveillance (Fig. 12.7).

The common femoral arteries are accessed via a cut down or percutaneous approach. Open exposure of the vessels allows direct visualization and evaluation of vessel quality, including the presence of calcific plaques, and selection of an appropriate arteriotomy site. In addition, passage of sheaths and devices may be facilitated by avoiding traversing through subcutaneous soft tissue and scars from previous surgical manipula-

tions. However, the use of ultrasound for guiding percutaneous access allows for evaluation of the femoral vessels, and may aid in achieving precise arterial access. If the percutaneous approach is chosen, large vessel closure device is used either in a preclose or a postclose fashion[44] (Fig. 12.8).

Once access to the common femoral arteries is established, stiff wires are placed into the descending aorta to "straighten out" the aortoiliac system. Aortography is performed with a calibrated catheter to identify the level of the renal arteries, as

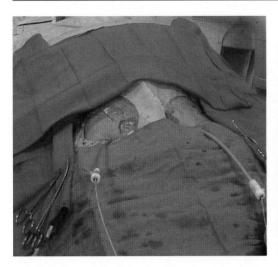

Fig. 12.8 Total percutaneous endovascular AAA repair. Preclose sutures placed in a preclose fashion are held with clamps, followed by sheath insertion into both common femoral arteries for endograft delivery

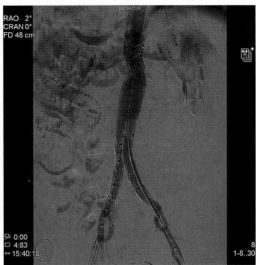

Fig. 12.9 Completion aortogram after successful EVAR. Note the patent bilateral renal and hypogastric arteries and the absence of endoleak

well as to confirm the diameters and lengths of the proximal neck, aorta, aneurysm sac, and aortic and iliac bifurcations. The appropriate endografts are selected and systemic anticoagulation with heparin or direct thrombin inhibitor is initiated. Adequate anticoagulation is ensured by keeping the activated clotting time greater than 250 seconds throughout the remainder of the case. The main body is inserted and positioned with the top portion of the fabric just inferior to the lowest renal artery. Oversizing the proximal neck of the main body can assist with proximal sealing through augmentation of radial force, but oversizing by greater than 20% can lead to fabric pleating and proximal endoleak.[45] Magnified views with proper gantry manipulation to obtain a perpendicular view to the proximal lowest renal artery allows for accurate proximal placement of the endograft. If a modular device is used, the contralateral gate must be oriented to allow for easy access. The exact orientation may vary depending on the anatomy of the aneurysm as well as the iliac arteries, but usually a lateral and slightly anterior positioning of the contralateral gate should suffice. The main body is deployed, and in some grafts, slight adjustment in positioning of the main body after partial deployment is

possible. The contralateral gate is then cannulated. Confirmation of access through the contralateral gate is crucial, and can be achieved via free rotation of a curved catheter in the proximal neck. Different curved catheters can be employed to assist with gate cannulation, and manipulating the C-arm to attain different anteroposterior and oblique views can assist in locating the gate in the three-dimensional. The distance from the main body to the iliac bifurcation, with appropriate overlap of the contralateral gate, is measured with a marking catheter and injection of contrast through the sheath. The contralateral limb is then deployed. Some devices require the deployment of an ipsilateral iliac limb, and the appropriate length graft is chosen through similar measurement techniques. Once all the pieces of the modular device are deployed, compliant balloons are used to mold the graft at the proximal, distal, and modular fixation sites. Completion arteriogram is required to check for exclusion of the aneurysm, presence of endoleaks, and patency of the renal and hypogastric arteries (Fig. 12.9).

If an iliac conduit was used for device delivery, distal anastomosis of the conduit to the common femoral artery is performed. All incisions are closed, and any applicable percutaneous closure

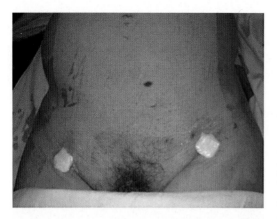

Fig. 12.10 Two small dressings are all that is required at the completion of a total percutaneous endovascular AAA repair

devices are deployed (Fig. 12.10). Anticoagulation is reversed. The patient can usually be extubated at the completion of the case, and brought to a monitored bed for recovery.

Intraoperative Complications

Numerous reports have documented the short-term benefits associated with endovascular treatment of aortic aneurysms when compared to open repair, including lower operative blood loss, earlier return to preoperative activity level, and shorter hospital stays,[46–48] but the endovascular approaches introduce unique potentials for complications.[49] Initial technical success, defined as the ability to deliver and deploy the endograft in the intended location, to avoid arterial injury, to provide secure fixation of the endograft without endoleak, and to reestablish end organ perfusion, has improved with operator experience[50] and the development of more flexible and smaller profile delivery systems.[51] Even with these advances, intraoperative complications can occur.

Access Vessel Injury

Dissection, rupture, and even avulsion of the access vessels can occur with passage of large caliber sheaths and devices.[52] This may manifest as diminished or absent flow through the femoral artery, extravasation of contrast on iliac angiogram, or visualization of the avulsed end of the distal artery around the introducer sheath. Severely calcified, tortuous, or small caliber vessels increase the risk of this complication. Women, owing to the smaller size of their access vessels, are at higher risk than men to develop this complication.[53] In addition, women have a higher prevalence of unfavorable aortic neck anatomy, and are less likely to be anatomic candidates for EVAR. Deterioration in vital signs may be rapid even in the absence of massive bleeding from the groin incisions, as bleeding from the iliac arteries tend to pool in the retroperitoneal space. Initial control should be gained with intraluminal balloon occlusion of the damaged vessel, followed by stent graft repair.[54] Occasionally, conversion to open repair may be required.

Renal Artery Exclusion

Coverage of the renal arteries with the stent graft fabric should be avoidable with precise endograft deployment and clear visualization of the renal artery orifice. However, the rate of renal artery exclusion has been reported to be 1% in published literature.[55] If the excluded renal artery can be accessed with a guide wire, stenting of the renal artery origin with extension of the stent into the uncovered proximal aorta can achieve renal salvage.[56]

Rupture of Aneurysm

Rupture of the aneurysm sac has been described during elective repair of aortic aneurysms.[57] Excessive manipulation and undue tension on the stent graft delivery device, stiff wires, and sheaths may lead to disturbance of mural thrombus, embolization, and even aortic wall trauma. Management of rupture is similar to that of endovascular repair of ruptured aortic aneurysms, as described later in this chapter. This potential for rapid hemorrhage from intraoperative aneurysm rupture or access vessel damage necessitates preoperative preparation for such events. These measures include the establishment of large bore intravenous accesses, central venous pressure monitoring, and preferably arterial pressure monitoring.

Embolization

Perfusion of the lower extremities can be compromised by dissection at the femoral access site or distal embolization.[55] Arteriotomy closure requires adequate visualization of the vessel lumen and avoidance of intimal flaps. Distal embolization can occur from disturbing luminal thrombus within the aneurysm sac or from rupture of atherosclerotic plaques in the iliofemoral arteries.[58] Excessive manipulation within the juxtarenal aorta should be avoided, as the renal arteries are also susceptible to embolic events.[59] Distal pulses should always be documented before and after the operation, and any change in the pulse exam should prompt the appropriate investigation, including examining the arteriotomy closure, performing an arteriogram, and embolectomy as indicated.

Postoperative Care

Postoperative care for these patients is usually less involved than for patients undergoing open repair of aortic aneurysms, but certain elements are critical. Distal pulses must be routinely checked for evidence of embolization, graft occlusion, or ilio-femoral vessel injury. Adequate fluid hydration provides for protection against contrast nephropathy, as a significant contrast load may be delivered during these procedures. The abdomen must be examined for evidence of peritonitis suggesting visceral ischemia. Groin access sites should be checked for hematoma or inadequate hemostasis. Oral intake can be resumed on the day of surgery or the first posto-perative day, and patients are typically discharged in 1 or 2 days.

Immediate Postoperative Complications

The most common problem in the immediate postoperative period is access site complication.[60] This includes hematoma, bleeding, or pseudoaneurysm formation. Attention to proper surgical technique is critical to reducing the incidence of this complication, including achieving hemostasis within the surgical field, meticulous closure of arteriotomies, and accurate placement of percutaneous access, if used. Access site complications are usually managed nonoperatively, but rarely surgical re-exploration for hematoma evacuation and arterial repair is required.

Coverage of the internal iliac arteries, when required to achieve adequate distal fixation, is usually preceded by embolization. Unilateral occlusion of the internal iliac artery should bear little consequence. However, if both hypogastric arteries are excluded, severe buttock claudication can result, and may progress to buttock necrosis.[61] Staged hypogastric occlusion may decrease this complication by allowing for the development of collateral circulation. Alternatively, one of the internal iliac arteries may be revascularized via bypass grafting from the external iliac artery.[18]

Occasionally, patients may present with fever and malaise for up to 10 days after endograft placement.[62] The symptoms usually resolve spontaneously, and treatment is limited to symptom control. This syndrome is thought to be due to the release of inflammatory cytokines from thrombosis within the excluded aneurysm sac,[63] but workup for infectious etiology is warranted.

Late Complications

The main issues associated with late complications from endograft treatment of aortic aneurysms include endoleaks (Fig. 12.11), graft migration, graft kinking, and device failure. It is because of these concerns that long-term postoperative surveillance should be employed in all

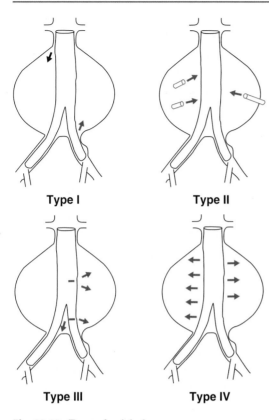

Fig. 12.11 Types of endoleaks

treated patients. Imaging modalities employed include CT scan, abdominal ultrasound, and plain abdominal radiograph.[64] The metallic stents allow for radiologic assessment of kinking or structural abnormalities, whereas tracking the size of the aneurysm sac over time provides an indirect measure of the adequacy of exclusion from arterial circulation. Although no universally agreed upon guidelines exist for the interval between surveillance studies, an initial period of frequent assessment followed by lengthening of the study interval should suffice in the absence of concerning findings. This allows for the possibility of reintervention before clinical failure. In both EVAR-1 and DREAM clinical trials, EVAR was associated with high reintervention rates compared to surgery. Routine surveillance of aneurysms treated with endograft is an important part of postoperative care, and any patient being considered for elective endovascular aneurysm repair should be willing and able to comply with follow-up protocols.[65,66]

Endoleaks

The most common etiology of treatment failure in the endovascular repair of aortic aneurysms is the presence of endoleak (20–30% in the early postoperative period). The persistence of blood flow within the aneurysm sac conveys a continued risk of aneurysm expansion and rupture.[67]

Types of Endoleaks

There are four defined types of endoleaks,[68] as outlined in the other chapters. Type I endoleak (8.2–18%) (Fig. 12.12) is the persistence of blood flow around the proximal (Ia) or distal (Ib) fixation sites. In type II endoleaks (8–45%), blood fills the aneurysm sac via retrograde flow from the excluded aortic branches, most commonly the inferior mesenteric artery and lumbar arteries, but can include accessory renal arteries, hypogastric arteries, or other small branches. Type III endoleaks (0.7–3.8%) result from inadequate sealing between modular components, or from tears or defects in the fabric of the stent graft. Type IV is rarely seen in modern-day devices, and is caused by excessive porosity of the graft fabric.

Early Endoleaks

Type I and III endoleaks observed intraoperatively are usually treated with additional procedures during the initial operation. This may include balloon dilatation of the proximal, intergraft, or distal fixation points to maximize graft apposition. The deployment of proximal extension cuffs or balloon-expandable bare metal giant stents can assist in resolution of proximal endoleaks.[69] Type Ib endoleaks can be managed with flared cuffs[19] or placement of extension limbs to the external iliac artery with coil embolization of the ipsilateral hypogastric artery. The diagnosis of a late type III endoleak can be managed with laying additional stent graft within the malfunctioning graft[70] (Fig. 12.13). Most type II endoleaks are treated with initial observation, as

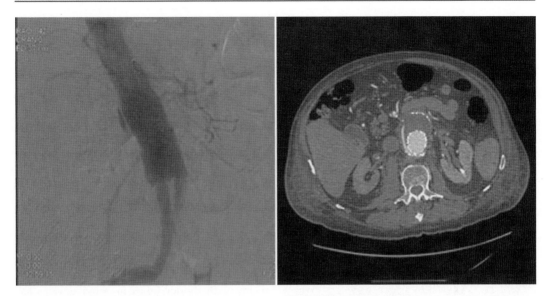

Fig. 12.12 Type I endoleak. Note the extravastion of contrast from the proximal fixation site into the aneurysm sac

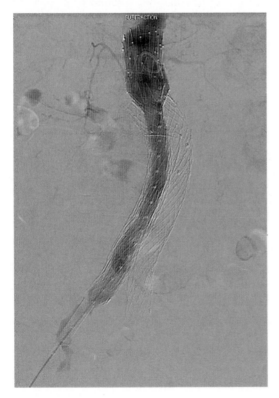

Fig. 12.13 Placement of an aorto-uni-iliac stent graft inside a bifurcated stent graft to repair a type I endoleak resulting from distal graft migration

most type II endoleaks resolve within the first month.[71] Intervention is reserved for continued aneurysm expansion. The diagnosis of type II

endoleaks can be made with CT angiography,[72] where a blush of contrast can be seen in the aneurysm sac associated with an aortic branch vessel, typically a lumbar artery or the inferior mesenteric artery. Occasionally, the offending vessel is not visualized, and continued aneurysm expansion leads to diagnostic angiography. Selective catheterization and arteriography of the internal iliac arteries and superior gluteal arteries can identify the contributing vessel, and coil embolization can be achieved in the same setting[73] (Fig. 12.14). The superior mesenteric artery also can be catheterized for access to the offending vessel. Additional access options include translumbar[74] or transperitoneal (open or laparoscopic[75]) approaches. Type IV endoleaks are becoming more rare with modern fabrics, but if present, should be observed, as the endoleak should resolve with graft incorporation.[76]

Late Onset Endoleaks

Two factors associated with late type I endoleaks are distal graft migration and aortic neck dilation.[77] Distal graft migration is defined as caudal movement of the most proximal portion of the graft by 5 mm or more, and accounts for the majority of late type I endoleaks. This situation arises when there is failure of the proximal graft

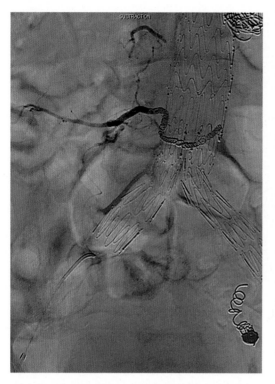

Fig. 12.14 Trans-hypogastric endoluminal coil embolization of lumbar arteries causing a type II endoleak

to maintain apposition to the aortic wall, either through failure of the fixation device or aortic neck dilation. Strategies to potentially decrease the incidence of distal migration include maximizing the length of proximal seal zones, increasing the strength of columnar support, applying suprarenal fixation, and using graft hooks or barbs.[78] Aortic neck dilation occurs either from proximal extension of the aneurysmal process or as a result of significant oversizing of the device,[79] leading to continued excessive exertion of radial force at the aortic neck. Late type I endoleaks tend to persist if not corrected, and persistent proximal type I endoleak is associated with a high risk of aneurysm rupture. The placement of a proximal cuff can often resolve the endoleak, and reestablish adequate sealing of the proximal graft.

Endotension (5%) (also classified as type V endoleak), is defined as persistent transmission of arterial pressure to the aneurysm sac and continued aneurysm growth without demonstrable leak on imaging studies. The exact mechanism and natural history are poorly defined. This poses diagnostic and therapeutic dilemma, as these patients may require intervention if the aneurys growth is persistent, since there is an increased risk of delayed aneurysm rupture.[80]

Kinking of Endograft

Exclusion of the aneurysm from arterial circulation leads to aortic remodeling. Sac shrinkage causes a reduction in not only the diameter but also the length of the native aorta.[81] This can lead to kinking (Fig. 12.15) or obstruction of the graft limbs. The use of external support and longer bodies with shorter limbs in newer devices has reduced the risk of kinking.[82] However, secondary procedures may be required to reopen the occluded graft and provide additional support for collapsed limbs.

Infection

Infection of aortic stent grafts is a catastrophic event. Although rare, this is thought to be due to intravascular seeding of the graft rather than primary graft infection.[83] Persistent positive blood cultures or CT scan finding of air around the graft suggest the diagnosis.[84] Definitive management requires complete excision of the implanted device and restoration of distal perfusion via extra-anatomic bypass[85] or in situ aortic reconstruction with autogenous femoral vein, antibiotic-soaked nonautogenous graft, or cryopreserved arterial allografts,[86] along with appropriate antibiotic treatment of accompanying bacteremia or sepsis.

Late Device Failure

Late device failure is associated with early generations of endografts (Fig. 12.16), and includes fabric disintegrations, stent fractures, suture breaks, and barb fractures.[87,88] Device failure may lead to repressurization of the aneurysm sac, imparting a

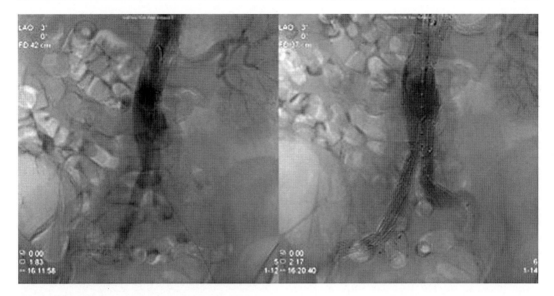

Fig. 12.15 Kinking of the right iliac limb due to vessel tortuosity. Placement of an additional stent within the iliac limb corrected the problem

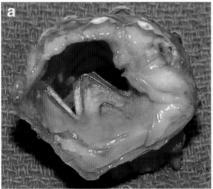

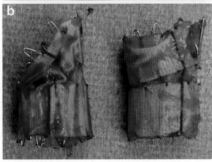

Fig. 12.16 (a, b) Long-term failure of endografts requiring open surgical removal of thoracic endografts and open aortic graft reconstruction

risk of rupture. However, barb fractures and suture breaks are usually benign, and may not represent any increased risk of rupture. Most device failures,

when indicated, can be addressed through endovascular techniques, including re-lining the failed graft with a new endograft, or placement of an aorto-uni-iliac graft with contralateral limb occluder and extra-anatomic bypass.[89] Rarely, open repair with explant of the failed endograft is required. Thus, long-term follow-up is required for all stent grafts to evaluate for device integrity, and timely appropriate management when such failures are detected.

Endovascular Repair of Ruptured Abdominal Aortic Aneurysms

The use of endografts in the management of acutely ruptured or symptomatic aortic aneurysms has been described in small series, and early results have been promising.[90,91] The advantages of the endovascular approach in the repair of ruptured abdominal aortic aneurysms includes avoiding laparotomy in an otherwise compromised patient, lower operative blood loss, and more rapid control of hemorrhage. Lower early mortality is anticipated by extrapolation of data from elective aneurysm repair, and has been supported in recent studies.[92,93] An additional advantage of starting with an endovascular approach is the ability to obtain rapid proximal aortic control without the need for open exposure of the supraceliac aorta. Even if conversion to an open repair is required, such as for a patient with unfavorable anatomy, the endovascular occlusion balloon allows for precise placement of the proximal "clamp," which may limit the degree of visceral or renal ischemia required during open aneurysm repair.

The applicability of the endovascular approach is dependant not only on anatomical considerations, but also on logistical factors involving device and treatment staff availability. Expeditious and successful treatment of ruptured abdominal aortic aneurysms requires a multidisciplinary team made up of the vascular surgeon, emergency department physicians, anesthesiologist, operating room staff, and x-ray technicians. An institutional protocol that directs the triaging of patients with ruptured abdominal aortic aneurysms should be established and rehearsed.[94] The preoperative process starts with a high index of suspicion in a patient presenting to the emergency department with an acutely symptomatic or ruptured aortic aneurysm. The treatment team is notified and activated. In patients with a maintainable blood pressure of >80 mmHg and not in immediate hemodynamic compromise, a CT scan should be obtained to determine suitability for endograft repair. The CT scan directs the choice of endografts through evaluation of the aortoiliac morphology and visualization of the aortic wall, which may be masked by luminal thrombus in angiographic images. Lloyd et al. suggest that patients who present with ruptured AAAs do have time to undergo expeditious imaging, with a majority of patients not undergoing treatment dying >2 h after diagnosis and admission.[95] Unstable patients, however, should be transported directly for operative repair without preoperative imaging (Fig. 12.17).

Early experiences with endovascular repair of ruptured AAAs involved the use of aorto-uniiliac devices,[96] but the use of modular bifurcated prosthesis is increasing.[97] An adequate inventory of commercially available stent-grafts, catheters, wires, balloons, and sheaths must be available,

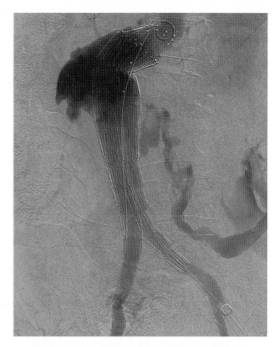

Fig. 12.17 Abdominal aortic aneurysm with free intraperitoneal rupture despite endograft deployment

and the vascular surgeon must be comfortable with using any of the available equipment. The ability to exclude the aneurysm sac from the arterial circulation depends on using endografts with proper diameter and lengths, and hybrid stent-grafts, combining pieces from different manufacturers, may be required to accomplish this task.

Once the decision to proceed has been made and the preoperative planning has been completed, the patient is brought into an operating room with interventional capabilities. The operating room setting is ideal, as it allows for conversion to open procedures as required. Appropriate lead shielding is worn or used by all personnel involved in the procedure. In a patient with a contained abdominal aortic aneurysm rupture, the muscular abdominal wall may provide an additional tamponade effect.[93] Therefore, prepping and draping the patient should be done before the induction of anesthesia. The patient is prepared as in an open aneurysm repair, from the xiphoid down to the knees, and to the table laterally. All lines, restraints, and monitoring equipment must be kept clear of the patient's chest, abdomen, and groin so as not to interfere with the acquisition of fluoroscopic images. Bilateral femoral access is obtained under local anesthesia. Simultaneously, the anesthesiologist places upper extremity arterial catheter and central venous catheter or sheath. For especially agitated or uncooperative patients, conscious sedation may be judiciously applied, but every attempt should be made to avoid neuromuscular blockade until femoral access has been attained. This allows for the placement of an aortic occlusion balloon for proximal control in the event of free rupture or hemodynamic instability on induction of general anesthesia. Stiff wires are passed into the thoracic aorta, followed by the endovascular balloon. A flush catheter is placed into the juxtarenal aorta, and an aortogram is performed. If a preoperative CT scan was not obtained, the feasibility of endograft repair and endograft selection, as applicable, is done based on the aortogram. In this scenario, oversizing of the endograft, particularly at the proximal neck, is recommended to allow for the presence of thrombus that may not be visualized on the arteriogram. The remainder of the operation is carried out similar to an elective repair. Postoperatively, the patient should be admitted to the intensive care unit, and if general anesthesia was used, the patient may be kept intubated for a short time to facilitate hemodynamic monitoring and manipulation. In these patients, special attention must be paid to the development of abdominal compartment syndrome, which has been reported to occur in 3–18% of patients.[98] The endovascular repair does not address the pressure effects exerted by the extravasated blood from the aneurysm rupture within either the retroperitoneum or the peritoneal cavity. High airway pressures, oliguria, or hypotension combined with supportive abdominal exam findings should raise suspicion to this syndrome, and decompressive laparotomy may be required to address these issues.

With the establishment of a well-defined protocol for the management of ruptured AAAs, Mehta et al. were able to achieve markedly improved mortality outcomes with endovascular techniques as compared to conventional open techniques.[94] The primary goal in the management of patients with ruptured AAAs is to exclude the aneurysm and stabilize the compromised patient. The endovascular approach, with its associated lower morbidity and mortality compared to open repair, is a logical first step to accomplishing that goal. Therefore, the anatomical inclusion criteria for elective EVAR should be expanded in the ruptured patient. This may require additional procedures or even open surgical repair to achieve a satisfactory long-term result, but these additional procedures are usually performed after the patient has been stabilized hemodynamically.

Endovascular Therapy for Thoracic Aortic Diseases

Thoracic Aortic Aneurysms

Most of the descending thoracic aneurysms are atherosclerotic and treatment is indicated for aneurysm diameter more than 5.5 cm or annual growth rate more than 1 cm. Endovascular therapy is particularly useful in localized or saccular aneurysms and focal anastomotic psueudoaneurysms. Clinical experience has shown that endovascular therapy is safe with lower mortality, morbidity, and paraplegia compared with conventional surgery.[99,100] Long-term durability is still unknown.

Thoracic Aortic Dissections

Endovascular treatment is indicated in complicated type B dissections. These include acute aortic rupture with pain, chronic dissection with false lumen enlargement, and branch vessel involvement (renal, mesenteric, iliac, and spinal vessels). The aim is to cover all entry and exit points or at least entry point in long aortic segment involvement. Results from several clinical series are promising[101] and current ongoing randomized trials should provide the answer (VIRTUE and ADSORB studies).

Traumatic Aortic Injuries

The endovascular approach may be particularly advantageous in patients who present with traumatic transections or acute rupture, as the presence of other injuries or comorbidities may make the risk of open thoracic repair prohibitively high.[102] Open thoracic aortic surgery is a morbid procedure, due to the need for thoracotomy, aortic cross-clamp, and cardiopulmonary bypass,[103] all of which are theoretically avoided through endovascular techniques.

Thoracoabdominal Aneurysms

Exclusion of aneurysm with the need to maintain branch vessel blood flow makes endovascular procedure difficult in these patients. Surgical debranching with hybrid endovascular procedure and fenestrated stents are two useful approaches. Barring the use of debranching procedures or branched endografts, only Crawford Type I thoracoabdominal aortic aneurysms can be repaired through purely endovascular techniques. Limited experience from few centers[104] does not allow any safe conclusions to be drawn.

Coarctation of Aorta

Current data suggest that endograft is a safe and effective alternative to open surgical treatment.[105] Re-intervention rate was 10–15% with catheter-based therapies. More long-term data are required before recommending endograft as the first-line treatment.

Aortic Arch Aneurysms

Endovascular graft technology is challenged with the need to preserve carotid and subclavian blood flow. Hybrid hemi or total arch transposition followed by aneurysm exclusion with stent graft (Fig. 12.18)[106] and fenestrated or branched stent grafts[107] has been employed. Clinical experience is limited to few centers.

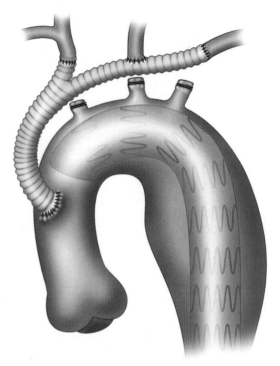

Fig. 12.18 Schematic of a hybrid procedure consisting of total arch transposition followed by aortic aneurysm exclusion with a stent graft

Technical Considerations

Spiral CT of the chest, abdomen, and pelvis is obtained for any patient being considered for endovascular repair of thoracic aortic aneurysms. The adequacy of proximal and distal seal zones, as well as access routes for the delivery of the endograft is evaluated. The most feared complication after endovascular repair of thoracic aortic aneurysms is spinal cord ischemia and paraplegia. However, studies have shown this incidence to be low, even in patients who have coverage of long aortic segments or the artery of Adamkiewicz supplying the anterior spinal artery.[108] Another complication that may arise is a type I endoleak, usually associated with distal graft migration.[109] The high velocity of blood traveling through the thoracic aorta causes high shear stress on the endograft. In addition, the graft itself may kink in the mid-portion of the aneurysm, which would contribute to distal migration of the proximal seal zone.[110] Therefore, most investigators recommend at least 2 cm of proximal landing zone.[111] To achieve adequate proximal fixation, coverage of the origin of the left subclavian artery may be required and is considered acceptable. However, the role of preoperative extra-anatomic revascularization of the left subclavian artery is unclear. Most patients who did not undergo preoperative left subclavian artery revascularization prior to coverage of its origin experienced only asymptomatic blood pressure differential between the two upper extremities.[112] However, strokes directly related to obstruction of left vertebral artery inflow have been described, usually in the setting of a concomitant right vertebral artery occlusion.[113,114] More recent studies have reported reduced risks of cerebrovascular accident and spinal cord ischemia when revascularization of the left subclavian artery is performed.[115] Therefore, detailed interrogation of the supra-aortic arteries is essential if coverage of the left subclavian artery is desired without preoperative bypass. Although more experience and long-term studies are required before meaningful conclusions can be drawn regarding the value of endovascular repair of thoracic aortic diseases, this approach may represent a less morbid and superior approach in patients considered too high risk for open repair.

Key Notes

1. The transfemoral endovascular repair of abdominal aortic aneurysms offers improved short-term survival compared to open repair, and this benefit is even greater in patients deemed high risk for surgery.
2. Eligibility for EVAR is based on a host of factors including size of aneurysm, risk of rupture, life expectancy, and patient anatomy. The proximal aortic neck is the most important anatomic consideration when considering endograft repair and a hostile neck can lead to inadequate exclusion of aneurysm sac from arterial circulation.
3. Personnel involved in EVAR must be conscious of radiation safety, and all efforts should be made on both a system as well as an individual level to monitor and minimize radiation exposure.
4. Operative planning includes consideration for possible complications, including aneurysm rupture, access vessel injury, and medical complications. The operative team must always be ready to convert to open repair.
5. Any patient being considered for EVAR must be able to comply with lifelong endograft surveillance. Graft endoleak is an ever-present threat, and early detection and treatment with secondary interventions address the threat of aneurysm enlargement and rupture.
6. Endovascular repair of ruptured abdominal aortic aneurysms offers an attractive alternative to open repair, with lower short-term mortality. Establishment of an institutional protocol for timely diagnosis and treatment of this highly morbid condition improves outcomes.
7. Indications for endovascular thoracic stenting continue to expand while the results of randomized clinical trials and long-term outcome studies are awaited.

References

1. Parodi JC, Palmaz JC, Barone HD. Transfemoral intraluminal graft implantation for abdominal aortic aneurysm. *Ann Vasc Surg*. 1991;5:491–499.
2. Huber TS, Wang JG, Derrow AE, et al. Experience in the United States with intact abdominal aortic aneurysm repair. *J Vasc Surg*. 2001;33:304–311.
3. Anderson PL, Arons RR, Moskowitz AJ, et al. A statewide experience with endovascular abdominal aortic aneurysm repair: rapid diffusion with excellent early results. *J Vasc Surg*. 2004;39:10–19.
4. Schermerhorn ML, O'Malley AJ, Jhaveri A, Cotterill P, Pomposelli F, Landon BE. Endovascular vs. open repair of abdominal aortic aneurysms in the Medicare population. *N Engl J Med*. 2008;358:464–474.
5. Zwolak RM, Sidawy AN, Greenberg RK, Schermerhorn ML, Shackelton RJ, Siami FS. *J Vasc Surg*. 2008;48(3): 511–518.
6. Prinssen M, Verhoeven EL, Buth J, et al. A randomized trial comparing conventional and endovascular repair of abdominal aortic aneurysms. *N Engl J Med*. 2004;351(16):1607–1618.
7. Greenhalgh RM, Brown LC, Kwong GP, Powell JT, Thompson SG. Comparison of endovascular aneurysm

repair with open repair in patients with abdominal aortic aneurysm (EVAR trial 1), 30-day operative mortality results: randomized controlled trial. *Lancet*. 2004;364:843–848.

8. Sajid MS, Desai M, Haider Z, Baker DM, Hamilton G. Endovascular aortic aneurysm repair has significantly lower perioperative mortality in comparison to open repair: a systematic review. *Asian J Surg*. 2008;31(3):119–123.

9. Giles KA, Pomposelli F, Hamdan A, Wyers M, Jhaveri A, Schermerhorn ML. Decrease in total aneurysm-related deaths in the era of endovascular aneurysm repair. *J Vasc Surg*. 2009;49(3):543–550. epub ahead of print.

10. Schermerhorn ML, Finlayson SR, Fillinger MF, Buth J, van Marrewijk C, Cronenwett JL. Life expectancy after endovascular versus open abdominal aortic aneurysm repair: results of a decision analysis model on the basis of data from EUROSTAR. *J Vasc Surg*. 2002;36(6):1112–1120.

11. The United Kingdom Small Aneurysm Trial Participants. Mortality results for randomized controlled trial of early elective surgery or ultrasonographic surveillance for small abdominal aortic aneurysms. *Lancet*. 1998;352(9141):1649–1655.

12. Ledele FA, Wilson SE, Johnson GR, et al. Immediate repair compared with surveillance of small abdominal aortic aneurysms. *N Engl J Med*. 2002;346: 1437–1444.

13. Schermerhorn ML. Should usual criteria for intervention in abdominal aortic aneurysms be "downsized", considering reported risk reduction with endovascular repair? *Ann NY Acad Sci*. 2006;1085:47–58.

14. Cambria RA, Gloviczki P, Stanson AW, et al. Outcome and expansion rate of 57 thoracoabdominal aortic aneurysms managed nonoperatively. *Am J Surg*. 1995;170:213–217.

15. Stanley BM, Semmens JB, Mai Q, et al. Evaluation of patient selection guidelines for endoluminal AAA repair with the Zenith stent-graft: the Australasian experience. *J Endovasc Ther*. 2001;8:457–464.

16. Choke E, Munneke G, Morgan R, et al. Outcomes of endovascular abdominal aortic aneurysm repair in patients with hostile neck anatomy. *Card Intervent Radiol*. 2006;29(6):975–980.

17. Parlani G, Zannetti S, Verzini F, et al. Does the presence of an iliac aneurysm affect outcome of endoluminal AAA repair? An analysis of 336 cases. *Eur J Vasc Endovasc Surg*. 2002;24:134–138.

18. Parodi JC, Ferreira M. Relocation of the iliac artery bifurcation to facilitate endoluminal treatment of abdominal aortic aneurysms. *J Endovasc Surg*. 1999;6:342–347.

19. Kritpracha B, Pigott JP, Russell TE, et al. Bell-bottom aortoiliac endografts: an alternative that preserves pelvic blood flow. *J Vasc Surg*. 2002;35:874–881.

20. Morrissey NJ, Faries PL, Carrocio A, et al. Intentional internal iliac artery occlusion in endovascular repair of abdominal aortic aneurysms. *J Invasive Cardiol*. 2002;14(12):760–763.

21. Peterson BG, Matsumura JS. Internal endoconduit: an innovative technique to address unfavorable iliac artery anatomy encountered during thoracic endovascular aortic repair. *J Vasc Surg*. 2008;47(2): 441–445.

22. Abu-Ghaida AM, Clair DG, Greenberg RK, et al. Broadening the application of endovascular aneurysm repair: the use of iliac conduits. *J Vasc Surg*. 2002;36:111–117.

23. Dalainas I, Moros I, Gerasimidis T, et al. Mid-term comparison of bifurcated modular endograft versus aorto-uni-iliac endograft in patients with abdominal aortic aneurysm. *Ann Vasc Surg*. 2007;21(3): 339–345.

24. Sakamoto S, Yamauchi S, Yamashita H, et al. Repair of an abdominal aortic aneurysm with a remarkably dilated meandering artery: report of a case. *Surg Today*. 2007;37(2):133–136.

25. Muhs BE, Verhoeven EL, Zeebregts CJ, et al. Mid term results of endovascular aneurysm repair with branched and fenestrated endografts. *J Vasc Surg*. 2006;44:9–15.

26. Klonaris C, Katsargyris A, Bastounis E. Endovascular therapy of aortic diseases. In: Boudoulas H, Stefanadis C, eds. *The Aorta, Structure, Function, Dysfunction and Diseases*. New York: Informa Health Care; 2009:228–240.

27. Allen RC, White RA, Zarins CK, et al. What are the characteristics of the ideal endovascular graft for abdominal aortic aneurysm exclusion? *J Endovasc Surg*. 1997;4:195–202.

28. Chuter TA, Faruqi RM, Reilly LM, et al. A Aortomonoiliac endovascular grafting combined with femorofemoral bypass: an acceptable compromise or a preferred solution? *Semin Vasc Surg*. 1999;12: 176–181.

29. Vlietstra RE, Wagner LK, Koenig T, Mettler F. Radiation burns as a severe complication of fluoroscopically guided cardiological interventions. *J Interv Cardiol*. 2004;17:131–142.

30. Vano E, Gonzalez L, Beneytez F, Moreno F. Lens injuries induced by occupational exposure in non-optimized interventional radiology laboratories. *Br J Radiol*. 1998;71:728–733.

31. MacKenzie I. Breast cancer following multiple fluoroscopies. *Br J Cancer*. 1965;19:1–8.

32. Koenig TR, Mettler FA, Wagner LK. Skin injuries from fluoroscopically guided procedures: part 2, review of 73 cases and recommendations for minimizing dose delivered to patient. *Am J Roentgenol*. 2001;177:13–20.

33. Nickoloff EL, Strauss KJ. Categorical course in diagnostic radiology physics: cardiac catheterization imaging. *Radiol Soc N Amer*. 1998; 222–230.

34. Wager LK, Archer BR. *Minimizing Risks from Fluoroscopic X-Rays*, 4th ed. 2004.

35. Moore RD, Villalba L, Petrasek PF, Samis G, Ball CG, Motamedi M. Endovascular treatment for aortic disease: is a surgical environment necessary? *J Vasc Surg*. 2005;42(4):645–649.

36. Longo GM, Matsumura JS. Endovascular repair of abdominal aortic aneurysms: technique and results. In: Moore WS, ed. *Vascular and endovascular surgery: a comprehensive review*. 7th ed. Philadelphia: Elsevier; 2006:383–395.

37. McCullough PA, Wolyn R, Rocher LL, Levin RN, O'Neil WW. Acute renal failure after coronary intervention: incidence, risk factors and relationship to mortality. *Am J Med*. 1997;103:368–375.

38. Mehran R, Aymong ED, Nikolsky E, et al. A simple risk score for prediction of contrast induced nephropathy after percutaneous coronary intervention: development and initial validation. *J Am Coll Cardiol*. 2004;44:1393–1399.

39. Stevens MA, McCullough PA, Tobin KJ, et al. A prospective randomized trial of prevention measures in patients at risk for contrast nephropathy: results of the P.R.I.N.C.E. study. Prevention of Radio Contrast Induced Nephropathy Clinical Evaluation. *J Am Coll Cardiol*. 1999;33:403–411.

40. Wong GTC, Irwin MG. Contrast induced nephropathy. *Br J Anaesth*. 2007;99:474–483.

41. McCullough P. Outcomes of contrast-induced nephropathy: experience in patients undergoing cardiovascular intervention. *Catheter Cardiovasc Interv*. 2006;67(3):335–343.

42. Criado E, Kabbani L, Cho K. Catheter-less angiography for endovascular aortic aneurysm repair: a new application of carbon dioxide as a contrast agent. *J Vasc Surg*. 2008;48:527–534.

43. Cavusoglu E, Chhabra S, Marmur JD, Kini A, Sharma SK. The prevention of contrast-induced nephropathy in patients undergoing percutaneous coronary intervention. *Minerva Cardioangiol*. 2004;52(5):419–432.

44. Rachel ES, Bergamini TM, Kinney EV, et al. Percutaneous endovascular abdominal aortic aneurysm repair. *Ann Vasc Surg*. 2002;16:43–49.

45. Sternbergh WC, Money SR, Greenbert RK, Chuter TA. Influence of endograft oversizing on device migration, endoleak, aneurysm shrinkage, and aortic neck dilation: results from the zenith multicenter trial. *J Vasc Surg*. 2004;39:20–26.

46. Hua HT, Cambria RP, Chuang SK, et al. Early outcomes of endovascular versus open abdominal aortic aneurysm repair in the National Surgical Quality Improvement Program-Private Sector (NSQIP-PS). *J Vasc Surg*. 2005;41(3):382–389.

47. EVAR trial participants. Endovascular aneurysm repair versus open repair in patients with abdominal aortic aneurysm (EVAR trial 1): randomised controlled trial. *Lancet*. 2005;365(9478):2179–2186.

48. Peterson BG, Matsumura JS, Brewster DC, Makaroun MS. Five-year report of a multicenter controlled clinical trial of open versus endovascular treatment of abdominal aortic aneurysms. *J Vasc Surg*. 2007;45(5):885–890.

49. Hertzer NR. Current status of endovascular repair of infrarenal abdominal aortic aneurysms in the context of 50 years of conventional repair. *Ann NY Acad Sci*. 2006;1085:175–186.

50. Troeng T. Volume versus outcome when treating abdominal aortic aneurysm electively—is there evidence to centralise? *Scand J Surg*. 2008;97(2):154–159.

51. Steingruber IE, Neuhauser B, Seiler R, et al. Technical and clinical success of infrarenal endovascular abdominal aortic aneurysm repair: a 10-year single-center experience. *Eur J Radiol*. 2006;59(3):384–392.

52. Cuypers PW, Laheij RJ, Buth J. Which factors increase the risk of conversion to open surgery following endovascular abdominal aortic aneurysm repair? The EUROSTAR collaborators. *Eur J Vasc Endovasc Surg*. 2000;20(2):183–189.

53. Wolf YG, Arko FR, Hill BB, et al. Gender differences in endovascular abdominal aortic aneurysm repair with the AneuRx stent graft. *J Vasc Surg*. 2002;35(5):882–886.

54. Fairman RM, Velazquez O, Baum R, et al. Endovascular repair of aortic aneurysms: critical events and adjunctive procedures. *J Vasc Surg*. 2001;33(6):1226–1232.

55. Gabrielli L, Baudo A, Molinari A, Domanin M. Early complications in endovascular treatment of abdominal aortic aneurysm. *Acta Chir Belg*. 2004;104(5):519–526.

56. Hedayati N, Lin PH, Lumsden AB, Zhou W. Prolonged renal artery occlusion after endovascular aneurysm repair: endovascular rescue and renal function salvage. *J Vasc Surg*. 2008;47(2):446–449.

57. Moskowitz DM, Kahn RA, Marin ML, Hollier LH. Intraoperative rupture of an abdominal aortic aneurysm during an endovascular stent-graft procedure. *Can J Anaesth*. 1999;46(9):887–890.

58. Maldonado TS, Ranson ME, Rockman CB, et al. Decreased ischemic complications after endovascular aortic aneurysm repair with newer devices. *Vasc Endovascular Surg*. 2007;41(3):192–199.

59. Walsh SR, Tang TY, Boyle JR. Renal consequences of endovascular abdominal aortic aneurysm repair. *J Endovasc Ther*. 2008;15(1):73–82.

60. Adriaensen ME, Bosch JL, Halpern EF, Myriam Hunink MG, Gazelle GS. Elective endovascular versus open surgical repair of abdominal aortic aneurysms: systematic review of short-term results. *Radiology*. 2002;224:739–747.

61. Zander T, Baldi S, Rabellino M, et al. Bilateral hypogastric artery occlusion in endovascular repair of abdominal aortic aneurysms and its clinical significance. *J Vasc Interv Radiol*. 2007;18(12):1481–1486.

62. Storck M, Scharrer-Pamler R, Kapfer X, et al. Does a postimplantation syndrome following endovascular treatment of aortic aneurysms exist? *Vasc Surg*. 2001;35(1):23–29.

63. Zimmer S, Heiss MM, Schardey HM, Weilbach C, Faist E, Lauterjung L. Inflammatory syndrome after endovascular implantation of an aortic stent—a comparative study. *Langenbecks Arch Chir Suppl Kongressbd*. 1998;115(Suppl 1):13–17.

64. Chaikof EL, Blankensteijn JD, Harris PL, et al. Reporting standards for endovascular aortic aneurysm repair. *J Vasc Surg*. 2002;35(5):1048–1060.

65. Kranokpiraksa P, Kaufman JA. Follow-up of endovascular aneurysm repair: plain radiography, ultrasound, CT/CT angiography, MR imaging/MR angiography, or what? *J Vasc Interv Radiol*. 2008;19(6 Suppl): S27-S36.

66. Van Herzeele I, Lefevre A, Van Maele G, Maleux G, Vermassen F, Nevelsteen A. Long-term surveillance is paramount after implantation of the Vanguard stent-graft for abdominal aortic aneurysms. *J Cardiovasc Surg*. 2008;49(1):59–66.

67. White GH, Yu W, May J, et al. Endoleak as a complication of endoluminal grafting of abdominal aortic aneurysms: classification, incidence, diagnosis, and management. *J Endovasc Surg*. 1997;4:152–168.

68. White GH, May J, Waugh RC, Chaufour X, Yu W. Type III and type IV endoleak: toward a complete definition of blood flow in the sac after endoluminal AAA repair. *J Endovasc Surg*. 1998;5(4): 305–309.

69. Barbiero G, Baratto A, Ferro F, Dall'Acgua J, Fitta C, Miotto D. Strategies of endoleak management following endoluminal treatment of abdominal aortic aneurysms in 95 patients: how, when, and why. *Radiol Med*. 2008;113(7):1029–1042.

70. Pozzi Mucelli F, Doddi M, Bruni S, Adovasio R, Pancrazio F, Cova M. Endovascular treatment of endoleaks after endovascular abdominal aortic aneurysm repair: personal experience. *Radiol Med*. 2007;112(3):409–419.

71. Warrier R, Miller R, Bond R, Robertson IK, Hewitt P, Scott A. Risk factors for type II endoleaks after endovascular repair of abdominal aortic aneurysms. *ANZ J Surg*. 2008;78(1–2):61–63.

72. AbuRahma AF. Fate of endoleaks detected by CT angiography and missed by color duplex ultrasound in endovascular grafts for abdominal aortic aneurysms. *J Endovasc Ther*. 2006;13(4):490–495.

73. Hobo R, Buth J. EUROSTAR collaborators. Secondary interventions following endovascular abdominal aortic aneurysm repair using current endografts. A EUROSTAR report. *J Vasc Surg*. 2006;43(5): 896–902.

74. Gorlitzer M, Mertikian G, Trnka H, et al. Translumbar treatment of type II endoleaks after endovascular repair of abdominal aortic aneurysm. *Interact Cardiovasc Thorac Surg*. 2008;7(5):781–784.

75. Feezor RJ, Nelson PR, Lee WA, Zingarelli W, Cendan JC. Laparoscopic repair of a type II endoleak. *J Laparoendosc Adv Surg Tech A*. 2006;16(3): 267–270.

76. Pitton MB, Schmiedt W, Neufang A, Duber C, Thelen M. Classification and treatment of endoleaks after endovascular treatment of abdominal aortic aneurysms. *Rofo*. 2005;177(1):24–34.

77. Litwinski RA, Donayre CE, Chow SL, et al. The role of aortic neck dilation and elongation in the etiology of stent graft migration after endovascular aortic

78. Tonnessen BH, Sternbergh WC 3rd, Money SR. Mid- and long-term device migration after endovascular abdominal aortic aneurysm repair: a comparison of AneuRx and Zenith endografts. *J Vasc Surg*. 2005;42(3):392–401.

79. Sampaio SM, Panneton JM, Mozes G, et al. Aortic neck dilation after endovascular abdominal aortic aneurysm repair: should oversizing be blamed? *Ann Vasc Surg*. 2006;20(3):388–345.

80. Gilling Smith GL, Martin J, Sudhindran S, et al. Freedom from endoleak after endovascular aneurysm repair does not equal treatment success. *Eur J Vasc Endovasc Surg*. 2000;19:421–425.

81. Harris PL, Brennan J, Martin J, et al. Longitudinal aneurysm shrinkage following endovascular aortic aneurysm repair: a source of intermediate and late complications. *J Endovasc Surg*. 1999;6:11–16.

82. Ouriel K, Clair DG, Greenberg RK, et al. Endovascular repair of abdominal aortic aneurysms: device-specific outcome. *J Vasc Surg*. 2003;37:991–998.

83. Heyer KS, Modi P, Morasch MD, et al. Secondary infections of thoracic and abdominal aortic endografts. *J Vasc Interv Radiol*. 2008;20(2):173–179. epub ahead of print.

84. Leon LR Jr. A diagnostic dilemma: does peri stent-graft air after thoracic aortic endografting necessarily imply infection? *Vasc Endovasc Surg*. 2007;41(5): 433–439.

85. Sharif MA, Lee B, Lau LL, et al. Prosthetic stent graft infection after endovascular abdominal aortic aneurysm repair. *J Vasc Surg*. 2007;46(3):442–448.

86. Zhou W, Lin PH, Bush RL, et al. In situ reconstruction with cryopreserved arterial allografts for management of mycotic aneurysms or aortic prosthetic graft infections: a multi-institutional experience. *Tex Heart Inst J*. 2006;33(1):14–18.

87. Norgren L, Jernby B, Engellau L. Aortoenteric fistula caused by a ruptured stent-graft: a case report. *J Endovasc Surg*. 1998;5:269–272.

88. Najibi S, Steinberg J, Katzen BT, et al. Detection of isolated hook fractures 36 months after implantation of the Ancure endograft: a cautionary note. *J Vasc Surg*. 2001;34:353–356.

89. Conners MS, Sternbergh WC, Carter G, et al. Secondary procedures after endovascular aortic aneurysm repair. *J Vasc Surg*. 2002;36:992–996.

90. Ohki T, Veith FJ, Sanchez LA, et al. Endovascular graft repair of ruptured aortoiliac aneurysms. *J Am Coll Surg*. 1999;189:102–113.

91. Hinchliffe RJ, Yusuf SW, Marcierewicz JA, et al. Endovascular repair of ruptured abdominal aortic aneurysm: challenge to open repair? Results of a single-center experience in 20 patients. *Eur J Vasc Endovasc Surg*. 2001;22:528–534.

92. Egorova N, Giacovelli J, Greco G, Gelijns A, Kent CK, McKinsey JF. National outcomes for the treatment of ruptured abdominal aortic aneurysm: comparison of open versus endovascular repairs. *J Vasc Surg*. 2008;48(5):1092–1100.

93. Lachat ML, Peammatter TH, Witzke HJ, et al. Endovascular repair with bifurcated stent-grafts under local anesthesia to improve outcome of ruptured aortoiliac aneurysms. *Eur J Vasc Endovasc Surg.* 2002;23:528–536.

94. Mehta M, Taggert J, Darling RC, et al. Establishing a protocol for endovascular treatment of ruptured abdominal aortic aneurysms: outcomes of a prospective analysis. *J Vasc Surg.* 2006;44(1):1–8.

95. Lloyd GM, Brown MJ, Norwood MGA, et al. Feasibility of preoperative computed tomography in patients with ruptured AAA: a time-to-death study in patients without operation. *J Vasc Surg.* 2004;39: 788–791.

96. Yilmaz N, Peppelenbosch N, Cuypers PW, et al. Emergency treatment of symptomatic or ruptured abdominal aortic aneurysms: the role of endovascular repair. *J Endovasc Ther.* 2002;9:729–735.

97. Verhoeven EL, Prins TR, van den Dungen JJAM, et al. Endovascular repair of acute AAAs under local anesthesia with bifurcated endografts: a feasibility study. *J Endovasc Ther.* 2002;9:729–735.

98. Veith FJ, Ohki T, Lipsitz EC, Suggs WD, Cynamon J. Endovascular grafts and other catheter-directed techniques in the management of ruptured abdominal aortic aneurysms. *Semin Vasc Surg.* 2003;16: 326–331.

99. Makaroun MS, Dillavou ED, Kee ST, et al. Endovascular treatment of thoracic aortic aneurysms: results of the phase II multicenter trial of the GORE TAG thoracic endoprosthesis. *J Vasc Surg.* 2005;41: 1–9.

100. Bavaria JE, Appoo JJ, Makaroun MS, et al. Endovascular stent grafting versus open surgical repair of descending thoracic aneurysms in low risk patients: a multicenter comparative trial. *J Thorac Cardiovasc Surg.* 2007;133:369–377.

101. Thompson M, Ivaz S, Cheshire N, et al. Early results of endovascular treatment of thoracic aorta using Valiant endograft. *Cardiovasc Inter Rad.* 2007;30:1130–1138.

102. Xenos ES, Minion DJ, Davenport DL, et al. Endovascular versus open repair for descending thoracic aortic rupture: institutional experience and meta-analysis. *Eur J Cardiothorac Surg.* 2008;35(2): 282–286. epub ahead of print.

103. Dillavou ED, Makaroun MS. Predictors of morbidity and mortality with endovascular and open thoracic aneurysm repair. *J Vasc Surg.* 2008;48(5):1114–1119.

104. Chutter TA, Reilly LM. Endovascular treatment of thoracoabdominal aneurysms. *J Cardiovasc Surg.* 2006;47:619–628.

105. Carr JA. The results of catheter based therapy compared with surgical repair of adult aortic coarctation. *J Am Coll Cardiol.* 2006;47:1101–1107.

106. Saleh HM, Inglese L. Combined surgical and endovascular treatment of aortic arch aneurysms. *J Vasc Surg.* 2006;44:460–466.

107. Inoue K, Hosokawa H, Iwase T, et al. Aortic arch reconstruction by transluminally placed endovascular branched stent graft. *Circulation.* 1999;100(19suppl): II316-II321.

108. Gravereaux E, Faries PL, Burks JA, et al. Risk of spinal cord ischemia after endograft repair of thoracic aortic aneurysms. *J Vasc Surg.* 2001;34:997–1003.

109. Milner R, Kasirajan K, Chaikof EL. Future of endograft surveillance. *Semin Vasc Surg.* 2006;19(2):75–82.

110. Resch T, Koul B, Dias NV, Lindblad B, Ivancev K. Changes in aneurysm morphology and stent-graft configuration after endovascular repair of aneurysms of the descending thoracic aorta. *J Thorac Cardiovasc Surg.* 2001;122(1):47–52.

111. Cambria PR, Brewster DC, Lauterbach SR, et al. Evolving experience with thoracic aortic stent-graft repair. *J Vasc Surg.* 2002;35:1129–1136.

112. Gawenda M, Brunkwall J. When is safe to cover the left subclavian and celiac arteries. Part I: left subclavian artery. *J Cardiovasc Surg (Torino).* 2008;49(4): 471–477.

113. Woo EY, Carpenter JP, Jackson BM, et al. Left subclavian artery coverage during thoracic endovascular aortic repair: a single-center experience. *J Vasc Surg.* 2008;48(3):555–560.

114. Manninen H, Tulla H, Vanninen R, Ronkainen A. Endangered cerebral blood supply after closure of left subclavian artery: postmortem and clinical imaging studies. *Ann Thorac Surg.* 2008;85(1):120–125.

115. Noor N, Sadat U, Hayes PD, Thompson MM, Boyle JR. Management of the left subclavian artery during endovascular repair of the thoracic aorta. *J Endovasc Ther.* 2008;15(2):168–176.

Anesthesia for Endovascular Aortic Surgery

13

Adam B. Lerner

Introduction

Endovascular aortic surgery presents unique challenges to the anesthesia care team. The ability to care for potentially complex vascular problems in patients with a wide range of comorbidities through a relatively noninvasive, percutaneous approach allows for a seemingly endless number of permutations of anesthetic interventions. This can allow for what might be thought of as "interesting" combinations of interventions such as the placement of invasive arterial catheters at multiple sites and/or pulmonary artery catheterization in a patient undergoing a procedure under monitored anesthesia care (MAC) with little or no sedation. Furthermore, while the hope is always for a quick and complication-free operative course, the anesthesia care team must be prepared for potential catastrophe given the nature and location of the inherent pathology.

A.B. Lerner (✉)
Department of Anesthesia, Critical Care, and Pain Medicine, Beth Israel Deaconess Medical Center, 330 Brookline Avenue, Boston, MA 02215, USA
and
Department of Anesthesia, Harvard Medical School, Boston, MA, USA
e-mail: alerner@bidmc.harvard.edu

Preoperative Evaluation

As with any anesthetic, preparation is paramount to success. Preparation starts with preoperative assessment. In addition to the standard preoperative evaluation of any patient undergoing endovascular aortic repair (EVAR), special attention needs to be paid to the assessment of the cardiac, pulmonary, and renal systems. Although the conversion rate to open repair is low in most modern series,[1] any patient undergoing EVAR needs to be evaluated for such a contingency. It is important to ascertain whether or not the patient's current condition can be optimized prior to surgery. This process needs to consider the urgency of the patient's need for surgery as well as the effectiveness of potential preoperative interventions in actually decreasing operative risk. Current guidelines can be helpful in making these determinations[2] (Fig. 13.1). Certainly patients with unstable coronary artery disease, decompensated heart failure, unstable arrhythmias, and severe valvular disease should be stabilized if at all possible prior to aortic endovascular procedures. However, the anesthetic caregiver will certainly be involved in situations where such time is not available. In these settings, intense anesthetic intervention will be required with attempts made to optimize patients in very short amounts of time. American Heart Association/American College of Cardiology (HA/ACC) recommendations consider EVAR as intermediate risk procedures as opposed to high-risk open vascular surgical

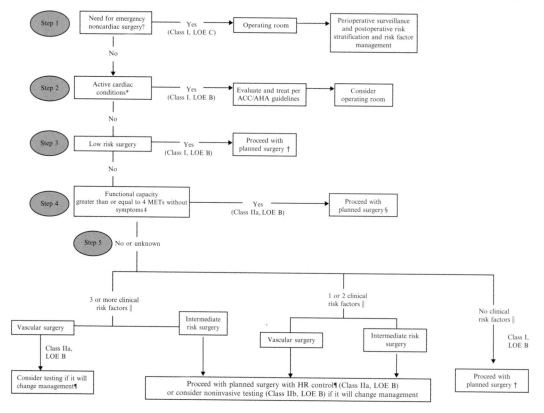

Fig. 13.1 Cardiac evaluation and care algorithm for noncardiac surgery based on active clinical conditions, known cardiovascular disease, or cardiac risk factors for patients 50 years of age or greater. *HR* heat rate, *MET*, metabolic equivalent (From Lee et al.[3] p. 1981, Figure 1. Reprinted with Permission, ©2007, American Heart Association, Inc.)

procedures based on mortality rates.[2] The type of surgery directs management only in patients with significant clinical risk factors (Fig. 13.1).

The most common medical issue in patients presenting for endovascular surgery is tobacco use (60–80%). It is not surprising that many of these patients have reactive airway disease and obstructive airway disease. EVAR is not postponed in these patients unless there is an acute exacerbation of their disease. Often, patients with stable disease are given bronchodilators and steroids on the day of surgery and, if possible, general anesthesia is avoided.[4]

Preoperative renal dysfunction is an important predictor of early mortality and long-term survival after endovascular abdominal aortic repair (EVAAR). Worsening of renal function can occur after EVAAR and it is often multifactorial. Approximately 6% of all patients undergoing EVAAR with normal preoperative renal function suffer a significant decrease in creatinine clearance, with 2% of patients requiring dialysis. The rate of significant worsening of renal function is four times more likely in patients with pre-existing renal insufficiency.[5] Measures should be taken to prevent deterioration of renal function perioperatively and they are described elsewhere in the book.

As EVAR is more often utilized nowadays in emergency and urgent situations, such as with dissections, trauma, and ruptured aneurysms, preoperative evaluation is often limited to eliciting relevant past medical history, focused physical examination (assessment of neurological status, hemodynamic condition, cervical spine, and associated injuries in trauma patients) and quick review of available laboratory tests (hematocrit, coagulation tests) and imaging studies (CT scanning).

Anesthesia Type

EVAR can be performed under general, regional, or local anesthesia. Spinal anesthesia, combined spinal-epidural, continuous epidural, continuous spinal, and bilateral paravertebral blocks are all described for EVAR.[6-11] Airway management during general anesthesia can be performed either with an endotracheal tube or a laryngeal mask airway. Balanced anesthesia with inhalational agents, intravenous anesthetics, and opioids are commonly used. Local anesthesia includes ilioinguinal and iliohypogastric nerve blocks along with skin infiltration. Loco-regional anesthetic techniques often require intravenous sedation with agents such as dexmedetomedine and/or propofol for patient comfort during long procedures.[7,12]

While knowing and understanding the surgical plan and approach are important to any successful anesthetic, it is even more critical in EVAR. Surgical plan can by itself determine the overall anesthetic plan, i.e. general anesthesia (GA) or regional anesthesia (RA) is required for iliac/retroperitoneal approach while local anes-thesia (LA) is adequate for femoral approach. Extensive inguinal exploration, previous inguinal scarring, and construction of femoral artery to femoral arterial conduit may also require regional or general anesthesia.[13] With regard to neuraxial anesthesia, it is always important to consider the fact that some form of anticoagulation, if not already being given to the patient preoperatively, will likely be introduced intraoperatively and, perhaps, continued postoperatively. Most commonly, this anticoagulation comes in the form of intraoperatively dosed, unfractionated heparin. The use of "single shot" neuraxial blocks as well as the placement and removal of neuraxial catheters must take this into consideration to prevent the rare complication of epidural hematoma and its potential catastrophic sequelae. American and European Societies of Regional Anesthesia and American College of Chest Physicians published guidelines for neuraxial anesthesia in the setting of anticoagulation.[14] Institutional protocols based on these guidelines are useful for planning the type of anesthesia for endovascular surgical patients (Table 13.1).

Table 13.1 Guidelines for neuraxial anesthesia in patients receiving antithrombotic therapy

Drugs	Recommendations for neuraxial anesthesia
NSAIDs (e.g., Aspirin)	No contraindication
Clopidogrel	Stop for 7 days before needle placement
Glycoprotein IIa/IIIb inhibitors	Discontinue for 8–48 h depending on the pharmacokinetics of the drug
Thrombolytics	Absolutely contraindicated
Direct thrombin inhibitors	Avoid regional anesthesia
Warfarin	Needle placement if INR is normal, catheter removal with INR ≤ 1.5
Subcutaneous unfractionated heparin (UFH) prophylaxis	No contraindication if total daily dose is less than 10,000 units; Delay the dose if technical difficulty is anticipated
Intravenous therapeutic UFH	Needle placement with minimal anticoagulation (normal PTT) Heparin can be given intraoperatively 1 h after needle placement Surgeons informed if there is a traumatic bloody tap, consider delay of subsequent anticoagulation Concomitant anticoagulation and postoperative epidural catheter analgesia requires careful monitoring for epidural hematoma and spinal cord function. Diagnostic imaging and surgery are needed if spinal hematoma is suspected Removal of catheter in the presence of normal PTT Restart heparin 1 h after removal of catheter
Low molecular weight heparin prophylaxis	Delay neuraxial block for 12 h after the last dose; Delay next dose for 2 h after needle placement and catheter removal
Therapeutic LMWH	Delay neuraxial block for 24 h after last dose

The potential for conversion from an endovascular to an open surgical approach should be discussed preoperatively with the surgical team and patients. Published rates of conversion are in the range of 0.6% to about 3%.[15–17] This suggests that in most situations the need for possible conversion should not be a major determinant of anesthetic plan.

Published Reports

The superiority of one technique over the others has not been clearly established. There have been several published studies that have attempted to address this issue. Unfortunately, all suffer from serious methodological issues that put their validity into question.

Ruppert et al. published the largest study to date that attempted to address the issue of anesthesia type for endovascular abdominal aortic aneurysm repair (EVAAR) and outcome.[18] This was a prospective, multicenter study of 5,557 patients included in the EUROSTAR registry. The authors found no mortality differences based on anesthesia but did see shorter procedures and shorter ICU and hospital stays in LA versus RA, LA versus GA, and RA versus GA comparisons. They also found a higher incidence of cardiac complications with GA versus both LA and RA groups. However, this was not a randomized study. The type of anesthetic was dictated by the care team and significant differences existed between patients in the different anesthetic groups. Furthermore, only 6% of the patient population had LA and the LA patients were more likely to have been cared for at the centers with the most experience with EVAAR. A more recent publication by the same group, which attempted to risk stratify these data, showed that high-risk patients who received LA and RA had less morbidity, mortality, systemic complications, and recovery times encouraging the use of loco-regional anesthesia in high-risk patients. But many of the same methodological flaws remain.[19]

Parra et al.[20] studied 424 EVAR patients having LA, RA, or GA at 13 different centers. There were 50 patients in the LA group. They found no mortality difference between the groups but did find a lower incidence of cardiac, renal, and wound healing complications in the LA group. Although this study was nonrandomized, risk factors did appear to be similar between the groups.

Verhoeven et al. prospectively studied 239 patients undergoing EVAR at a single center.[21] All patients received LA unless there was a technical reason not to or if the patient preferred GA or RA (170 patients received LA in this study). LA patients had shorter ICU and hospital stays as well as a lower complication rate. This study was, as pointed out by the authors themselves, more of a feasibility study for the use of LA. The study's nonrandom structure prevents a true comparison between anesthetic types.

Bettex et al. studied 91 patients undergoing EVAR and compared LA to epidural anesthesia (EA), and GA.[22] They found less use of vasopressor support, lower percentage of ICU admission, and shorter hospital stays in LA compared to EA and GA. There were no differences in mortality or significant complications between the groups. This was a small study wherein the type of anesthesia was dependent on location of the incision (femoral versus iliac) and the anesthesia team's preference.

De Virgilio et al. retrospectively reviewed 229 patients undergoing EVAR with LA or GA[23] (71 patients were in the LA group). They found no difference between the groups in terms of mortality or cardiopulmonary complications. However, the two patient groups differed significantly with LA patients being older and having more risk factors while GA patients had larger aneurysms. Furthermore, patients included from the first 2 years of the study when the procedure was relatively new all had GA whereas LA was provided for the latter patients. This has serious implications to the interpretation of the results.

In summary, published literature gives the sense that patients who receive loco-regional anesthesia tend to have improved postoperative outcomes by reducing hospital stay, ICU stay, mortality, and morbidity.[24] However, until appropriately powered, prospective, randomized trials are performed, there will be no certainty provided to the

Table 13.2 Local and regional anesthesia in endovascular aortic surgery

Advantages
Greater hemodynamic stability, less requirement of intravenous fluids, inotropes, and vasopressors (Applies to epidural block only if high sympathectomy is avoided)
Minimal changes in pulmonary mechanics
Ability to detect complications early while awake (i.e. anaphylaxis to dye, persistent pain indicating rupture of vessel into retroperitoneum)
Decreased hospital stay and recovery times

Disadvantages
Patient discomfort in supine position during long operations (inexperienced surgeon, technical difficulties, patients with back pain, symptomatic patients with compromised cardiopulmonary illnesses, patients with obesity)
Need to convert to general anesthesia if the procedure is converted to open procedure
It is imperative that the patient be able to comply with breath holding and remain immobile during image acquisition to allow for adequate visualization of anatomic landmarks to avoid potential problems with endograft positioning such as inadvertent coverage of the renal arteries or the hypogastric arteries, or excessive distal deployment of the endograft, increasing the risk of type I endoleaks

Table 13.3 General anesthesia for endovascular aortic surgery

Advantages
Airway secured for the procedure duration and allows better crisis management in cases of aneurysm rupture or rupture of access vessel or graft migrations
Hemodynamics can be controlled and easily manipulated with medications under general anesthesia
Better patient tolerance of longer procedures in supine position
Reduced patient movement during critical phases of procedure (e.g., stent deployment)
Control of respiration during fluoroscopy
Placement of invasive lines and transfusions easier if required

Disadvantages
More hypotensive episodes
Increased fluids and vasopressor requirement
Longer recovery and more intensive care unit requirement

question of anesthetic superiority in terms of patient outcomes. Until then, the appropriate choice depends on an assessment of individual patient characteristics as well as personnel and procedural aspects. Published literature certainly lends support to the feasibility of any of these anesthetic methods. While it is certainly intuitive to think that less anesthetic intervention is always better for patients, individual circumstances should always serve as an important backdrop for developing the most appropriate anesthetic plan. The advantages and drawbacks of GA and locoregional anesthesia are summarized in Tables 13.2 and 13.3.

Special Considerations for Preparation, Equipment, and Monitoring

The need for significant hemodynamic manipulation as well as the potential for hemodynamic compromise exists in all EVAR cases. With this as a background, the following suggestions for preparation are appropriate for most anesthetic plans.

Monitoring above and beyond the American Society of Anesthesiologists (ASA) standards for basic monitoring (Standards for Basic Anesthesia Monitoring, ASA House of Delegates, October 21, 1986, and last amended on October 25, 2005) are determined by patient and procedural issues. For appropriate patients undergoing anticipated "straightforward" procedures, no other monitoring may be necessary. However, the presence of significant comorbidities, the possibility of hemodynamic compromise, and the need for the assessment of technical success and/or complications will dictate the need for further monitoring.

The placement of devices and cables that are radio opaque, e.g. ECG leads, pulse oximetry cables, etc., must be considerate of likely fluoroscopic views (Fig. 13.2). Lengthwise and arched movements of the table are necessary. Invasive monitoring cables and lines as well as respiratory circuit tubing should be of sufficient length to prevent disconnections.

Invasive Arterial Pressure Monitoring

Invasive arterial monitoring will be useful in most situations given the frequency of cardiovascular comorbidities and because of the potential for

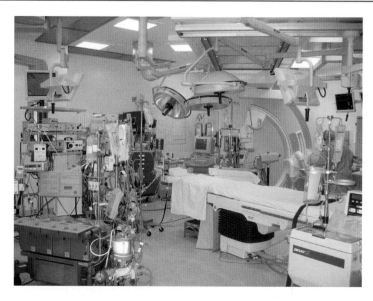

Fig. 13.2 Picture of the modern endovascular operating room suite. These facilities provide for the use of integrated radiographic and angiographic equipment in an environment that maintains the capabilities present in a fully functional cardiac surgical operating room

hemodynamic compromise. In addition, there exists the potential need for frequent laboratory analysis of arterial blood. Sick patients under monitored anesthesia care (MAC) and sedation can develop significant blood gas and acid–base abnormalities after long tedious procedures in the supine position. Arterial blood gas (ABG) monitoring is helpful in such situations and aids in making early decisions such as the need for endotracheal intubation, controlled ventilation, and conversion to GA. Blood loss during EVAR can be significant and often concealed. In one series, the average blood loss was 662 ml (range; 100–2,500 ml).[25] Duration of these procedures varies from 2 to 4 h and average crystalloid administration typically ranges in the 2–3 liter range. Serial electrolytes and hematocrit measurements can guide fluid therapy and blood transfusions. The use of an intraoperative activated clotting time (ACT) monitoring system may also be helpful in ensuring adequate levels of heparin anticoagulation. Individual patient responses to fixed heparin doses can be unpredictable.[26,27] Furthermore, a significant number of the subset of patients that come for EVAR procedures will have acute or chronic exposure to heparin. Therefore, there is the finite potential for heparin resistance due to low levels of antithrombin III (ATIII). In addition, resistance from other, non-ATIII-related issues have been suggested to occur in as many as 11% of cardiac surgical patients deemed as heparin-resistant.[28] The optimum ACT goal for EVAR is not well established. Martin et al. suggest that a goal of more than 200 s be set for peripheral vascular surgery, but it is not clear whether or not this correlates with EVAR.[27] One may argue that EVAR induces less of an inflammatory/coagulation response than open procedures and therefore would require less anticoagulation, but this remains to be studied. Monitoring of ACTs every 30 min during the time necessary for anticoagulation allows for guidance of repeat heparin dosing. Furthermore, if protamine reversal is used, ACT after neutralization can help to ensure adequate effect.

It is also important to establish which sites will be incorporated into the surgical field and potentially unavailable for access or monitoring. Some of the more complex endovascular surgeries may require prior bypass procedures to allow for blood flow to vital organs where normal "feeding" vessels are to be obstructed by an endovascular stent. An example would be the need to perform a left subclavian artery to left common

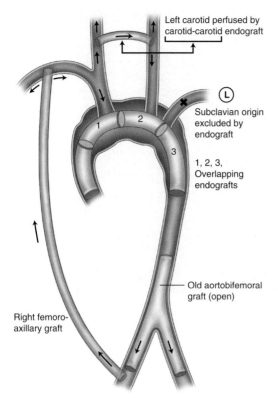

Left carotid perfused by carotid-carotid endograft

Ⓛ

Subclavian origin excluded by endograft

1, 2, 3, Overlapping endografts

Old aortobifemoral graft (open)

Right femoro-axillary graft

Fig. 13.3 Example of complex endovascular surgery requiring several prior bypass procedures that allow for endovascular stent placement over critical arterial ostia. This can have tremendous impact on anesthetic plan and arterial monitoring sites (From Subramaniam et al.[29], with permission)

carotid bypass in a patient wherein an aortic endovascular stent overlies the origin of the left subclavian (Fig. 13.3). Such a plan has enormous implications to overall anesthetic plan as well as planned monitoring sites and should be discussed with the surgical team.

The number of sites for placement of arterial catheters requires some forethought. In most situations, one catheter placed in a location that will remain unobstructed both during and after placement of endovascular aortic stents is sufficient. However, complex surgical procedures may require multiple cannulations. For example, if an endovascular aortic stent is to be placed in proximity to the takeoff of the left subclavian artery from the aorta, the placement of arterial catheters in the left and right upper extremities will allow for comparisons that may help detect obstruction of flow. In a similar fashion, comparisons between arterial catheters in the upper and lower extremities can help to diagnose potential partial aortic, iliac, or femoral arterial obstruction. This information can be used as a supplement to angiographic imaging to determine the need for further intervention.

Central Venous and Pulmonary Wedge Pressure Monitoring

In general, large bore intravenous catheter or catheters should be inserted given the potential for blood loss inherent in many of these procedures. In addition, appropriate blood product reserve and support should be confirmed. Access to the central venous circulation and the pulmonary arterial circulation may be helpful for resuscitation in situations of hemodynamic instability as well as for monitoring. Once again, the need for monitoring some combination of central venous pressure, pulmonary artery pressure, cardiac output, or mixed venous oxygen saturations should be guided by unique patient and/or procedural issues. The value of the assessment of these parameters correlates directly with an understanding of the limitations of these measurements as well as the complications that can be associated with the placement of these catheters.

Transesophageal Echocardiography

As will be discussed in detail in another chapter, the use of transesophageal echocardiography (TEE) during EVAR has been advocated by several groups.[30-32] Most of the uses of TEE during endovascular aortic surgery are in category II indications. Should complications such as extension of dissection or aneurysm rupture occur and result in significant hemodynamic compromise, the use of TEE becomes a category I indication to diagnose the cause of hemodynamic deterioration. The use of TEE during thoracic endovascular aortic repair (TEVAR) confirms the diagnosis of aortic pathology, aids fluoroscopy and angiography in the placement of guidewires and stent grafts, and can help in the detection of endoleaks

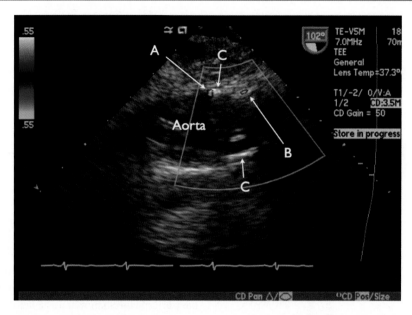

Fig. 13.4 Intraoperative TEE imaging of endoleaks. In this long axis view of the descending thoracic aorta, two different endoleaks are visible. Point *A* represents a small type 1A endoleak wherein points *C* represent the proximal edges of an aortic endograft. Point *B* represents a likely type IV endoleak representing simple graft wall porosity

in the postdeployment phase[32,33] (Fig. 13.4). TEE is a very sensitive modality in the diagnosis of endoleaks.[30,34,35] There are four different types of endoleaks, each with differing levels of clinical importance.[30] The assessment and classification of endoleaks at the time of the initial procedure allows for, when necessary, immediate revision. Intravascular ultrasound (IVUS) is also utilized to analyze the intraluminal pathology and assist in placement of endografts along with TEE and fluoroscopy.

Cerebral Monitoring

Postoperative stroke is a major complication of TEVAR with an incidence (2.3–8.2%) comparable to open thoracic aortic surgery. This complication is associated with a high mortality.[36] Two different etiologies exist. Direct coverage of subclavian or carotid artery by stent graft may result in stroke in anatomically predisposed patients. Stent graft coverage of the left subclavian artery can impair vertebral artery blood supply resulting in stroke affecting the brainstem and cerebellum in patients with a dominant left vertebral artery or an incomplete circle of Willis. It can also result in spinal cord ischemia (SCI) in patients with poor

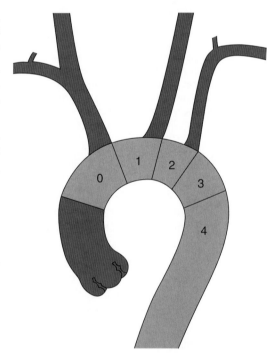

Fig. 13.5 Endograft landing zones of thoracic aorta

segmental collaterals. Stent coverage of the common carotid artery can result in hemispheric stroke. TEVAR involving the ascending aorta and arch (zones 0–2, Fig. 13.5) is associated with higher

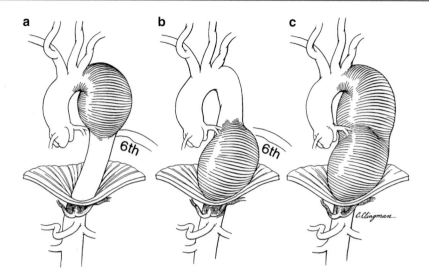

Fig. 13.6 The incidence of stroke after endovascular repair is related to the extent of descending thoracic aortic aneurysm. The extent coverage (**a**, **b**, or **c**) of the descending thoracic aortic aneurysm (Reprinted with permission from Gutsche et al.[36])

stroke risk compared to zone 3–4.[37] Proximal descending thoracic aorta (extent A and C) stenting is associated with higher stroke risk than extent B repairs (Fig. 13.6).[36]

Manipulation of guidewires, angiographic catheters, and stent-grafts in the setting of severely atherosclerotic aortic disease is another potential source of postoperative neurological dysfunction. History of prior stroke, obesity, and advanced atheromatous disease were identified as risk factors for neurological dysfunction after EVAR.[36,38] The stroke risk varies according to the aortic pathology for which EVAR was performed. Patients who had EVAR for fusiform aneurysms associated with atherosclerosis had a higher incidence of stroke (5.5%) compared to patients with traumatic disruption of the aorta (3.7%).[38] Prolonged procedures, higher blood loss, and intraoperative hypotension have also been associated with the risk of postoperative stroke.[37,39] These types of issues are often associated with more difficult stent-graft placement and, therefore, increased intra-aortic manipulations, which can increase stroke risk. Intraoperative echocardiography may aid in minimizing the manipulations of intra-aortic devices and in avoiding areas, where severe and mobile atheromas may reside.

Intraoperative cerebral monitoring and its role in the reduction of neurological dysfunction after TEVAR have not been well studied. Somatosensory evoked potential (SSEP) monitoring predicted stroke in one patient undergoing TEVAR.[36] Intraoperative transcranial Doppler (TCD) is being utilized in some institutions to detect embolic events. TCD monitoring detected accidental partial coverage of left common carotid artery and prevented stroke even when angiography failed to detect this complication in a patient with Stanford type B dissection treated with TEVAR.[40] While the use of cerebral oximetry in endovascular aortic surgery has not been specifically studied, it may also have some utility in procedures involving aortic arch vessels. It can also be used to help guide hemodynamic interventions to improve cerebral perfusion pressure and oxygen delivery. The benefits of this modality are its ease of use and interpretation as well as its continuous nature. Certainly, the ability of the cerebral oximeter to impact neurologic and clinical outcomes is still highly debated.[41-43] With the advent of newer generation fenestrated and branched grafts and hybrid procedures for the treatment of thoracic aortic pathology, intraoperative cerebral monitoring may have an expanded role to play.

More research is needed on the various available monitoring modalities and their usefulness in preventing neurological dysfunction after endovascular surgery.

Spinal Cord Monitoring

Published rates of paraplegia after TEVAR vary from 0% to 12%. It is possible that underreporting may have impact on the actual rate. The true risk of paraplegia with endovascular therapy is not insignificant. It appears that the incidence may be comparable or less than open surgery.[44] The advantages of endovascular procedures over open repairs in maintaining perfusion to the spinal cord comes from the following factors[1]; avoidance of aortic cross-clamping, proximal aortic hypertension, and their negative effects on cerebrospinal perfusion,[2] maintenance of continuous distal aortic perfusion,[4] lack of reperfusion injury from reimplantation of segmental arteries,[5] less intraoperative blood loss and hypotension.[45]

The main mechanism of spinal cord ischemia (SCI) after TEVAR is ill defined and the proposed mechanisms include direct coverage of intercostal arteries, compromise of collateral segmental spinal cord blood supply, and atherosclerotic embolization.[46] Amabile et al. found that a length of stent coverage of the aorta exceeding 205 mm was the only predictor of SCI after stent-graft repair.[47] Previous or concomitant abdominal aortic repair, perioperative hypotension (<70 mmHg), hypogastric artery interruption, subclavian artery coverage, and emergent repair were other risk factors associated with increased risk of SCI.[46] SCI after EVAAR has also been reported but certainly appears to be relatively uncommon.[48]

It is not clear whether stent coverage of artery of Adamkiewickz alone will result in paraplegia. In the study of Amabile et al., coverage of distal third of thoracic aorta was not a predictor of SCI.[47] Griepp et al. routinely ligated the presumed origin of this vessel without clinical consequence.[49] Though anatomical considerations would suggest major importance for this artery, clinical significance is probably overstated. Additional collateral arterial networks involving

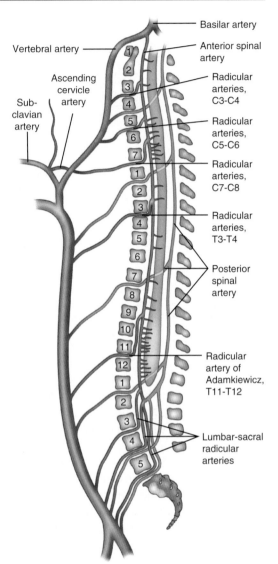

Fig. 13.7 Anatomy of spinal cord blood flow (From Smith and Grichnik,[50] with kind permission from Current medicine Group, LLC)

the pelvic circulation may be more relevant in maintaining cord perfusion in patients undergoing TEVAR (Fig. 13.7).[51,52] Disruption of this network in patients who have had previous abdominal aortic surgery may be the reason for the dependence of spinal cord perfusion on segmental intercostal arteries and the higher incidence of SCI after thoracic endograft coverage of those segmental vessels.[53] Perioperative hypotension significantly increases the risk of SCI because higher blood pressure is needed to drive blood through these collateral networks.

Neurophysiologic intraoperative monitoring (NIOM) such as somatosensory evoked potentials (SSEP) and transcranial motor evoked potentials (tcMEP) can be utilized for identification of SCI. Baseline recordings of both potentials are obtained after the induction of GA for comparison with intraoperative recordings. Weigang et al. observed alterations in evoked potentials in 75% (tcMEP) and 90% (SSEP) of patients who had open thoracoabdominal repair compared to 22% of patients who underwent EVAR. In their study, detection of NIOM changes lead to interventions and those interventions reversed the abnormalities in NIOM.[54] Interventions included increases in mean arterial pressure (MAP)>80 mmHg, decreases in central venous pressure (CVP) < 12 mmHg, and cerebrospinal fluid (CSF) drainage (for CSF pressure > 15 mmHg). They also noticed that SSEP showed delayed alterations in latency, amplitude, and recovery after tcMEP. In another study published by the same group, 35% of patients exhibited NIOM changes after thoracic endograft deployment and changes reversed with interventions in 91% of those patients.[55]

Studies by Weigang et al. showed a very high incidence of SCI by NIOM. In contrast, none of the patients in Husain et al.'s study developed significant NIOM changes during TEVAR suggestive of SCI.[56] Husain et al. monitored both peripheral and cortical ulnar and tibial SSEP and tcMEP from all extremities during TEVAR. They used a 90% decrease in tcMEP amplitude as a threshold for defining presumed SCI unlike Weigang et al. who used a 50% decrease. This could have reduced the false-positive results. Also, unilateral loss of both peripheral and cortical impulses could be related to limb ischemia due to an endovascular sheath placed in the femoral artery and the changes in NIOM should disappear after femoral sheath removal in this case. A guide to Interpretation of SSEP and tcMEP changes is described in Table 13.4.[56]

When NIOM is being used to monitor for SCI, the effects of anesthetic agents on SSEP and tcMEP potentials must be considered.[57,58] TcMEP is very sensitive to inhalational anesthetics and they are often avoided.[59,60] Total intravenous anesthetic (TIVA) techniques with propofol and remifentanil infusions, with or without nitrous oxide, are often preferred.[61] Ketamine and dexmedetomidine use have also been described.[57,62] With tcMEP monitoring, the use of neuromuscular blocking drugs should be carefully titrated as complete blockade will prevent effective monitoring.[63] Irrespective of the anesthetic technique employed, communication between surgeon, anesthesiologist, neurophysiologist, and monitoring personnel is extremely important in determining whether the changes in evoked potential are related to surgical interruption of spinal cord

Table 13.4 Interpretation of neurophysiologic intraoperative monitoring

	SSEP				tcMEP	
	Ulnar		Tibial			
	Erb point	N20 cortical	Popliteal fossa	P37 cortical	Upper limb	Lower limb
Technical	–	–	–	–	–	–
Cerebral ischemia, hypotension, anesthesia	+	–	+	–	–	–
Spinal cord ischemia	+	+	+	–	+	–
Lower limb ischemia	+	+	–	–	+	±
Brachial plexus injury	–	–	+	+	–	+
Scalp edema	+	+	+	+	–	–

Reprinted with permission from Lippincoat Williams and Wilkins; Husain et al.[56]
Erb point and popliteal fossa are peripheral SSEP waveforms, N20 and P37 are cortical SSEP waveforms.

blood supply, anesthetic medications, hemodynamic changes, or other reasons (endovascular femoral sheath).

Placement of a CSF catheter for monitoring and drainage can be done in the immediate preoperative period or the day before planned surgery. The question as to whether or not a CSF drain should be placed for all TEVAR procedures has not been adequately addressed by the existing randomized trials. It appears that relatively few centers insert CSF catheters in all TEVAR subjects while it appears that most selectively use them in patients at high risk for SCI. Hnath et al.[46] retrospectively reviewed 121 patients undergoing TEVAR, 46% had a CSF drain placed. None of the patients in the group with a CSF drain developed SCI whereas 8% of patients in the group without a CSF drain developed SCI. They also found that 60% of patients with SCI responded to blood pressure augmentation and CSF drainage. The patients who developed SCI were all high-risk patients (previous AAA repair, emergent surgery, longer aortic coverage, and higher vasopressor use).[46] There are several common practical situations (emergency surgery such as polytrauma and ruptured aneurysm, documented coagulopathy, failed procedure, and CSF catheter malfunction) in which the anesthesia team may not be able to provide CSF drainage even in high-risk patients. When possible, these patients should be carefully monitored intraoperatively by NIOM and postoperatively by periodic neurologic examination. In the event that patients are unable to be assessed adequately after the procedure, e.g., if they are unable to be awakened, consideration of postoperative neurophysiologic monitoring may be reasonable. CSF catheter insertion may be necessary during the course of the procedure or postoperatively. Neurosurgical consultation and/or interventional radiology consultation for fluoroscopy-guided CSF catheter insertion are reasonable in cases of difficult spinal catheter placement. Published algorithms for management of spinal cord ischemia can be extremely useful[64] (Fig. 13.8).

CSF drainage can lead to complications such as spinal headache, epidural and subdural hematoma, as well as infections. Published rates of such complications are in the range of 1–3%.[46] The reported incidence of SDH with open descending aortic surgeries is in the range of 3.5%.[65,66] In a multivariate analysis, Dardik et al. found that the amount of CSF drained was the only variable predictive of SDH.[65] Based on review of available evidence, it has been suggested that setting a lower limit of CSF pressure at 10 mmHg and limiting CSF drainage to no more than 10 ml/h and 240 ml/day represent justifiable management goals.[29]

Temperature Control

Although many of these procedures occur through very limited incisions, the use of GA or neuraxial anesthesia attenuates normal temperature regulatory responses and consideration should be given to the use of appropriate warming devices.[67] Frequent movements of the table may hinder upper body propelling air systems. Warmed blankets and fluids are frequently used.

Techniques for Precise Endograft Placement

Particular consideration must be given to the strategy which will be utilized to help prevent malposition of aortic stents during their deployment as ultimate success depends on meticulous positioning. Most available prostheses cannot be repositioned after deployment. Qu et al. demonstrated that a combination of debranching in order to extend the proximal landing zone, clear definition of target location, and related anatomy by markers on magnified angiographic screens, avoidance of movement of the table and patient during deployment, and induced hypotension or temporary cardiac asystole by adenosine bolus can result in precise endograft placement.[68]

There are two basic designs of aortic stents: they are either self-expanding or they require balloon expansion. Most of the current devices used are of the self-expanding class. Although certainly more of an issue for stents requiring balloon expansion, all of these devices are prone to significant movement during their deployment as pulsatile blood flow causes the stent and related

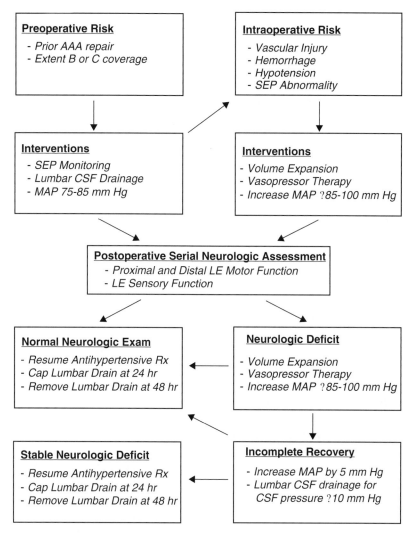

Fig. 13.8 A proposed algorithm for the management of spinal cord ischemia. *AAA* abdominal aortic aneurysm, *CSF* cerebrospinal fluid, *hr* hours, *LE* lower extremity, *MAP* mean arterial pressure, *Rx* drug therapy, *SEP* somatosensory evoked potential (From Cheung et al.[64], with permission)

catheters to move to and fro.[69] Distal migrations likely constitute the majority of malpositions. They occur as a result of the force of forward blood flow on the stent and/or the deployment balloon as well as the "windsock" effect caused by the retraction of the sheath used with self-expanding stents.[70] These malpositions can be clinically significant and can certainly require further intervention. Related to the use of a balloon expander for stent deployment is the potential for significant proximal hypertension and afterload increase as a result of balloon inflation in the thoracic aorta. Generally, balloon inflation is short (less than 30 s) but in situations where the balloon is inflated in the proximal descending thoracic aorta or for prolonged periods, this may represent a significant hemodynamic issue.

Several strategies have been proposed and employed to decrease the force of forward blood flow so as to reduce some of the elements involved in malpositions.

Induced Hypotension

Blood pressure rise should be avoided during deployment. In the modern era of abdominal aortic endograft procedures and simple descending thoracic aortic endografts with adequate proximal landing zone, a temporary reduction of systolic BP to the 80 mmHg range is generally all that is required to avoid migration of these prostheses. Medications for systemic blood pressure control that allow for rapid onset and offset are most sensible. They include nitroglycerine, nitroprusside, and calcium channel blockers such as nicardipine and clevidipine. A recent prospective study comparing these agents in 1,512 cardiac patients demonstrated the relative safety and efficacy of all of these agents.[71] Each agent has a side-effect profile that should be considered in the context of the particular patient/procedure situation. Practitioner experience is also an important factor that should be considered.

Measures other than induced hypotension may be needed with complicated thoracic endograft procedures with projected landing zones in the ascending aorta or aortic arch. Regardless of the type of endograft (self-expanding or balloon expandable), any method to eliminate or reduce the propulsive aortic flow force is helpful for precise intrathoracic endograft placement.[68] Once again, it is very likely that institutional and practitioner's choice will play an important role in determining the best strategy to be employed.

Adenosine Cardiac Arrest

Adenosine is an endogenous glycoside analog that exerts negative dromotropic and chronotropic effects at both the sinoatrial and atrioventricular nodes. Adenosine, given by rapid IV administration, produces temporary cardiac asystole as the half life of adenosine is 10 s. Qu et al. described four cases of distal migration requiring the placement of an additional proximal cuff when adenosine cardiac arrest was not used in thoracic stenting compared with no need for such intervention in an adenosine asystole cohort.[68] Other studies with adenosine have also demonstrated its effectiveness.[69,72–74] Adenosine use has been described in patients undergoing GA, RA, and MAC.[75]

Darros et al. administered trial doses of IV adenosine in the predeployment phase after anesthesia induction until a period of asystole greater than

20 s was recorded.[69] This predetermined dose was then administered to produce asystole during deployment. At doses less than 1 mg/kg, a linear relationship between dose and duration of cardiac arrest was observed.[76] Clinically, adenosine has been used for this purpose in the dose range of 20–90 mg. Failure to produce asystole and the requirement for repeat dosing are common at lower doses (less than 30 mg IV).[77,78] Sporadic ventricular contractions that occur with lower doses may interfere with accurate endograft placement.[75] Higher doses (60–90 mg) are often required during thoracic endograft procedures to achieve reliable asystole lasting 20–30 s.[68] These higher doses of adenosine also produce significant peripheral vasodilatation and may help to minimize the clinical significance of isolated ventricular contractions on stent placement should they occur.[76] Adenosine is avoided in patients with conduction block, severe coronary artery disease, and reactive airway disease. The impact of adverse effects on awake patients, such as facial flushing, light headedness, dizziness, nausea, shortness of breath, and palpitations can be attenuated by sedation with propofol (1–2 mg/kg) or etomidate (0.1–0.3 mg/kg). Transient hypotension lasting 1–2 min, transient left bundle branch block, and ST changes that require no further treatment have been reported.[72] Complications requiring intervention occurred in 6.2% of patients in one series.[75] These included the need for temporary external transthoracic pacing or transvenous pacing to treat prolonged asystolic response and external synchronized cardioversion for atrial fibrillation. Plaschke et al. studied EEG changes and neurological function after adenosine asystole for thoracic endografting. EEG changes were transient, reversible, and short in nature and no neurological dysfunction occurred postoperatively.[76]

Rapid Ventricular Pacing

Rapid ventricular pacing decreases left ventricular preload, cardiac output, and stroke volume because of loss of atrioventricular synchrony and decreased ventricular filling time. Ventricular pacing can be obtained with pacing Swan Ganz pulmonary artery catheters or transvenous bipolar or quadpolar cardiac pacing.[79,80] Ventricular pacing rates between 120 and 200/min have been used. Ventricular pacing rate 130–180/min generally produce systolic blood pressures between 40 and 60 mmHg whereas rates in the 160–200/min range can decrease systolic blood pressures to 20–30 mmHg.[68] General anesthesia was used in all the reports using this technique.

The effect on blood pressure is immediate and recovers immediately after discontinuation of pacing. This can be repeated if necessary during additional stent placements or during postdeployment ballooning when hypertension is commonly observed. Complications are rare but induction of serious ventricular arrhythmias and atrial or ventricular perforation can occur. Temporary pacing may be needed in patients with LBBB.

Other Methods

The induction of ventricular fibrillation by an alternating current transformer attached to the heart by temporary transvenous pacing wires followed by external defibrillation has also been described.[81] This technique also requires GA and is somewhat cumbersome and risky. The temporary occlusion of the right atrial inflow (superior or inferior vena cava) by using a balloon inserted percutaneously from the jugular or femoral vein has also been described as an effective method to reduce cardiac preload, cardiac output, and blood pressure during stent deployment.[70,82] These techniques are invasive and add more interventions, equipment, and time to TEVAR procedures and are not routinely practiced. Valsalva maneuver with IV nitroglycerine bolus has also been used to achieve the same result.[83,84]

In a retrospective review, Nienaber et al. compared rapid ventricular pacing, adenosine cardiac arrest, and induced hypotension with sodium nitroprusside during thoracic endograft procedures.[85] Patients who had rapid RV pacing had rapid onset and offset of hypotension, the lowest instantaneous flow velocities in the aorta, and achieved more precise positioning of the device, compared to the other methods. No difference in neurological function was noticed postoperatively between the three groups.

Postoperative Considerations in Endovascular Aortic Surgery

In uncomplicated endovascular aortic surgeries, postoperative management generally does not require the use of ICU. Patients are advanced to regular diet and ambulation on the first postoperative day and the average length of stay is usually less than 5 days.[86] However, complicated thoracic stent procedures, stents for ruptured aneurysms, and traumatic dissections may require extended monitoring in ICU depending on individual patient- and procedure-related issues.

Percutaneous approaches and associated smaller incisions generally make pain management much easier. Long-acting local anesthetics placed at the surgical sites or sites intraoperatively can certainly help in providing postoperative analgesia. In addition to parenteral opioids, oral opioids and nonopioid analgesics, such as nonsteroidal medications, can be very useful wherever appropriate. Neuraxial opioids and local anesthetics should be used with caution since their use may delay or prevent the diagnosis of a new neurologic deficit.

Surveillance for bleeding and for ischemia of other organ beds (e.g., renal, mesenteric, spinal cord, and leg ischemia) that may have been impacted by endovascular stent placement should continue into the postoperative period. Clinical signs, serial laboratory evaluations, and diagnostic imaging can assist in diagnosing these problems. Surgery should be consulted promptly if there is a need for re-exploration or revision of the surgical intervention.

Postimplantation Syndrome

A postimplantation syndrome consisting of some combination of fever, leukocytosis, coagulopathy, and peri-graft air has been described after EVAR. This syndrome is believed to result from the release of inflammatory mediators, in particular C-reactive protein, released as a result of endothelial injury during the procedure. Peri-aortic inflammation that represents a "healing response" is also responsible.[87] Contact activation caused by the stent itself has also been suggested as a possible mechanism.[88] This inflammatory response is usually moderate and subsides over a few days. Nonsteriodal anti-inflammatory drugs may be necessary to attenuate symptoms. Hyperthermia can cause hypoxemia, tachyarrhythmias, and angina in patients with cardiopulmonary illnesses. Oxygen supplementation and treatment with antipyretics, antiarrhythmics, and antianginal drugs may be needed in those patients.[89] Thrombus in the excluded aneurysm sac may initiate fibrinolysis and can, potentially, cause disseminated intravascular coagulation.[90]

It is still not completely clear that the components of this syndrome are truly unique to EVAR or in anyway different to those seen after open repair.[91] While some suggest that the responses to EVAR are greater than with open procedures,[92] measurements of inflammatory mediators have demonstrated lower postoperative levels in EVAR versus open aortic procedures.[93] What appears more likely is that these signs and symptoms of inflammation can mimic those seen with infection making for a difficult postoperative dilemma in some patients.

Summary

In conclusion, endovascular aortic surgery presents unique challenges to the anesthesia care team. The typical patient brings along a host of significant comorbidities. While the procedures are less invasive, the potential for significant morbidity and mortality remains. This combination requires a level of planning and vigilance that equals that necessary for even the most demanding open procedures.

Key Notes

1. Endovascular aortic surgery encompasses procedures for several types of aortic pathology that can be managed with stents
2. Although the procedures are typically performed percutaneously through limited incisions, the combination of patient comorbidi-

ties, procedural issues, and potential for complications makes them very demanding for the anesthesia care team
3. Preoperative assessment should follow current guidelines, and discussion with the surgical team is extremely important in developing the anesthetic plan
4. Any anesthetic is feasible so long as patient and procedural issues are accounted for
5. Patient and procedural issues influence monitoring decisions
6. Special consideration should be given to monitoring for the obstruction of critical arterial beds by endovascular stents, for spinal cord ischemia, for the diagnosis of endoleaks, and for the adequacy of heparinization
7. Medications that allow for rapid blood pressure control should be available
8. Strategies for the prevention of stent malpositions during deployment should be considered and ready
9. Postoperative care for uncomplicated procedures is relatively straightforward
10. Complications related to endovascular surgery, including bleeding, stent malpositions, and postimplantation syndrome can make postoperative care difficult

References

1. May J, White GH, Yu W, et al. Endovascular grafting for abdominal aortic aneurysms: changing incidence and indications for conversion to open operation. *Cardiovasc Surg.* 1998;6:194–197.
2. Fleisher LA, Beckman JA, Brown KA, et al. ACC/AHA 2006 guideline update on perioperative cardiovascular evaluation for noncardiac surgery: focused update on perioperative beta-blocker therapy–a report of the American College of Cardiology/American Heart Association Task Force on Practice Guidelines (Writing Committee to Update the 2002 Guidelines on Perioperative Cardiovascular Evaluation for Noncardiac Surgery). *Anesth Analg.* 2007; 104:15–26.
3. Lee AF, Joshua AB, Kenneth AB, et al. ACC/AHA 2007 Guidelines on Perioperative Cardiovascular Evaluation and Care for Noncardiac Surgery. *Circulation.* 2007;116:1971–1996.
4. Riddel JM, Black JH, Brewster DC, Dunn PF. Endovascular abdominal aortic repair. *Int Anesthesiol Clin.* 2005;43:79–91.

5. Walker SR, Yusuf SW, Wenham PW, Hopkinson BR. Renal complications following endovascular repair of abdominal aortic aneurysms. *J Endovasc Surg.* 1998;5:318–322.

6. Leykin Y, Rubulotta FM, Mancinelli P, Tosolini G, Gullo A. Epidural anaesthesia for endovascular stent graft repair of a ruptured thoracic aneurysm. *Anaesth Intensive Care.* 2003;31:455–460.

7. Falkensammer J, Hakaim AG, Klocker J, et al. Paravertebral blockade with propofol sedation versus general anesthesia for elective endovascular abdominal aortic aneurysm repair. *Vascular.* 2006;14:17–22.

8. Grabowska-Gaweł A, Molski S, Porzych K. Effects of combined spinal-epidural anesthesia in patients undergoing abdominal aorta aneurysms stent-grafting. *Wiad Lek.* 2006;59:110–112.

9. Kim SS, Leibowitz AB. Endovascular thoracic aortic aneurysm repair using a single catheter for spinal anesthesia and cerebrospinal fluid drainage. *J Cardiothorac Vasc Anesth.* 2001;15:88–89.

10. Mathes DD, Kern JA. Continuous spinal anesthetic technique for endovascular aortic stent graft surgery. *J Clin Anesth.* 2000;12:487–490.

11. Aadahl P, Lundbom J, Hatlinghus S, Myhre HO. Regional anesthesia for endovascular treatment of abdominal aortic aneurysms. *J Endovasc Surg.* 1997;4:56–61.

12. Brown BJ, Zakhary S, Rogers L, Ellis-Stoll C, Gable D, Ramsay MA. Use of dexmedetomidine versus general anesthesia for endovascular repair of abdominal aortic aneurysms. *Proc (Bayl Univ Med Cent).* 2006; 19:213–215.

13. Kahn RA, Moskowitz DM. Endovascular aortic repair. *J Cardiothorac Vasc Anesth.* 2002;16:218–233.

14. Horlocker TT, Wedel DJ, Rowlingson JC, et al. Regional Anesthesia in the Patient Receiving Antithrombotic or Thrombolytic Therapy: American Society of Regional Anesthesia and Pain Medicine Evidence-Based Guidelines (Third Edition). *Reg Anesth Pain Med.* 2010;35:64–101.

15. EVAR trial participants. Endovascular aneurysm repair and outcome in patients unfit for open repair of abdominal aortic aneurysm (EVAR trial 2): randomised controlled trial. *Lancet.* 2005;365: 2187–2192.

16. Greenhalgh RM, Brown LC, Kwong GP, Powell JT, Thompson SG. Comparison of endovascular aneurysm repair with open repair in patients with abdominal aortic aneurysm (EVAR trial 1), 30-day operative mortality results: randomised controlled trial. *Lancet.* 2004;364:843–848.

17. Prinssen M, Verhoeven EL, Buth J, et al. A randomized trial comparing conventional and endovascular repair of abdominal aortic aneurysms. *N Engl J Med.* 2004;351:1607–1618.

18. Ruppert V, Leurs LJ, Steckmeier B, Buth J, Umscheid T. Influence of anesthesia type on outcome after endovascular aortic aneurysm repair: an analysis based on EUROSTAR data. *J Vasc Surg.* 2006;44:16–21. discussion.

19. Ruppert V, Leurs LJ, Rieger J, Steckmeier B, Buth J, Umscheid T. Risk-adapted outcome after endovascular aortic aneurysm repair: analysis of anesthesia types based on EUROSTAR data. *J Endovasc Ther.* 2007;14:12–22.

20. Parra JR, Crabtree T, McLafferty RB, et al. Anesthesia technique and outcomes of endovascular aneurysm repair. *Ann Vasc Surg.* 2005;19(1):123–129.

21. Verhoeven EL, Cina CS, Tielliu IF, et al. Local anesthesia for endovascular abdominal aortic aneurysm repair. *J Vasc Surg.* 2005;42:402–409.

22. Bettex DA, Lachat M, Pfammatter T, Schmidlin D, Turina MI, Schmid ER. To compare general, epidural and local anaesthesia for endovascular aneurysm repair (EVAR). *Eur J Vasc Endovasc Surg.* 2001;21: 179–184.

23. De Virgilio C, Romero L, Donayre C, et al. Endovascular abdominal aortic aneurysm repair with general versus local anesthesia: a comparison of cardiopulmonary morbidity and mortality rates. *J Vasc Surg.* 2002;36:988–991.

24. Sadat U, Cooper DG, Gillard JH, Walsh SR, Hayes PD. Impact of the type of anesthesia on outcome after elective endovascular aortic aneurysm repair: literature review. *Vascular.* 2008;16:340–345.

25. Henretta JP, Hodgson KJ, Mattos MA, et al. Feasibility of endovascular repair of abdominal aortic aneurysms with local anesthesia with intravenous sedation. *J Vasc Surg.* 1999;29:793–798.

26. Stelmach WS, Myers KA, Scott DF, Devine TJ, Lee L. In vivo heparin response and consumption in patients before and during arterial reconstructive surgery. *J Cardiovasc Surg (Torino).* 1991;32:166–173.

27. Martin P, Greenstein D, Gupta NK, Walker DR, Kester RC. Systemic heparinization during peripheral vascular surgery: thromboelastographic, activated coagulation time, and heparin titration monitoring. *J Cardiothorac Vasc Anesth.* 1994;8:150–152.

28. Avidan MS, Levy JH, Scholz J, et al. A phase III, double-blind, placebo-controlled, multicenter study on the efficacy of recombinant human antithrombin in heparin-resistant patients scheduled to undergo cardiac surgery necessitating cardiopulmonary bypass. *Anesthesiology.* 2005;102:276–284.

29. Subramaniam B, Panzica PJ, Pawlowski JB, et al. Epidural blood patch for acute subdural hematoma after spinal catheter drainage during hybrid thoracoabdominal aneurysm repair. *J Cardiothorac Vasc Anesth.* 2007;21:704–708.

30. Swaminathan M, Lineberger CK, McCann RL, Mathew JP. The importance of intraoperative transesophageal echocardiography in endovascular repair of thoracic aortic aneurysms. *Anesth Analg.* 2003;97:1566–1572.

31. Van der Starre P, Guta C, Dake M, Ihnken K, Robbins R. The value of transesophageal echocardiography for endovascular graft stenting of the ascending aorta. *J Cardiothorac Vasc Anesth.* 2004;18:466–468.

32. Rapezzi C, Rocchi G, Fattori R, et al. Usefulness of transesophageal echocardiographic monitoring to

improve the outcome of stent-graft treatment of thoracic aortic aneurysms. *Am J Cardiol.* 2001;87: 315–319.

33. Moskowitz DM, Kahn RA, Konstadt SN, Mitty H, Hollier LH, Marin ML. Intraoperative transoesophageal echocardiography as an adjuvant to fluoroscopy during endovascular thoracic aortic repair. *Eur J Vasc Endovasc Surg.* 1999;17:22–27.

34. Koschyk DH, Nienaber CA, Knap M, et al. How to guide stent-graft implantation in type B aortic dissection? Comparison of angiography, transesophageal echocardiography, and intravascular ultrasound. *Circulation.* 2005;112:I260–I264.

35. Rocchi G, Lofiego C, Biagini E, et al. Transesophageal echocardiography-guided algorithm for stent-graft implantation in aortic dissection. *J Vasc Surg.* 2004;40:880–885.

36. Gutsche JT, Cheung AT, McGarvey ML, et al. Risk factors for perioperative stroke after thoracic endovascular aortic repair. *Ann Thorac Surg.* 2007;84: 1195–1200.

37. Feezor RJ, Martin TD, Hess PJ, et al. Risk factors for perioperative stroke during thoracic endovascular aortic repairs (TEVAR). *J Endovasc Ther.* 2007;14: 568–573.

38. Khoynezhad A, Donayre CE, Bui H, Kopchok GE, Walot I, White RA. Risk factors of neurologic deficit after thoracic aortic endografting. *Ann Thorac Surg.* 2007;83:S882–S889.

39. Buth J, Harris PL, Hobo R, et al. Neurologic complications associated with endovascular repair of thoracic aortic pathology: Incidence and risk factors. a study from the European Collaborators on Stent/Graft Techniques for Aortic Aneurysm Repair (EUROSTAR) registry. *J Vasc Surg.* 2007;46:1103–1110.

40. Khoynezhad A, Kruse MJ, Donayre CE, White RA. Use of transcranial Doppler ultrasound in endovascular repair of a type B aortic dissection. *Ann Thorac Surg.* 2008;86:289–291.

41. Hong SW, Shim JK, Choi YS, Kim DH, Chang BC, Kwak YL. Prediction of cognitive dysfunction and patients' outcome following valvular heart surgery and the role of cerebral oximetry. *Eur J Cardiothorac Surg.* 2008;33:560–565.

42. Taillefer MC, Denault AY. Cerebral near-infrared spectroscopy in adult heart surgery: systematic review of its clinical efficacy. *Can J Anaesth.* 2005;52: 79–87.

43. Murkin JM, Adams SJ, Novick RJ, et al. Monitoring brain oxygen saturation during coronary bypass surgery: a randomized, prospective study. *Anesth Analg.* 2007;104:51–58.

44. Anyanwu A, Spielvogel D, Griepp R. Spinal cord protection for descending aortic surgery. Clinical and scientific basis for contemporary surgical practice. In: Rosseau H, Verhoye JP, Heautot JF, eds. *Thoracic Aortic Diseases.* 1st ed. Berlin: Springer; 2006:81–98.

45. Weigang E, Hartert M, Siegenthaler MP, et al. Neurophysiological monitoring during thoracoabdominal aortic endovascular stent graft implantation. *Eur J Cardiothorac Surg.* 2006;29:392–396.

46. Hnath JC, Mehta M, Taggert JB, et al. Strategies to improve spinal cord ischemia in endovascular thoracic aortic repair: outcomes of a prospective cerebrospinal fluid drainage protocol. *J Vasc Surg.* 2008;48: 836–840.

47. Amabile P, Grisoli D, Giorgi R, Bartoli JM, Piquet P. Incidence and determinants of spinal cord ischaemia in stent-graft repair of the thoracic aorta. *Eur J Vasc Endovasc Surg.* 2008;35:455–461.

48. Maldonado TS, Rockman CB, Riles E, et al. Ischemic complications after endovascular abdominal aortic aneurysm repair. *J Vasc Surg.* 2004;40:703–709.

49. Griepp RB, Ergin MA, Galla JD, Klein JJ, Spielvogel D, Griepp EB. Minimizing spinal cord injury during repair of descending thoracic and thoracoabdominal aneurysms: the Mount Sinai approach. *Semin Thorac Cardiovasc Surg.* 1998;10:25–28.

50. Smith MS, Grichnik KP. Anesthetic considerations for lung transplantation and thoracic aortic surgery. In: Miller RD, Reves JG, eds. *Atlas of Anesthesia*, Cardiothoracic Anesthesia, vol. VIII. Philadelphia: Current Medicine (Churchill Livingstone); 1999:6.1–18.

51. Jacobs MJ, de Mol BA, Elenbaas T, et al. Spinal cord blood supply in patients with thoracoabdominal aortic aneurysms. *J Vasc Surg.* 2002;35:30–37.

52. Griepp RB, Ergin MA, Galla JD, et al. Looking for the artery of Adamkiewicz: a quest to minimize paraplegia after operations for aneurysms of the descending thoracic and thoracoabdominal aorta. *J Thorac Cardiovasc Surg.* 1996;112:1202–1213.

53. Martin DJ, Martin TD, Hess PJ, Daniels MJ, Feezor RJ, Lee WA. Spinal cord ischemia after TEVAR in patients with abdominal aortic aneurysms. *J Vasc Surg.* 2009;49(2):302–306.

54. Weigang E, Sircar R, von Samson P, et al. Efficacy and frequency of cerebrospinal fluid drainage in operative management of thoracoabdominal aortic aneurysms. *Thorac Cardiovasc Surg.* 2007;55:73–78.

55. Weigang E, Hartert M, Siegenthaler MP, et al. Perioperative management to improve neurologic outcome in thoracic or thoracoabdominal aortic stent-grafting. *Ann Thorac Surg.* 2006;82:1679–1687.

56. Husain AM, Swaminathan M, McCann RL, Hughes GC. Neurophysiologic intraoperative monitoring during endovascular stent graft repair of the descending thoracic aorta. *J Clin Neurophysiol.* 2007;24: 328–335.

57. Kawaguchi M, Furuya H. Intraoperative spinal cord monitoring of motor function with myogenic motor evoked potentials: a consideration in anesthesia. *J Anesth.* 2004;18:18–28.

58. Ku AS, Hu Y, Irwin MG, et al. Effect of sevoflurane/nitrous oxide versus propofol anaesthesia on somatosensory evoked potential monitoring of the spinal cord during surgery to correct scoliosis. *Br J Anaesth.* 2002;88:502–507.

59. Reinacher PC, Priebe HJ, Blumrich W, Zentner J, Scheufler KM. The effects of stimulation pattern and sevoflurane concentration on intraoperative motor-evoked potentials. *Anesth Analg.* 2006;102: 888–895.

60. Ubags LH, Kalkman CJ, Been HD. Influence of iso-flurane on myogenic motor evoked potentials to single and multiple transcranial stimuli during nitrous oxide/opioid anesthesia. *Neurosurgery.* 1998;43:90–94.

61. Hans P, Bonhomme V. Why we still use intravenous drugs as the basic regimen for neurosurgical anaesthesia. *Curr Opin Anaesthesiol.* 2006;19:498–503.

62. Bala E, Sessler DI, Nair DR, McLain R, Dalton JE, Farag E. Motor and somatosensory evoked potentials are well maintained in patients given dexmedetomidine during spine surgery. *Anesthesiology.* 2008;109:417–425.

63. Van Dongen EP, ter Beek HT, Schepens MA, et al. Within-patient variability of myogenic motor-evoked potentials to multipulse transcranial electrical stimulation during two levels of partial neuromuscular blockade in aortic surgery. *Anesth Analg.* 1999;88:22–27.

64. Cheung AT, Pochettino A, McGarvey ML, et al. Strategies to manage paraplegia risk after endovascular stent repair of descending thoracic aortic aneurysms. *Ann Thorac Surg.* 2005;80:1280–1288.

65. Dardik A, Perler BA, Roseborough GS, Williams GM. Subdural hematoma after thoracoabdominal aortic aneurysm repair: an underreported complication of spinal fluid drainage? *J Vasc Surg.* 2002;36:47–50.

66. Weaver KD, Wiseman DB, Farber M, Ewend MG, Marston W, Keagy BA. Complications of lumbar drainage after thoracoabdominal aortic aneurysm repair. *J Vasc Surg.* 2001;34:623–627.

67. Sessler DI. Temperature monitoring and perioperative thermoregulation. *Anesthesiology.* 2008;109: 318–338.

68. Qu L, Raithel D. Techniques for precise thoracic endograft placement. *J Vasc Surg.* 2009;49: 1069–1072.

69. Dorros G, Cohn JM. Adenosine-induced transient cardiac asystole enhances precise deployment of stent-grafts in the thoracic or abdominal aorta. *J Endovasc Surg.* 1996;3:270–272.

70. Marty B, Morales CC, Tozzi P, Ruchat P, Chassot PG, von Segesser LK. Partial inflow occlusion facilitates accurate deployment of thoracic aortic endografts. *J Endovasc Ther.* 2004;11:175–179.

71. Aronson S, Dyke CM, Stierer KA, et al. The ECLIPSE trials: comparative studies of clevidipine to nitroglycerin, sodium nitroprusside, and nicardipine for acute hypertension treatment in cardiac surgery patients. *Anesth Analg.* 2008;107:1110–1121.

72. Kahn RA, Moskowitz DM, Marin ML, et al. Safety and efficacy of high-dose adenosine-induced asystole during endovascular AAA repair. *J Endovasc Ther.* 2000;7:292–296.

73. Fang TD, Lippmann M, Kakazu C, et al. High-dose adenosine-induced asystole assisting accurate deployment of thoracic stent grafts in conscious patients. *Ann Vasc Surg.* 2008;22:602–607.

74. Lippmann M, Kakazu C, Fang TD, Bui H, Donayre C, White RA. Adenosine's usefulness in vascular surgery. *Tex Heart Inst J.* 2007;34:258–259.

75. Kahn RA, Moskowitz DM, Marin M, Hollier L. Anesthetic considerations for endovascular aortic repair. *Mt Sinai J Med.* 2002;69:57–67.

76. Plaschke K, Böckler D, Schumacher H, Martin E, Bardenheuer HJ. Adenosine-induced cardiac arrest and EEG changes in patients with thoracic aorta endovascular repair. *Br J Anaesth.* 2006;96:310–316.

77. Yasuda S, Tateoka K, Sakurai K, Takahata O, Iwasaki H. Anesthetic management of endovascular stent graft placement for thoracic aortic aneurysm using induction of transient cardiac asystole by ATP. *Masui.* 2002;51:1023–1025.

78. Tanito Y, Endou M, Koide Y, Okumura F. ATP-induced ventricular asystole and hypotension during endovascular stenting surgery. *Can J Anaesth.* 1998;45:491–494.

79. Pornratanarangsi S, Webster MW, Alison P, Nand P. Rapid ventricular pacing to lower blood pressure during endograft deployment in the thoracic aorta. *Ann Thorac Surg.* 2006;81:e21–e23.

80. Yamagishi A, Kunisawa T, Katsumi N, Nagashima M, Takahata O, Iwasaki H. Anesthesic management of thoracic aortic stent graft deployment using rapid ventricular pacing. *Masui.* 2008;57:983–986.

81. Kahn RA, Marin ML, Hollier L, Parsons R, Griepp R. Induction of ventricular fibrillation to facilitate endovascular stent graft repair of thoracic aortic aneurysms. *Anesthesiology.* 1998;88:534–536.

82. Hata M, Tanaka Y, Iguti A, Saito H, Ishibashi T, Tabayashi K. Endovascular repair of a descending thoracic aortic aneurysm: a tip for systemic pressure reduction. *J Vasc Surg.* 1999;29:551–553.

83. Bernard EO, Schmid ER, Lachat ML, Germann RC. Nitroglycerin to control blood pressure during endovascular stent-grafting of descending thoracic aortic aneurysms. *J Vasc Surg.* 2000;31:790–793.

84. Diethrich EB. A safe, simple alternative for pressure reduction during aortic endograft deployment. *J Endovasc Surg.* 1996;3:275.

85. Nienaber CA, Kische S, Rehders TC, et al. Rapid pacing for better placing: comparison of techniques for precise deployment of endografts in the thoracic aorta. *J Endovasc Ther.* 2007;14:506–512.

86. Mordecai MM, Crawford CC. Intraoperative management: endovascular stents. *Anesthesiol Clin North America.* 2004;22:319–332.

87. Velazquez OC, Carpenter JP, Baum RA, et al. Perigraft air, fever, and leukocytosis after endovascular repair of abdominal aortic aneurysm. *Am J Surg.* 1999; 178:185–189.

88. Storck M, Scharrer-Pamler R, Kapfer X, et al. Does a postimplantation syndrome following endovascular treatment of aortic aneurysms exist? *Vasc Surg.* 2001;35:23–29.

89. Meites G, Sellin M. Anesthetic management of the endovascular thoracic aorta. In: Rosseau H, Verhoye JP, Heautot JF, eds. *Thoracic Aortic Diseases.* 1st ed. Berlin: Springer; 2006:81–98.

90. Cross KS, Bouchier-Hayes D, Leahy AL. Consumptive coagulopathy following endovascular stent repair of abdominal aortic aneurysm. *Eur J Vasc Endovasc Surg.* 2000;19:94–95.

91. Storck M, Scharrer-Pamler R, Kapfer X, et al. Does a postimplantation syndrome following endovascular treatment of aortic aneurysms exist? *Vasc Surg.* 2001;35:23–29.

92. Baril DT, Kahn RA, Ellozy SH, Carroccio A, Marin ML. Endovascular abdominal aortic aneurysm repair: emerging developments and anesthetic considerations. *J Cardiothorac Vasc Anesth*. 2007; 21:730–742.

93. Bolke E, Jehle PM, Storck M, et al. Endovascular stent-graft placement versus conventional open surgery in infrarenal aortic aneurysm: a prospective study on acute phase response and clinical outcome. *Clin Chim Acta*. 2001;314:203–207.

Anesthesia for Open Abdominal Aortic Aneurysm Repair

14

Theresa A. Gelzinis and Kathirvel Subramaniam

Abdominal aortic aneurysms (AAAs) are the 13th leading cause of death in the United States[1] and approximately 40,000 patients undergo elective AAA repair each year.[2] With the population aging, this number is expected to increase. Although the use of endovascular AAA repair is becoming more common, open repair, first reported by Dubost et al. in 1951 remains the gold standard.[2] This chapter will review the etiology, risk factors, diagnosis, pathophysiology, operative technique, perioperative management, and postoperative complications of patients undergoing open AAA repair.

Definition

The International Society for Cardiovascular Surgery/Society for Vascular Surgery defines an abdominal aortic aneurysm as a focal dilation of the aorta leading to a diameter at least 50% larger than normal.[3] Normal abdominal aortic diameter ranges from 17 to 24 mm and this depends on several factors such as age, gender, and body habitus. AAA is defined as an aorta with a diameter more than 30 mm.[3]

T.A. Gelzinis (✉)
Department of Anesthesiology,
University of Pittsburgh, 1 200 Lothrop Street,
15213, Pittsburgh, PA, USA
e-mail: gelzinista@anes.upmc.edu

True abdominal aortic aneurysms affect all three layers of the aortic wall and are characterized by their shape and location. Fusiform aneurysms, the most common type, involve the entire circumference of the aorta while saccular aneurysms involve only part of the circumference of the aorta.[1] The most common location for these aneurysms is infrarenal, usually located several centimeters below the renal arteries, extending to the aortic bifurcation, and frequently involve the iliac arteries. When the aneurysm involves the renal ostia, it is defined as pararenal.

Pararenal AAAs are characterized by the absence of normal aortic tissue between the upper extent of the aneurysm and the renal arteries.[4] Approximately 8–20% of AAAs are pararenal, which includes both juxtarenal and suprarenal AAAs. Juxtarenal AAAs are infrarenal aneurysms that involve the lower margin of the origin of the renal arteries. Suprarenal aneurysms are defined as an aneurysm that involved the aorta above the renal arteries and they require reconstruction of renal arteries.[5]

Etiology

The majority of AAAs are due to atherosclerotic disease, but there are other causes (Table 14.1). Inflammatory aneurysms deserve a special mention and are defined by a thickened aneurysmal wall, perianeurysmal and retroperitoneal fibrosis,

Table 14.1 Etiology of abdominal aortic aneurysms

1. Atherosclerosis
2. Cystic medial necrosis
3. Connective Tissue Disorders
   a. Marfan's syndrome
   b. Ehler–Danlos syndrome type IVs
   c. Turner's syndrome
   d. Polycystic kidney disease
4. Arteritis
   a. Giant cell arteritis
   b. Takayasu's disease
   c. Relapsing polychondritis
5. Infectious
   a. Acute
      i. Syphilis
      ii. Salmonella
      iii. Staphylococcus
      iv. Brucellosis
   b. Chronic
      i. Tuberculosis
   c. Fungal (mycotic)
6. Posttraumatic
7. Inflammatory

Table 14.2 Risk factors for the development of abdominal aortic aneurysms

- Age > 60 years
- Male
- Family history
- Hyperlipidemia
- Hypertension
- Chronic obstructive pulmonary disease
- Smoking
- Diabetes
- Caucasian race
- Sedentary life style
- Coronary artery disease
- Peripheral vascular disease

and dense adhesions to adjacent abdominal organs.[1] They represent between 3 and 10% of all AAAs. They are more common in males and patients with long history of tobacco use. They tend to present in the sixth decade of life and are associated with increased surgical risk.[6] They have a genetic component and are seen in patients with a familial history of AAAs. Inflammatory aneurysms are thought to arise from an immune response to an antigen in the adventitial wall. This antigen is unknown but is thought to be viral, a lipid, or a product of lipid peroxidation from atherosclerosis.[7] Herpes simplex virus and cytomegalovirus have been identified in the aortic wall in patients with inflammatory AAAs.[6] Patients with inflammatory AAAs are very symptomatic (back, flank, and abdominal pain) and have an elevated erythrocyte sedimentation rate.

Risk Factors

Abdominal aortic aneurysms occur predominantly in the elderly, with the average age of 70 years, with its incidence increasing with advancing age. The prevalence of AAAs is

estimated to be 2–5% in patients over 65 years. AAAs are uncommon in patients under 50 years of age unless the aneurysm is familial, posttraumatic, or mycotic. Additional risk factors for the development of AAAs are listed in Table 14.2. There is a strong association between smoking and AAA formation. Not only is the rate of AAA formation fourfold higher in smokers, aneurysm growth is more rapid. AAAs can be familial and first-degree relatives of patients with a history of AAAs are prone to develop aneurysms at a younger age with a more frequent rupture rate.

In the United States, approximately 150,000 patients die from ruptured AAAs each year. The most important risk factor for rupture is aneurysm diameter. Patients with aneurysm diameters ≥6 cm have a 10–20% chance of rupture per year.[8] Other risk factors for rupture include female gender, uncontrolled diastolic hypertension, familial history, severe chronic obstructive pulmonary disease (COPD), current tobacco use, and rapid expansion of the aneurysm.

Pathogenesis

The two main determinants of the mechanical properties of the aorta are elastic fibers and fibrillar collagens. Elastin in the media is responsible for the viscoelastic properties of the aorta while collagen present in both media and adventitia provides tensile strength to help maintain the structural integrity of the aortic wall. Early in aneurysm formation, there is fragmentation of elastic fibers, and, as the aneurysm develops, there is degradation of collagen, which is the ultimate cause of rupture. This process is mediated by proteolytic enzymes such as the matrix metalloproteins (MMPs) and plasmin-generated plasminogen activators.[9] There is also a reduction in smooth muscle cells in the media, which participate in vascular wall remodeling and have a protective role against inflammation and proteolysis.[10]

AAAs may be associated with mural thrombus formation. Since the thrombus is continuously exposed to blood flow, there is constant remodeling of the thrombus. This leads to ongoing coagulation and fibrinolytic activity as measured by increased serum thrombin–antithrombin III complex and D-dimer levels.[11] Although the thrombus may reduce wall stress, its increasing thickness may lead to local hypoxia at the inner layer of the media, which can induce medial neovascularization and inflammation.

Most AAAs are infrarenal because of hemodynamic differences in the distal aorta. These include a higher peripheral vascular resistance, increased oscillary wall shear stress, and reduced flow.[8] There is also increased MMP-9 expression in the infrarenal aorta. These conditions can predispose the distal aorta to inflammation and aneurysm formation.

Clinical Presentation and Diagnosis

Unruptured AAAs

The majorities of unruptured AAAs are asymptomatic and are diagnosed as an incidental finding in patients with concurrent coronary, peripheral, or cerebrovascular disease or during population screening. Patients may experience chronic vague symptoms of back and abdominal pain, which result from direct pressure or distention of adjacent structures. The average rate of aneurysm expansion is approximately 3–5 mm per year. AAAs are prone for rupture and recent onset of severe lumbar pain may indicate impending rupture.

Rarely, unruptured AAAs can be diagnosed after complications such as distal embolization or acute thrombosis. Ureterohydronephrosis may occur with inflammatory aneurysms or aneurysms involving the iliac bifurcation.

AAAs can be diagnosed by palpating for a pulsatile mass in the supraumbilical area, but this is a poor screening tool with a sensitivity of approximately 68%. Sensitivity of abdominal palpation increases with the diameter of the lesion and decreases with abdominal girth.[12] Radiologic imaging techniques such as abdominal ultrasound, computed tomography (CT), or magnetic resonance imaging (MRI) are the preferred modalities to diagnose AAAs. An AAA may be diagnosed on a lateral abdominal x-ray if calcifications are present, which may allow visualization of the dilated aorta. Abdominal ultrasonography is the simplest and least expensive diagnostic modality. It can accurately measure aortic size and can be used for diagnosis, follow-up surveillance, and screening.[13] If there is an aneurysm detected on screening, the next step is to perform an abdominal CT to determine the type of treatment.[14] Information that can be elicited from a CT includes visualization of the proximal neck, extension to the iliac arteries, patency of the visceral arteries, and the presence and thickness of a mural thrombus. CT can also detect anatomic variants such as a left vena cava, posterior left renal vein, or horseshoe kidney that may interfere with the procedure, and can reveal blood within the mural thrombus called the crescent sign, which may be a predictive marker of imminent rupture.[15] In patients with inflammatory aneurysms, CT can estimate the thickness of the aortic wall and determine the presence of para-aortic fibrosis. CT can also be used to determine the suitability for placement of endovascular devices. (Figs. 14.1 and 14.2).

MR angiography is useful in patients with suspected renal involvement because the gadolinium contrast material is less nephrotoxic than CT contrast. CT and MRI provide the same information, and the choice of study depends on the preference of the surgeon and radiologist, the availability of the study at the medical center, the patient's hemodynamic status, the ability of

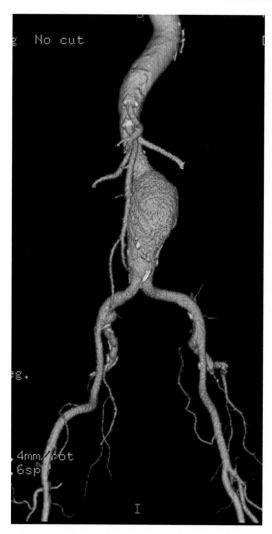

Fig. 14.1 CT reconstruction of infrarenal abdominal aortic aneurysm

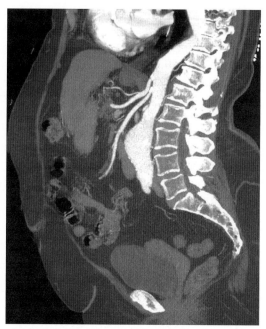

Fig. 14.2 CT angiography of infrarenal abdominal aorta

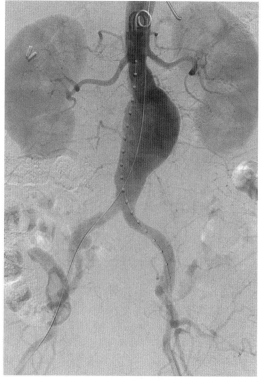

Fig. 14.3 Angiogram of abdominal aorta showing infrarenal AAA

the patient to lie still for an MRI examination, and the presence of renal dysfunction.

Angiography, the gold standard for the diagnosis of abdominal AAAs, is reserved for patients with inconclusive CT or MRI studies, in patients with more extensive aneurysms, such as those which involve the kidneys or viscera and require a more accurate determination of branch anatomy, in patients with peripheral occlusive disease, and in patients with renal abnormalities such as horseshoe or pelvic kidneys (Fig. 14.3).[16]

Ruptured AAA (RAAA)

A total of 50–60% of AAAs will rupture in 5 years. Larger aneurysms are more prone for rupture and 98% of the ruptured AAAs occur infrarenally. Rupture of the anterolateral wall of the aneurysm into the peritoneal wall carries mortality between 60 and 97% (Fig. 14.4 and 14.5). Most patients (88%) present with a rupture of the posterolateral wall into the retroperitoneum where the rupture can be sealed by clot formation, retroperitoneal hematoma, and abdominal muscle tone, and hemorrhage is limited by hypotension. This event is followed within hours by a larger rupture. The period between the two ruptures is called the intermediate period and is

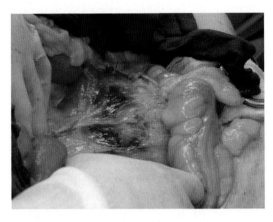

Fig. 14.4 Intraoperative image of ruptured abdominal aneurysm

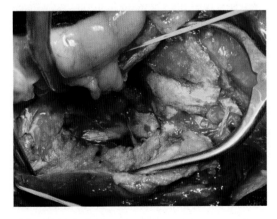

Fig. 14.5 Severe atherosclerotic ruptured abdominal aorta opened after cross-clamping

the time where the diagnosis and emergency repair can be accomplished.[1] The triad of symptoms of an RAAA include sudden onset of mid-abdominal or flank pain radiating to the scrotum, circulatory shock, and the presence of a pulsatile abdominal mass. The presence of flank ecchymosis (Grey Turner sign) represents retroperitoneal hemorrhage. Diagnosis is mostly clinical, but ultrasound, CT or MRI scanning, or aortagraphy can also be helpful depending on hemodynamic stability. Contrast CT shows extravasation of contrast material, which is diagnostic of rupture. Early diagnosis reduces mortality by 50%. In rare cases, the first episode of rupture can be contained to become a chronic pulsatile extra-aortic hematoma or aneurysms can rupture into another structure, such as the duodenum, producing an aorto-duodenal fistula or the vena cava, which can lead to lower extremity edema.[17]

Surgical Management

Indications for Open Repair

Open AAA repair is recommended for aneurysms associated with an aortic neck >28 mm or significant angulation defined as >45° from midline, or those associated with laminated thrombus at the proposed site of stent-graft attachment. Open AAA repair is also recommended for the majority of pararenal aneurysms because endovascular repair with fenestrated grafts is a long complicated procedure, with the potential for failure, and is reserved for elderly or high-risk patients.[18] Patients with atherosclerotic disease of the femoral, iliac, or renal arteries may be difficult to treat endovascularly.

Open Versus Endovascular AAA Repair

The recent endovascular aneurysm repair (EVAR-1) and Dutch Randomized Endovascular Aneurysm Management (DREAM) trials addressed management of AAAs larger than 5.5 cm in diameter. They randomized patients appropriate for open repair between endovascular repair (EVAR) and open repair (OR). EVAR decreased perioperative complications, including myocardial events, and was associated with decreased recovery times. In patients with large AAAs who are fit for OR, EVAR offers an initial mortality advantage over OR, with a persistent reduction in AAA-related death at 4 years. However, EVAR offers no overall survival benefit, is more costly, and requires more interventions and indefinite surveillance with only a brief Quality of Life (QOL) benefit.[19] Open repair is more durable and does not require the extensive surveillance unlike endovascular repairs. This may lead to a better quality of life. The DREAM trial patients received QOL questionnaires preoperatively, then at 3 weeks, 6 months, and at 1 year. Preoperative scores were similar. At 3 weeks, the patients undergoing endovascular repair had a better quality of life, but at 6 months and 1 year, the patients undergoing the open repair reported a better quality of life.[20]

Techniques of Infrarenal AAA Repair

There are two surgical approaches for open AAA repair, midline transperitoneal approach, or a left retroperitoneal approach. Both can be performed either by laparotomy or by laparoscopic-assisted technique.

Transperitoneal Approach

With this approach, a midline incision is performed, the transverse colon and omentum are covered with moist towels and packed in the upper abdomen. The small bowel is reflected to the right side of the peritoneal cavity and a retractor is placed to maintain exposure (Fig. 14.6). The retroperitoneal lining is excised and the aorta is dissected until the renal artery is exposed proximally and the common iliac arteries are exposed distally. During the proximal dissection, bleeding can occur from injury to the left lumbar, gonadal, adrenal, or renal veins, especially when the retroperitoneum has inflammatory or fibrotic changes. Injury to the ureters or iliac veins can occur during distal dissection.

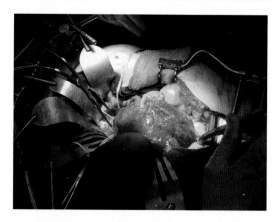

Fig. 14.6 Transperitoneal approach to the abdominal aortic aneurysm

The aneurysm is mobilized at the neck and the common iliac arteries are controlled at their bifurcations to prepare for clamping. Intravenous heparin is administered, vascular clamps are applied, and the aneurysmal sac is opened. Atherosclerotic debris and thrombi are removed, and back-bleeding from the lumbar and inferior mesenteric arteries is controlled with sutures within the sac. The aortotomy is extended to the aneurysmal neck and the aorta transected. A tube graft repair is performed, first with the proximal anastomosis to the aorta. After the proximal anastomosis is completed, a second clamp is placed on the graft to assess the strength of the anastomosis under pressure. The distal anastomosis is then performed either to the distal aorta or iliac arteries. The iliac artery anastomosis is preferred over the common femoral artery anastomosis because the femoral anastomosis is more prone to infection. The aneurysm sac is then closed over the graft, the retroperitoneum is approximated, and then the abdominal wall and skin are closed.

Retroperitoneal Approach

It is the technique of choice in patients with prior abdominal surgery, urinary or enteric stomas, previous abdominal or pelvic radiation, ascites, patient who are on peritoneal dialysis, morbid obesity, inflammatory aneurysms, aneurysms associated with horseshoe kidneys, and juxta- or suprarenal aneurysms. This approach is indicated in the presence of accessory renal arteries and when removing an infected aortic graft. The retroperitoneal approach may be associated with lesser blood loss, fluid and blood transfusion, better pain control, improved pulmonary function, earlier return of bowel function, and reduced incidence of wound dehiscence.[21] Disadvantages of this approach are that it may be difficult to access or control the right iliac artery and that the intraperitoneal contents cannot be inspected. Aortobifemoral grafts for aorto-occlusive disease also require transperitoneal approach.

Pararenal AAA Repair

Juxtarenal AAA repair requires suprarenal clamping, but the aortic reconstruction is performed infrarenally. Most juxtarenal AAAs can be approached by a retroperitoneal approach.[5] For suprarenal AAAs and type IV thoracoabdominal aortic aneurysms, the patient is placed in the right lateral decubitus position with the patient's shoulders raised to 60° and the torso should be rotated so that the hips are as parallel to the table as possible. The retroperitoneal dissection is extended to the diaphragmatic hiatus, and the left crus is divided to expose the supraceliac aorta. The proximal clamp is then placed above the celiac axis or between the renal and superior mesenteric arteries. The inferior mesenteric artery is tied close to the aortic wall to keep it collateral to the superior mesenteric artery. In some cases, the inferior mesenteric artery is reimplanted into the aortic prosthesis to maintain blood flow to the sigmoid colon and rectum. Reimplantation is required if there is significant stenosis of the superior mesenteric artery and celiac trunk or if internal iliac flow cannot be restored after abdominal aortic surgery.[22] If the left renal artery cannot be directly included into the anastomosis, it has to be reimplanted into the graft after primary reconstruction has been completed. The surgical risks of pararenal repair are greater because of renal and possibly mesenteric ischemia, increased alterations in cardiovascular physiology due to the higher aortic cross-clamp, and atheroembolization.

Laparascopic Approach

Ferrari et al. described a laparoscopically assisted approach to AAA repair that is associated with less morbidity and mortality than a standard laparotomy approach.[23] This technique can be used to treat elective infrarenal and pararenal aneurysms. Contraindications for this approach include previous abdominal or aortic surgery, bilateral diffuse common iliac and/or internal iliac aneurysms, massive aortoiliac calcifications, inflammatory aneurysms, and severe underlying cardiac or pulmonary disease. The main advantage of this procedure is a decreased length of stay. Coggia et al.[24] described a total laparoscopic infrarenal aneurysm repair. This technique has the potential for faster wound healing and decreased discomfort.

Systemic Inflammatory Response Syndrome (SIRS)

Systemic inflammatory response is considered to be the precursor of morbidity and mortality after open repair.[25] The inflammatory response is higher in patients presenting for RAAA repair compared to patients presenting for elective AAA repair and the levels of inflammatory mediators correlate with the development of acute respiratory distress syndrome and multiorgan failure (MOF). Operative mortality following ruptured AAA repair may be divided into early and late deaths. The most frequent cause of early death is hemorrhagic shock while up to 90% of deaths after 24 h are caused by MOF. SIRS arises from the response to extensive surgical trauma, the release of vasoactive agents due to bowel manipulation and mesenteric traction, response to graft material, intestinal ischemia from intraoperative hypotension, aortic clamping and ligation of inferior mesenteric artery, ischemia-reperfusion injury, blood transfusions, which alter cytokine production, and cytokines released from the mural thrombus.

Endotoxin, which has been implicated as the trigger for the inflammatory response, can be released directly from bowel ischemia-reperfusion or indirectly through the release of inflammatory mediators after lower limb reperfusion.[26]

The clinically significant cytokines that are released include TNF-α, IL-1β, IL-6, and neutrophil CB 11b. IL-1β is a locally acting cytokine, which acts as a pyrogen, induces hypotension, activates and promotes leukocyte adherence, induces acute phase protein synthesis, and stimulates the secretion of IL-6. Increased IL-6 is the most consistent response to aortic surgery. It enables the neutrophils to release TNF-α and neutrophil CD11b, which, along with IL-6, have been implicated as mediators of SIRS and MOF.[27] A study by Vasdekis et al.[25] demonstrated higher levels of endotoxin, IL-6, and neutrophil CD11b in patients who developed postoperative complications. Excessive manipulation in AAAs with intramural thrombi can lead to a clinical response similar to SIRS that is not seen in patients with small or no mural thrombi.

Risk Stratification and Perioperative Mortality

The operative mortality for elective AAA repair has been reported to range from 1.1% to 7%.[2] Risk assessment methods have become an essential part of preoperative evaluation and consent process for any surgical procedure. For unruptured AAAs, various risk-scoring systems have been tested to predict the risk of postoperative mortality and morbidity. Glasgow Aneurysm Scale (GAS), Vascular-Physiologic and Operative Severity Score for the enUmeration of Mortality and Morbidity (V-POSSUM), and Vascular Biochemical and Hematological Outcome Model (VBHOM) score are few of the risk-scoring methods (Table 14.3).

GAS is simple and easier to use compared to other scoring systems and has been validated numerous times and predicts mortality in elective and ruptured AAA. GAS does not reliably identify individual high-risk patients and does not predict morbidity. The V-POSSUM score is an equation based on 12 preoperative variables each scored and a total score obtained. This is a complex scale with numerous perioperative variables and several subjective-based parameters. The use of physiologic

Table 14.3 Risk stratification scores for abdominal aortic surgery

Glasgow Aneurysm Scale = Age + (17 for shock) + (7 for myocardial disease) + (10 for cerebrovascular disease) + (14 for renal disease)
V-POSSUM physiology-only score = ln (R/1 _ R) = 6.0386 + 0.1539 (physiology score) Physiologic parameters Age Cardiac and pulmonary signs and symptoms Systolic blood pressure Heart rate Serum sodium and potassium Blood urea Hemoglobin level White cell count Electrocardiography Intraoperative variables Grading of operation Number of procedures Total blood loss Peritoneal soiling Presence of malignancy Timing of surgery VBHOM = ln (R/1 _R) = −2.257 + 0.1511(gender)
+0.9940(mode of admission) + 0.05923(age on admission) +0.001401(urea) +0.01303(sodium) +0.03585(potassium) +0.2278(Hb) _ 0.02059(WBC).
Hardman Index Preoperative Hb < 9gm/dl Serum creatinine >1.9 mg/dl ECG evidence of ischemia In-hospital loss of consciousness Age > 76 years

scores yielded inconsistent results when used to predict outcome after AAA repair. One reason for this outcome was that missing variables were scored as normal, which can overestimate the mortality in low-risk patients. The VHBOM score predicts mortality based on single biochemical and hematologic tests and is simple and suitable for collection in both emergency and elective situations. This model is yet to be validated.

Patterson et al. in a systematic review comparing different scoring systems concluded that GAS is the most useful and consistently validated scoring method for elective AAA repair.[28] A risk score that determined an individual patient's predicted risk in specific hospitals would be useful in the consent process because the hospital volume of AAA cases and experience of the surgeons and staff influence the outcome significantly. Center-specific mortality has to be taken into consideration in addition to the patient and operative variables.

The intraoperative mortality for RAAAs ranges from 50% to 70% and various scoring systems have been evaluated to predict mortality after ruptured AAA. The Hardman system is the most well-known scoring system with five independent variables (Table 14.3). The mortality rate was 100% with three or more risk factors, 48% with two risk factors, 28% with one risk factor, and 18% with no risk factors.[1] POSSUM-RAAA score (combined operative and physiologic variables), the GAS, and Vancouver scoring systems are some other models studied in RAAA.

Irrespective of the scoring system used, the following parameters predict poor outcome: advanced age, cardiac arrest with cardiopulmonary resuscitation, hypotension (systolic BP < 80 mmHg on admission and <100 mmHg at the end of surgery), loss of consciousness, low hematocrit, increased creatinine, ischemic heart disease, free intraperitoneal rupture, operating time >4 h, the administration of more than 7 L of fluid, blood loss >11 L, and blood transfusion of more than 17 units.[29] Tambyraja et al. in a review of published evidence revealed that none of the current scores has the ability to accurately predict outcomes during ruptured AAA repairs. The decision to operate or not in an individual patient is based on the subjective evaluation of the experienced surgeon until further evidence is available.[30]

For patients who survived 48 h after RAAA surgery, Laukontaus et al. demonstrated that the best predictors of 30 day mortality include the preoperative Glasgow score, the need for suprarenal clamping, and the sequential organ failure assessment score (SOFA).[31] The SOFA score uses the PaO_2/FiO_2 ratio, the platelet count, and presence of hypotension, serum bilirubin levels, the Glasgow Coma Scale, and the renal creatinine to predict the likelihood of developing MOF.

Preoperative Evaluation and Preparation

Clinical evidence of coronary artery disease (CAD) is reported in 25–69% of patients by various investigators. The rate of cardiac-related mortality ranges from 0 to 8% and cardiac complications account for 62% of all deaths after AAA repair.[17] Hertzer et al.[32] in their series from Cleveland Clinic revealed that in patients with AAAs undergoing coronary angiography, 6% had normal coronaries, 29% had mild to moderate coronary artery disease (CAD), 31% had correctable CAD, 12–15% had severe correctable CAD, and 5% had inoperable CAD. In their series, 44% with clinical indicators of CAD and 15% without clinical indicators had angiographic demonstration of severe CAD.

According to American Heart Association/American College of Cardiology (AHA/ACC) recommendations, patients with active cardiac conditions, such as unstable or severe angina, recent ST elevation or non-ST elevation MI, decompensated cardiac failure, or significant ischemic cardiac arrhythmias should undergo coronary angiography and revascularization before elective AAA repair. Coronary revascularization is also indicated in patients with stable angina with left main disease, stable angina with 3-vessel disease, and stable angina with 2-vessel disease and proximal left anterior descending (LAD) stenosis with low left ventricular ejection fraction (LVEF) less than 0.50 where the survival benefits are proven.[33]

Preoperative treatment of patients with no active cardiac conditions but with significant clinical risk factors, such as a history of CAD, stable angina, treated stable or past history of heart failure, cerebrovascular disease, age more than 70 years, renal insufficiency, and diabetes mellitus is more complex. It is controversial whether these patients benefit from preoperative testing and subsequent revascularization. Few clinical trials addressed this issue.

Mcfalls et al. randomized their vascular surgical patients into revascularization group ($n=258$) and no-revascularization group ($n=225$) and found a similar incidence of 30-day mortality, myocardial infarction (MI), and mortality after 2.7 years (Coronary Artery Revascularization Prophylaxis study-CARP). Though they excluded patients with unstable angina, left main coronary artery stenosis, and a low left ventricular ejection fraction (LVEF), 74% of their patients had 2 or more clinical risk factors or moderate or large reversible perfusion defects on nuclear stress testing.[34]

The DECREASE-2 (Dutch Echocardiographic Cardiac Risk Evaluation Applying Stress Echo) clinical trial evaluated the value of preoperative cardiac stress testing in intermediate risk (1–2 risk factors) patients. Patients ($n=770$) were randomly assigned to testing ($n=386$) and no testing. All patients received beta-blockers. Tested and nontested patients had similar 30-day cardiovascular mortality and nonfatal myocardial infarction after vascular surgery. Limited ischemia was detected in 17% and extensive ischemia (>3 walls in stress perfusion scintigraphy or >5 segments in dobutamine stress echocardiography) in 8.8% of tested patients. Of 33 patients with extensive ischemia, only 12 were suitable for revascularization, which did not improve 30-day outcome. However, the cardiovascular death or MI was higher in patients with extensive ischemia (odds ratio, OR = 107) and limited ischemia (OR = 42), compared to patients with no ischemia.[35]

The same group of investigators followed up with the DECREASE V clinical trial in which they randomized high-risk (> 2 clinical risk factors) patients with extensive ischemia during cardiac testing into revascularization ($n=49$) and no-revascularization groups ($n=51$). Revascularization did not improve 30-day or 1-year composite outcomes (cardiovascular death or nonfatal myocardial infarction) after the intended vascular surgery.[36]

The results from these studies indicate that high or intermediate risk patients with stable CAD may undergo AAA repair without preoperative revascularization if medical therapy is expected to yield similar protection. The lack of benefit of revascularization is not fully understood, though plaque rupture induced by the perioperative stress response in nonsignificant

coronary lesions, which are not revascularized, may be the culprit.[37]

Noninvasive stress testing has a low positive predictive value and is not routinely recommended in intermediate and low-risk groups. High risk (>2 risk factors) with poor functional status may be referred for stress testing for risk stratification, though the benefits of revascularization in patients with extensive ischemia are not well demonstrated.

The recommendation for coronary angiography (CAG) is similar to the nonoperative setting and it is the clinician's responsibility to take patient-specific factors into account before sending the patients for CAG before AAA surgery. Routine CAG is not advised before AAA repair because of its inherent risk, cost, and manpower.[37] Risk of CAG, mortality of revascularization procedure before AAA repair, hazards of AAA rupture during the waiting period, and risk of AAA surgery, all these put together do not justify routine CAG in all patients presenting for AAA repair.

Among the revascularization methods, percutaneous coronary intervention (PCI) was associated with increased risk of MI compared to coronary artery bypass grafting (CABG) in DECREASE V and CARP trials. Several other studies raised similar concerns. The increased risk could be related to stent thrombosis after PCI, especially if dual antiplatelet therapy (aspirin and clopidogrel) is discontinued perioperatively. The type of PCI planned will depend on the interval between PCI and planned noncardiac surgery. If AAA repair is planned within a month, bare metal stent implantation or balloon angioplasty are the most recommended options. With bare metal stents, after the month of dual antiplatelet therapy, the clopidogrel may be discontinued but aspirin should be continued. If discontinued, the clopidogrel should be restarted as soon as possible in the postoperative period. Drug-eluting stents require 12 months of uninterrupted dual antiplatelet therapy before discontinuing clopidogrel to prevent stent thrombosis.[33]

In patients with unstable CAD and AAA, the options for treatment include a combined CABG/AAA repair or a staged approach with shorter interval (2 weeks) between revascularization and AAA repair. The disadvantage of the staged procedure is postoperative rupture of the AAA, which can occur in up to 30% of patients.[38] The staged approach is therefore appropriate when aneurysm rupture is not imminent, such as with nontender aneurysms between 5 and 8 cm in diameter.[39] The combined approach has been adopted in patients when rupture of the aneurysm is imminent in the immediate postoperative period, which includes tender aneurysms, large aneurysms > 8 cm, rapidly enlarging aneurysms, and aneurysms with recent contained leaks. The advantages of the combined procedure are a reduced total anesthesia time, convalescence, hospital stay, and total costs.[40,41] The CABG can be done on or off cardiopulmonary bypass (CPB).[42–47] In pump cases, both CABG and AAA repair were done while on CPB in some patients while in others, AAA resection was performed after weaning from CPB.[47] CABG on CPB is known to activate inflammatory mediators, produce coagulopathy and embolic phenomenon leading to end organ damage. Operative mortality is high in these patients and ranges from 6% to 33%.[48] Off-pump CABG is a safe and effective alternative to on-pump CABG in these patients. In selected patients, endovascular AAA repair with CABG is an option and can be done either as combined or staged procedure.[48]

The anesthetic management of the combined procedure is similar to that for CABG alone. When the AAA is performed following the CABG, the initial heparinization required for CPB is reversed with protamine and then an additional smaller dose of heparin (5,000 U) is administered prior to aneurysm clamping. In patients who are hemodynamically unstable or who have large aneurysms, the surgeon may elect to perform the repair on CPB. This technique is associated with longer bypass times, which can be complicated by post-bypass coagulopathy, myocardial dysfunction due to long ischemic times, and hemodynamic instability.[49]

In patients with diffuse small-vessel CAD and poor ventricular function, preoperative medical optimization with aspirin, statins, and beta-blockers and intensive perioperative monitoring may reduce the risk of AAA repair. Other options for these patients include serial three-monthly observations with abdominal ultrasound or internal iliac ligation with axillobifemoral bypass.[50]

Besides CAD, the preoperative evaluation should detect and determine the extent of other comorbid diseases including diabetes, hypertension with left ventricular diastolic dysfunction, COPD, chronic renal insufficiency, and cerebrovascular disease. Medications that are commonly prescribed to these patients include antihypertensive agents, oral hypoglycemic agents, insulin, diuretics, inhaled bronchodilators and steroids, antianginal agents, antiplatelet agents, and anticoagulants. Except for diuretics and possibly angiotensin-converting enzyme inhibitors, patients should continue their antihypertensive regimen up to the time of surgery.

Preoperative laboratory tests should include the baseline hematocrit, white cell with differential count to assess for occult infection, platelet and coagulation studies when epidural anesthesia is planned, electrolyte, renal, and hepatic panels, and urine analysis to rule out the presence of a urinary tract infection since a prosthetic graft is used. Blood should be typed and cross-matched. Fresh frozen plasma and platelets are obtained if the patient has a baseline coagulopathy or is taking antiplatelet and anticoagulant agents at the time of surgery. Since the majority of patients undergoing open AAA repair smoke or have COPD, pulmonary function tests and arterial blood gases may be useful in determining the extent of the patient's pulmonary dysfunction.

Monitoring

Standard ASA monitoring (ECG, noninvasive blood pressure, pulse oximetry, capnography, temperature), invasive arterial blood pressure, central venous pressure (CVP) or pulmonary artery catheter (PAC), urine output, and transesophageal echocardiogram (TEE) are used in these patients. Lead V_5 in ECG alone has the ability to idenify approximately 75% of ischemic episodes and the combination of leads II, V4, and V_5 have been demostrated to have 96% sensitivity in detecting myocardial ischemia.[51] Arterial catheterization may be performed prior to the induction of anesthesia to monitor the hemodynamic changes during induction. In patients with peripheral vascular disease, difficult arterial cannulation should be anticipated. Arterial blood gases are monitored frequently and any acid base, electrolyte, blood glucose, and hematocrit disturbances are corrected accordingly. A blood gas is always sent before unclamping and any abnormalities corrected.

Central venous catheterization is performed after induction for venous access to administer fluids, blood and vasoactive medications, and to monitor filling pressures. In patients with normal ventricular function, CVP and pulmonary artery wedge pressures (PCWP) correlate and the use of PAC is not required. PACs may be indicated in patients with pre-existing left ventricular dysfunction, active ischemic heart disease, pulmonary disease with pulmonary hypertension, and renal insufficiency. PACs are especially useful in patients requiring a higher aortic cross-clamp and those with the potential for massive fluid losses. PAC can be used to detect ischemia but poor specificity makes it less useful than ECG and TEE. Ischemia manifests as increases in PCWP and ischemic mitral regurgitation produces large V waves in the pulmonary capillary waveform. PACs with capability to monitor mixed venous oxygen saturation and continuous cardiac output may be useful in patients with extensive SIRS, sepsis, and RAAA.

TEE is used in most of the open AAA repairs at our institution. TEE allows early recognition of evolving myocardial ischemia and facilitates immediate fluid and specific pharmacologic interventions to reduce perioperative cardiac complications. However, all RWMA are not ischemic and not all RWMA detected by TEE correlate with postoperative complications.[52] TEE, the most sensitive monitor of myocardial ischemia, can also be used to evaluate volume status and valvular function. Cardiac output measured by TEE correlates very well with thermodilution cardiac output derived from PAC in the absence of significant mitral regurgitation.[53] Myocardial performance index (MPI), uses measurements taken during the cardiac cycle, from end-diastole to the next end-diastole, is calculated using isovolumetric contraction time (IVCT), isovolumetric relaxation time (IVRT), and ejection time (ET). This index is believed to describe both systolic and diastolic performance of the myocardium. An elevated MPI has been shown to predict poor outcomes (congestive and ventilatory failure) in patients undergoing AAA repair.[54]

Cardiac output can be measured from continuous analysis of pulse pressure waveform by the insertion of a catheter with manometer into axillary or brachial artery. These pulse contour cardiac output (PiCCO; Pulsion Medical Inc, East Brunswick, NJ, USA) devices can also measure transpulmonary thermodilution cardiac output, but require insertion of central venous catheter in addition to arterial catheter.[55] Echo-esophageal Doppler (Hemosonic 100; Arrow, Reading, PA), which measures cardiac output through mean blood velocity in the descending aorta and diameter of descending aorta, have been found to be useful in infrarenal abdominal aortic surgery.[56] These could be potential alternatives for PAC in these patients, although these devices need further evaluation and validation during different periods of aortic surgery such as clamping and unclamping.

Aortic Cross-Clamping

The effects of cross-clamping depend on the level of the clamp, the patient's baseline myocardial function and presence of CAD, the type of aortic disease, the degree of collateralization, volume status, and anesthetic technique.

While infrarenal clamping is well tolerated in most patients, suprarenal clamping produces more hemodynamic changes and is associated with an increased 30-day mortality after RAAA. This can be explained by the effect of the level of cross-clamp on blood volume redistribution and myocardial function as described in the chapter on anesthesia for open descending aortic surgery.[57,58]

Left ventricular hypertrophy and diastolic dysfunction are not uncommon in AAA surgical patients. The impact of aortic cross-clamping on diastolic dysfunction and the resultant hemodynamic changes in patients with diastolic dysfunction are not well studied. Infrarenal clamping is associated with a change in ventricular compliance and PCWP did not correlate with left ventricular end-diastolic area (LVEDA) during aortic cross-clamping.[59] Mahmood et al., using transmitral flow propagation velocity in 35 patients undergoing elective AAA surgery, reported an increase in diastolic dysfunction after aortic cross-clamping, which returned to baseline after unclamping. They did not report any hemodynamic parameters, so the impact of the diastolic dysfunction is not clear.[60] Meierhenrich et al. reported a 50% baseline incidence of diastolic dysfunction in patients undergoing AAA repair. Aortic cross-clamping was not associated with impairment of diastolic dysfunction and the hemodynamic changes were similar in patients with or without diastolic dysfunction.[61] Shuetz et al. have shown that the treated hypertensive patients had significant increase in mean arterial pressure (MAP), PCWP, and mean peak A/peak E velocity after cross-clamping, compared to normotensive controls, but these disturbances normalized after unclamping and the intraoperative management did not differ in both groups.[62] Fayed et al. reported acute diastolic dysfunction after high aortic clamping in six of nine patients with normal E/A ratios before clamping in thoracoabdominal surgery and three of those patients developed myocardial infarction.[63] The level of aortic cross clamp again has an influence on diastolic dysfunction and its effect on outcome.

Patients with CAD and a reduced LVEF experience more hemodynamic changes compared to patients without CAD and a normal ejection fraction.[64] Attita et al. reported a 30% incidence of myocardial ischemia after infrarenal cross-clamping in patients with known severe CAD.[65] Gooding et al. studied the effect of CAD on hemodynamic response to infrarenal aortic cross-clamping in 25 patients undergoing either aortofemoral bypass or abdominal aortic aneurysmectomy. Ten patients had evidence of CAD and 15 did not. They concluded that patients with preexisting CAD had significantly lower cardiac indices and increased PCWP, which may suggest that this subgroup is at greater risk for perioperative myocardial dysfunction.[66]

Patients with aortic occlusive disease may experience less hemodynamic changes compared to AAA patients to clamping and unclamping. Johnston et al. compared hemodynamics in patients with aneurysmal and aorto-occlusive disease and found that patients in the aorto-occlusive group had an increased stroke volume and less of an increase in SVR during aortic cross-clamping compared to patients with aneurysmal disease.[67] These findings could be explained by persistent para-aortic collateral circulation to the lower extremities in chronic occlusive disease and minimal metabolite and lactate accumulation.[68,69] This accounts for the stable hemodynamics that occurs during aortic cross-clamping in patients undergoing repair of aorto-occlusive disease.

The management of the hemodynamic changes associated with aortic cross-clamping center on decreasing afterload, normalizing preload, and maintaining coronary blood flow and contractility. Volume status should be monitored and optimized throughout the clamping period. TEE is very useful in discriminating between hypovolemia and myocardial dysfunction as the cause of hemodynamic compromise. Vasodilators and inotropes may be necessary in some patients. Blood pressure proximal to the clamp should be maintained at preoperative basal level so that the blood flow through collateral circulation to the viscera distal to the clamp is maintained.

Aortic Unclamping

The major hemodynamic response to aortic unclamping is hypotension. The etiology of this hypotension is multifactorial. During clamping of infrarenal aorta, the lower extremities undergo ischemic vasodilatation and vasomotor paralysis. Release of the clamp causes blood sequestration in the previously ischemic lower extremities, central hypovolemia, and decreased blood flow to the critical coronary, renal, and hepatic circulations (Fig. 14.7). The use of vasopressors to increase the blood pressure without restoring blood volume may further decrease blood flow to these critical organs. Adequate volume loading prior

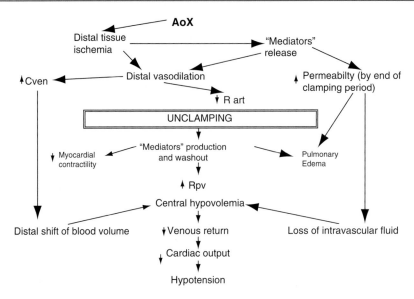

Fig. 14.7 Hemodynamic effects of aortic unclamping (Reprinted with permission from Gelman[58])

to release of the clamp to a higher PCWP than the baseline value is recommended.[70] Ueda et al.[71] used volume loading with 10 ml/kg of albumin before unclamping during AAA repair and have shown that albumin did not prevent systemic hypotension, but significantly increased pulmonary artery pressure and right ventricular afterload causing RV dilatation. Cautious fluid administration is recommended in patients with cardiac dysfunction. Bitoh et al.[72] reported left ventricular diastolic dysfunction, measured using the mitral annular velocity by tissue Doppler method, after unclamping in eight patients undergoing infrarenal AAA repair and the dysfunction persisted until the end of the surgery. Pulmonary edema occurred in two of their patients with the lowest tissue Doppler mitral annular velocity. Gradual release of the clamp is recommended to prevent adverse events after unclamping in such cases. Close communication with surgical team is essential.

Hypotension may also be the result of the accumulation and release of vasodilating and myocardial depressant metabolites. This response involves adenosine, inosine, hypoxanthine, lactate, oxygen free radicals, and prostaglandins, and the activation of neutrophils and the complement system (Fig. 14.7).[70] The correction of metabolic acidosis may be required but may not completely correct arterial hypotension indicating persistent tissue acidosis. The degree and duration of hypotension depends on the level of the aortic clamp and duration of ischemia. Minimizing ischemic time is the goal to prevent severe hemodynamic disturbances. If hypotension is persistent or severe, the aorta may have to be reclamped.[50]

Anesthesia for Ruptured Abdominal Aortic Aneurysms

The initial evaluation of these patients takes place in the operating room. Relevant history, comorbid conditions, details of resuscitation, and the results of laboratory tests and diagnostic imaging should be obtained from the patient, relatives, emergency medical service (EMS) providers, or primary care providers, such as the surgeon or the emergency medicine physician. A quick evaluation of the patient's hemodynamic status is desirable. This should occur quickly because the most important determinant of survival is time to aortic cross-clamping.

Usually, some intravenous access is already established in the emergency room or by EMS. If needed, additional large bore intravenous access should be obtained to allow for adequate fluid resuscitation. Rapid infuser systems with warming capability should be set up and connected to large bore IVs for blood and fluid administration. Blood is also sent for cross-matching from the emergency room. Ten units of packed red cells, 10 units of fresh frozen plasma, and platelets are ordered and should be available by the time the patient reaches the operating room. Type-specific cross-matched blood is preferred. If cross-matching is not done, type-specific blood can be used. Upper extremity invasive arterial lines are placed while the patient is preoxygenated. In patients with hypovolemic shock, axillary or brachial arterial cannulation may be necessary. Ultrasound can be used to quickly cannulate the axillary artery. Fluid and blood administration should continue during induction to the target systolic blood pressure between 50 and 100 mmHg systolic in patients with severe hypovolemic shock.

Patients are induced only when the surgeon is prepared for incision because of the tamponade effect of tight abdominal muscles, which is lost with induction and can precipitate catastrophic hemorrhage. Typically, rapid sequence induction is done with etomidate and succinylcholine. All other medications, such as fentanyl, midazolam, and inhalational anesthetics, should be titrated very carefully in these patients. Scopolamine can be used to produce amnesia in hemodynamically unstable patients. Vasopressors and fluids should be administered cautiously before clamping, as aggressive resuscitation may unplug the hemostatic clot and cause bleeding. Several animal studies using an abdominal aortotomy model of ruptured AAA have demonstrated improved tissue perfusion, decreased blood loss, and improved survival associated with hypotensive resuscitation compared with aggressive resuscitation.[73] There are human studies advocating delayed rather than immediate resuscitation in trauma patients,[74,75] but there are no prospective studies of hypotensive resuscitation in patients with ruptured AAAs. Minimal fluid resuscitation seems to be a logical option provided rapid surgical control of bleeding could be achieved. After induction, a PAC is inserted and TEE can be used along with the PAC to monitor volume status and contractility. Arterial blood gases should be obtained to determine the presence of acidosis, electrolyte abnormalities, and hematocrit. A normal hematocrit may be indicative of hemoconcen-tration. If massive blood transfusion is required, a 1:1 mixture of packed red blood cells (PRBCs) and fresh frozen plasma (FFP) should be administered to prevent dilutional coagulopathy. Autotransfusion may also be useful. Platelets and cryoprecipitate should be available if multiple units of PRBCs and FFP are administered or if the patient is taking antiplatelet agents. Once the aneurysm is clamped, the goal is to maintain hemodynamics and to preserve cardiac function. Hypotension during maintenance is multifactorial and includes the loss of sympathetic tone, hypovolemia, and cardiac dysfunction. If the patient is hypotensive despite adequate fluid resuscitation, vasopressor agents, such as vasopressin or norepinephrine, may be required if the patient has normal cardiac function and inotropic agents, such as epinephrine or dopamine, may be required if the patient has decreased cardiac function. If massive transfusions have been administered, the patient may have citrate toxicity and calcium chloride should be administered. Unclamping shock can be profound and is related to the duration of clamping, degree of shock prior to clamping, the speed with which clamps are released, and the patient's volume status and cardiovascular reserve.

After the repair, the patient may be coagulopathic despite administration of FFP, cryoprecipitate, and platelets. Further transfusion should be guided by the use of thromboelastography (TEG) or coagulation studies such as prothrombin time, activated partial thromboplastin time, platelet count, and thrombin time. If the bleeding continues despite massive transfusion of blood products, activated Factor VII may be considered. Maintenance of normothermia is difficult and should be accomplished during and after the operation to prevent coagulopathy and arrhythmias.

Fluid and Transfusion Management

Open resection of AAA subjects the patient to a laparotomy incision, third space loss that follows

T.A. Gelzinis and K. Subramaniam

extensive tissue trauma, manipulation, exposure and retraction, systemic inflammatory response with increased microvascular permeability, major retroperitoneal edema, hemorrhage, ischemia-reperfusion of lower extremities, and hemodynamic effects of epidural anesthesia. Manipulation of the bowel can lead to the generation and release of vasoactive agents, including substance P, vasoactive intestinal peptide, prostacyclin, and nitric oxide, which can induce splanchnic ischemia and increased intestinal permeability. Fluid management should take all this into consideration. Typically, 2–4 L of intravenous crystalloids are infused for these procedures. Restrictive fluid strategy has been shown to reduce postoperative complications in abdominal surgery.[76,77] McArdle et al.[77] in a retrospective study demonstrated that patients with positive fluid balance had an

increased incidence of adverse postoperative cardiac and respiratory complications and increased ICU and overall hospital stays after open AAA surgery (Fig. 14.8). Adesanya et al.[78] in another retrospective study on patients undergoing major vascular surgery have shown that fluid restriction less than 3 L decreased ICU stay and duration of mechanical ventilation and the benefits of fluid restriction were similar to those seen with major abdominal surgery.

A systematic review on the choice of fluid therapy indicates that there is no advantage of using any specific fluid over another in the management of aortic aneurysm surgery.[79] Lactated Ringer (LR) solution, normal saline, 5% dextrose, 5% dextrose in 0.45% saline, 5% dextrose in LR, mannitol, 1.8% saline, human albumin in LR, human albumin in water, 5% dextrose with human

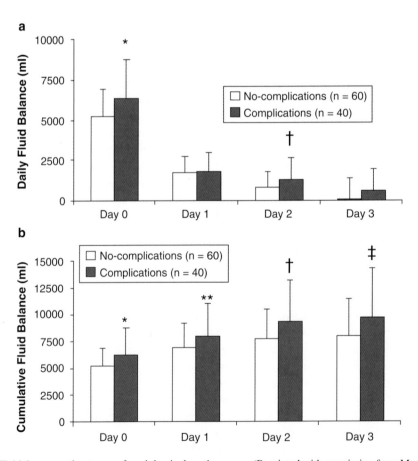

Fig. 14.8 Fluid therapy and outcome after abdominal aortic surgery (Reprinted with permission from McArdle[77])

albumin, Dextran, Isotonic hydroxyethyl starch (HES), and hypertonic HES (6% HES 7.2% saline) were some of the fluid types studied.

The blood loss during AAA surgery can occur from the lumbar arteries when aneurysm is opened or at the proximal and distal anastomotic site. Bleeding may be related to inadequate hemostasis, coagulopathy, or excess heparinization. Techniques to reduce homologous blood transfusion are employed to reduce the transfusion risks and prevent the adverse effects associated with extensive stored blood therapy. Preadmission autologous blood donation (PABD) in combination with intraoperative autotransfusion (IAT) has been shown to eliminate the need for homologous transfusion in two thirds of elective AAA patients.[80] Similar efficacy of PABD with IAT was demonstrated in aortic surgery when compared with IAT alone or with no conservation technique.[81,82] Erythropoietin has also been used in patients undergoing preoperative blood donation.[83] The routine use of IAT in all elective AAA patients is controversial. A meta-analysis of four randomized controlled trials examining the efficacy of IAT reported 37% reduction in risk of allogenic blood transfusion.[84] Few other studies reported lack of efficacy and found this practice to be not cost-effective when applied to all AAA patients.[85,86] While some surgeons use IAT routinely, few others consider it in selected operations where blood loss is likely to be high, such as RAAA, complex reconstructions, thoracoabdominal aneurysms and suprarenal aneurysm surgery, or in patients with religious concerns.[87] The disadvantages of the washed red cells are that they do not contain platelets or coagulation factors. TEG is utilized intraoperatively to detect and treat coagulopathy. Acute normovolemic hemodilution (ANH) has been used in combination with intraoperative cell savage (ICS) and found to be an effective strategy for AAA patients.[88] Wolowczyk et al.[89] in a randomized controlled clinical trial compared ANH with ICS to ICS alone in patients undergoing elective AAA repair and concluded that ANH did not reduce transfusion requirements and had no impact on systemic inflammatory response or overall outcome. Even without ANH, the large volumes of fluid infused as part of standard fluid management in these patients produced hemodilution, which is the reason why additional ANH is ineffective in saving bank blood.[90]

Pain Management

Intravenous opioid patient-controlled analgesia (PCA) with hydromorphine or morphine is the standard method of pain relief after abdominal aortic surgery to which other methods are compared. Compared to intravenous opioids, epidural analgesia provided superior pain control, reduced duration of tracheal intubation and mechanical ventilation by 20%, reduced the overall incidence of cardiovascular complications, acute respiratory failure, gastrointestinal complications, and renal insufficiency.[91] Patients presenting for AAA resection have associated thromboembolic and cardiovascular disease and may take antiplatelet agents and anticoagulants. Medication and preoperative coagulation studies, such as the platelet count, bleeding time, prothrombin time, and partial thromboplastin time should be reviewed before insertion of epidural catheters. Lower thoracic epidural catheters are used in AAA surgery.

Combined epidural and general anesthesia may attenuate the increased systemic resistance with aortic cross-clamping and may produce stable cardiovascular dynamics following cross-clamp release if intravascular volume is maintained.[92-94] The intraoperative use of epidural anesthesia in combination with general anesthesia is favored by some clinicians for these reasons while others elect not to use the epidural analgesia intraoperatively as they feel it causes more hypotension and necessitates increased infusion of intravenous fluids and vasopressors.[95] Intravenous fentanyl is used for intraoperative analgesia in such cases. Epidural analgesia with ropivacaine 0.1% or bupivacaine 0.125%, with hydromorphine 10 μg/cc is initiated before abdominal wound closure to facilitate extubation and pain relief in the immediate postoperative period. Initiation of epidural also controls the hypertensive response associated with extubation.

Typically, epidural analgesia is continued for 3–5 days. The superior analgesia by epidural is especially useful in patients with chronic obstructive pulmonary disease.[96] In these patients, epidural analgesia decreases the duration of mechanical ventilation and the incidence of pulmonary complications.[97] Epidural catheter insertion is not without risk. Epidural hematoma with paraparesis and iliopsoas hematoma with lumbosacral plexopathy have been reported with epidural analgesic use after AAA repair.[98,99] Though these complications are rare when appropriate precautions are taken, the prognosis of these neurological complications can be serious. Postoperative monitoring of neurological dysfunction is an essential part of epidural analgesia. Anticoagulants should be discontinued and normal coagulation studies should be documented before the removal of epidural catheters.

Bilateral paravertebral blocks (PVB) offer an alternate effective method of pain relief with infrequent neurologic and hemodynamic effects. Paravertebral catheters are placed outside the central neuraxis making the possibility of central neuraxial hematoma unlikely. Compared to epidural analgesia, PVB was also associated with better pulmonary function, less hypotension, urinary retention, and postoperative nausea and vomiting (PONV) after thoracic surgical procedures.[100] There are no clinical trials comparing PVB and epidural analgesia in abdominal vascular surgery. Richardson et al.[101] reported their experience of bilateral PVB as a part of balanced analgesia, with intravenous morphine and diclofenac, in eight patients undergoing abdominal vascular surgery. They noted satisfactory intraoperative hemodynamic stability and good quality of postoperative analgesia without any significant pain-related complications. Randomized trials comparing epidural and paravertebral analgesia are needed in abdominal aortic surgery.

Intrathecal opioids can also be utilized to provide effective postoperative analgesia. Low-dose (0.2 mg) intrathecal morphine decreased pain scores and IV morphine consumption compared to controls in patients undergoing abdominal aortic surgery.[102] In another study using intrathecal sufentanil (1 µg/kg) with intrathecal morphine (8 µg/kg), intense analgesia was produced in the first 24 h with intrathecal regimen compared to control group.[103] Improvement in analgesia was not associated with decrease in cardiovascular, respiratory, and renal complications. Intrathecal opioids can be used as an alternate method in selected patients in whom continuous epidural or PVB catheters cannot be utilized.

Wound infiltration of local anesthetics has not been shown to be effective in improving pulmonary function or decreasing opioid consumption after aortic surgery.[104] Other analgesic adjuvants that can be used include ketorolac, acetaminophen, and ketamine, especially in opioid-dependent patients.

Optimal pain management is important when the patient is considered a candidate for fast track AAA repair. Mukherjee et al. described a multidisciplinary technique involving anesthesiologists, surgeons, and nurses, which allows patients to be ambulatory and to eat by postoperative day 1, and to be discharged, on average, by postoperative day 3.6. "Fast-tracking" involves the use of a limited retroperitoneal incision, with minimal bowel manipulation, an anesthetic that allows extubation in the operating room and postoperative pain control with epidural anesthesia, and metoclopramide to facilitate gastric emptying.[105] By postoperative day 1, patients are encouraged to ambulate and are offered a clear liquid diet, which is advanced as tolerated. By the third postoperative day, all intravenous catheters are removed and oral analgesics are started. If tolerated, the patient is discharged by postoperative day 3 or 4. In a limited series of 30 patients, there was one death and one ureteral injury, which had similar morbidity and mortality to the standard procedure.

Blunt Aortic Trauma

Blunt injury of the abdominal aortic is rare and results from direct mechanical forces that compress the aorta against the lumbar spine. The injuries that result include contusions, intimal disruption, intramural hematoma, false aneurysm, and rupture.[106] Since aortic injuries tend to progress from the intima to the adventitia, the most common injury from blunt aortic trauma is intimal tearing. This injury occurs predominantly in males and the majority are caused by automobile accidents including steering wheel and seat belt injuries. Early clinical signs include acute arterial insufficiency, acute abdomen, and neurologic manifestations, such as paraplegia and sensory loss and late clinical signs include claudication, an abdominal mass or bruit, and persistent abdominal pain. The diagnostic modality of choice is a helical CT with aortography for inconclusive CTs[107] and treatment depends on the injury and includes open or endovascular repair, flap suture of intimal tears, and thromboembolectomy.[108]

Postoperative Management

The postoperative care of these patients is usually in the intensive care unit where the patient can be closely monitored. The management of these patients includes monitoring for and treating myocardial ischemia and ventricular dysfunction, treating hypertension by continuing preoperative antihypertensive regimens, including beta-blocking agents, optimizing pulmonary function, through the use of inhaled bronchodilators, incentive spirometry, and early extubation, providing analgesia either with regional or parenteral analgesia, and monitoring for bleeding, bowel, and renal dysfunction. Renal dysfunction is treated by avoiding nephrotoxins and maintaining adequate renal perfusion through the use of fluids and inotropic agents.

Postoperative Complications

Cardiac Complications

Postoperative myocardial infarction (MI) is the most common cause of death following AAA repair. Predisposing factors for myocardial ischemia include pre-existing coronary artery disease, pain, mobilization of third-space fluid into central circulation, stress and hypermetabolism, sympathetic overactivity, anemia, and hypothermia. Added to

the hemodynamic stress is hypofibrinolysis and thrombin activation leading to prothrombotic state and myocardial injury.[109,110]

Identifying perioperative MI is difficult because chest pain is infrequent (fewer than 50% of ischemic episodes are symptomatic) and disguised by analgesics. ECG is the mainstay of the diagnosis, but the changes may be subtle and transient. Most of the postoperative MIs are of the non-Q wave variety. Moderate elevations of creatinine kinase myocardial band fraction can occur in aortic surgical patients. Cardiac troponin (TnI) elevation may be more specific. Elevated TnI has been demonstrated in 46% of the patients who survived RAAA repair and was associated with increased cardiac dysfunction and death.[111] Ali et al.[112] studied 43 patients undergoing elective AAA repair for evidence of myocardial injury. Elevated TnI was seen in 20 (47%) patients. Clinical evidence MI and myocardial events occurred in 11 patients. Survival free of cardiac events was seen in 55% of patients who had elevated CnI compared to 81% who did not have elevated CnI at 1.5 years after discharge. In doubtful cases of perioperative MI, echocardiography and nuclear scans may help in diagnosis.

Therapy of non-ST elevation MI includes oxygen, analgesics, nitrates, beta-blockers, angiotensin-converting enzyme inhibitors, and anticoagulation with aspirin and heparin, when approved by the surgeon. An increased bleeding risk precludes the use of thrombolytics in the immediate postoperative period. Cardiology consultation is initiated immediately for percutaneous interventions, such as cardiac catheterization, angioplasty, stenting, or surgery in patients who still have ischemia despite maximal medical therapy. Intervention is required in all cases of ST elevation MI. Treatment of cardiogenic shock require invasive monitoring, such as a PAC with continuous cardiac output and mixed venous saturation monitoring and inotropic support.

Pulmonary Complications

Various perioperative factors influence the development of respiratory failure after AAA repair.

Preoperative factors: Advanced age, cigarette smoking, history of COPD, morbid obesity, and

ASA IV status are risk factors for postoperative pulmonary complications. Abnormal pulmonary function tests (FEVI or FVC < 70% predicted, Expiratory flow rate less than 200 ml/min) and arterial blood gas (PCO2 > 45 mmHg on room air) also increase the incidence of postoperative pulmonary complications.

Intraoperative factors: Prolonged surgery, large volume infusion, large midline vertical incision, and transperitoneal approach are cited as risk factors for pulmonary complications.

Postoperative factors: Abdominal distension from ileus, inadequate analgesia, large doses of parenteral narcotic administration, hypothermia, bed rest in supine position all prolong weaning and early extubation

Respiratory failure is caused by a restrictive defect with decreased functional residual capacity, altered secretions, impaired cough and mucociliary clearance, bronchospasm, atelectasis, exacerbation of chronic lung disease, and pneumonia. Respiratory failure prolongs the hospital stay. Pneumonia is usually caused by pseudomonas aeruginosa and staphylococcus aureus and associated with mortality of 21%.[113]

Pulmonary complications can be minimized by tobacco cessation several weeks before the procedure, aggressive perioperative pulmonary toilet, lung expansion maneuvers, such as deep breathing exercises and incentive spirometry, antibiotics for pneumonia, and epidural or paravertebral analgesia, which allow for early extubation and mobilization.[17]

Renal Insufficiency

Pre-existing renal dysfunction with creatinine levels higher than 2 mg/dl is associated with operative mortality of 19% versus 4.2% mortality if the creatinine was less than 2 mg/dl.[114] Patients with creatinine levels more than 4 mg/dl require preoperative initiation of hemodialysis.[115] AAA may be associated with renal artery stenosis or ureteric obstruction, which should be evaluated preoperatively by renal ultrasound and excretory urography, respectively.[116]

The incidence of new onset of renal failure after infrarenal clamping is 3% and the rates for suprarenal occlusion are five times greater. Transient renal insufficiency is more common and patients who develop renal insufficiency have longer periods of intubation, ICU, and hospital length of stay. Aortic cross-clamping increases renal vascular resistance and decreases renal cortical blood flow and increases renin–angiotensin secretion and decreases glomerular filtration rate (GFR). Suprarenal clamping decreases blood flow by 80% and infrarenal clamping decreases by 38%.[117,118]

The incidence of renal failure following ruptured AAA repair ranges from 8 to 46% and is associated with a mortality of 57–97%.[1] Additional perioperative factors that contribute to the development of renal insufficiency include pre-existing cardiac disease, advanced age, contrast studies without proper hydration, suprarenal clamping, ischemic time > 30 min, hypovolemia (due to fasting, bowel preparation, and blood loss), hypotension, large volume transfusion, rhabdomyolysis, early reoperation, and atheromatous plaque embolization.

Urine output does not correlate with GFR and oliguria does not predict postoperative renal insufficiency.[119] The incidence of postoperative renal insufficiency may be decreased by preventing hypovolemia, maintaining cardiac output, and by diagnosing and treating oliguria early.

Neurologic Complications

The two major neurologic complications include spinal cord ischemia and postoperative cognitive dysfunction. Benoit et al. studied the incidence of postoperative delirium following AAA repair and found that delirium occurs in up to one third of patients within the first 6 postoperative days. Risk factors for postoperative delirium include advanced age, being unmarried and living alone, preoperative depression and psychoactive medication use, a lower education, and a history of prolonged tobacco abuse.[120]

Spinal cord ischemia (SCI) is a rare (0.3%) but potentially devastating complication after abdominal aortic surgery.[121] SCI has been reported to occur in both elective repairs and ruptured AAAs.

Ruptured aneurysms produce significant hypotension, require supraceliac cross-clamping, and usually heparin is not used; all these factors predispose to SCI. SCI can occur with infrarenal and suprarenal aortic cross-clamps and with both surgery for AAA and aorto-iliac occlusive disease.[122]

The low incidence of paraplegia after elective AAA surgery may be explained by the low level of clamping relative to the origin of arteria radicularis magna and the presence of adequate pelvic collaterals. In general, when the greater radicular artery is open and of normal size, the pelvic blood supply is of minor importance. When greater radicular artery is compromised, the pelvic blood supply becomes critically important. Interference of pelvic blood supply has to be avoided preventing significant hypotension, revascularization of internal iliac artery with a separate graft, and gentle surgical techniques to avoid embolization.[21] SCI after infrarenal AAA and iliac surgery has a poor prognosis and may be reversed by spinal fluid drainage.

Gastrointestinal Complications

The most common complication is paralytic ileus, which is due to bowel manipulation and fluid sequestration. The return of GI function depends on the technique employed and the level of the clamp. GI function returns more rapidly with the retroperitoneal technique and infrarenal cross-clamping. Infrarenal cross-clamping produces little effect on splanchnic blood flow compared to suprarenal or supraceliac cross-clamping.

A rare (0.6–1%) but more devastating complication is ischemic colitis, which is associated with a higher mortality rate (50–75%). RAAA repair, ligation of a patent inferior mesenteric artery, marginal collateral circulation, and perioperative low flow state are risk factors. Inferior mesenteric stump pressure less than 40 mmHg and loss of mesenteric Doppler signals are predictors of the development of colonic ischemia. The risk is reduced by IMA revascularization and ensuring the circulation is preserved through at least one internal iliac artery.[21]

Signs and symptoms of ischemic colitis include excessive fluid requirements, abdominal pain, fever, leukocytosis, diarrhea, and bloody stools. Nonsurgical treatment includes bowel rest, aggressive fluid resuscitation, and antibiotics. Surgical treatment is indicated for full thickness bowel necrosis.[17]

Hemorrhage

Hemorrhage is the second most common postoperative complication and is almost always the result of technical error. Continued hemorrhage increases transfusion requirements and mortality. Surgical causes include persistent retroperitoneal bleeding, anastomotic disruption, and injury to adjacent venous structures while nonsurgical causes include dilutional coagulopathy, disseminated intravenous coagulation, and preoperative anticoagulants, such as antiplatelet agents. If the administration of platelets and clotting factors fail to improve the bleeding or if the TEG and coagulation studies are normal, the patient may require a reoperation to search for a surgical bleeding. Patients undergoing repair of a ruptured AAA have a higher incidence of postoperative bleeding and hence re-explorations.

Disseminated Intravascular Coagulation (DIC)

Activation of fibrinolysis and consumptive coagulopathy can present in AAA patients preoperatively or develop during and after operation.[123,124] Though DIC can occur in both ruptured and unruptured cases, clinically manifesting DIC is more common in RAAA.[125] Clinical presentation can range from bleeding to thrombotic complications and MOF. Heparin therapy may be needed preoperatively and if this is not effective, immediate surgical treatment is curative.[126,127]

Limb Ischemia

Limb ischemia is usually associated with anastomotic complications or distal thromboembolism. Thromboembolism can be micro or macroembolization.[128] Placing the iliac clamp before aortic cross-clamp minimizes distal embolization. Peripheral pulses are evaluated before leaving the operating room. Management includes thrombolytic, anticoagulant, and antiplatelet therapy. Macroembolism can be treated either surgically or by thrombolysis or amputation.[129]

Key Notes

1. An abdominal aortic aneurysm is a focal dilation of the aorta, is defined as an aortic diameter of at least 50% larger than normal or a diameter of greater than 30 mm.
2. The majority of AAAs are infrarenal and are located several centimeters below the renal arteries. Pararenal AAAs are aneurysms that involve the renal ostia and include juxtarenal AAAs, which involve the renal artery origin and suprarenal AAAs, which involve the aorta above the renal arteries.
3. AAAs associated with mural thrombi have increased coagulation and fibrinolytic activity, produce local hypoxia in the media, which can lead to neovascularization and inflammation.
4. The majority of AAAs are asymptomatic and are discovered during routine screening. Ultrasound is the recommended screening modality CT or MRI are used to delineate the anatomy of the aneurysm, and aortography, the gold standard, is reserved for patients with inconclusive studies.
5. For ruptured AAAs, the triad of symptoms include sudden onset of mid-abdominal or flank pain radiating to the scrotum, circulatory shock, and a pulsatile abdominal mass.
6. Open AAA repair is recommended for the majority of pararenal aneurysms, aneurysms with an enlarged neck or significant angulation, and those with laminated thrombus at the stent-graft attachment. Open AAA repair does not require yearly surveillance as with endovascular techniques and is associated with improved patient quality of life as compared with endovascular repair.

7. The surgical approaches to open AAA include the transperitoneal and retroperitoneal approach, including total and assisted laparoscopic techniques. The retroperitoneal approach is associated with decreased pain and perioperative complications, and is the approach of choice for pararenal aneurysms.
8. SIRS, more common in patients with RAAAs, is associated with the release of endotoxin, which causes the release of inflammatory cytokines, such as IL-6, TNFα, and IL-6β, leading to the development of ARDS and MOF.
9. Advanced age, cardiac arrest with cardiopulmonary resuscitation, hypotension, loss of consciousness, low hematocrit, and elevated creatinine are associated with a poor outcome.
10. Since up to half of patients with AAAs have underlying coronary artery disease and perioperative cardiac complications are the major cause of morbidity and mortality, these patients should be evaluated according to the 2007 ACC/AHA guidelines.
11. Monitoring for patients with uncomplicated AAAs includes standard ASA monitors, along with arterial blood pressure, central venous pressure, and urine output. For high-risk patients, additional monitoring may include pulmonary artery catheterization and transesophageal echocardiography.
12. The effects of aortic cross-clamping depends on the level of the clamp, the baseline myocardial function and presence of CAD, the type of aortic disease and degree of collateralization, volume status, and anesthetic technique.
13. Aortic unclamping produces hypotension and acidosis, which is due to the release of vasodilating and myocardial depressant metabolites from ischemia and reperfusion. This can be treated with vasopressors, fluid administration, and reclamping, if necessary.
14. The most important determinant of survival in patients with RAAA is time to aortic cross-clamp. The goals of anesthetic management in these include performing a rapid evaluation, including hemodynamic status, obtaining large bore intravenous access, obtaining blood

and blood products for transfusion, and maintaining hemodynamic stability, with vasoactive agents

15. Fluid and transfusion management for these patients should include fluid restriction and blood conservation techniques, including cell salvage. Patients with coagulopathy during AAA repair should be monitored with TEG and treated with blood products and factor VIIa, if necessary.

16. Postoperative pain management in these patients is diverse and includes neuraxial analgesia with spinal opioids or epidural anesthesia, paravertebral analgesia, and intravenous patient-controlled analgesia.

17. Although the most common perioperative complication is cardiovascular, other complications during AAA repair include renal, pulmonary, neurological, gastrointestinal, hemorrhage, DIC, and limb ischemia.

References

1. Sakalihasan N, Limet R, Defawe OD. Abdominal aortic aneurysm. *Lancet.* 2005;365:1577–1589.
2. Krupski WC, Rutherford RB. Update on open repair of abdominal aortic aneurysms: the challenges for endovascular repair. *J Am Coll Surg.* 2004;199:946–960.
3. Shames ML, Thompson RW. Abdominal aortic aneurysms: surgical treatment. *Cardiol Clin.* 2002;20:563–578.
4. West CA, Noel AA, Bower TC, et al. Factors affecting outcomes of open surgical repair of pararenal aortic aneurysms: a 10 year experience. *J Vasc Surg.* 2006;43:921–928.
5. Chiesa R, Marone EM, Brioschi C, et al. Open repair of pararenal aortic aneurysms: operative management, early results, and risk factor analysis. *Ann Vasc Surg.* 2006;20:739–746.
6. Tang T, Boyle JR, Dixon K, et al. Inflammatory abdominal aortic aneurysms. *Eur J Vasc Endovasc Surg.* 2005;29:353–362.
7. Hellman DB, Grand DJ, Freischlag JA. Inflammatory abdominal aortic aneurysm. *JAMA.* 2007;297:395–400.
8. Dalman RL, Tedesco MM, Myers J, et al. AAA disease: mechanism, stratification, and treatment. *Ann NY Acad Sci.* 2006;1085:92–105.
9. Shah PK. Inflammation, metalloproteinases, and increased proteolysis: an emerging pathophysiological paradigm in aortic aneurysm. *Circulation.* 1997;96:2115–2117.
10. Annambhotla S, Bourgeois S, Wang X, et al. Recent advances in molecular mechanisms of abdominal aortic aneurysm formation. *World J Surg.* 2008;32:976–986.
11. Aho PS, Niemi T, Pililonen A, Lassila R. Interplay between coagulation and inflammation in open and endovascular abdominal aortic aneurysm repair – impact of intra-aneurysmal thrombus. *Scand J Surg.* 2007;96:229–235.
12. Lynch RM. Accuracy of abdominal examination in the diagnosis of non-ruptured abdominal aortic aneurysm. *Accid Emerg Nurs.* 2004;12:99–107.
13. Quill DS, Colgan MP, Sumner DS. Ultrasonic screening for the detection of abdominal aortic aneurysms. *Surg Clin North Am.* 1989;69:713–720.
14. Barkin AZ, Rosen CL. Ultrasound detection of abdominal aortic aneurysm. *Emerg Med Clin N Am.* 2004;22:675–682.
15. Schwartz SA, Taljanovic MS, Smyth S. CT findings of rupture, impending rupture, and contained rupture of abdominal aortic aneurysms. *Am J Roentgenol.* 2007;188:W57–W62.
16. Sanders C. Current role of conventional and digital aortography in the diagnosis of aortic disease. *J Thorac Imaging.* 1990;5:48–59.
17. Ghansah JN, Murphy JT. Complications of major aortic and lower extremity vascular surgery. *Semin Cardiothorac Vasc Anesth.* 2004;8:335–361.
18. Chuter TAM. Fenestrated and branched stent-grafts for thoracoabdominal, pararenal, and juxtarenal aortic aneurysm repair. *Semin Vasc Surg.* 2007;2:90–96.
19. EVAR trial participants. Endovascular aneurysm repair versus open repair in patients with abdominal aortic aneurysm (EVAR trial 1): randomized controlled trial. *Lancet.* 2005;365(9478):2179–2186.
20. Prinssen M, Buskens E, de Jong SE, et al. DREAM trial participants. Cost-effectiveness of conventional and endovascular repair of abdominal aortic aneurysms: results of a randomized trial. *J Vasc Surg.* 2007;46:883–890.
21. Cambria RP, Brewster DC, Abbott WM, et al. Transperitoneal versus retroperitoneal approach for aortic reconstruction: a randomized prospective study. *J Vasc Surg.* 1990;11:314–324.
22. Connolly JE, Ingegno M, Wilson SE. Preservation of the pelvic circulation during infrarenal aortic surgery. *Cardiovasc Surg.* 1996;4:65–70.
23. Ferrari M, Adami D, Del Corso A, et al. Laparoscopy-assisted abdominal aortic aneurysm repair. Early and middle term results of a consecutive series of 122 cases. *J Vasc Surg.* 2006;43:695–700.
24. Coggia M, DeCenti I, Javerliat I, et al. Total laparoscopic infrarenal aortic aneurysm repair: preliminary results. *J Vasc Surg.* 2004;40:448–454.
25. Vasdekis SN, Argentou M, Kakisis JD, et al. A global assessment of the inflammatory response elicited upon open abdominal aortic aneurysm repair. *Vasc Endovasc Surg.* 2008;42:47–53.
26. Swartbol P, Truedsson L, Norgren L. The inflammatory response and its consequence for the clinical

outcome following aortic aneurysm repair. *Eur J Vasc Endovasc Surg*. 2001;21:393–400.

27. Bown MJ, Nicholson ML, Bell PR, Sayers RD. The systemic inflammatory response syndrome, organ failure, and mortality after abdominal aortic aneurysm repair. *J Vasc Surg*. 2003;37:600–606.

28. Patterson BO, Holt PJ, Hinchliffe R, Loftus IM, Thompson MM. Predicting risk in elective abdominal aortic aneurysm repair: a systematic review of current evidence. *Eur J Vasc Endovasc Surg*. 2008;36:637–645.

29. Brimacombe J, Berry A. Hemodynamic management in ruptured abdominal aortic aneurysm. *Postgrad Med J*. 1994;70:252–256.

30. Tambyraja AL, Murie JA, Chalmers RT. Prediction of outcome after abdominal aortic aneurysm rupture. *J Vasc Surg*. 2008;47:222–230.

31. Laukontaus SJ, Lepantalo M, Hynninen M, et al. Prediction of survival after 48-h of intensive care following open surgical repair of ruptured abdominal aortic aneurysm. *Eur J Vasc Endovasc Surg*. 2005; 30:509–515.

32. Hertzer NR, Beven EG, Young JR, et al. Coronary artery disease in peripheral vascular patients: a classification of 1000 coronary angiograms and results of surgical management. *Ann Surg*. 1984;199:223–233.

33. Fleisher LA, Beckman JA, Brown KA, et al. ACC/AHA 2007 Guidelines on Perioperative Cardiovascular Evaluation and Care for Noncardiac Surgery: Executive Summary: A Report of the American College of Cardiology/American Heart Association Task Force on Practice Guidelines (Writing Committee to Revise the 2002 Guidelines on Perioperative Cardiovascular Evaluation for Noncardiac Surgery): Developed in Collaboration With the American Society of Echocardiography, American Society of Nuclear Cardiology, Heart Rhythm Society, Society of Cardiovascular Anesthesiologists, Society for Cardiovascular Angiography and Interventions, Society for Vascular Medicine and Biology, and Society for Vascular Surgery. *Circulation*. 2007; 116:1971–1996.

34. McFalls EO, Ward HB, Moritz TE, et al. Coronary-artery revascularization before elective major vascular surgery. *N Engl J Med*. 2004;351:2795–2804.

35. Poldermans D, Bax JJ, Schouten O, Dutch Echocardiographic Cardiac Risk Evaluation Applying Stress Echo Study Group, et al. Should major vascular surgery be delayed because of preoperative cardiac testing in intermediate-risk patients receiving beta-blocker therapy with tight heart rate control? *J Am Coll Cardiol*. 2006;48:964–969.

36. Poldermans D, Schouten O, Vidakovic R, DECREASE Study Group, et al. A clinical randomized trial to evaluate the safety of a noninvasive approach in high-risk patients undergoing major vascular surgery: the DECREASE-V Pilot Study. *J Am Coll Cardiol*. 2007; 49(17):1763–1769.

37. Parent MC, Rinfret S. The unresolved issues with risk stratification and management of patients with coro-

nary artery disease undergoing major vascular surgery. *Can J Anaesth*. 2008;55:542–556.

38. Ruddy JM, Yarbrough W, Brothers T, Robison J, Elliott B. Abdominal aortic aneurysm and significant coronary artery disease: strategies and options. *South Med J*. 2008;101(11):1113–1116.

39. Mazer CD. Con: Combined coronary and vascular surgery is not better than separate procedures. *J Cardiothorac Vasc Anesth*. 1998;12:228–230.

40. Finegan BA, Kashkari I. Pro: Combined coronary and vascular surgery is better than separate procedures. *J Cardiothorac Vasc Anesth*. 1998;12:225–227.

41. King RC, Parrino PE, Hurst JL, Shockey KS, Tribble CG, Kron IL. Simultaneous coronary artery bypass grafting and abdominal aneurysm repair decreases stay and costs. *Ann Thorac Surg*. 1998;66:1273–1276.

42. Autschbach R, Falk V, Walther T, et al. Simultaneous coronary bypass and abdominal aortic surgery in patients with severe coronary disease–indication and results. *Eur J Cardiothorac Surg*. 1995;9:678–683.

43. Ruby ST, Whittemore AD, Couch NP, et al. Coronary artery disease in patients requiring abdominal aortic aneurysm repair. Selective use of a combined operation. *Ann Surg*. 1985;201:758–764.

44. Gade PV, Ascher E, Cunningham JN, et al. Combined coronary artery bypass grafting and abdominal aortic aneurysm repair. *Am J Surg*. 1998;176:144–146.

45. Morimoto K, Taniguchi I, Miyasaka S, Aoki T, Kato I, Yamaga T. Usefulness of one-stage coronary artery bypass grafting on the beating heart and abdominal aortic aneurysm repair. *Ann Thorac Cardiovasc Surg*. 2004;10:29–33.

46. Minami H, Mukohara N, Obo H, et al. Simultaneous operation of off pump coronary artery bypass and abdominal aortic aneurysm repair. *Jpn J Thorac Cardiovasc Surg*. 2005;53:133–137.

47. Blackbourne LH, Tribble CG, Langenburg SE, et al. Optimal timing of abdominal aortic aneurysm repair after coronary artery revascularization. *Ann Surg*. 1994;219:693–696.

48. Onwudike M, Barnard M, Singh-Ranger R, Raphael M, Adiseshiah M. For debate: concomitant critical coronary arterial disease and abdominal aortic aneurysm–timing of corrective procedures. *Cardiovasc Surg*. 2000;8:333–339.

49. O'Connor MS, Licina MG, Kraenzler EJ, et al. Perioperative management and outcome of patients having cardiac surgery combined with abdominal aortic aneurysm resection. *J Cardiothor Vasc Anesth*. 1994; 8:519–526.

50. Cunningham AJ. Anaesthesia for abdominal aortic surgery–a review (Part I). *Can J Anaesth*. 1989;36: 426–444.

51. London MJ, Hollenberg M, Wong MG, et al. Intraoperative myocardial ischemia: localization by continuous 12-lead electrocardiography. *Anesthesiology*. 1988;69:232–241.

52. Mark JB. Multimodal detection of perioperative myocardial ischemia. *Tex Heart Inst J*. 2005;32:461–466.

53. Ryan T, Page R, Bouchier-Hayes D, Cunningham AJ. Transoesophageal pulsed wave Doppler measurement of cardiac output during major vascular surgery: comparison with the thermodilution technique. *Br J Anaesth*. 1992;69:101–104.

54. Mahmood F, Matyal R, Maslow A, et al. Myocardial performance index is a predictor of outcome after abdominal aortic aneurysm repair. *J Cardiothorac Vasc Anesth*. 2008;22:706–712.

55. Antonini M, Meloncelli S, Dantimi C, et al. The PiCCO system with brachial-axillary artery access in hemodynamic monitoring during surgery of abdominal aortic aneurysm. *Minerva Anestesiol*. 2001;67:447–456.

56. Lafanechère A, Albaladejo P, Raux M, et al. Cardiac output measurement during infrarenal aortic surgery: echo-esophageal Doppler versus thermodilution catheter. *J Cardiothorac Vasc Anesth*. 2006;20:26–30.

57. Roizen MF, Beaupre PN, Alpert RA, et al. Monitoring with two-dimensional transesophageal echocardiography. Comparison of myocardial function in patients undergoing supraceliac, suprarenal-infraceliac, or infrarenal aortic occlusion. *J Vasc Surg*. 1984;1:300–305.

58. Gelman S. The pathophysiology of aortic cross-clamping and unclamping. *Anesthesiology*. 1995;82: 1026–1060.

59. Gillespie DL, Connelly GP, Arkoff HM, et al. Left ventricular dysfunction during infrarenal abdominal aortic aneurysm repair. *Am J Surg*. 1994;168: 144–147.

60. Mahmood F, Matyal R, Subramaniam B, et al. Transmitral flow propagation velocity and assessment of diastolic function during abdominal aortic aneurysm repair. *J Cardiothorac Vasc Anesth*. 2007;21: 486–491.

61. Meierhenrich R, Gauss A, Anhaeupl T, Schütz W. Analysis of diastolic function in patients undergoing aortic aneurysm repair and impact on hemodynamic response to aortic cross-clamping. *J Cardiothorac Vasc Anesth*. 2005;19:165–172.

62. Schuetz W, Radermacher P, Goertz A, Georgieff M, Gauss A. Cardiac function in patients with treated hypertension during aortic aneurysm repair. *J Cardiothorac Vasc Anesth*. 1998;12:33–37.

63. Fayad A, Yang H, Nathan H, Bryson GL, Cina CS. Acute diastolic dysfunction in thoracoabdominal aortic aneurysm surgery. *Can J Anaesth*. 2006;53: 168–173.

64. Wozniak MF, LaMuraglia GM, Musch G. Anesthesia for open abdominal aortic surgery. *Int Anesthesiol Clin*. 2005;43:61–78.

65. Attia RR, Murphy JD, Snider M, Lappas DG, Darling RC, Lowenstein E. Myocardial ischemia due to infrarenal aortic cross-clamping during aortic surgery in patients with severe coronary artery disease. *Circulation*. 1976;53:961–965.

66. Gooding JM, Archie JP Jr, McDowell H. Hemodynamic response to infrarenal aortic cross-clamping in patients with and without coronary artery disease. *Crit Care Med*. 1980;8:382–385.

67. Johnston WE, Balestrieri FJ, Plonk G, D'Souza V, Howard G. The influence of periaortic collateral vessels on the intraoperative hemodynamic effects of acute aortic occlusion in patients with aorto-occlusive disease or abdominal aortic aneurysms. *Anesthesiology*. 1987;66:386–389.

68. O'Toole DP, Broe P, Bouchier-Hayes D, Cunningham AJ. Perioperative haemodynamic changes during aortic vascular surgery: comparison between occlusive and aneurysm disease states. *Br J Anaesth*. 1988; 60:322.

69. Walker PM, Johnston KW. Changes in cardiac output during major vascular surgery. *Am J Surg*. 1980; 140:602–605.

70. Ueda N, Dohi S, Akamatsu S, et al. Pulmonary arterial and right ventricular responses to prophylactic albumin administration before aortic unclamping during abdominal aortic aneurysmectomy. *Anesth Analg*. 1998;87:1020–1026.

71. Bitoh H, Nakanishi K, Takeda S, Kim C, Mori M, Sakamoto A. Repair of an infrarenal abdominal aortic aneurysm is associated with persistent left ventricular diastolic dysfunction. *J Nippon Med Sch*. 2007;74: 393–401.

72. Roberts K, Revell M, Youssef H, Bradbury AW, Adam DJ. Hypotensive resuscitation in patients with ruptured abdominal aortic aneurysm. *Eur J Vasc Endovasc Surg*. 2006;31:339–344.

73. Bickell WH, Wall MJ, Pepe PE, et al. Immediate versus delayed fluid resuscitation for hypotensive patients with penetrating torso injuries. *N Engl J Med*. 1994;331:1105–1109.

74. Mattox KL, Bickell WH, Pepe PE. Prospective, randomized evaluation of antishock MAST in post traumatic hypotension. *J Trauma*. 1986;26:779–786.

75. Nisanevich V, Felsenstein I, Almogy G, Weissman C, Einav S, Matot I. Effect of intraoperative fluid management on outcome after intraabdominal surgery. *Anesthesiology*. 2005;103:25–32.

76. Joshi GP. Intraoperative fluid restriction improves outcome after major elective gastrointestinal surgery. *Anesth Analg*. 2005;101:601–605.

77. McArdle GT, Price G, Lewis A, et al. Positive fluid balance is associated with complications after elective open infrarenal abdominal aortic aneurysm repair. *Eur J Vasc Endovasc Surg*. 2007;34:522–527.

78. Adesanya A, Rosero E, Timaran C, Clagett P, Johnston WE. Intraoperative fluid restriction predicts improved outcomes in major vascular surgery. *Vasc Endovasc Surg*. 2008–2009;42(6):531–536.

79. Zavrakidis N. Intravenous fluids for abdominal aortic surgery. *Cochrane Database of Systematic Reviews*. 2000, Issue 3. Art. No.: CD000991. DOI: 10.1002/14651858.CD000991

80. O'Hara PJ, Hertzer NR, Krajewski LP, Cox GS, Beven EG. Reduction in the homologous blood requirement for abdominal aortic aneurysm repair by the use of preadmission autologous blood donation. *Surgery*. 1994;115:69–76.

81. Tedesco M, Sapienza P, Burchi C, et al. Preoperative blood storage and intraoperative blood recovery in elective treatment of abdominal aorta aneurysm. *Ann Ital Chir.* 1996;67:399–403.

82. Kawano D, Komori K, Furuyama T, et al. Usefulness of preadmission autologous blood donation and intraoperative autotransfusion using the "cell saver" for the patients with abdominal aortic aneurysm repair. *Fukuoka Igaku Zasshi.* 2000;91:165–169.

83. Komai H, Naito Y, Iwasaki Y, Iwahashi M, Fujiwara K, Noguchi Y. Autologous blood donation with recombinant human erythropoietin for abdominal aortic aneurysm surgery. *Surg Today.* 2000;30:511–515.

84. Takagi H, Sekino S, Kato T, Matsuno Y, Umemoto T. Intraoperative autotransfusion in abdominal aortic aneurysm surgery: meta-analysis of randomized controlled trials. *Arch Surg.* 2007;142:1098–1101.

85. Serrano FJ, Moñux G, Aroca M. Should the cell saver autotransfusion system be routinely used in elective aortic surgery? *Ann Vasc Surg.* 2000;14:663–668.

86. Huber TS, McGorray SP, Carlton LC, et al. Intraoperative autologous transfusion during elective infrarenal aortic reconstruction: a decision analysis model. *J Vasc Surg.* 1997;25:984–993.

87. Suding PN, Wilson SE. Intraoperative autotransfusion in abdominal aortic aneurysm surgery: meta-analysis of randomized controlled trials—invited critique. *Arch Surg.* 2007;142:1102.

88. Torella F, Haynes SL, Kirwan CC, Bhatt AN, McCollum CN. Acute normovolemic hemodilution and intraoperative cell salvage in aortic surgery. *J Vasc Surg.* 2002;36:31–34.

89. Wolowczyk L, Nevin M, Day A, Smith FC, Baird RN, Lamont PM. The effect of acute normovolaemic haemodilution on the inflammatory response and clinical outcome in abdominal aortic aneurysm repair–results of a pilot trial. *Eur J Vasc Endovasc Surg.* 2005;30:12–19.

90. Wolowczyk L, Nevin M, Smith FC, Baird RN, Lamont PM. Haemodilutional effect of standard fluid management limits the effectiveness of acute normovolaemic haemodilution in AAA surgery–results of a pilot trial. *Eur J Vasc Endovasc Surg.* 2003;26:405–411.

91. Nishimori M, Ballantyne JC, Low JH. Epidural pain relief versus systemic opioid-based pain relief for abdominal aortic surgery. *Cochrane Database Syst Rev.* 2006;19:3. CD005059.

92. Her C, Kizelshteyn G, Walker V, Hayes D, Lees DE. Combined epidural and general anesthesia for abdominal aortic surgery. *J Cardiothorac Anesth.* 1990;4:552–557.

93. Lunn JK, Dannemiller FJ, Stanley TH. Cardiovascular responses to clamping of the aorta during epidural and general anesthesia. *Anesth Analg.* 1979;58:372–376.

94. Reiz S, Nath EP, Freidman A, Backlund U, Olsson B, Rais O. Effects of thoracic epidural block and beta-1 adrenoceptor agonist prenalterol on the cardiovascular response to infrarenal aortic cross clamping in man. *Acta Anaesth Scand.* 1979;23:395–403.

95. Bunt TJ, Manczuk M, Varley K. Continuous epidural anesthesia for aortic surgery: thoughts on peer review and safety. *Surgery.* 1987;101:706–714.

96. Bush RL, Lin PH, Reddy PP, et al. Epidural analgesia in patients with chronic obstructive pulmonary disease undergoing transperitoneal abdominal aortic aneurysmorraphy—a multi-institutional analysis. *Cardiovasc Surg.* 2003;11:179–184.

97. Kalko Y, Ugurlucan M, Basaran M, et al. Epidural anaesthesia and mini-laparotomy for the treatment of abdominal aortic aneurysms in patients with severe chronic obstructive pulmonary disease. *Acta Chir Belg.* 2007;107:307–312.

98. Allen D, Dahlgren N, Nellgård B. Risks and recommendations in Bechterew disease. Paraparesis after epidural anesthesia. *Lakartidningen.* 1997;10(94): 4771–4774.

99. Crosby ET, Reid DR, DiPrimio G, Grahovac S. Lumbosacral plexopathy from iliopsoas haematoma after combined general-epidural anaesthesia for abdominal aneurysmectomy. *Can J Anaesth.* 1998; 45:46–51.

100. Shine TS, Greengrass RA, Feinglass NG. Use of continuous paravertebral analgesia to facilitate neurologic assessment and enhance recovery after thoracoabdominal aortic aneurysm repair. *Anesth Analg.* 2004;98:1640–1643.

101. Richardson J, Vowden P, Sabanathan S. Bilateral paravertebral analgesia for major abdominal vascular surgery: a preliminary report. *Anaesthesia.* 1995; 50:995–998.

102. Blay M, Orban JC, Rami L, et al. Efficacy of low-dose intrathecal morphine for postoperative analgesia after abdominal aortic surgery: a double-blind randomized study. *Reg Anesth Pain Med.* 2006;31: 127–133.

103. Fléron MH, Weiskopf RB, Bertrand M, et al. A comparison of intrathecal opioid and intravenous analgesia for the incidence of cardiovascular, respiratory, and renal complications after abdominal aortic surgery. *Anesth Analg.* 2003;97:2–12.

104. Pfeiffer U, Dodson ME, Van Mourik G, Kirby J, McLoughlin GA. Wound instillation for postoperative pain relief: a comparison between bupivacaine and saline in patients undergoing aortic surgery. *Ann Vasc Surg.* 1991;5:80–84.

105. Mukherjee D. "Fast-Track" abdominal aortic aneurysm repair. *Vasc Surg.* 2003;37(5):329–334.

106. Lassonde J, Laurendeau F. Blunt injury of the abdominal aorta. *Ann Surg.* 1981;194:745–748.

107. Crabb GM, McQuillen KK. Subtle abdominal aortic injury after blunt chest trauma. *J Emerg Med.* 2006;31:29–31.

108. Roth SM, Wheeler JR, Gregory RT, et al. Blunt injury of the abdominal aorta: a review. *J Trauma.* 1997;42:748–755.

109. Adam DJ, Ludlam CA, Ruckley CV, Bradbury AW. Coagulation and fibrinolysis in patients undergoing operation for ruptured and nonruptured infrarenal abdominal aortic aneurysms. *J Vasc Surg.* 1999; 30:641–650.

110. Skagius E, Siegbahn A, Bergqvist D, Henriksson AE. Fibrinolysis in patients with an abdominal aortic

aneurysm with special emphasis on rupture and shock. *J Thromb Haemost.* 2008;6:147–150.

111. Tambyraja AL, Dawson AR, Murie JA, Chalmers RT. Cardiac troponin I predicts outcome after ruptured abdominal aortic aneurysm repair. *Br J Surg.* 2005;92:824–827.

112. Ali ZA, Callaghan CJ, Ali AA, et al. Perioperative myocardial injury after elective open abdominal aortic aneurysm repair predicts outcome. *Eur J Vasc Endovasc Surg.* 2008;35:413–419.

113. Greenway CA, Embil J, Orr PH, et al. Nosocomial pneumonia on general and surgical wards in a tertiary care hospital. *Infect Control Hosp Epidemiol.* 1997;18:749–756.

114. Sladen RN, Endo E, Harrison T. Two hour versus 22-hour creatinine clearence in critically ill patients. *Anesthesiology.* 1987;67:1013–1016.

115. Luft FC, Hamburger RJ, Dyer JK, Szwed JJ, Kleit SA. Acute renal failure following operation for aortic aneurysm. *Surg Gynecol Obstet.* 1975;141:374–378.

116. Darling RC, Brewster DC. Elective treatment of abdominal aortic aneurysms. *World J Surg.* 1980;4:661–667.

117. Gamulin Z, Forster A, Morel D, et al. Effect of infrarenal crossclamping on renal hemodynamics in humans. *Anesthesiology.* 1984;61:394–399.

118. Berkowitz HD, Shetty S. Renin release and renal cortical ischemia following aortic cross clamping. *Arch Surg.* 1974;109:612–617.

119. Knos GB, Berry AJ, Isaacson IJ, Weitz FI. Intraoperative urinary output and postoperative blood urea nitrogen and creatinine levels in patients undergoing aortic reconstructive surgery. *J Clin Anesth.* 1989;1:181–185.

120. Benoit AG, Campbell BL, Tanner JR, et al. Risk factors and prevalence of perioperative cognitive dysfunction in abdominal aneurysm patients. *J Vasc Surg.* 2005;42:884–890.

121. Szilagyi DE, Hageman JH, Smith RF, et al. Spinal cord damage in surgery of the abdominal aorta. *Surgery.* 1978;83:38–56.

122. Rosenthal D. Risk factors for spinal cord ischemia after abdominal aortic operations. Is it preventable? *J Vasc Surg.* 1999;30:391–399.

123. Mulcare RJ, Royster TS, Weiss HJ, Phillips LL. Disseminated intravascular coagulation as a complication of abdominal aortic aneurysm repair. *Ann Surg.* 1974;180:343–349.

124. Goto H, Kimoto A, Kawaguchi H, et al. Surgical treatment of abdominal aortic aneurysm complicated with chronic disseminated intravascular coagulopathy. *J Cardiovasc Surg (Torino).* 1985;26:280–282.

125. Aboulafia DM, Aboulafia ED. Aortic aneurysm-induced disseminated intravascular coagulation. *Ann Vasc Surg.* 1996;10:396–405.

126. Rowlands TE, Norfolk D, Homer-Vanniasinkam S. Chronic disseminated intravascular coagulopathy cured by abdominal aortic aneurysm repair. *Cardiovasc Surg.* 2000;8:292–294.

127. Oba J, Shiiya N, Matsui Y, Goda T, Sakuma M, Yasuda K. Preoperative disseminated intravascular coagulation (DIC) associated with aortic aneurysm—does it need to be corrected before surgery? *Surg Today.* 1995;25:1011–1014.

128. Imparato AM. Abdominal aortic surgery: prevention of lower limb ischemia. *Surgery.* 1983;93:112–116.

129. Kuhan G, Raptis S. Trash foot following operations involving abdominal aorta. *Aust N Z J Surg.* 1997;67:21–24.

Renal Protection Strategies

15

Mark Stafford-Smith, Chad Hughes,
Andrew D. Shaw, and Madhav Swaminathan

Introduction

The well-known quote from the renal physiologist Dr. Homer Smith as he proposed that "...the composition of the blood is determined not by what the mouth ingests but by what the kidneys keep.."[1] highlights not only the kidneys' domain of influence, but why even the smallest functional perturbations can have widespread effects. The kidney plays a central role in homeostasis, including keeping extracellular composition and fluid volume constant, while excreting toxins and metabolic waste in the urine. Acute kidney injury (AKI) is a major complication of aortic surgery and highly associated with poor outcome.

As a collection of procedures, there are probably no interventions more associated with postoperative AKI or dialysis than those involving the treatment of aortic pathology. This is due not only to the character of aortic interventions, which are often emergent and commonly involve disease close to the origin of the renal vessels, but also to the numerous kidney insults that are unavoidable as part of these procedures. Finally, the medical conditions that typically contribute to aortic disease make these patients vulnerable to perioperative AKI.

This chapter reviews renal physiology and pathophysiologic states as they relate to aortic surgery practice, and then addresses strategies for recognizing and managing patients at risk for renal failure.

Renal Anatomy and Physiology

Gross Anatomy/Ultrastructure (Fig. 15.1a and b)

The normal kidney is a reddish-brown ovoid organ measuring approximately 10 cm long, 5 cm wide, and 2.5 cm thick with a medial margin deeply indented and concave at its middle. The hilus is the vertical cleft in the medial aspect that lies at the level of the first lumbar vertebra and transmits structures entering and leaving the kidney. The kidneys are retroperitoneal; the right is "crowded" by the liver and slightly lower than the left. Embryologically, the kidneys derive from the mesoderm and form below the pelvic rim, passing up and along the paravertebral gutters to lie in their adult position by the ninth week of gestation. During each kidney's ascent, its blood supply comes from successive sources, and a residual accessory artery sometimes enters the lower pole of the kidney from the aorta. The rudimentary organs are adjacent and occasionally join forming a single large fused kidney, the ascent of which is presumably impeded by the inferior mesenteric artery; hence, the pelvic position of the adult "horseshoe" kidney. A thick fibrous capsule

M. Stafford-Smith (✉)
Department of Anesthesiology,
Duke University Medical Center, Durham,
NC 27710, USA
e-mail: STAFF002@mc.duke.edu

K. Subramaniam et al. (eds.), *Anesthesia and Perioperative Care for Aortic Surgery*,
DOI 10.1007/978-0-387-85922-4_15, © Springer Science+Business Media, LLC 2011

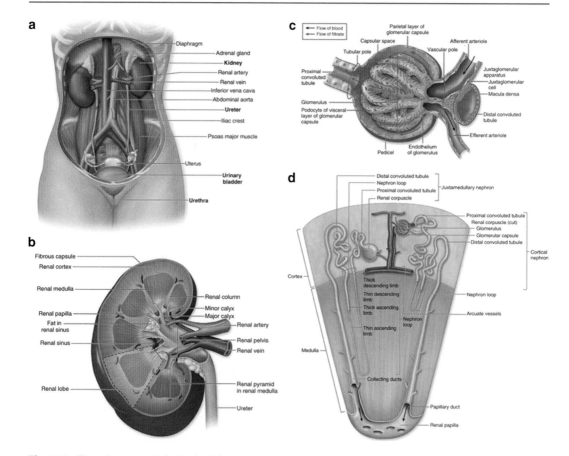

Fig. 15.1 The urinary tract includes the kidneys, ureters, urinary bladder, and urethra (**a**). A coronal section of the right kidney demonstrates the highly organized renal parenchyma and vasculature (**b**). Approximately 20% of plasma entering each glomerulus will be filtered into the renal tubule (**c**). The functional unit of the kidney is the nephron (**d**), which will pass through the specialized capillary wall into Bowman's capsule and enter the tubule to be processed and generate urine (From: (**a–d**) used with permission from http://academic.kellogg.cc.mi.us/herbrandsonc/bio201_McKinley/Urinary%20System.htm - site accessed March 10, 2009)

surrounds each kidney separated from the more loosely applied renal fascia by a fatty layer.

Inspection of the cut surface of a kidney reveals an outer capsule surrounding a paler cortex, which in turn encircles the darker, conical pyramids of the renal medulla. Visible in each pyramid are radial striations (medullary rays) that converge towards the hilus forming renal columns. The funnel-like spaces separating medullary pyramids are termed calyces, and these merge in the hilus forming the renal pelvis, which exits the kidney quickly narrowing to become the ureter that conveys urine on to the bladder. Each lobe of the kidney (pyramid and its covering of cortex) produces collecting tubules that discharge urine via renal papillae at the entrance of each

pyramid into the calyceal system. The collecting tubules carry urine from deep within the radial striations where it is generated by the functional units of the kidney, the nephrons.

Usually, a single renal artery enters the hilum anterior to the renal pelvis and divides many times to produce arcuate arteries that travel along the boundary between cortex and outer medulla. Arcuate arteries give rise to interlobular arteries that produce large numbers of afferent arterioles, which supply each glomerulus with a capillary tuft, efferent arteriole, and peritubular capillaries. The glomerular capillary tuft is the porous barrier where plasma elements filter from the vascular to tubular space. An approximately parallel venous system conveys blood back to the renal vein and inferior vena cava. The renal arteries usually lie posterior to the veins at the hilum, and the right renal artery passes behind the inferior vena cava to reach the aorta.

Renal sympathetic innervation is provided by preganglionic fibers from T8-L1 including sensation (colic). Parasympathetic innervation comes from the vagus nerve while the ureters are supplied through spinal segments S2–S4.

Ultrastructure (Fig. 15.1c and d)

A single kidney contains approximately 1×10^6 tightly packed nephrons. Each nephron consists of a tuft of leaky capillaries and a tubule. At its proximal end in the cortex, an expanded portion of the tubule (Bowman's capsule) envelopes the capillary tuft to form a specialized structure for filtering plasma (the glomerulus), while at its distal end in the medulla this tube delivers processed urine to the collecting ducts. The vascular–tubular filtration interface within the glomerulus is highly specialized including fenestrated negatively charged capillary endothelial cells and tubular epithelial cells (podocytes) separated by a basement membrane. As effluent filters into the tubule, it enters the highly metabolically active proximal convoluted tubule. This serpentine segment then merges with the loop of Henle, a straighter portion that courses directly toward the medulla, with a hairpin turn, then away from the medulla. Nephrons are classified by the location of their glomeruli into juxtamedullary (15%) and cortical (85%) types; these have differing functions due to their different loops of Henle. Only loops of Henle from juxtamedullary nephrons course deep enough into the medulla to significantly participate in countercurrent exchange, a mechanism that facilitates the formation of highly concentrated urine. Effluent continues through the loops of Henle back to the cortex into the distal convoluted tubule and finally the collecting duct. Each collecting duct accepts effluent from numerous distal convoluted tubules. Feedback control of tubular function comes in part from a cluster of cells derived from the distal convoluted tubule and afferent arteriole known as the juxtaglomerular apparatus. It is the combined actions of the specialized segments of the nephron that forms urine and returns the vast majority of glomerular filtrate to the circulation.

Cells and proteins larger than 60–70 kDa are prevented from crossing the selectively permeable barrier of the glomerulus, and typically only 25% of the plasma elements pass into Bowman's capsule. Notably, abnormalities of this barrier can occur with disease that permit much larger proteins and even red blood cells to enter the tubule; nephrotic syndrome (proteinuria >3.5 g/24 h) or glomerulonephritis (hematuria and proteinuria) may result. The peritubular capillaries derive from an efferent arteriole, which itself is generated from the convergence of glomerular capillaries; this arrangement involving two capillary beds connected in series by arterioles is unusual in the body. Peritubular capillaries that follow the loops of Henle deep into the medulla are known as vasa recta.

Correlation of Structure and Function

Renal tissues constitute only 0.4% of body weight but receive 25% of cardiac output making them by far the most highly perfused of any major organ. For comparison, this flow is eightfold higher per gram of tissue than heavily exercising muscle and is key to plasma filtration rates as high as 125–140 ml/min in adults. Such filtration generates a huge volume of tubular effluent, equivalent to a can of soda every 3 min, but reabsorption allows only 1% of this (approximately 4 ml per 12 oz soft drink) to emerge from the kidney as urine. Beyond volume control, tubular processing also closely regulates solute homeostasis (extracellular sodium, potassium, hydrogen ion, bicarbonate, and glucose) and clearance of nitrogenous and other waste products (e.g., creatinine, urea, bilirubin, toxins, and many classes of drugs). Finally, the kidneys also serve endocrine, exocrine, immune, and metabolic functions.

A common measure to reflect the overall yield of water and solutes from filtration is the glomerular filtration rate (GFR), expressed as the volume of plasma filtered per minute (mL/min). Plasma filtration from the vascular space into Bowman's capsule varies based on surface area and permeability characteristics of the glomerular barrier (ultrafiltration constant – Kf) and gradients between capillary (P_{GC}) and oncotic pressures (π_{GC}). P_{GC} is directly influenced by renal artery pressure, particularly by changes in arteriolar tone, both upstream (afferent) and downstream (efferent) from the glomerulus. A major increase in afferent arteriolar tone, as occurs with angiotensin II or sympathetic stimulation, causes a fall in filtration pressure and thus GFR. Milder angiotensin or sympathetic effects lead to selective efferent arteriolar vasoconstriction, which increases filtration pressure and GFR. Afferent arteriolar dilatation enhances glomerular flow and increases GFR by raising glomerular capillary pressure. The π_{GC} is directly dependent on plasma oncotic pressure.

Renal vasculature autoregulation maintains relatively constant rates of blood flow and filtration over a range of arterial blood pressures; however, since perfusion far exceeds oxygen demand for the whole kidney, it is unclear whether this response facilitates limiting excessive flow to the delicate glomeruli or optimization of oxygen delivery. The myogenic reflex theory holds that increasing arterial pressure causes afferent arteriolar stretch that triggers reflex vasoconstriction; likewise, pressure decreases cause afferent arteriolar dilatation. The other autoregulatory mechanism involves tubuloglomerular feedback through the juxtaglomerular apparatus – when renal blood flow and GFR decrease, the juxtaglomerular apparatus, sensing a decrease in chloride delivery, responds by effecting afferent arteriolar dilatation and increased glomerular barrier perfusion pressure, thus returning GFR to previous levels. Tubular chloride concentration also constitutes a feedback signal for control of efferent arteriolar tone. Declining chloride delivery to the distal convoluted tubule is sensed by the juxtaglomerular apparatus triggering the release of renin and the formation of angiotensin II.

The energy consuming Na+/K+ATPase pump actively transports sodium from the nontubular (serosal) surface of cells and chloride ions follow. Also strongly coupled to proximal sodium reabsorption are reuptake of glucose, amino acids, and other organic compounds, but water movement is passive and osmotically linked. Interestingly, higher peritubular capillary pressures (e.g., related to inferior vena cava obstruction) oppose water reuptake and increase urine output. The proximal tubule accounts for approximately two thirds of reabsorption, and a further 15% comes from the loop of Henle. Beyond the proximal tubule, no further active sodium transport occurs until the loop of Henle medullary thick ascending limb (mTAL). When fluid intake is limited, maximum water retention and solute excretion rely on the kidney's ability to produce a concentrated urine. Although water follows osmotic gradients out of the descending loop of Henle, the thin ascending and mTAL portions are relatively water-impermeable and prevent water return. The remaining effluent passes to the distal tubule and the collecting duct where water reuptake is entirely controlled by antidiuretic hormone (ADH). ADH increases permeability allowing passive water diffusion back to the circulation (under considerable osmotic pressure). The posterior pituitary responds to increased extracellular sodium concentration or osmolality by releasing ADH. Absolute or relative reductions in intravascular fluid volume also trigger ADH release through arterial and atrial baroreceptors. "Inappropriate" ADH release can occur in response to physiologic stresses such as surgery and cause renal cortical vasoconstriction producing a shift in blood flow to the hypoxia-prone renal medulla.

Drops in blood pressure, sympathetic stimulation, and increased tubular chloride trigger renin release from the juxtaglomerular apparatus. Sympathetic stimulation also causes aldosterone release. Renin converts circulating angiotensinogen to angiotensin I, which is then converted to angiotensin II (ATII) in the lungs; this potent vasoconstrictor raises blood pressure and hence renal flow rates. ATII also promotes proximal tubular sodium reabsorption and ADH and aldosterone release. Aldosterone and ADH contribute to intravascular volume expansion by facilitating sodium and water reabsorption from the distal tubule and collecting duct.

Volume expansion and vasoconstrictor effects are balanced by the actions of atrial natriuretic peptide (ANP), nitric oxide, and the renal prostaglandin system. Under volume expansion conditions, atrial stretch triggers ANP release. ANP inhibits renin and aldosterone release, opposes the actions of angiotensin II,[2] and blocks sodium reabsorption in the distal tubule and collecting duct. ANP also increases GFR and urine output through renal artery vasodilation. Nitric oxide and prostaglandin production within the kidney also opposes renal sympathetic and angiotensin II effects, promoting sodium and water excretion and participating in tubuloglomerular feedback.[3] Renal ischemia and other stress states including a drop in blood pressure stimulate renal prostaglandin production through cyclooxygenase and phospholipase A_2 enzymes.[4]

Although the reflex phenomenon known as ischemic preconditioning that involves a brief exposure to ischemia that attenuates injury due to subsequent ischemic episodes is present in the kidney, the clinical relevance of this adenosine receptor-mediated phenomenon remains unclear.[3]

Clinical Assessment and Definitions of AKI

Most agree that urine output correlates poorly as a measure of perioperative renal function (Fig. 15.2)[5]; however, much can be learned assessing clearance of circulating substances and urine inspection.

Filtration is the most clinically assessed kidney function. Filtration function guides drug dosing and aids in preoperative risk stratification, but acute perioperative declines are also important since they indicate AKI and predict a more complicated postoperative course.[6] GFR normally ranges between 90 and 140 mL/min and refers to the plasma volume filtered by the kidneys per unit time. As a rule of thumb, GFR is 10 mL/min greater in men than women and declines 1% per year after age 30. In addition to gender and age, GFR is related to body weight and to some extent ethnicity. GFR values below 60 mL/min are considered impaired and rates below 15 mL/min often require dialysis.

Although more "ideal" substances exist to assess GFR, the most inexpensive and practical

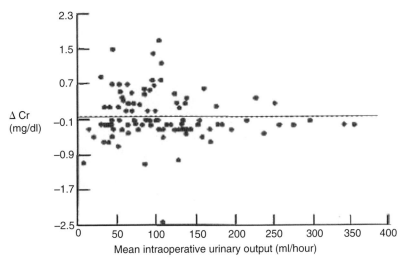

Fig. 15.2 Perioperative urine flow is commonly reported in renal preservation studies, and monitored by clinicians to assess kidney function despite questionable evidence that this variable is a meaningful assessment of perioperative AKI. Data from a study contrasting postoperative rises in serum creatinine (Δ Cr) with urine output after aortic surgery highlights that lack of correlation between these two variables (Used with permission from Alpert et al.[2])

test involves creatinine. Despite creatinine's limitations, its proven usefulness in numerous clinical settings cannot be disputed relative to other currently available markers. Although more "ideal" substances and other "early biomarkers" of AKI are being evaluated as clinical tools, none is yet ready to replace creatinine.

Using urine and blood creatinine tests, estimates of GFR (eGFR) can be made from creatinine clearance (CrCl) determination. Two-hour urine collections are sufficient in stable, critically ill patients to calculate CrCl[4] using the following formula:

$$CrCl(mL/min) = \left(U_{Cr}(mg/dL) \times V(mL)\right) / \left(P_{Cr}(mg/dL) \times time(min)\right)$$

where U_{Cr} = urine creatinine, V = total volume of urine collected P_{Cr} = plasma creatinine, time = collection time

Clinical use of GFR estimation from a single steady-state serum creatinine value is commonly used. Notably, predictive formulas are vulnerable to factors such as fluid shifts, hemodilution, and hemorrhage that may add "unsteadiness" to perioperative GFR estimates from a serum creatinine value. Nonetheless, serum creatinine remains unsurpassed particularly to reflect *trends* of change in renal filtration and to predict outcome even during the perioperative period.[7–9] The Cockroft–Gault equation is one of the most durable predictive formulas,[10] using patient gender, age (years), weight (kg), and serum creatinine (mg/dL) as follows:

$$Cockroft - Gault\ eGFR(mL/min)$$
$$= (140 - age) \times weight(kg) / (Cr \times 72)$$
$$(\times 0.85\ for\ females)$$

A more recent method developed from the Modification of Diet in Renal Disease (MDRD) study that adds other factors including ethnicity (black versus nonblack) has also gained popularity.[11] However, even a detailed MDRD eGFR under ideal conditions often correlates poorly with a "gold standard"-determined GFR.[11]

Several consensus definitions for significant perioperative renal dysfunction exist. The Society of Thoracic Surgeons define postoperative renal failure as new dialysis or creatinine rise beyond 2.0 mg/dL involving at least a 50% increase above baseline.[12] Another definition requires creatinine to rise more than 25% or 0.5 mg/dL (44 µmol/L) within 48 h.[13] The AKIN (AKI Network) definition, a 1.5-fold or 0.3 mg/dL (≥ 26.4 µmol/L) creatinine rise within a 48 h period or more than 6 h of oliguria (less than 0.5 mL/kg/h), is a modification of its predecessor, the Acute Dialysis Quality Initiative (ADQI) Group so-called "RIFLE" criteria.[2]

Disappointment in the ability of traditional tests, such as creatinine, to allow sufficiently early intervention to improve the care of AKI has fueled a rebirth of interest in old indicators, and a search for new "early biomarkers." These include markers of renal adaptive responses to stress, impaired filtration, tubular dysfunction (tubular proteinuria), or cell damage (tubular enzymuria). Although preliminary studies give hope that better tools will become available, serum creatinine continues to be the mainstay of most renal function monitoring strategies.

Risk Factors for Surgery-Related AKI

Numerous factors have been linked with an increased likelihood of postoperative AKI; some are quite specific to aortic surgical procedures and relate primarily to patient and procedural characteristics (Table 15.1, Fig. 15.3). The role of preexisting renal disease as a risk factor is complicated. It is undeniable that patients with severe baseline renal disease need only have a small additional renal insult to lose sufficient renal function to require dialysis thus having acute renal failure. Postoperative patients requiring new dialysis are more likely to have preexisting renal dysfunction. However, although patients with preexisting renal dysfunction as a group have more associated comorbidities, interestingly they *are not* more likely to sustain a perioperative renal injury, described as a relative change in renal function perioperatively (e.g., 50% rise in serum creatinine).

Table 15.1   Summary of renal risk factors and dialysis risk by procedure and surgical strategy

Procedure[a]	Strategy	Procedural renal risk factors					Dialysis risk (x to xxxx)
		Contrast dye[b] (x to xxxx)	Warm renal isch[c] (x to xxxx)	CPB duration (x to xxxx)	Suprarenal AO × Clamp (x to xxxx)	DHCA (approx mins)	
Ascending aortic aneurysm repair	Open	o/x	o	xxx	o	0	x
Ascending hemiarch aortic aneurysm repair	Open	o/x	o	xxxx	o	15	xx
Total aortic arch aneurysm repair							
Arch only	Open	o/x	o	xxxx	o	15	xxx
	Hybrid	xxx	o	o	o	0	xx
Arch and ascending aorta	Open	o/x	o	xxxx	o	15	xx
Open -2 stage	Step 1 (open)	o/x	o	xxxx	o	15	xxx
	Step 2 (stent-graft)	o	xxxx	o	o	0	xx
'Elephant trunk' procedure	Step 1 (open)	o/x	o	xxxx	o	45–60	xxx
	Step 2 (stent-graft)	xxx	o	o	o	0	xx
Descending hemiarch aortic aneurysm repair	Open	o/x	xxxx	o	o	0	xx
	Hybrid	xxxx	o	o	o	0	xx
Descending thoracic aortic aneurysm repair	Open	o/x	xxxx	o	o	0	xx
	Clamp and sew	o/x	xxxx	o	xxx	0	xx
	Gott shunt	o/x	o	o	o	0	xx
	Partial left heart bypass	o/x	o	xxx	o	0	xx
	Stent-graft	xxxx	o	o	o	0	x/xx?
Thoraco-abdominal aortic aneurysm repair	Open	o/x	xxxx	o	xxxx	0	xxx
	Clamp and sew	o/x	o	xxx	o	0	xxx
	Gott shunt	o/x	o	xxxx	o	45	xxx
	Partial left heart bypass	o/x	o	xxxx	o	0	xx/xxx?
	Hybrid	xxxx	xxx	o	o	0	
Abdominal aortic aneurysm repair (± abdominal branch involvement)	Open	o/x	o/xxx	o	o/xxxx	0	xx
	Hybrid	xxxx	o/xxx	o	o	0	xx
	Stent-graft	xxxx	o	o	o	0	x

[a] Emergent procedures typically add renal risk
[b] Preoperative contrast dye administration for imaging is often part of emergent aortic surgery
[c] Debranching reimplantation of a renal artery involves 7–15 min warm renal ischemia

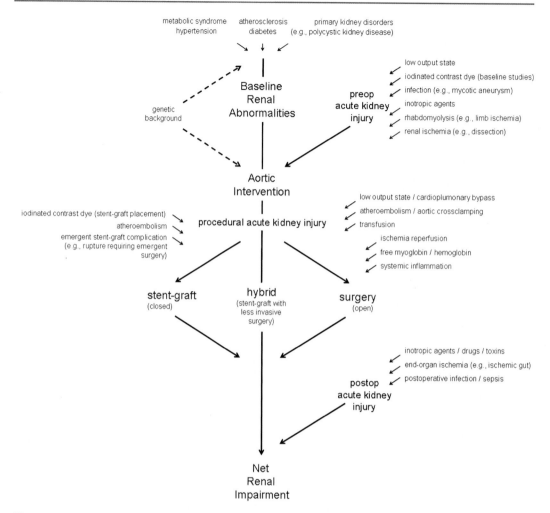

Fig. 15.3 Contributors to perioperative change in renal function are factors influencing baseline renal function and renal vulnerability (e.g., genetic background), numerous perioperative sources of renal insult. *preop*–preoperative, *intraop*–intraoperative, *postop*–postoperative

Mechanisms of Surgery-Related AKI

The diverse sources of perioperative renal insult are extensively reviewed elsewhere (Fig. 15.3).[14] Commonly, perioperative AKI represents a cumulative burden of insult from diverse sources including exacerbation of preexisting disease, ischemia/reperfusion, nephrotoxins, oxidative stress, and inflammation. Hypoperfusion, inflammation, and atheroembolism are well studied contributors to aortic surgery-related AKI. Contrast dye is also an important insult as part of some hybrid procedures,[15] and a variety of other contributors such as rhabdomyolysis related to an ischemic limb may be important for some patients. In addition, particular surgeries add renal risk due to the nature of the procedure, such as those involving circulatory arrest or temporary renal artery occlusion. In general, each patient assumes a cumulative burden of renal insult that combine with factors that influence vulnerability to injury such as genetic makeup[16] to predict the kidney's response. Unfortunately, preoperative risk assessment alone anticipates only a small fraction of the variability observed in postoperative AKI. Two common primary pathways are thought to enact AKI-related renal cell death; these are irreversible injury due to ischemia-reperfusion and apoptosis related to activation of caspase "executioner" enzymes.

Low output states, cardiopulmonary bypass, hypovolemic shock, vasoconstrictor use, and circulatory arrest all may contribute to the renal ischemic burden of a surgery. Tissue disruption, endotoxemia from infectious or septic complications, transfusion, and cardiopulmonary bypass can serve as triggers for release of pro-inflammatory cytokines such as tumor necrosis factor alpha [TNFα] and interleukin 6 [IL-6].

Clamp occlusion and cannulation of the aorta are actions that can cause embolization by disrupting atheromatous plaque. Measures of aortic atherosclerosis and intraoperative arterial emboli counts are strong independent predictors of AKI after cardiac surgery.[17,18] Embolic occlusion of renal vessels from dislodgement of atheromatous plaque can lead to segmental necrosis of an affected kidney (Fig. 15.4). Surgical procedures on atherosclerotic vessels are known to have high

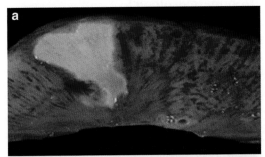

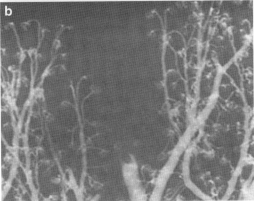

Fig. 15.4 Organization of the renal vasculature means that embolic arterial obstruction is poorly compensated for by collateral flow. Examples in a gross kidney specimen (**a**) and by 30× angiography (**b**) demonstrate the typical "pizza-slice" pattern of an embolic renal infarct. (Figure 15.4a used with permission from http://www-medlib.med.utah.edu/WebPath/CINJHTML/CINJ015.html. Figure 15.4b used with permission from Bookstein and Clark[127])

particulate emboli rates (57–77%),[19,20] and emboli showers are predictably high, for example, at the time of aortic unclamping.[21]

Aortic stent-graft technology is rapidly changing the treatment of aortic disease. Some recent studies suggest that the reduced invasiveness of endovascular stent-graft or hybrid (surgery plus stent-graft) interventions may be associated with less AKI and acute dialysis compared to open procedures. However, while stent-graft procedures require less aortic manipulation and avoid the stress of surgery, the imaging required currently obliges a potentially nephrotoxic contrast dye load, and thus benefits of reduced invasiveness may be traded for other renal insults. Moreover, it is unclear whether the AKI rate is best predicted by repair technique or the unique vulnerability of specific patients related to their vascular anatomy.

In a prospective nonrandomized study of 279 elective abdominal aortic aneurysm repair by stent-graft or open surgery, Greenberg and colleagues found that stent-graft patients were less likely to develop AKI before hospital discharge (creatinine rise >30% or creatinine >2.0 mg/dL; 5/198 vs. 8/79, p=0.01), but in this study only one patient from each group required postoperative dialysis, and there was no difference between groups at 30 days, 6 months, or 12 months postoperatively with regard to renal function.[22] A second retrospective study involving 22,830 matched pairs of Medicare patients undergoing open and endovascular abdominal aortic aneurysm procedures found a twofold greater incidence of perioperative acute renal failure (p<0.001) after open procedures.[23] Fewer studies are available reporting outcomes from thoracic aortic procedures. In a retrospective study of 30 open and hybrid thoracoabdominal aortic aneurysm procedures, Murphy and colleagues noted a reduced incidence of renal failure (0 vs. 42%, p=0.002) despite a greater incidence of renal risk factors in the endovascular group.[24] In contrast, a review of several case series by Chiesa and colleagues noted a 9.9% renal failure rate in 107 patients undergoing hybrid thoracoabdominal aortic aneurysm repair, and these authors suggest that the rate of acute renal failure has not been significantly affected by the advent of endovascular stent-graft and debranching.[25]

Ten percent of all in-hospital AKI is attributed to contrast-induced nephropathy. Garwood and colleagues found elevated urine markers of tubular injury in a group of 27 cardiac surgery patients presenting within 5 days of cardiac catheterization.[26] In a prospective study of 649 cardiac surgery patients, Provenchere and colleagues found radiocontrast agent administration <48 h before surgery to be an independent predictor of AKI.[27] Delaying elective surgery to permit recovery from contrast-associated nephropathy would seem prudent. Patients with chronic kidney disease who undergo interventional cardiology procedures have reduced risk of contrast-nephropathy with low osmolar contrast media accompanied by aggressive prestudy hydration.[15]

Sodium bicarbonate for AKI prophylaxis may be effective for contrast-induced nephropathy. In animal AKI models, pretreatment with sodium bicarbonate is more protective than sodium chloride.[28] In a randomized trial of 119 angiography patients receiving either sodium chloride or sodium bicarbonate (154 mEq/L), as a bolus (3 mL/kg per hour for 1 h) prior to receiving iopamidol contrast, followed by a 6 h postprocedure infusion (1 mL/kg/h), contrast-induced nephropathy was noted in eight patients (13.6%) receiving sodium chloride but only one (1.7%) with sodium bicarbonate (p=0.02).[29] Haase and colleagues made similar observations in a similarly designed study in cardiac surgery patients.[30] Whether renal benefit resulted from receiving sodium bicarbonate or from the potentially deleterious effect of sodium chloride was not explored in these studies.

Pigmenturia either from hemolysis sufficient to exceed the adsorptive capacity of circulating haptoglobin and renal tubular reuptake mechanisms (hemoglobinuria) or with muscle cell necrosis (myoglobinuria) is a potent kidney insult. The mechanisms underlying myoglobin- and hemoglobin-related AKI are similar (renal vasoconstriction, tubular obstruction by casts, and direct cytotoxicity).[31] Nonsteroidal anti-inflammatory drugs (NSAIDs) have potent nephrotoxic effects causing renal vasoconstriction through inhibition of local synthesis of vasodilator prostaglandins. Aminoglycoside antibiotics, aprotinin,[32] and cyclosporin are other nephrotoxic agents that can have effects on renal function.

Despite steadily improving understanding of the time course and consequences of renal insults related to aortic and cardiac surgeries (Fig. 15.5), there has been very little progress in improving renal protection for these procedures.

Renal Preservation Strategies

Clinical management decisions may reduce AKI,[3,6,33–48] and pharmacologic interventions have been studied for their renoprotective properties. These factors are reviewed below.

Modifiable Clinical Factors (Nonpharmacologic)

Preoperative Management

Contrast-induced nephropathy has been discussed above. Decisions about chronic preoperative medications are relevant, although there are no clear guidelines due to the very few studies available in this area. Angiotensin-converting enzyme inhibitors (ACEIs) and angiotensin I receptor blockers may precipitate AKI when angiotensin is critical to renal filtration regulation, such as with acute volume depletion or renal artery stenosis.[49,50] In a prospective study of 249 aortic surgery patients, Cittanova and colleagues observed a link between chronic ACEI therapy and postoperative AKI.[51] However, Weightman and colleagues did not confirm preoperative ACEI as a risk factor for mortality in a retrospective analysis of 1,800 cardiac surgery procedures.[52] Preoperative loop diuretic therapy was an independent risk factor for postoperative complications in a retrospective study of 248 cardiac surgery patients.[53]

Intraoperative Management

Fluid choices have been attributed risk based on data from some postoperative AKI studies. Several retrospective reports have linked the use of hydroxyethyl starch (HES) preparations for

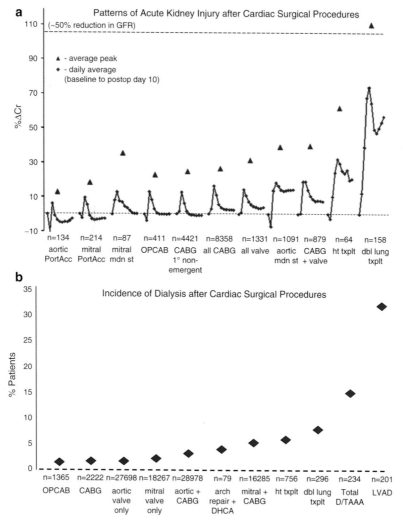

Fig. 15.5 Average peak (*triangles*) and average daily (*diamonds*) serum creatinine values represented relative to baseline for the first 10 days (**a**) and average (new) dialysis rates (**b**) for various surgical procedures. Peak creatinine values considerably exceed the highest daily average value since peaks occur on different days for different patients. Abbreviations: %ΔCr – peak fractional serum creatinine rise, *PortAcc* – port access mitral valve surgery, *OPCAB* – off-pump coronary artery bypass surgery, *CABG* – coronary artery bypass graft surgery, *DHCA* – deep hypothermic circulatory arrest, *mdn st* – median sternotomy, *ht txplt* – heart transplant, *dbl lung txplt* – double lung transplant, *D/TAAA* – descending/thoracoabdominal aortic aneurysm, *LVAD* – left ventricular assist device, *1°* – nonemergent, *postop* – postoperative, *aortic PortAcc* – minimally invasive parasternotomy aortic valve replacement. (Used with permission from Stafford-Smith et al.[128])

volume expansion with perioperative AKI.[54–57] In a randomized study of 129 septic patients receiving either 6% HES or 3% gelatin, the frequency of AKI and oliguria was higher in the HES group.[58] In this study, HES was also an independent predictor of acute renal failure. In contrast, there was no evidence of increased renal risk in a smaller randomized study of 30 major abdominal surgery patients receiving either gelatin or 6% HES.[59] The solutions supporting HES preparations and their potential to promote the onset of metabolic hyperchloremic acidosis may influence renal outcome.

Metabolic hyperchloremic acidosis is commonly observed in postoperative patients with the exclusive use of saline or saline-based colloid solutions. In a randomized study of 47 elderly patients receiving 6% HES in either 0.9% sodium chloride (HESPAN®, B. Braun Medical, Inc., Irvine, CA) or a balanced salt solution (Hextend®, BioTime, Inc., Berkeley, CA), none of the balanced salt-based solution patients, but two thirds of those receiving the sodium chloride, developed hyperchloremic metabolic acidosis (p<0.0001).[60] Some have speculated that this acid–base abnormality may modify perioperative renal vulnerability.[61] Hyperchloremia and acidosis influences renin release, increases afferent arteriolar tone, and reduces renal blood flow and glomerular filtration rate.[62,63] An appropriate clinical trial to address this question has not yet been reported.

Although CPB involves a small fraction of the perioperative period, this mode of circulatory support involves renal risk. Changes that occur with initiation of CPB include a disproportionate reduction of renal compared to systemic perfusion, and stress hormone and inflammatory responses known to be harmful to the kidney.[64–66] In numerous studies, the duration of CPB predicts postcardiac surgery AKI.[3,6,40,41]

Low CPB perfusion pressures associated with low flow rates were linked with AKI and dialysis in one case control analysis.[67] Although notably when low CPB perfusion pressures are associated with *normal* flow rates, no such relationship has been demonstrated.[46,48,68,69] Interestingly, neither the presence nor severity of renal artery stenosis has been associated with postcardiac surgery AKI.[70]

Hemodilution is a controversial CPB management issue. Although extreme CPB hemodilution (hematocrit <20%) is often tolerated, this practice has recently been linked to adverse outcomes.[71–73] Several large, retrospective studies have linked lowest hematocrit levels during CPB with postoperative acute renal injury and failure.[74–77] Ironically, one alternative to tolerating extreme CPB hemodilution, transfusion has also been considered risky.[74,77] Although optimal hematocrit management during CPB is difficult to define, it is well accepted that transfusion during CPB may contribute to postoperative AKI and should be avoided until other strategies to avoid hemodilution have been exhausted.

Hypothermia reduces metabolism and is essential to renal preservation during ischemia for kidney transplant surgery. Although it would seem logical that CPB hypothermia during CPB would be renoprotective, three prospective randomized studies have not confirmed renal protection from mild CPB hypothermia[78–80]; nonetheless, direct cooling appears to be renoprotective in the setting of renal artery occlusion.[81]

A possible explanation for the link between intraoperative hyperglycemia and AKI in cardiac surgery patients (regardless of diabetes history) may involve the greater likelihood of an exaggerated resistance to insulin in high-risk patients rather than inadequate insulin therapy.[3,74] Aggressive postoperative control of serum glucose (target <150 mg/dL) with insulin therapy reduces the occurrence of acute renal failure,[82] but an equivalently aggressive intraoperative glucose management strategy does not confer further benefit and may even portend harm.[83]

Infusion of vasoactive agents may compound indirect hemodynamic, humoral, and autonomic effects that typically influence perioperative renal blood flow.[84,85] Retrospective studies identify inotropic agents as predictors of postoperative AKI, independent of other markers of low cardiac output[35,40,47]; however, the differences among vasoactive agents are not well understood.

Postoperative Management

Many intraoperative issues remain pertinent to the postoperative period. Notably, the renoprotective benefits of insulin are most evident in the postoperative period. Patients at high risk for postoperative AKI are not good candidates for "fast track" recovery protocols. One study found an increased incidence of moderate and severe renal failure in high renal-risk patients[86] that resolved when high-risk patients were returned to standard recovery protocols.

Pharmacologic Interventions

DA1 Agonist Agents (Dopamine, Fenoldopam, Dopexamine)

Selective stimulation of mesenteric dopamine-1 (DA1) receptors by intravenous dopamine (<5 µg/kg/min) and fenoldopam increases renal blood flow, decreases renal vascular resistance, and induces natriuresis and diuresis. Unfortunately, numerous randomized trials and meta-analyses of randomized trials have failed to support dopamine as a renoprotective agent in many different surgical and nonsurgical settings.[87–90] In a meta-analysis of 3,359 patients randomized to "low-dose" dopamine versus control from 61 trials, there was no benefit regarding mortality, dialysis, or adverse events[91]; although, on the 1st day of dopamine therapy, there was a 24% increase in urine output, 4% reduction in serum creatinine, and 6% increase in creatinine clearance, which had disappeared by the following day.

Fenoldopam mesylate is a more selective agonist of DA1 receptors than dopamine. There is currently no consensus regarding the effectiveness of fenoldopam as a renoprotective agent. A study involving 80 high-risk cardiac surgery patients found no benefit.[92] A study of 160 cardiac surgery patients with baseline renal dysfunction noted lower postoperative serum creatinine values and higher creatinine clearance values compared to baseline with fenoldopam but not with placebo; no long-term outcome was evaluated in this study.[93] A double-blind study of 155 post-cardiac surgery and other critically ill patients with established renal injury found no benefit and even discussed possible increased adverse outcomes in diabetic patients.[94,95] In 28 aortic surgery patients, Halpenny and colleagues found a decline in creatinine clearance with aortic cross-clamp application and higher postoperative day 1 serum creatinine values in patients receiving placebo but not in the fenoldopam group.[96] Although a recent meta-analysis of 1,059 patients from 13 randomized and case-matched studies suggested benefit,[97] there is clearly a need for larger randomized trials to better assess this agent.

Dopexamine hydrochloride is a DA-1 receptor and beta 2-adrenoceptor agonist that is notable in that its metabolism is significantly reduced with liver dysfunction. A systematic review of 21 randomized-controlled dopexamine trials found insufficient evidence to support the use of dopexamine for renoprotection.[98]

Diuretic Agents

Diuretics increase urine by reducing tubular reuptake of glomerular filtrate; this can occur through blocking active solute reuptake (e.g., loop diuretics), altering osmotic gradients to favor filtrate remaining in the tubule (e.g., mannitol), or through exogenous hormonal effects (e.g., ANP). The general rationale underpinning diuretic renoprotection involves the "flushing" of tubular casts to prevent obstruction by increased solute flow, thus avoiding oligo/anuria and the need for dialysis. Importantly, despite the irresistibly satisfying full urine bag, increased perioperative urine volume from diuretics has never been linked with improved renal function.[5]

Loop diuretics (furosemide, ethacrynic acid, and bumetanide) increase urine by inhibiting active reabsorption in the mTAL of the loop of Henlee. Furosemide also induces renal cortical vasodilation. Notably, early treatment with loop diuretics has demonstrated renoprotective benefit in some types of AKI, including those where tubular obstruction is a primary concern, and evidence indicates that forced diuresis is therapeutic. This includes conditions such as myoglobinuric and hemoglobinuric AKI, tumor lysis syndrome, and nephrotoxic drug effects such as lithium, theophylline, and salicylates.[99] However, there is little evidence to support the use of loop diuretics as routine perioperative renoprotective agents and reasonable evidence that these agents may even aggravate most perioperative AKI. Numerous retrospective studies report no renal benefit and even harm with loop diuretics in critically ill and surgical patients.[100–102] Several randomized trials have also found no renoprotective benefit. Hager and colleagues found no renoprotection from an extended postoperative furosemide infusion compared to placebo in a randomized study of 121 major thoracoabdominal or vascular surgery procedures.[100] Notably, a similar study in 126 cardiac surgery patients indicated worsened renal outcome in those receiving furosemide compared to dopamine or placebo.[103] A study of 78 angiography patients with chronic renal dysfunction receiving either prehydration alone, with furosemide or mannitol, found more contrast nephropathy with mannitol (11 vs. 28%) and furosemide (40%; $p = 0.05$) compared to prehydration alone.[104]

Mannitol augments renal blood flow and increases glomerular filtration and urine output and is often used in priming the cardiopulmonary bypass circuit. A study involving 30 supra- and infrarenal aortic surgeries with cross-clamping found no benefit of mannitol.[105] Other cardiac surgery studies report no benefit with a range of doses (0.5–1.0 g/kg).[78,106] In addition, inappropriately high-dosing of mannitol may cause harm to the kidney particularly in patients with impaired renal function.[107] Unless a forced diuresis is desirable, there is little evidence to support the perioperative use of mannitol for renal preservation.

The natriuretic peptides are normally secreted in response to volume expansion, and their primary effects include receptor-mediated vasodilation and natriuresis. Three natriuretic peptides have received most of the attention in human trials: ANP (Anaritide), urodilantin (Ularitide), and BNP (Nesiritide).[108] ANP increases urinary output and glomerular filtration by dilating the afferent and constricting the efferent arterioles.[109] Human renoprotective trials of ANP have been inconclusive. In secondary analysis of data from a randomized trial of 504 critically ill patients with established AKI, a 24-h intravenous infusion of ANP (0.2 μg/kg/min) was associated with improved dialysis-free survival in oliguric patients (8 vs. 27%, p=0.008) but not in nonoliguric patients (59 vs. 48%; p = 0.03).[110] Unfortunately, a second study of 222 critically ill patients designed to reproduce the favorable findings of the first did not find any benefit.[111] Fewer studies have evaluated urodilatin, another natriuretic peptide, but these have also provided inconclusive results.[112]

Finally, BNP is generated in response to ventricular dilatation and has potent vasodilating properties. Although recent evidence suggests that BNP treatment may worsen renal function in heart failure patients,[113,114] two randomized studies in cardiac surgery patients have indicated renoprotective benefit from this agent.[115,116]

N-Acetylcysteine

N-acetylcysteine is a vasodilator that enhances endogenous glutathione scavenging and has antioxidant properties. Numerous contrast nephropathy studies suggest renoprotective studies, although complicating interpretation of these studies is the inconvenient fact that N-acetylcysteine may affect circulating serum creatinine levels independent of any renal effects.[117] Two meta-analyses of contrast nephropathy trials concluded that N-acetylcysteine renoprotective findings were inconsistent.[118,119] In a similar evaluation of patients with baseline renal dysfunction, N-acetylcysteine was felt to reduce the risk for contrast nephropathy.[120] A study of 30 abdominal aortic surgery patients receiving either N-acetylcysteine, mannitol, or placebo suggests benefit.[121] However, two large randomized comparisons with placebo in cardiac surgery patients did not indicate renoprotective benefit.[122,123]

Alpha 2 Adrenergic Agonist Agents

Alpha 2 adrenergic agonists mediate renal vasodilation, inhibit renin release, and cause a water diuresis. Clonidine (an alpha 2 agonist) may counteract the adverse effects of vasoconstrictors that are known to contribute to the pathophysiology of AKI and attenuate AKI. Two randomized studies involving 204 cardiac surgery patients have described early renal benefit from clonidine therapy.[124] A 23 studies meta-analysis of 3,395 patients receiving perioperative alpha 2 agonists (clonidine, dexmedetomidine, or mivazerol) also identified a survival benefit with these agents.[125]

Calcium Channel Blockers

Calcium channel blockers decrease renal vascular resistance and increase glomerular filtration. Although there have been many randomized renoprotection investigations of the three major classes of calcium antagonists (benzothiazepines - e.g., diltiazem, phenylalkylamines - e.g., verapamil, and dihydropyridines - e.g., nifedipine, nimodipine), a meta-analysis of randomized cardiac surgery studies comparing perioperative use of these agents with placebo or other agents (e.g., nitroglycerin, dopamine) found overall inconclusive evidence of calcium antagonist blocker-mediated renal preservation.[126]

Summary

Thoracic aortic disease often presents as an emergent life-threatening condition, but, even when interventions are elective, many surgeries historically have involved sufficient physiologic trespass that rates of morbidity and mortality considered intolerable for other operations have been accepted. Whether renal perfusion was preserved or not as part of these procedures, they have involved a high risk of AKI, and the highest rates of postoperative dialysis observed for any type of surgery. It is, therefore, with great enthusiasm that the advent of stent-graft technology has been embraced into the treatment of thoracic aortic pathology, offering the possibility of stenting alone or in combination with less invasive surgery (i.e., hybrid procedures) as a viable less invasive alternative for most conditions. While the proximity of the renal blood supply and the requirements for these new thoracic aortic procedures, such as a contrast dye load, assure continued risk to the kidneys, there is significant hope that a reduction in postoperative complications will include better renal preservation, and that improved long-term outcomes will result.

Key Notes

1. Acute kidney injury is a common complication of aortic surgery, and its occurrence in any degree is associated with higher morbidity and mortality rates.
2. Factors related to perioperative AKI in aortic surgical patients are numerous and diverse, but can be primarily grouped into categories that influence renal vulnerability, or ischemia/reperfusion, inflammation, and toxin-mediated renal insult.
3. Indirect tools such as observing serum creatinine trends are the best practical currently available perioperative tools to assess for changes in renal function.
4. Specific definitions for AKI have been described that primarily involve serum creatinine rise exceeding a certain threshold.
5. Urine formation during aortic surgery procedures depends on numerous factors and is an unreliable and insensitive method to assess risk of postoperative AKI.
6. Markers for earlier recognition of AKI hold promise and are a current focus of much

research that may soon lead to new tests able to provide prompt clinical information. Notably, these tools have yet to be validated for their association with major adverse outcomes associated with AKI (e.g., mortality).
7. Although much research has been directed towards identifying renoprotective strategies, there has been very little success in improving the course of established AKI. Avoidance of renal insult, however, through such adjustments as procedure modification (e.g., stent-graft vs. open) may offer significant renal benefit in high-risk aortic surgery candidates.

References

1. Smith HW. *Lectures on the Kidney*. Lawrence: University Extension Division, University of Kansas; 1943.
2. Bellomo R, Ronco C, Kellum JA, Mehta RL, Palevsky P. Acute renal failure - definition, outcome measures, animal models, fluid therapy and information technology needs: the Second International Consensus Conference of the Acute Dialysis Quality Initiative (ADQI) Group. *Crit Care*. 2004;8(4):R204–212.
3. Mora-Mangano C, Diamondstone LS, Ramsay JG, Aggarwal A, Herskowitz A, Mangano DT. Renal dysfunction after myocardial revascularization: risk factors, adverse outcomes, and hospital resource utilization. The Multicenter Study of Perioperative Ischemia Research Group. *Ann Intern Med*. 1998;128(3):194–203.
4. Sladen RN, Endo E, Harrison T. Two-hour versus 22-hour creatinine clearance in critically ill patients. *Anesthesiology*. 1987;67(6):1013–1016.
5. Alpert RA, Roizen MF, Hamilton WK, et al. Intraoperative urinary output does not predict postoperative renal function in patients undergoing abdominal aortic revascularization. *Surgery*. 1984;95(6):707–711.
6. Conlon PJ, Stafford-Smith M, White WD, et al. Acute renal failure following cardiac surgery. *Nephrol Dial Transplant*. 1999;14(5):1158–1162.
7. Bloor GK, Welsh KR, Goodall S, Shah MV. Comparison of predicted with measured creatinine clearance in cardiac surgical patients. *J Cardiothorac Vasc Anesth*. 1996;10(7):899–902.
8. Gowans EM, Fraser CG. Biological variation of serum and urine creatinine and creatinine clearance: ramifications for interpretation of results and patient care [see comments]. *Ann Clin Biochem*. 1988;25(Pt 3): 259–263.
9. Morgan DB, Dillon S, Payne RB. The assessment of glomerular function: creatinine clearance or plasma creatinine? *Postgrad Med J*. 1978;54(631):302–310.

10. Cockcroft DW, Gault MH. Prediction of creatinine clearance from serum creatinine. *Nephron*. 1976; 16(1):31–41.

11. Levey AS, Bosch JP, Lewis JB, Greene T, Rogers N, Roth D. A more accurate method to estimate glomerular filtration rate from serum creatinine: a new prediction equation. Modification of Diet in Renal Disease Study Group. *Ann Intern Med*. 1999;130(6): 461–470.

12. Ferguson TB Jr, Dziuban SW Jr, Edwards FH, et al. The STS National Database: current changes and challenges for the new millennium. Committee to Establish a National Database in Cardiothoracic Surgery, The Society of Thoracic Surgeons. *Ann Thorac Surg*. 2000;69(3):680–691.

13. Barrett BJ, Parfrey PS. Prevention of nephrotoxicity induced by radiocontrast agents. *N Engl J Med*. 1994;331(21):1449–1450.

14. Stafford-Smith M. Perioperative renal dysfunction: implications and strategies for protection. In: Newman MF, ed. *Perioperative Organ Protection*. Baltimore: Lippincott Williams and Wilkins; 2003:89–124.

15. Porter GA. Contrast-associated nephropathy: presentation, pathophysiology and management. *Miner Electrolyte Metab*. 1994;20(4):232–243.

16. Stafford-Smith M, Podgoreanu M, Swaminathan M, et al. Association of genetic polymorphisms with risk of renal injury after coronary artery bypass graft surgery. *Am J Kidney Dis*. 2005;45(3):519–530.

17. Davila-Roman VG, Kouchoukos NT, Schechtman KB, Barzilai B. Atherosclerosis of the ascending aorta is a predictor of renal dysfunction after cardiac operations. *J Thorac Cardiovasc Surg*. 1999;117(1):111–116.

18. Sreeram GM, Grocott HP, White WD, Newman MF, Stafford-Smith M. Transcranial Doppler emboli count predicts rise in creatinine after coronary artery bypass graft surgery. *J Cardiothorac Vasc Anesth*. 2004;18(5): 548–551.

19. Thurlbeck W, Castleman B. Atheromatous emboli to the kidneys after aortic surgery. *N Engl J Med*. 1957;257:442–447.

20. Reichenspurner H, Navia JA, Berry G, et al. Particulate emboli capture by an intra-aortic filter device during cardiac surgery. *J Thorac Cardiovasc Surg*. 2000;119(2):233–241.

21. Barbut D, Yao FS, Lo YW, et al. Determination of size of aortic emboli and embolic load during coronary artery bypass grafting. *Ann Thorac Surg*. 1997;63(5): 1262–1267.

22. Greenberg RK, Chuter TA, Lawrence-Brown M, Haulon S, Nolte L. Analysis of renal function after aneurysm repair with a device using suprarenal fixation (Zenith AAA Endovascular Graft) in contrast to open surgical repair. *J Vasc Surg*. 2004;39(6):1219–1228.

23. Schermerhorn ML, O'Malley AJ, Jhaveri A, Cotterill P, Pomposelli F, Landon BE. Endovascular vs. open repair of abdominal aortic aneurysms in the Medicare population. *N Engl J Med*. 2008;358(5):464–474.

24. Murphy EH, Beck AW, Clagett GP, DiMaio JM, Jessen ME, Arko FR. Combined aortic debranching and thoracic endovascular aneurysm repair (TEVAR) effective but at a cost. *Arch Surg*. 2009;144(3): 222–227.

25. Chiesa R, Tshomba Y, Melissano G, Logaldo D. Is hybrid procedure the best treatment option for thoraco-abdominal aortic aneurysm? *Eur J Vasc Endovasc Surg*. 2009;38(1):26–34.

26. Garwood S, Mathew J, Hines R. Renal function and cardiopulmonary bypass: does time since catheterization impact renal performance? *Anesthesiology*. 1997;87:A90.

27. Provenchere S, Plantefeve G, Hufnagel G, et al. Renal dysfunction after cardiac surgery with normothermic cardiopulmonary bypass: incidence, risk factors, and effect on clinical outcome. *Anesth Analg*. 2003; 96(5):1258–1264.

28. Atkins JL. Effect of sodium bicarbonate preloading on ischemic renal failure. *Nephron*. 1986;44(1):70–74.

29. Merten GJ, Burgess WP, Gray LV, et al. Prevention of contrast-induced nephropathy with sodium bicarbonate: a randomized controlled trial. *JAMA*. 2004; 291(19):2328–2334.

30. Haase M, Haase-Fielitz A, Bellomo R, et al. Sodium bicarbonate to prevent increases in serum creatinine after cardiac surgery: a pilot double-blind, randomized controlled trial. *Crit Care Med*. 2009;37(1):39–47.

31. Corwin HL, Schreiber MJ, Fang LS. Low fractional excretion of sodium: occurrence with hemoglobinuric- and myoglobinuric-induced acute renal failure. *Arch Intern Med*. 1984;144(5):981–982.

32. Shaw AD, Stafford-Smith M, White WD, et al. The effect of aprotinin on outcome after coronary-artery bypass grafting. *N Engl J Med*. 2008;358(8):784–793.

33. Stafford-Smith M, Phillips-Bute B, Reddan DN, Milano C, Newman MF, Winn M. The association of postoperative peak and fractional change in serum creatinine with mortality after coronary bypass surgery. *Anesthesiology*. 2000;93:A240.

34. Chertow GM, Lazarus JM, Christiansen CL, et al. Preoperative renal risk stratification. *Circulation*. 1997;95(4):878–884.

35. Zanardo G, Michielon P, Paccagnella A, et al. Acute renal failure in the patient undergoing cardiac operation: prevalence, mortality rate, and main risk factors. *J Thorac Cardiovasc Surg*. 1994;107(6):1489–1495.

36. Yeh T, Brackney E, Hall D, Ellison R. Renal complications of open-heart surgery: predisposing factors, prevention and management. *J Thorac Cardiovasc Surg*. 1964;47:79–95.

37. Porter GA, Kloster FE, Herr RJ, Starr A, Griswold HE, Kimsey J. Renal complications associated with valve replacement surgery. *J Thorac Cardiovasc Surg*. 1967;53(1):145–152.

38. McLeish KR, Luft FC, Kleit SA. Factors affecting prognosis in acute renal failure following cardiac operations. *Surg Gynecol Obstet*. 1977;145(1):28–32.

39. Mangos GJ, Brown MA, Chan WY, Horton D, Trew P, Whitworth JA. Acute renal failure following cardiac surgery: incidence, outcomes and risk factors. *Aust N Z J Med*. 1995;25(4):284–289.

40. Llopart T, Lombardi R, Forselledo M, Andrade R. Acute renal failure in open heart surgery. *Ren Fail.* 1997;19(2):319–323.

41. Hilberman M, Myers BD, Carrie BJ, Derby G, Jamison RL, Stinson EB. Acute renal failure following cardiac surgery. *J Thorac Cardiovasc Surg.* 1979; 77(6):880–888.

42. Heikkinen L, Harjula A, Merikallio E. Acute renal failure related to open-heart surgery. *Ann Chir Gynaecol.* 1985;74(5):203–209.

43. Gailiunas P Jr, Chawla R, Lazarus JM, Cohn L, Sanders J, Merrill JP. Acute renal failure following cardiac operations. *J Thorac Cardiovasc Surg.* 1980;79(2):241–243.

44. Doberneck RC, Reiser MP, Lillehei CW. Acute renal failure after open-heart surgery utilizing extracorporeal circulation and total body perfusion. *J Thorac Cardiovasc Surg.* 1962;43:441–452.

45. Corwin HL, Sprague SM, DeLaria GA, Norusis MJ. Acute renal failure associated with cardiac operations: a case-control study. *J Thorac Cardiovasc Surg.* 1989;98(6):1107–1112.

46. Bhat JG, Gluck MC, Lowenstein J, Baldwin DS. Renal failure after open heart surgery. *Ann Intern Med.* 1976;84(6):677–682.

47. Andersson LG, Ekroth R, Bratteby LE, Hallhagen S, Wesslen O. Acute renal failure after coronary surgery–a study of incidence and risk factors in 2009 consecutive patients. *Thorac Cardiovasc Surg.* 1993;41(4):237–241.

48. Abel RM, Buckley MJ, Austen WG, Barnett GO, Beck CH Jr, Fischer JE. Etiology, incidence, and prognosis of renal failure following cardiac operations: results of a prospective analysis of 500 consecutive patients. *J Thorac Cardiovasc Surg.* 1976;71(3):323–333.

49. Mimran A, Ribstein J. Angiotensin converting enzyme inhibitors and renal function. *J Hypertens Suppl.* 1989;7(5):S3–9.

50. Kamper AL, Nielsen AH, Baekgaard N, Just S. Renal graft failure after addition of an angiotensin II receptor antagonist to an angiotensin-converting enzyme inhibitor: unmasking of an unknown iliac artery stenosis. *J Renin Angiotensin Aldosterone Syst.* 2002;3(2):135–137.

51. Cittanova ML, Zubicki A, Savu C, et al. The chronic inhibition of angiotensin-converting enzyme impairs postoperative renal function. *Anesth Analg.* 2001;93(5):1111–1115.

52. Weightman WM, Gibbs NM, Sheminant MR, Whitford EG, Mahon BD, Newman MA. Drug therapy before coronary artery surgery: nitrates are independent predictors of mortality and beta-adrenergic blockers predict survival. *Anesth Analg.* 1999;88(2):286–291.

53. Charlson M, Krieger KH, Peterson JC, Hayes J, Isom OW. Predictors and outcomes of cardiac complications following elective coronary bypass grafting. *Proc Assoc Am Physicians.* 1999;111(6):622–632.

54. Cittanova ML, Leblanc I, Legendre C, Mouquet C, Riou B, Coriat P. Effect of hydroxyethylstarch in brain-dead kidney donors on renal function in kidney-transplant recipients. *Lancet.* 1996;348(9042):1620–1622.

55. Peron S, Mouthon L, Guettier C, Brechignac S, Cohen P, Guillevin L. Hydroxyethyl starch-induced renal insufficiency after plasma exchange in a patient with polymyositis and liver cirrhosis. *Clin Nephrol.* 2001;55(5):408–411.

56. Winkelmayer WC, Glynn RJ, Levin R, Avorn J. Hydroxyethyl starch and change in renal function in patients undergoing coronary artery bypass graft surgery. *Kidney Int.* 2003;64(3):1046–1049.

57. De Labarthe A, Jacobs F, Blot F, Glotz D. Acute renal failure secondary to hydroxyethylstarch administration in a surgical patient. *Am J Med.* 2001;111(5):417–418.

58. Schortgen F, Lacherade JC, Bruneel F, et al. Effects of hydroxyethylstarch and gelatin on renal function in severe sepsis: a multicentre randomised study. *Lancet.* 2001;357(9260):911–916.

59. Kumle B, Boldt J, Piper S, Schmidt C, Suttner S, Salopek S. The influence of different intravascular volume replacement regimens on renal function in the elderly. *Anesth Analg.* 1999;89(5):1124–1130.

60. Wilkes NJ, Woolf R, Mutch M, et al. The effects of balanced versus saline-based hetastarch and crystalloid solutions on acid-base and electrolyte status and gastric mucosal perfusion in elderly surgical patients. *Anesth Analg.* 2001;93(4):811–816.

61. Parekh N. Hyperchloremic acidosis. *Anesth Analg.* 2002;95:1821.

62. Wilcox C. Regulation of renal blood flow by plasma chloride. *J Clin Invest.* 1983;71:726–735.

63. Hansen PB, Jensen BL, Skott O. Chloride regulates afferent arteriolar contraction in response to depolarization. *Hypertension.* 1998;32(6):1066–1070.

64. Andersson LG, Bratteby LE, Ekroth R, et al. Renal function during cardiopulmonary bypass: influence of pump flow and systemic blood pressure. *Eur J Cardiothorac Surg.* 1994;8(11):597–602.

65. Reves JG, Karp RB, Buttner EE, et al. Neuronal and adrenomedullary catecholamine release in response to cardiopulmonary bypass in man. *Circulation.* 1982;66(1):49–55.

66. Laffey J, Boylan J, Cheng D. The systemic inflammatory response to cardiac surgery: implications for the anesthesiologist. *Anesthesiology.* 2002;97:215–252.

67. Fischer UM, Weissenberger WK, Warters RD, Geissler HJ, Allen SJ, Mehlhorn U. Impact of cardiopulmonary bypass management on postcardiac surgery renal function. *Perfusion.* 2002;17(6):401–406.

68. Urzua J, Troncoso S, Bugedo G, et al. Renal function and cardiopulmonary bypass: effect of perfusion pressure. *J Cardiothorac Vasc Anesth.* 1992;6(3):299–303.

69. Swaminathan M, Knauth K, Phillips-Bute B, Smith P, Stafford-Smith M. Lowest CPB Hematocrit is inversely associated with creatinine rise after coronary bypass surgery. *Anesth Analg.* 2002;94:S70.

70. Conlon PJ, Crowley J, Stack R, et al. Renal artery stenosis is not associated with the development of acute renal failure following coronary artery bypass grafting. *Ren Fail.* 2005;27(1):81–86.

71. DeFoe G, Ross C, Olmstead E, et al. Group NNECDS: lowest hematocrit on bypass and adverse outcomes associated with coronary artery bypass grafting. *Ann Thorac Surg*. 2001;71:769–776.

72. Fang WC, Helm RE, Krieger KH, et al. Impact of minimum hematocrit during cardiopulmonary bypass on mortality in patients undergoing coronary artery surgery. *Circulation*. 1997;96(9 Suppl):II-194–199.

73. Ranucci M, Pavesi M, Mazza E, et al. Risk factors for renal dysfunction after coronary surgery: the role of cardiopulmonary bypass technique. *Perfusion*. 1994;9(5):319–326.

74. Swaminathan M, Phillips-Bute BG, Conlon PJ, Newman S, Smith PK, Stafford-Smith M. The association of lowest hematocrit during cardiopulmonary bypass with acute renal injury after coronary bypass surgery. *Ann Thorac Surg*. 2003;76(3):784–791.

75. Karkouti K, Beattie WS, Wijeysundera DN, et al. Hemodilution during cardiopulmonary bypass is an independent risk factor for acute renal failure in adult cardiac surgery. *J Thorac Cardiovasc Surg*. 2005; 129(2):391–400.

76. Habib RH, Zacharias A, Schwann TA, et al. Role of hemodilutional anemia and transfusion during cardiopulmonary bypass in renal injury after coronary revascularization: implications on operative outcome. *Crit Care Med*. 2005;33(8):1749–1756.

77. Kincaid EH, Ashburn DA, Hoyle JR, Reichert MG, Hammon JW, Kon ND. Does the combination of aprotinin and angiotensin-converting enzyme inhibitor cause renal failure after cardiac surgery? *Ann Thorac Surg*. 2005;80(4):1388–1393.

78. Ip-Yam PC, Murphy S, Baines M, Fox MA, Desmond MJ, Innes PA. Renal function and proteinuria after cardiopulmonary bypass: the effects of temperature and mannitol. *Anesth Analg*. 1994;78(5):842–847.

79. Regragui IA, Izzat MB, Birdi I, Lapsley M, Bryan AJ, Angelini GD. Cardiopulmonary bypass perfusion temperature does not influence perioperative renal function. *Ann Thorac Surg*. 1995;60(1):160–164.

80. Swaminathan M, East C, Phillips-Bute B, et al. Report of a substudy on warm versus cold cardiopulmonary bypass: changes in creatinine clearance. *Ann Thorac Surg*. 2001;72(5):1603–1609.

81. Bakirtas H, Eroglu M, Naldoken S, Akbulut Z, Tekdogan UY. Nephron-sparing surgery: the effect of surface cooling and temporary renal artery occlusion on renal function. *Urol Int*. 2009;82(1):24–27.

82. Van den Berghe G, Wouters P, Weekers F, et al. Intensive insulin therapy in the critically ill patients. *N Engl J Med*. 2001;345(19):1359–1367.

83. Gandhi GY, Nuttall GA, Abel MD, et al. Intensive intraoperative insulin therapy versus conventional glucose management during cardiac surgery: a randomized trial. *Ann Intern Med*. 2007;146(4): 233–243.

84. Burchardi H, Kaczmarczyk G. The effect of anaesthesia on renal function. *Eur J Anaesthesiol*. 1994;11(3): 163–168.

85. Sladen RN, Landry D. Renal blood flow regulation, autoregulation, and vasomotor nephropathy. *Anesthesiol Clin N Am*. 2000;18(4):791–807. ix.

86. Page US, Washburn T. Using tracking data to find complications that physicians miss: the case of renal failure in cardiac surgery. *Jt Comm J Qual Improv*. 1997;23(10):511–520.

87. Bellomo R, Chapman M, Finfer S, Hickling K, Myburgh J. Low-dose dopamine in patients with early renal dysfunction: a placebo- controlled randomised trial. Australian and New Zealand Intensive Care Society (ANZICS) Clinical Trials Group. *Lancet*. 2000;356(9248):2139–2143.

88. Marik PE. Low-dose dopamine: a systematic review. *Intensive Care Med*. 2002;28(7):877–883.

89. Kellum JA, Decker JM. Use of dopamine in acute renal failure: a meta-analysis. *Crit Care Med*. 2001;29(8):1526–1531.

90. Prins I, Plotz FB, Uiterwaal CS, van Vught HJ. Low-dose dopamine in neonatal and pediatric intensive care: a systematic review. *Intensive Care Med*. 2001;27(1):206–210.

91. Friedrich JO, Adhikari N, Herridge MS, Beyene J. Meta-analysis: low-dose dopamine increases urine output but does not prevent renal dysfunction or death. *Ann Intern Med*. 2005;142(7):510–524.

92. Bove T, Landoni G, Grazia Calabro M, et al. Renoprotective action of Fenoldopam in high-risk patients undergoing cardiac surgery: a prospective, double-blind, randomized clinical trial. *Circulation*. 2005;111(24):3230–3235.

93. Caimmi PP, Pagani L, Micalizzi E, et al. Fenoldopam for renal protection in patients undergoing cardiopulmonary bypass. *J Cardiothorac Vasc Anesth*. 2003;17(4):491–494.

94. Tumlin J, Finckle K, Murray P, Shaw A. Dopamine receptor 1 agonists in early acute tubular necrosis: a prospective, randomized, double blind, placebo-controlled trial of fenoldopam mesylate. *J Am Soc Nephrol*. 2003;14:PUB001.

95. Tumlin JA, Finkel KW, Murray PT, Samuels J, Cotsonis G, Shaw AD. Fenoldopam mesylate in early acute tubular necrosis: a randomized, double-blind, placebo-controlled clinical trial. *Am J Kidney Dis*. 2005;46(1):26–34.

96. Halpenny M, Rushe C, Breen P, Cunningham AJ, Boucher-Hayes D, Shorten GD. The effects of fenoldopam on renal function in patients undergoing elective aortic surgery. *Eur J Anaesthesiol*. 2002; 19(1):32–39.

97. Landoni G, Biondi-Zoccai GG, Marino G, et al. Fenoldopam reduces the need for renal replacement therapy and in-hospital death in cardiovascular surgery: a meta-analysis. *J Cardiothorac Vasc Anesth*. 2008;22(1):27–33.

98. Renton MC, Snowden CP. Dopexamine and its role in the protection of hepatosplanchnic and renal perfusion in high-risk surgical and critically ill patients. *Br J Anaesth*. 2005;94(4):459–467.

99. Albright RC Jr. Acute renal failure: a practical update. *Mayo Clin Proc.* 2001;76(1):67–74.

100. Hager B, Betschart M, Krapf R. Effect of postoperative intravenous loop diuretic on renal function after major surgery. *Schweiz Med Wochenschr.* 1996; 126(16):666–673.

101. Shilliday IR, Quinn KJ, Allison ME. Loop diuretics in the management of acute renal failure: a prospective, double-blind, placebo-controlled, randomized study. *Nephrol Dial Transplant.* 1997;12(12):2592–2596.

102. Nuutinen L, Hollmen A. The effect of prophylactic use of furosemide on renal function during open heart surgery. *Ann Chir Gynaecol.* 1976;65(4):258–266.

103. Lassnigg A, Donner E, Grubhofer G, Presterl E, Druml W, Hiesmayr M. Lack of renoprotective effects of dopamine and furosemide during cardiac surgery. *J Am Soc Nephrol.* 2000;11(1):97–104.

104. Solomon R, Werner C, Mann D, D'Elia J, Silva P. Effects of saline, mannitol, and furosemide to prevent acute decreases in renal function induced by radiocontrast agents. *N Engl J Med.* 1994;331(21): 1416-20. 331:1416–1420.

105. Myers BD, Miller DC, Mehigan JT, et al. Nature of the renal injury following total renal ischemia in man. *J Clin Invest.* 1984;73(2):329–341.

106. Carcoana OV, Mathew JP, Davis E, et al. Mannitol and dopamine in patients undergoing cardiopulmonary bypass: a randomized clinical trial. *Anesth Analg.* 2003;97(5):1222–1229.

107. Visweswaran P, Massin EK, Dubose TD Jr. Mannitol-induced acute renal failure. *J Am Soc Nephrol.* 1997;8(6):1028–1033.

108. Joffy S, Rosner MH. Natriuretic peptides in ESRD. *Am J Kidney Dis.* 2005;46(1):1–10.

109. Deegan PM, Ryan MP, Basinger MA, Jones MM, Hande KR. Protection from cisplatin nephrotoxicity by A68828, an atrial natriuretic peptide. *Ren Fail.* 1995;17(2):117–123.

110. Allgren RL, Marbury TC, Rahman SN, et al. Anaritide in acute tubular necrosis. Auriculin Anaritide Acute Renal Failure Study Group. *N Engl J Med.* 1997;336(12):828–834.

111. Lewis J, Salem MM, Chertow GM, et al. Atrial natriuretic factor in oliguric acute renal failure. Anaritide Acute Renal Failure Study Group. *Am J Kidney Dis.* 2000;36(4):767–774.

112. Meyer M, Pfarr E, Schirmer G, et al. Therapeutic use of the natriuretic peptide ularitide in acute renal failure. *Ren Fail.* 1999;21(1):85–100.

113. Sackner-Bernstein JD, Skopicki HA, Aaronson KD. Risk of worsening renal function with nesiritide in patients with acutely decompensated heart failure. *Circulation.* 2005;111(12):1487–1491.

114. Teerlink JR, Massie BM. Nesiritide and worsening of renal function: the emperor's new clothes? *Circulation.* 2005;111(12):1459–1461.

115. Mentzer RM Jr, Oz MC, Sladen RN, et al. Effects of perioperative nesiritide in patients with left ventricular dysfunction undergoing cardiac surgery: the NAPA trial. *J Am Coll Cardiol.* 2007;49(6):716–726.

116. Chen HH, Sundt TM, Cook DJ, Heublein DM, Burnett JC Jr. Low dose nesiritide and the preservation of renal function in patients with renal dysfunction undergoing cardiopulmonary-bypass surgery: a double-blind placebo-controlled pilot study. *Circulation.* 2007;116(11 Suppl):I-134–138.

117. Hoffmann U, Fischereder M, Kruger B, Drobnik W, Kramer BK. The value of N-acetylcysteine in the prevention of radiocontrast agent-induced nephropathy seems questionable. *J Am Soc Nephrol.* 2004;15(2): 407–410.

118. Kshirsagar AV, Poole C, Mottl A, et al. N-acetylcysteine for the prevention of radiocontrast induced nephropathy: a meta-analysis of prospective controlled trials. *J Am Soc Nephrol.* 2004;15(3): 761–769.

119. Pannu N, Manns B, Lee HH, Tonelli M. Systematic review of the impact of N-acetylcysteine n contrast nephropathy. *Kidney Int.* 2004;65(4):1366–1374.

120. Alonso A, Lau J, Jaber BL, Weintraub A, Sarnak MJ. Prevention of radiocontrast nephropathy with N-acetylcysteine in patients with chronic kidney disease: a meta-analysis of randomized, controlled trials. *Am J Kidney Dis.* 2004;43(1):1–9.

121. Kretzschmar M, Klein U, Palutke M, Schirrmeister W. Reduction of ischemia-reperfusion syndrome after abdominal aortic aneurysmectomy by N-acetylcysteine but not mannitol. *Acta Anaesthesiol Scand.* 1996;40(6):657–664.

122. Cote G, Denault A, Belisle S, Martineau R, Perrault L. N-acetylcysteine in the preservation of renal function in patients undergoing cardiac surgery. *ASA Annual Meeting Abstracts.* 2003;99(3A):A420.

123. Burns KE, Chu MW, Novick RJ, et al. Perioperative N-acetylcysteine to prevent renal dysfunction in high-risk patients undergoing cabg surgery: a randomized controlled trial. *JAMA.* 2005;294(3): 342–350.

124. Kulka PJ, Tryba M, Zenz M. Preoperative alpha2-adrenergic receptor agonists prevent the deterioration of renal function after cardiac surgery: results of a randomized, controlled trial. *Crit Care Med.* 1996;24(6):947–952.

125. Wijeysundera DN, Naik JS, Beattie WS. Alpha-2 adrenergic agonists to prevent perioperative cardiovascular complications: a meta-analysis. *Am J Med.* 2003;114(9):742–752.

126. Wijeysundera DN, Beattie WS, Rao V, Karski J. Calcium antagonists reduce cardiovascular complications after cardiac surgery: a meta-analysis. *J Am Coll Cardiol.* 2003;41(9):1496–1505.

127. Bookstein JJ, Clark RL. Renal microvascular disease: angiographic-microangiographic correlates. In: HL A, ed. *Library of Radiology.* 1st ed. Boston: Little, Brown and Company; 1980.

128. Stafford-Smith M, Patel UD, Phillips-Bute BG, Shaw AD, Swaminathan M. Acute kidney injury and chronic kidney disease after cardiac surgery. *Adv Chronic Kidney Dis.* 2008;15:257–277.

Comprehensive Management of Patients with Traumatic Aortic Injury

16

Charles E. Smith and Donn Marciniak

Thoracic Aortic Trauma

Thoracic aortic trauma frequently occurs in the setting of chest trauma. As such, victims of aortic trauma may have multiple life-threatening thoracic injuries involving the chest wall, trachea, bronchus, lungs, pleura, heart, diaphragm, esophagus, and great vessels (Table 16.1). Multisystem injuries such as head, face, abdomen, spine, and extremities frequently co-exist in patients sustaining thoracic aortic trauma (Table 16.2).[1,2] The purpose of this chapter is to provide an up-to-date clinical review of the anesthetic management of adult patients with thoracic aortic trauma. The incidence, pathophysiology, surgical options, and preoperative issues will be discussed, following which the anesthetic considerations will be explored.

Incidence and Pathophysiology

Trauma is the third leading cause of death in the United States and the leading cause of death in individuals under the age of 40 years. Thoracic trauma accounts for 20–25% of traumatic deaths, and traumatic aortic rupture (TAR) is one of the commonest causes of death by motor vehicle

accidents, accounting for 8,000 deaths per year in the United States.[3] Blunt aortic injury accounts for 20% of fatal motor vehicle accidents with extremely high prehospital mortality (80–90%).[4] In the classic study of Parmley, of those who survived for 1 h (e.g., aortic rupture contained by

Table 16.1 Type and incidence of thoracic injuries in patients with blunt chest trauma presenting to the operating room for emergency surgery

Type of injury	Incidence (%)
Rib fractures	67
Pulmonary contusion	65
Pneumothorax	30
Hemothorax	26
Flail chest	23
Diaphragmatic injury	9
Myocardial contusion[a]	5.7
Blunt aortic injury (traumatic aortic dissection)	4.8
Tracheobronchial injury	0.8
Laryngeal injury	0.3

Modified and reprinted from Devitt et al.[67]
[a]Diagnosed by radionuclide angiography or at autopsy

Table 16.2 Extrathoracic injuries in patients with chest trauma

Injury	Incidence (%)
Head injury	49
Cervical spine	12
Facial injuries	29.8
Abdomen and pelvis	49
Extremities including bony pelvis	72.6

Modified and reprinted from Devitt et al.[67]

C.E. Smith (✉)
Department of Anesthesia, MetroHealth Medical Center, Case Western Reserve University, 2500 MetroHealth Drive, Cleveland, OH 44109, USA
e-mail: csmith@metrohealth.org

K. Subramaniam et al. (eds.), *Anesthesia and Perioperative Care for Aortic Surgery*, DOI 10.1007/978-0-387-85922-4_16, © Springer Science+Business Media, LLC 2011

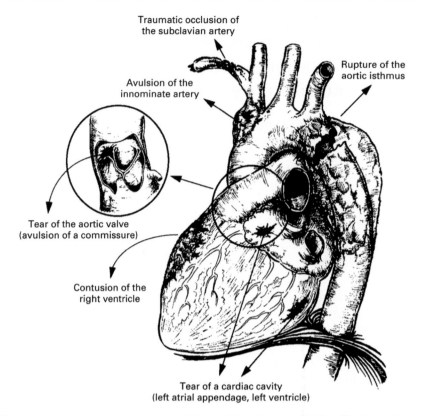

Fig. 16.1 Blunt trauma to the great vessels and heart (Reprinted from Pretre and Chilcott[123] with permission from New England Journal of Medicine: Copyright c [1997] Massachusetts Medical Society. All rights reserved)

adventitia), 30% died within 6 h, 40% within 24 h, 72% by 8 days, 83% by 3 weeks, and 90% died by 10 weeks if the lesion was not diagnosed and treated.[5]

High-speed motor vehicle collisions involving frontal and side impacts or occupant ejection, and motorcycle crashes are frequent causes of blunt aortic injury (BAI).[6] Other causes of aortic injury include autopedestrian collisions, falls, blast injuries, airplane and train crashes, and penetrating chest injuries. The mechanisms associated with BAI involve sudden and violent deceleration as well as a crushing mechanical load on the organs within the thorax. Trauma associated with a rapid deceleration and stress mostly affects the aortic isthmus, which is the junction between the relatively fixed descending aorta and relatively mobile aortic arch (Fig. 16.1).[3] The deceleration response is also associated with deformation in the spine and thoracic cage due to their flexibility, which can transfer a crushing mechanical load on organs within the chest. Direct loading of the

pressurized descending thoracic aorta resulted in isthmus injury secondary to aortic wall strain in an animal model.[7] A critical load is required to cause transection and exsanguination.

Shearing and bending stresses are most likely responsible for BAI at the isthmus, whereas torsion stress and stress from the water–hammer effect (high pressure wave reflected back along the aorta when flow of blood is suddenly occluded due to mechanical compression) are more likely to affect the ascending aorta.

Pathology

Aortic ruptures occur at isthmus in 80% of cases in pathological series versus 95% in clinical series. Ascending aorta is involved in 10–20% of autopsy series versus 5% in clinical series.[5,8,9] This indicates the high prehospital mortality. Other sites involved are distal descending aorta (12%) and infrarenal abdominal aorta (4.7%). Blunt trauma may also result in injuries to the brachiocephalic vessels, most commonly the base of the innominate artery.[10]

According to the study by Parmley et al.,[5] TAR can be classified pathologically as: intimal hemorrhage with or without laceration, medial laceration, complete laceration, false aneurysm formation, and periaortic hemorrhage. Intimal hemorrhage and tears may heal spontaneously. When the lesion involves media and intima, false aneurysm formation occurs, which is fusiform in circumferential lesions and saccular in partial lesions. Complete rupture of the aorta including adventitia and periadventitial connective tissue lead to immediate death, unless the rupture is contained by the formation of hematoma in periaortic and mediastinal tissues (15% of cases). In a few cases of TAR, the intima and media tears form a flap, which acts as a ball-valve, partial aortic obstruction occurs, with upper extremity hypertension reported as pseudocoarctation (10%).[11]

Prehospital Care

Improved prehospital care and rapid transportation have increased survival, but mortality from thoracic aortic injury still remains high. In patients with aortic injury and hemorrhagic shock, control of the bleeding in the operating room is the goal. Efforts to stabilize with rapid intravenous fluids and pneumatic antishock trousers may dislodge the clot or hematoma at the aortic injury site and worsen the situation.[12,13] Rapid transport to the appropriate facility after initial airway control with cervical stabilization is advised.

Emergency Room Care

Once the patient arrives at the emergency room, evaluation and resuscitation following principles of the American College of Surgeons Advanced Trauma Life Support® (ATLS®) are done.[14] Teamwork between trauma surgeons, emergency department personnel, anesthesiologists, radiologists, nurses, and specialists is essential. Management begins with the primary survey together with resuscitation of vital functions (oxygen supplementation, tracheal intubation, large bore intravenous (IV) access, fluid resuscitation, control of bleeding, and chest decompression), followed by adjuncts to the primary survey such as chest x-ray (CXR), fast-focused abdominal sonography for trauma, a detailed secondary survey, and definitive care. Immediate life-threatening aortic and other injuries are identified during primary survey since they present with massive bleeding. The patient may require emergency surgery at this point, and should be transported immediately to the operating room for exploration by a qualified surgeon. Another group of patients with aortic injuries are identified during the secondary survey and are stable enough to undergo further diagnostic imaging. Further management is planned based on the results of the tests.

Clinical Presentation and Preoperative Evaluation

The degree of external trauma may not fully predict the severity of injury; thus, clinical suspicion of pulmonary, cardiac, and great vessel trauma should be heightened in patients who have sustained high-energy decelerating trauma. Patients who sustained TAR should be screened for associated other organ system injuries as they are frequent (90%). Long bone, pelvic and spine fractures, pulmonary contusion, cardiac injury, closed head injury and abdominal visceral injuries (especially liver and spleen) often dominate the clinical picture.

Respiratory distress and hemodynamic instability are common presenting features. Loss of consciousness may be present. Back pain, midscapular pain, and retrosternal pain are reported in 20–75% of patients.[15] Dysphagia, hoarseness, upper extremity ischemia, and paraplegia (6%) are other presenting features. Difference in the blood pressure between the two upper extremities and between lower and upper extremities may be present.[15] Upper extremity hypertension can be attributed to pseudo-coarctation or compression by aortic hematoma. Loss of lower extremity pulses may also indicate embolization. Systemic hypertension (17%) may occur due to reflex induced by stretching and stimulation of cardiac plexus at isthmus.[15] Negative physical examination is reported in 5–14% of cases[15] Signs of rupture or impending rupture include recurrent bleeding into pleural space, hypotension below 90 mmHg in spite of adequate fluid resuscitation, vocal cord palsy, tracheal or superior vena cava compression.[15,16] Finally, substance abuse may be a contributing factor in many instances, and a history of intoxication should be documented.

All laboratory and diagnostic imaging should be reviewed with particular emphasis on hemoglobin, hematocrit, electrolytes, arterial blood gases, coagulation studies, toxicology, electrocardiogram (ECG), and imaging studies (CXR, pelvic X-ray, abdominal ultrasound, transthoracic echocardiogram (TTE), Computerized Tomographic (CT) scan of head, neck, chest, and abdomen). Prior interventions during the prehospital, emergency department, and other phases of resuscitation such as radiology and intensive care unit (ICU) should be noted including the primary and secondary trauma surveys. Interventions preceding diagnostic studies may include definitive airway control, cardiorespiratory resuscitation, blood transfusion, tube thoracostomy, and in some cases craniotomy, thoracotomy, laparotomy, and pelvic fixation.[17]

Identification of any head injuries and interventions to resuscitate and stabilize these patients following initial presentation take priority.

Diagnostic Imaging of Aortic Trauma

Chest Roentgenography (Fig. 16.2a and b)

Suggestive radiological signs are evident on the CXR and they are not specific (Table 16.3).[18] Most of these signs are valuable by their absence, rather than by their presence as indicators of rupture. True erect CXR has high negative predictive value (98%) and has been utilized in the past as a screening test for identifying subjects who will require further imaging studies.[19]

Computerized Tomography (Fig. 16.3a–c)

Chest CT is more commonly used in the acute setting as it allows concurrent evaluation of other thoracic trauma.[20] Improvements in CT

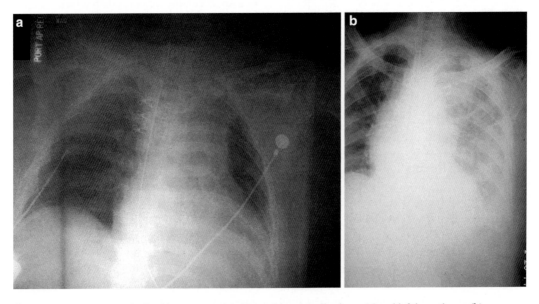

Fig. 16.2 Chest radiograph after blunt trauma showing a widened mediastinum (**a**) and left hemothorax (**b**)

Table 16.3 Chest radiographic evidence suggestive of aortic injury

Widened mediastinum >8.0 cm
Mediastinum:chest ratio >0.25
Opacification of aorto-pulmonary window
Irregular aortic knob
Blurred aortic contour
Deviation of nasogastric tube
Tracheal deviation to patient's right
Depressed left main bronchus
Elevation and rightward shift of right bronchus
Pulmonary contusion
Widened left paraspinal stripe
Left apical cap
Fractures (rib, thoracic spine, clavicle, and scapula)

Modified from Aydin et al.[18]

technology with helical and multirow detector CT, and multiplanar reformation and volume rendering techniques have resulted in CT being the definitive screening test for major thoracic vascular injury.[21] In the AAST2 (American Association for the Surgery of Trauma 2) study, there was nearly complete elimination of aortography and TEE as the method of definitive diagnosis of BAI.[22] Both the contrast-enhanced and non-contrast-enhanced CT scans are used to maximize the ability to identify the aortic pathologies such as dissection and intramural hematoma. Findings suggestive of aortic disruption include wall thickening, filling defects, aortic hematoma (para-aortic and intramural),

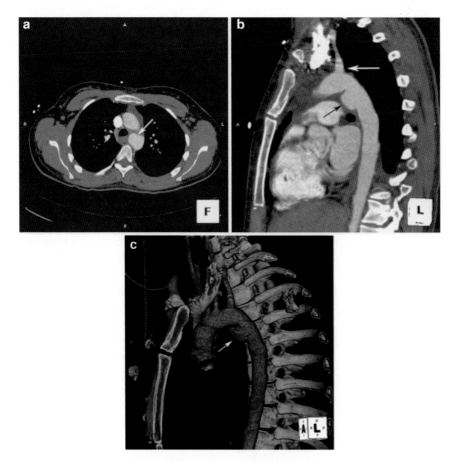

Fig. 16.3 (**a–c**) Traumatic disruption of the aorta. (**a**) Axial image of a chest *CT* that demonstrates posttraumatic aortic wall disruption (*arrow*) in a young patient with a normal aorta. (**b**) Multiplanar reconstruction view in the same patient demonstrates the bulging of the aorta (*black arrow*) just distal to the *left* subclavian artery (*white arrow*). (**c**) Volumetric 3D reconstruction of the same *CT* scan demonstrates the aortic transection just distal to the origin of the left subclavian artery. The heart and pulmonary artery have been removed to facilitate visualization of the aortic arch and descending thoracic aorta (Reprinted with permission from Aydin et al.[18])

intimal flaps, and contrast extravasation. CT imaging is crucial in determining the suitability of an endovascular repair and for procedural planning. Important information for endovascular repair consists of proximal and distal landing zones, access vessels, and device sizing. Injuries to the brachiocephalic vessels will also be identified with CT imaging. Because CT provides high-quality images with reduction in artifacts and acquisition time, CT is the method of choice to evaluate polytrauma patients with suspected BAI.

Aortagraphy

Aortography has been used as a standard in the past to diagnose BAI. Linear filling defect at the level of isthmus with focal bulge with delayed washout are highly specific for aortic rupture (Fig. 16.4). Several cases of mortality (without cause and effect relationship) and the high rate of complications (10.5%) make aortography not a recommended procedure in this era of high resolution noninvasive modalities in polytrauma patients with suspected BAI.[23,24] Aortography still has a role, where new-generation CT is not available. In addition, aortic arch and branch vessel injuries are difficult to

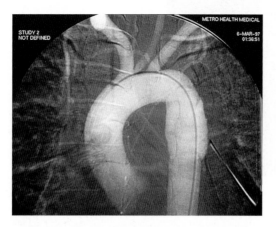

Fig. 16.4 Aortography showing extravasation of contrast material distal to the left subclavian artery

diagnose by CT, and this information may be important in surgical planning.

Transesophageal Echocardiography (Fig. 16.5)

TEE does have specific advantages, especially portability[25,26] (Table 16.4). TEE is valuable for diagnosing BAI (intraluminal thick stripes, intramural hematoma, intimal flap, disruption, aneurysm, dissection, and increased aorta-probe distance) and can be used to grade BAI according to therapeutic implications[27] (Table 16.5). However, TEE may miss injuries in the distal ascending aorta, proximal aortic arch, and branch vessels. Moreover, TEE cannot be done in patients with esophageal injury. In a study of 121 trauma patients admitted to the emergency room with a diagnosis of possible BAI, TEE could not be completed in 28 patients due to lack of available equipment or operators to perform the study (20 patients), difficulty in achieving sedation (six patients), refusal of consent (one patient), and mandibular fracture (one patient).[28] Compared with helical chest CT, multiplane TEE was more sensitive for the detection of superficial thoracic aortic injuries involving the aortic intimal or medial layers and blunt cardiac trauma.[29] The key to TEE diagnosis is to understand that imaging of the descending thoracic aorta is normally excellent, but when the aorta is disrupted and surrounded by hematoma, there is echocardiography "dropout" leading to poor imaging. Furthermore, the aorta decreases in size as it travels distally. If the aortic diameter increases in size from the arch to the descending, then BAI must be suspected. Finally, severe aortic atheroma is very uncommon in patients less than 50 years old. Disruption to the intima can appear like severe aortic atheroma, and, in the setting of a young person with a deceleration injury, then this points to aortic transection. TEE also allows the diagnosis of associated cardiac injuries. TEE evaluation of aortic trauma is further described in detail in the chapter on echocardiography of aorta.

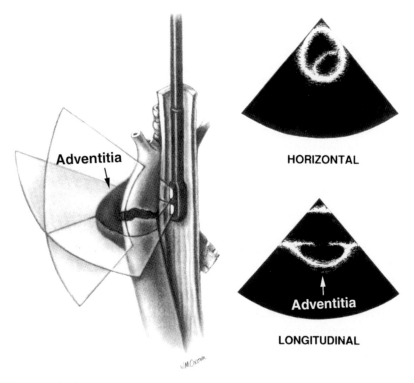

Fig. 16.5 *TEE* exam of the descending thoracic aorta showing aortic disruption with adventitial containment (Reprinted with permission from Oxorn et al.[124])

Table 16.4 Advantages and disadvantages of transesophageal echocardiography in aortic trauma

Advantages	Disadvantages
Portability	Requires experienced specialist (operator-dependent)
Ease of performance	Contraindicated in esophageal pathology
Ease of follow-up examinations	Potential to exacerbate unstable cervical spine injuries
No perceptible delay in primary or secondary survey	Potential airway problems if not tracheally intubated
Excellent imaging of descending thoracic aorta, proximal ascending aorta, distal aortic arch, right and left heart chambers, valves, interatrial septum, and intracardiac lesions	Unable to visualize portions of the ascending aorta, aortic arch, and brachiocephalic branches due to the tracheal air column
	Decreased diagnostic ability if pneumomediastinum

Modified and reprinted with permission from Ben-Menachem[26]

Table 16.5 Transesophageal echocardiography findings and possible management of blunt aortic injury

Severity and characteristic finding	Therapy
Grade 1: Intramural hematoma or limited intimal flap	Medical follow-up
Grade 2: Subadventitial rupture or modification of the geometric shape of the aorta	Open or endovascular repair. Urgent vs. Delayed
Grade 3: Aortic transection with active bleeding or aortic obstruction with ischemia	Emergency repair

Modified and reprinted with permission from Goarin[27]

Magnetic Resonance Imaging

MRI has high diagnostic accuracy (100%) in BAI and can differentiate circumferential and partial lesions, hematomas, and aneurysms. Patient access and the imaging time are limitations. In the era of stabilization and delayed surgery, MRI can be utilized in the subacute phase to monitor the aortic lesion before surgery because of its noninvasiveness, high accuracy, and reproducibility.

Modern Therapeutic Strategies for BAI

Three types of clinical presentations are described for patients with aortic injuries. The first group has massive injuries and dies at the scene or on transport. A second group presents to the hospital in a hemodynamically unstable condition, but may have time for diagnostic imaging and operative intervention. Their mortality is high despite immediate surgery. Endovascular stenting is another therapeutic option in unstable patients. A third group presents to the hospital with stable hemodynamics and have contained aortic rupture as diagnosed by chest CT or aortography. Aortic injury related death is very rare in this group. Mortality is usually dependent on associated other major injuries. **Life-threatening conditions (liver injury, spleen rupture, and intracranial bleeding) should be treated first to prevent hypovolemic shock and multiorgan failure.** Pulmonary contusions increase the chance of ARDS postoperatively. Lesions such as open fractures and major burns are prone to develop sepsis and should be stabilized. Systemic heparinization, which may be required to repair the aorta early, may precipitate fatal hemorrhage in the brain, abdomen, lungs, and elsewhere. Persistent systolic blood pressure above 140 mmHg is associated with increased risk of aortic rupture, mandating medical therapy with antihypertensives such as beta-blockers and vasodilators.

The concept of medical therapy with delayed definitive repair has gained wide acceptance.[22] Delayed surgical approach consists of serial imaging and monitoring of the aortic lesion.[30] A management algorithm of modern therapeutic strategy of BAI is shown in Fig. 16.6.[31]

Open Surgery for Aortic Trauma

Ascending aortic tears require sternotomy, and may necessitate replacement/repair of the aortic valve and reimplantation of coronary arteries. A period of deep hypothermic circulatory arrest with antegrade cerebral perfusion (axillary artery cannulation) may be used, especially if the distal ascending aorta, arch, and arch vessels are involved. The average duration of circulatory arrest was 31 min in one study of acute and chronic traumatic great vessel injuries.[32] Injuries involving the origin of innominate and left carotid can be bypassed with a graft to ascending aorta. Partial occluding clamp without cardiopulmonary bypass (CPB) can be done.[33,34]

Open surgical repair of descending thoracic aorta injury requires left thoracotomy. Overall surgical mortality in a meta-analysis was 21.3% ranging from 0 to 54.2%.[35] In a more recent review, the mortality decreased and ranged from 8 to 15%.[36] Advances in surgical and anesthesia techniques, perfusion management, neuromonitoring, neuroprotection strategies, and postoperative management have contributed to significant reductions in morbidity and mortality over the past 50 years.[37–40]

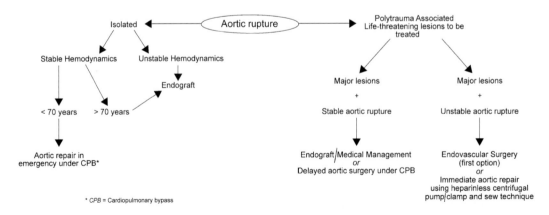

Fig. 16.6 Management Algorithm for traumatic aortic injury (Modified with permission from Langanay et al.[31])

Nonetheless, open repair has the potential to induce major hemodynamic, respiratory, and physiologic stresses on trauma patients with complex injuries. Considerations include the potential for massive blood loss; hemodynamic alterations induced by aortic cross-clamping; requirement for one-lung ventilation; spinal cord and visceral ischemia during cross clamp; hypothermia, and coagulopathy.

The patient is positioned in right lateral decubitus position with hips rolled back towards a supine position to get access to femoral vessels. One lung ventilation is required to facilitate access to the aorta. Distal perfusion technique using left atrial to femoral artery partial bypass is employed.

One of the significant issues is anticoagulation for partial or full bypass in the setting of head injury or other severe trauma. In such cases, left heart bypass with centrifugal pump can be performed either without heparin, with heparin-coated extracorporeal circuits, or with low-dose heparin, thus reducing bleeding complications.[41] Distal perfusion techniques attenuate proximal hypertension, provide blood flow to the lower body, prevent metabolic acidosis and hypotension after unclamping, and may possibly decrease the incidence of renal failure and paraplegia.[42]

Adequate blood products are made available and cell-saver device is used to suck the blood from the chest for autotransfusion. Femoral artery cannulation is done before thoracotomy if the chances of rupture of false aneurysm and bleeding are high during thoracotomy and dissection. Fibrosis around the lesions make the late repair difficult compared to fresh cases. Proximal control is achieved between left carotid and left subclavian arteries because efforts to clamp will result in release of false aneurysm and exsanguination. Patients with left internal mammary artery graft may require CPB and circulatory arrest. The vertebral artery, a branch of the left subclavian artery (SCA), also perfuses the spinal cord. Clamps proximal to the left SCA may decrease collateral flow to the cord. If this is recognized, the clamp should be moved beyond the left SCA. The distal clamp is applied as close to

the aneurysm to preserve perfusion to the spinal cord by intercostals. Low placement of the distal aortic clamp may interfere with the artery of Adamkiewiz arising from T5-T8 in 12–15% of patients. After excision of the aortic lesion, direct continuity is reestablished by end-to-end suture or a graft interposition.

Spinal cord ischemia remains unpredictable and a major cause of morbidity after open repair of descending aortic tears.[43] The increased risk of paraplegia is heightened during repair of TAR because of the lack of preformed collaterals. Risk factors for developing paraplegia after aortic surgery include duration of aortic cross-clamping, intraoperative hypotension, and surgical technique. Limiting the aortic cross-clamp time to ≤30 min is crucial in determining the frequency of postoperative spinal cord injury after descending thoracic aortic surgery.[44] The incidence of paraplegia is decreased from 16 to 14% by using some form of distal perfusion.[36,45] Von Opell et al. found that paraplegia was 19% with clamp and sew, 11% with passive shunts, and 2.3% with distal circulatory support.[35] The hypothesis that decreasing cerebrospinal fluid (CSF) pressures with the use of intrathecal catheters will prevent postoperative neurologic deficit after aortic repair for TAR has yet to be adequately studied in humans. Use of nitroprusside to control proximal aortic pressure during cross-clamp may result in lower distal aortic pressures, higher CSF pressures, lower spinal cord perfusion pressures, and an increased incidence of postoperative paraplegia.[46] Other complications after open aortic repair include respiratory failure, pneumonia, renal failure, suture line failure, stroke, coagulopathy, worsening of pre-existing injuries, and recurrent nerve palsy.

Endovascular (Endoluminal) Stenting

In recent years, delayed aortic surgery has represented one of the advances in the treatment of polytrauma with BAI.[47,48] Delaying surgery is not without risk. Studies quote 5% risk of rupture.[4,49,50] Repeated hemothorax and uncontrolled blood pressure are signs of impending rupture. In these patients, endovascular repair is a suitable alternative to operative repair. Endovascular stent grafting can also be employed in acute aortic trauma patients and in the treatment of chronic posttraumatic false aneurysms. Endovascular stent grafts may enable definitive repair or serve as a bridge until the patient is stable enough to undergo an operation, if necessary.[18]

Endovascular stent grafting is a technology where patient comorbidities have driven this therapeutic option (Fig. 16.7). Experience gained from endovascular abdominal aortic repair has allowed the successful treatment of aortic pathology involving the distal aortic arch and thoracic aorta including aneurysms, dissection, pseudoaneurysms, and trauma rupture. Endovascular repair has replaced open repair in many centers,

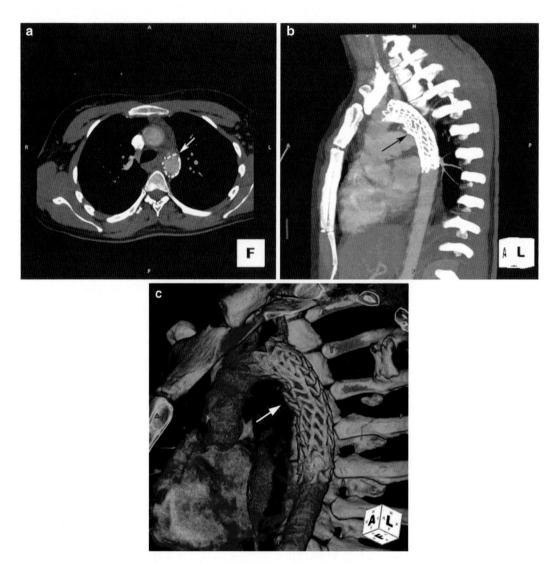

Fig. 16.7 (**a**) Axial *CT* scan in the same patient as in Fig. 16.9 following endovascular stent graft placement (*arrow*), which demonstrates exclusion of the transected portion of the thoracic aorta with no evidence of extravasation of contrast. (**b**) Multiplanar reconstruction in the same patient showing the stent graft placed in the proximal descending thoracic aorta just distal to the origin of the left subclavian artery. Note contrast filling of the left subclavian artery demonstrating patency. (**c**) Volumetric 3D reconstruction of the postprocedure *CT* scan demonstrating a thoracic stent graft in situ with successful exclusion of the aortic transection (Reprinted with permission Aydin et al.[18])

resulting in a major reduction of mortality and procedure-related paraplegia.[51–54] Endovascular stenting of BAI has been shown to have excellent mid-term results and acceptable rates of morbidity and mortality.[55–58] Potential benefits include the option to perform this procedure under local and regional anesthesia and nonrequirement for thoracotomy, one-lung ventilation, aortic cross-clamping, and cardiopulmonary bypass. Avoidance of a thoracotomy minimizes post-operative pain, and associated respiratory compromise. Endovascular exclusion of an aortic disruption reduces blood pressure shifts and surgical blood loss, and minimizes visceral organ ischemic time. Requirement for anticoagulation is minimal, which is desirable in patients with intracranial, orthopedic, and abdominal injuries.

Limitations of endovascular repair include rigorous anatomic criteria as to the suitability of endograft procedure, development of an endoleak, lack of long-term outcome data, nonavailability of the stent grafts in many centers, lack of trained personnel, and access issues.[59,60] During stent-graft deployment, complications may arise from use of vasodilators, adenosine, or controlled ventricular fibrillation. Temporary pacing may be required along with vasopressors. Collapsed graft with aortic coarctation has been reported in one patient at 3-month follow-up.[61]

Adequate proximal and distal landing zones must be present for fixation of the stent graft in the thoracic aorta. Anatomic criteria for endovascular graft include proximal neck of the lesion should be more than 10 mm in length, distance of more than 5 mm from the left subclavian artery, and absence of thrombus, calcification, and hemorrhage on the aortic wall on the neck site. CT imaging is done along with postimaging analysis to ensure that the anatomy is appropriate for an endovascular repair. Analysis must also include an assessment of the femoral and iliac access vessels. Patients with access vessels of inadequate size, significant calcification, or tortuosity may require the creation of an iliac conduit, or distal aortic conduit to permit delivery of the stent graft.

Endoleaks are uncommon after treatment of BAI with endograft. Healthy aorta proximally and distally from rupture site means a satisfactory seal can be easily accomplished without type 1 leak. Since the rupture is at the isthmus and few intercostal arteries arise from this pathologic segment, there is minimal risk of type 2 endoleak. Furthermore, as a single stent graft is used, the risk of type 3 endoleak is also minimized.[62]

Given that the majority of the traumatic aortic disruptions are in proximity to the left SCA, consideration must be given to SCA coverage. The safety of overstenting of the SCA was demonstrated in different series.[62,63] Since prophylactic carotid to SCA bypass itself carries the risk of stroke, a bypass procedure can be done if symptoms of vertebral insufficiency or upper extremity ischemia develop postoperatively. Recent literature and imaging studies suggest that the risk of vertebrobasilar and spinal cord ischemia is low.[64] In the unusual setting of the patient who has had the left internal thoracic artery utilized as a coronary bypass graft, coverage of the left SCA orifice may lead to coronary ischemia and myocardial infarction.

The incidence of paraplegia following stent-graft repair approaches zero, which is in stark contrast to the incidence following open repair.[4,18] In a retrospective study of 74 patients with acute traumatic aortic rupture, hospital mortality was lower in the endovascular group compared with the open surgical repair group (7.7% vs. 20%).[65] In the 39 patients in the endovascular group, one patient required conversion to conventional surgery, while stent-graft implantation was successful in the remaining cases, without peri-interventional complications or procedure-induced paraplegia. In nine patients, the left subclavian artery was covered with the device. Two patients underwent surgical repair 15 days and 4 months after endografting because of injury of the aortic wall by the stent and development of an aneurysm.

In a retrospective analysis of the New Zealand stent database, 27 patients had endovascular repair of acute thoracic aortic injuries between 2001 and 2007.[66] Primary technical success was achieved in 26 patients, endoleaks occurred in 4, maldeployment occurred in 1 (stent graft covered the left vertebral artery arch origin with partial occlusion of the left common carotid artery), and common femoral artery thrombosis occurred in one. No deaths occurred during the endovascular procedure and no patient developed paraplegia. Mean length of stay was 24 days. Other complications were related to multiple trauma and consisted of pulmonary contusion with collapse/consolidation, chest infection, atrial fibrillation, confusion, oliguria, intra-abdominal bleeding, and bile leak. Two patients died after stent grafting- one from intra-abdominal hemorrhage (1 day after stenting) and one from sepsis and head injury (59 days post-procedure).

In a comparative study of patients with similar lesions and severity scores, endovascular grafting ($n = 29$) was associated with no mortality and paraplegia, compared to 21% mortality and 7% of paraplegia associated with open repair ($n = 35$). Mean follow-up period was 46 months.[62]

Endovascular management of BAI represents a major advance in the care of trauma patients, and has achieved excellent technical success, low mortality, and a very low incidence of paraplegia. The technical expertise and knowledge required to successfully treat BAI in an endovascular manner requires endovascular skills and advanced imaging equipment. Careful follow-up in patients undergoing endovascular repair of aortic trauma is necessary to prove the long-term efficacy of this treatment modality.

Intraoperative Monitoring

Standard Monitoring

Standard monitoring includes ECG, noninvasive blood pressure, pulse oximetry, end-tidal CO_2, precordial or esophageal stethoscope, and temperature. A peripheral nerve stimulator is used to assess the degree of neuromuscular blockade. Electroencephalogram, evoked potentials, and cerebral oximetry are useful, especially for patients undergoing cardiopulmonary bypass and DHCA (see section on neurologic monitoring). Peak and plateau airway pressures are continuously monitored during mechanical ventilation. Tidal volumes of 6 ml/kg are generally employed. Peak airway pressures are maintained at ≤ 30 cm

H_2O. Any sudden increases in pressure during volume-controlled ventilation may signify tension pneumothorax. Similarly, any sudden decrease in tidal volume using pressure-controlled ventilation must be critically investigated. If a chest tube has been placed, ongoing blood loss from the affected hemithorax can be monitored.[67]

Invasive Monitoring

Direct measurement of arterial blood pressure is routine. Insertion of an arterial catheter allows for precise beat-to-beat measurement of blood pressure. The arterial catheter also facilitates sampling of arterial blood gases, blood chemistry, hematocrit, hemoglobin, and coagulation parameters. A left radial (or brachial) arterial line is used for ascending and arch repairs, which may require circulatory arrest. In these cases, right axillary cannulation with antegrade cerebral perfusion can be done together with EEG and cerebral oximetry monitoring. A right radial (or brachial) and right femoral arteries are cannulated to monitor the blood pressures above and below aortic cross-clamp during open descending thoracic aorta surgery. Right radial arterial line is also recommended for endovascular cases where the left SCA may be covered by endograft.

Arterial pulse contour analysis provides useful information in the form of pulse pressure and systolic pressure variation (SPV).[68] Systolic pressure variation (SPV) and pulse pressure variation (PPV) can be valuable tools in assessing volume status. Arterial pulse contour changes stem from changes in preload during the respiratory cycle. The patient must be mechanically ventilated and in sinus rhythm to derive meaningful data. When pleural and transpulmonary pressures are increased during mechanical ventilation of the lung, systemic venous return is impaired, causing a decrease in right ventricular (RV) filling and an increase in RV afterload and, thus, a transient decrease in RV ejection.[69,70] Reduced RV stroke volume results in a preload reduction of the left ventricle (LV). This cyclical respiratory variation in LV stroke volume can be observed in arterial pressure throughout the respiratory cycle.[71,72]

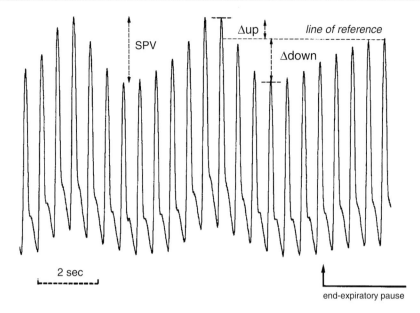

Fig. 16.8 Respiratory changes during mechanical ventilation. The difference between maximal and minimal values of systolic blood pressure over a single respira-tory cycle is the systolic pressure variation (*SPV*) (Adapted from Michard and Teboul[125] (Permission from Springer))

Systolic pressure variation (SPV) is the difference in minimum and maximum systolic BP over one respiratory cycle (Fig. 16.8). SPV is divided into two components, Δup and Δdown. These values represent the maximum and minimum variation in systolic blood pressure during one respiratory cycle compared to a reference value. These changes represent changes in LV stroke volume by a combination of changes in LV preload and afterload, or extramural aortic pressure. SPV ≥ 12 mmHg is considered a threshold value for volume responders versus nonresponders.[73]

PPV variation is the change in the difference between the diastolic and systolic BP, with a peak and trough over a single respiratory cycle (Fig. 16.9). Pulse pressure variation depends on changes in aortic transmural pressure, and is directly proportional to LV stroke volume and inversely related to arterial compliance. Pulse pressure variation is not directly influenced by changes in pleural pressure, since the increase in pleural pressure by positive pressure ventilation will influence both systolic and diastolic pressures. In patients undergoing coronary artery bypass grafting, a pulse pressure variation ≥11% was found to have a sensitivity of 100% and a specificity of 93% as an indicator for an increase in cardiac output after volume administration.[74]

SPV has been evaluated in assessing the effects of hemorrhage on pulse contour in humans and animals and has been compared to pulse pressure variation in conditions of severe hemorrhage in an animal study.[75-79] Data supports using these measures as assessors of intravascular depletion. A particular advantage of pulse pressure variation and SPV in the trauma setting is that it is a dynamic estimate of volume status. A practical advantage to using arterial waveform analysis as a guide to fluid resuscitation in trauma is that it is relatively safe, is less prone to complications, and is typically much faster than placing a central venous line or a pulmonary artery catheter.

Central venous pressure catheters provide secure access for fluid therapy, drug infusions, and for CVP monitoring. Trends in CVP are useful in managing patients requiring massive fluid resuscitation and in those patients requiring infusion of vasopressors and inotropes. With pericardial tamponade, there is elevation and equalization of diastolic filling pressures. The x descent is preserved and the y descent is dampened because of restricted early right ventricular filling. With pulmonary contusion, CVP

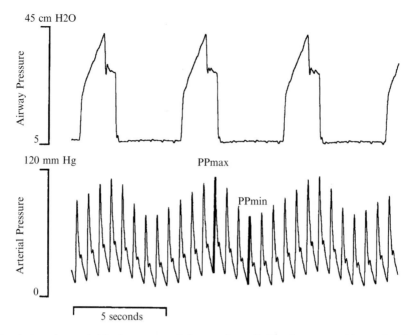

Fig. 16.9 Respiratory changes in blood pressure and airway pressure during mechanical ventilation. Pulse pressure (*PP*) variation is the difference between the diastolic and systolic blood pressure, with a peak and trough over a single respiratory cycle (Adapted from Michard and Teboul[125] (Permission from Springer))

may be a better estimate of cardiac preload compared with pulmonary capillary wedge pressure, due to increased pulmonary vascular resistance, airway resistance, and dead space ventilation.[80]

The pulmonary artery (PA) catheter allows for accurate hemodynamic assessment and modification of therapy. It is a useful monitor in patients with impaired cardiac function who require vasoactive drug therapy to maintain perfusion and/or pressure. Although it is reasonable to assume that more precise knowledge of cardiovascular parameters will permit more appropriate treatment, there are many well-known risks of PA catheter monitoring.

Transesophageal Echocardiography (TEE)

TEE monitoring of ventricular function and preload are useful in the management of open repair, especially during cross-clamp and reperfusion periods.[81,82] TEE can assess preload more accurately than PA catheters. TEE is also used to

Table 16.6 Sensitivity and specificity of various modalities in diagnosing blunt aortic injury (aortic transaction)

	Sensitivity (%)	Specificity (%)
Contrast-enhanced CT	100	100
Transesophageal echocardiography	63–100	84–100
Aortography	100	100

From Aydin et al.[18]

monitor RV function after myocardial contusions. TEE is an excellent diagnostic tool for valvular disease, pericardial effusion and tamponade, hemothorax, and mediastinal hematoma. TEE may be the only imaging technique readily available in trauma patients undergoing surgery in the operating room. In these patients, TEE can be used to define the presence and extent of aortic injury to guide further management (immediate versus delayed surgical repair of BAI/surgical versus endovascular repair). The sensitivity and specificity of TEE in comparison to other diagnostic modalities are given in Table 16.6. TEE can also be used during endograft procedures to evaluate the landing zone, guide the wire placement, assess for endoleaks immediately after endograft deployment, and evaluate any procedure-related injuries after the procedure.[83] TEE has also been used to prevent the unintentional entry of the stent introducer into a descending aorta psuedoaneurysm with potential disruption of a contained aortic transection.[84]

Neurologic Monitoring

Electroencephalogram (EEG)

Several monitors are available, which convert select EEG signals into a single number that reflects the patient's level of consciousness. This number is used to guide pharmacologic therapy and depth of anesthesia. In trauma, depth of anesthesia monitors would be predicted to behave normally. The brain-injured patient potentially presents a special case. Several studies have taken place trying to correlate Glasgow Coma Scale score (GCS) and observational sedation scales with BIS levels in the brain-injured patient. A correlation exists between GCS score and BIS so that the higher the GCS score, the higher the BIS. This relationship was maintained both with and without sedation, validating the use of BIS in brain-injured patients.[85,86] Use of a processed EEG monitor does not guarantee lack of awareness.[87,88]

Evoked Potentials

Evoked potentials measure nervous system electrical activity that has been elicited by a stimulus. Evoked potentials are described in terms of amplitude, latency, and morphology. The most common evoked potentials used in the operating room are sensory and motor.

Somatosensory Evoked Potentials (SSEPs)

The somatosensory system relays vibration, proprioception, and light touch information from the periphery to the central nervous system. Electrical stimuli are applied to peripheral nerves (most commonly the median, ulnar, common peroneal, and posterior tibial nerves) and signals are assessed along the path of the nerve to the cortex. Typically, electrical potentials are assessed at the level of the cortex by scalp electrodes. Many signals are averaged from repeated stimulation to obtain a clinically useful waveform.[89] SSEP signals are carried mostly in the posterior spinal column; thus, anterior damage due to aortic cross-clamping may not be recorded by the SSEP. Anesthetic agents have variable effects on the signal.

Motor Evoked Potentials (MEPs)

Transcranial or spinal cord electrical stimulation produces a descending signal that can be recorded over the spinal cord, peripheral nerve, or muscle. Damage to anterior spinal tracts (motor tracts) not identified by SSEPs might be recognized by MEPs. MEPs are sensitive to inhaled anesthetic agents and a total intravenous anesthetic approach is commonly employed without neuromuscular blockade.[90]

Cerebral Oximetry

Cerebral oximetry is a noninvasive measure of cerebral perfusion. Regional cerebral saturation monitors use near-infrared spectroscopy, similar to pulse oximetry, to measure tissue saturation (rSO2). Regional cerebral saturation is measured noninvasively using cutaneous patches placed on the forehead. The alteration of regional cerebral perfusion and thus rSO2 can be detected by the sensors. Cerebral oximetry is used in patients requiring bypass and circulatory arrest.

Studies have shown improvements in stroke rates and major organ morbidity and mortality when cerebral saturation is measured and interventions performed to keep the saturation within 75% of baseline.[91] Cerebral oxygen saturation can be improved by various anesthetic and perfusion interventions in a stepwise approach (Table 16.7). Cerebral oximetry is also useful in head trauma patients. Cerebral blood flow depends on cerebral perfusion pressure (CPP). Therapy in head trauma patients is guided towards improving CPP and,

Table 16.7 Cerebral desaturation treatment algorithm

1. Increase inspired oxygen to 100%
2. Check head and cannula position to ensure adequate venous drainage
3. If PaCO2 <40 mmHg, increase PaCO2 to >40 mmHg
4. If MAP <50, increase MAP to >60 mmHg
5. If hematocrit <20%, transfuse PRBC's
6. If none of the above interventions improve cerebral saturation, decrease cerebral oxygen consumption by increasing anesthesia depth

Reprinted with permission from www.scahq.org (May and Greilich[127]).

MAP mean arterial blood pressure, *PRBCs* packed red blood cells.

thus, cerebral perfusion in the setting of elevated intracranial pressure (ICP). In the past, many patients needed to have invasive ICP monitors placed in order to determine CPP. A study showed a correlation of CPP to cerebral saturation. Cerebral oxygen saturation greater than 75% suggested that CPP was adequate to meet metabolic demands whereas rSO2 < 55 suggested inadequate CPP.[92] A follow-up study showed a correlation of cerebral hypoxia (rSO2 < 60%) with lower GCS scores, lower CPP, more severe head computed tomography score, and decreased survival.[93]

Limitations of cerebral oximetry include effect of temperature on near-infrared absorption spectrum, contamination of the signal by chromophores in the skin, and differences between the various manufacturer's devices. Despite these limitations, cerebral oximetry together with BIS is routinely used during hypothermic circulatory arrest.

Specific Anesthetic Agents

While open surgical repair requires general anesthesia with OLV and extensive monitoring, endovascular procedures can be done using monitored anesthesia care (MAC), local, regional, or general anesthesia. The selection of specific agents for induction and maintenance of anesthesia and neuromuscular blockade is less important than applying appropriate physiological and pharmacological principles to the patient.

Induction Agents

The hemodynamically compromised patient is especially susceptible to the cardiovascular suppression of bolus doses of propofol and thiopental. Opioids enjoy a wide therapeutic margin in the presence of blood loss. Etomidate is better tolerated in patients with hemodynamic instability.

Maintenance of Anesthesia

Anesthesia can be maintained with inhalational agents or propofol infusion together with opioid supplementation. During aortic surgery with suprarenal cross-clamp, propofol anesthesia was superior to sevoflurane as evidenced by less neutrophil infiltration, lower plasma proinflammatory cytokine levels, lower production of oxygen free radicals, less lipid peroxidation, and reduced nitric oxide synthase activity during reperfusion.[94] Sevoflurane has been shown to attenuate hemodynamic sequelae of ischemia reperfusion injury induced by thoracic aorta occlusion.[95]

Low-dose ketamine can be infused together with propofol and midazolam, often in a TIVA combination.[96] Ketamine produces bronchodilatation, maintains hypoxic pulmonary vasoconstriction, confers hemodynamic stability, and has neuroprotective, analgesic, and anti-inflammatory effects. The incidence of psychomimetic effects when combined with propofol is 0–2%. When subjects are controlled for arterial carbon dioxide, there was no increase in intracranial pressure (ICP). There is no human in vivo evidence of myocardial depression. S(+)-ketamine is thought to have a lower incidence of side effects (psychotropic effects, salivation) and more rapid metabolism, yet produce more intense analgesia at an equimolar dose in comparison to R(-)-ketamine.

Ketamine may increase the heart rate. The advantages of ketamine in trauma patients outweigh the disadvantages.

All volatile agents produce dose-dependent decreases in myocardial function. Isoflurane, enflurane, and halothane blunt coronary autoregulation. Hypoxic pulmonary vasoconstriction (HPV) is impaired by the volatile agents in a concentration-dependent fashion, which can be clinically significant in patients with respiratory problems requiring one-lung ventilation. All inhalational agents are respiratory depressants. They also result in dose-dependent decreases in renal and hepatic blood flow. With general anesthesia, nitrous oxide is avoided because of the risk of expanding air-filled spaces.

In hypotensive unstable patients requiring general anesthesia, midazolam 1–2 mg or scopolamine 0.4 mg may be given for amnesia. Low-dose isoflurane (0.4%) together with synthetic opioids are generally well tolerated in most instances following shock resuscitation. Hemodynamic instability during low-dose volatile-opioid anesthesia is generally the result of other causes rather than anesthetic agents. Neuromuscular blocking drugs are used to facilitate tracheal intubation and provide surgical relaxation. Complete paralysis is necessary during placement and manipulation of double lumen endobronchial tubes (DLTs) and bronchial blockers to avoid excessive coughing due to the proximity to the carina.

Adjuncts to Anesthesia

With transluminal techniques, the self-expanding stent arm vascular endoprosthesis is passed retrograde into the aorta. Current-generation endografts can be deployed using controlled hypotension (systolic BP 80 mmHg) to prevent distal migration of the device as a result of the forward flow during systole.[97-99] There is variability of stent-graft deployment times related to the complexity of the anatomy within the vascular segment being repaired. A duration of 55–172 s has been reported by Kahn et al. for stent-graft repair of descending thoracic aneurysms using controlled ventricular fibrillation.[99] Complex thoracic stent cases may require adenosine cardiac arrest or rapid ventricular pacing. Anesthesiologists should be familiar with such methods. The bolus dose of adenosine necessary to produce a 20–30-s period of asystole varies widely (12–45 mg), but after the dosage is determined, the action of adenosine is predictable and reproducible. Therefore, the minimum dose of adenosine to produce transient asystole of >20 s

has to be established for each patient.[100] When the stent-graft device is in position, this bolus dose of adenosine is administered, and the device is deployed after the occurrence of cardiac arrest.

One-Lung Ventilation for Open Surgical Repair

One-lung ventilation (OLV) is indicated for open repair of descending thoracic aortic tears. OLV facilitates surgical exposure in the left thoracotomy incision. OLV may not be well tolerated in the presence of right-sided pulmonary contusion or pneumo-hemothorax. Surgery may be delayed until the contusion resolves. The optimal technique for providing OLV depends on patient factors, available equipment, and skills and training of the anesthesiologist.[101] Preferred methods for OLV and each of their advantages and disadvantages are shown in Table 16.8. A left-sided double-lumen tube (DLT) is the authors' first choice for providing OLV for open repairs because of experience of the anesthesia and surgical teams with this tube. In patients requiring postoperative mechanical ventilation, the DLT is usually changed to a single-lumen tube. In patients with difficult airways where insertion of DLT is difficult or anticipated difficulty in exchanging to single-lumen tube at the end of the procedure (e.g., c-spine injury, maxillofacial trauma, laryngeal or pharyngeal edema), a Univent tube or single-lumen tube with bronchial blockers are used.

Fluid and Transfusion Management

The degree of exsanguination determines the type and volume of fluid and blood therapy[102] (Table 16.9). Patients with estimated blood loss >30% of blood volume require resuscitation with blood and crystalloid. Patients with lesser degrees of blood volume deficit may be managed more conservatively. Use of large quantities of crystalloid before hemorrhage has been controlled may decrease resistance to flow around a partially formed thrombus due to increased BP and dilute clotting factors (Fig. 16.10). In a randomized,

Table 16.8 Methods for lung isolation during open repair of descending thoracic aorta injury

Options	Advantages	Disadvantages
Double lumen tube Can be placed via laryngos-copy, tube exchanger, and/or fiber-optically	– quickest to place successfully – repositioning rarely required – bronchoscopy to isolated lung – suction to isolated lung – CPAP easily added – can alternate 1LV to either lung easily – placement still possible if bronchos-copy not available	– size selection more difficult – difficult to place in patients with difficult airways or abnormal tracheas – nonoptimal postoperative 2 lung ventilation – laryngeal trauma – bronchial trauma
Bronchial Blockers 1. Arndt 2. Cohen 3. Fuji 4. Fogarty catheter	– size selection rarely an issue – easily added to regular ETT – allows ventilation during placement – easier placement in patients with difficult airways and in children – postoperative two lung ventilation easily accomplished by withdrawing blocker – selective lobar lung isolation possible – CPAP to isolated lung possible	– more time needed for positioning – repositioning needed more often – bronchoscope essential for positioning – bronchoscopy to isolated lung impossible – minimal suction to isolated lung – difficult to alternate 1LV to either lung
Univent	– same as bronchial blockers – less repositioning compared to bronchial blockers	– same as bronchial blockers – ETT portion has higher air flow resistance than regular ETT – ETT portion has larger diameter than regular ETT
ETT advanced into right mainstem bronchus	– easier placement in patients with difficult airways	– does not allow for bronchoscopy, suctioning, or CPAP to isolated lung – cuff not designed for lung isolation – difficult right lung 1LV due to obstruction of right upper lobe

Modified from Kanellakos and Slinger.[101]
ETT endotracheal tube, *DLT* double lumen tube, *CPAP* continuous positive airway pressure, *1LV* one lung ventilation.

Table 16.9 Asanguinous fluid options for aortic trauma

Lactated Ringers (LR)	Preferred isotonic crystalloid solution for most trauma resuscitations. Do not mix with blood or use in blood lines because it contains calcium
0.9% Saline	Preferred isotonic crystalloid solution for head trauma. Only solution used in blood transfusion lines and to dilute PRBCs. May cause hyperchloremic metabolic acidosis [with normal anion gap] due to excess chloride displacing serum HCO3
Hespan (6% hetastarch in 0.9% saline)	High MW hetastarch. Not recommended because of adverse effects on hemostasis, Half-life 30 h. Abandoned at author's institution in favor of Hextend
Hextend (6% hetastarch in balanced electrolyte solution)	High MW hetastarch. Half-life 30 h. Less coagulopathy+platelet dysfunction compared with Hespan. Maximum dose 10–15 ml/kg
Low+medium MW hetastarch	Colloid solutions with less coagulopathy+platelet dysfunction compared with high MW hetastarch. Low MW hetastarch associated with improved muscle oxygen tension, lower markers of inflammation+endothelial activation compared with LR. Available in Europe+Canada. Not currently available in US

(continued)

Table 16.9 (continued)

Albumin (5%)	Little effect on coagulation. May pass into interstitial compartment if impaired vascular integrity with resultant endothelial swelling + impaired microcirculatory perfusion. Increased mortality after head trauma in SAFE study (vs. 0.9% saline)[140]
Hypertonic saline	Variety of solutions/concentrations. May be combined with colloid to prolong duration of action. Efficiently restores intravascular volume + decreases extravascular volume + tissue edema. Decreases ICP + increases CPP. Especially advantageous in prehospital situations + in head trauma with refractory increased ICP. Not associated with improved neurological outcomes

Modified From Novikov and Smith.[103]

MW molecular weight, *ICP* intracranial pressure, *CPP* cerebral perfusion pressure, *PRBC* packed red blood cells.

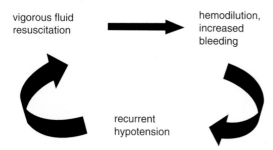

Fig. 16.10 Vicious cycle of vigorous crystalloid fluid resuscitation may lead to hemodilution and increased bleeding (Reprinted with permission from Dutton[126])

Table 16.10 Approach to transfusing red blood cells (RBCs)

1. Transfuse RBCs if hemoglobin <6 g/dl
2. Do not transfuse RBCs if hemoglobin >10 g/dl

3. Decision to transfuse RBCs should be individualized based on
  – presence of organ ischemia (altered mental status, myocardial ischemia, acidosis, low mixed venous oxygen saturation)
  – rate of bleeding
  – magnitude of bleeding
  – intravascular volume status and cardiopulmonary reserve

Modified From Novikov and Smith.[103]

prospective trial of immediate versus delayed fluid resuscitation in patients with penetrating trauma, there was increased mortality, length of stay, and postoperative complication rate in the immediate versus the delayed group.[12]

Goals of fluid and blood include maintenance of normovolemia, oxygen delivery, and hemostasis. Arterial pressure contour analysis is extremely useful. Measurement of SPV is routine. Manifestations of improved perfusion and organ function after aortic trauma include improved mental status, increased pulse pressure, decreased HR, increased urine output, resolution of acidosis and base deficit, brisk capillary refill, and improvement in mixed venous oxygen saturation.[103]

Decisions about transfusion should take into account cardiovascular and pulmonary status, blood loss, and hemoglobin concentration[104] (Table 16.10). A hemoglobin level of 8.0 g/dl appears to be an appropriate threshold for transfusion in patients with no risk for myocardial ischemia, cardiac injuries, or pulmonary contusion. Hematocrit, arterial blood gas, and thromboelastography are used to guide transfusion of blood products. A higher goal may be targeted if active hemorrhage is occurring.[105] Massive transfusion guidelines are followed in patients who have experienced severe blood loss (Table 16.11). In addition to surgery and anesthesia, this entails the close cooperation of blood bank, nursing, and transport. Recombinant factor (RF) VIIa and cryoprecipitate may be given after the 2nd shipment of blood products using the massive transfusion protocol according to attending physician preference. RF VIIa has been used for hemostasis in cases of persistent and excessive bleeding that is unresponsive to other means.[106]

Other Intraoperative Problems

Other intraoperative problems such as hypoxemia, hypotension, hypothermia, and coagulopathy are common in patients with aortic trauma, especially with open repair.

Table 16.11 Massive transfusion protocol at MetroHealth Medical Center for trauma

PRINCIPLE
The policy has been developed to assist the trauma team in the resuscitation of the injured patient. The protocol is designed to achieve volume support, increased oxygen-carrying capacity, and stabilization of the coagulation process for the trauma patient undergoing emergency surgery. Massive transfusion is defined as
- One blood volume loss in 24 h or four or more units replaced in 1 h with continued bleeding
- 50% blood volume loss in 3 h
- 50 units blood lost in 48 h
- 20 units blood lost in 24 h
- Blood loss exceeding 150 ml/min

Adapted from Repine et al.[128]
The trauma team will utilize the massive transfusion protocol when one the following circumstances occur
1. 5 units of blood loss in 1 h (50% blood volume) or
2. 10 units blood loss anticipated in the case or within 12–24 h of observation (one blood volume) or
3. Hypovolemic hypotension uncorrected by crystalloid and packed red blood cell resuscitation during ongoing hemorrhage

ACTIVATION
The clinician contacts the Blood Bank and activates the MTP. The Massive Transfusion Protocol is then followed

SPECIMEN
Pre- or posttransfusion blood sample (signed, 7 mL pink top tube) from massively transfused patient

PROCEDURE
When clinician contacts Blood Bank on the distinct-ring, MTP Hot-line phone and gives a verbal order to begin the MTP on a patient, complete a pink verbal PHONE ORDER form. Record two patient identifiers, the date, location, the physician's name and identification number, and the person calling and initiating the MTP
A runner will come to the Blood Bank to obtain the products. Do NOT tube the blood

FIRST MTP PACK – Collect the 4 O Negative RBCs and 2 AB plasma units already set up for emergency release. Pack in a blood bank insulated cooler. Complete the ALERT label for the insulated cooler, the INSULATED COOLER – BLOOD STORAGE TRACKING SHEET, and the INSULATED COOLER SIGN-OUT SHEET
As soon as the 1st MTP pack is issued, begin preparing the 2nd MTP pack
If a sample has not yet been submitted, contact the blood bank medical director and inquire as to whether the patient should be switched to O Rh Positive

SECOND MTP PACK – 6 units of RBCs (O Neg/Pos or type-specific if sample has been submitted) 4 units of Plasma (AB or type-specific if sample has been submitted), second insulated cooler, necessary emergency release/insulated cooler paperwork
As soon as the 2nd MTP pack is issued, begin preparing the 3rd MTP pack
Third and subsequent packs should have the RBCs crossmatched using an abbreviated crossmatch procedure since 10 RBCs will at that point be issued in less than a 24 h period

THIRD AND ALL SUBSEQUENT MTP PACKS CONSIST OF THE FOLLOWING
6 units of RBCs (O Neg or type-specific if sample has been submitted)
4 units of plasma (AB or type-specific if sample has been submitted)
6 random A/AB platelets (or one five-day pool or one apheresis platelet product)
Insulated cooler (Do NOT place platelets in cooler, for RBCs/Plasma only)
Necessary emergency release/insulated cooler paperwork
Continue with preparing an MTP pack after an MTP pack has been issued until the blood bank has been notified by a clinician to discontinue the MTP. Record on a verbal phone order the two patient identifiers, the date, location, the physician's name and ID #, and the person calling to inactivate the MTP order

RBC red blood cells, *MTP* massive transfusion protocol

Hypoxemia

Frequent causes of hypoxemia include DLT or endotracheal tube malposition, hypoventilation, airway obstruction, aspiration, lung contusion, pneuomothorax, hemothorax, pulmonary edema, pulmonary embolism, bronchospasm, and hemoglobinopathies. Hypoxemia can also be caused by accidental administration of a low F_1O_2 or from problems related to the anesthesia breathing circuit. Increased oxygen consumption, low cardiac output, and decreased oxygen content can also produce hypoxemia.

Rarely, lung torsion can occur.[107] Signs and symptoms of intraoperative pulmonary torsion such as hypoxemia, hypotension, and increased airway pressures may be attributable to other processes. Bronchoscopy may show obliterated left mainstem bronchial lumen, the differential diagnosis for which includes extrinsic compression of the bronchus, endobronchial mass, or bronchial wall edema. Re-exploration of the chest and detorsion of the lung are mandatory. Spillage of necrotic material from the torsed lung tissue into adjacent lung tissue may occur. Detorsion may lead to profound hemodynamic consequences even in the absence of hemorrhagic bronchorrhea due to flow into the left atrium of deeply hypoxemic and acidotic blood released from the pulmonary veins of the torsioned lung or showering of emboli from the pulmonary veins.

Hypotension

Hemorrhage and hypovolemia are the most common causes of hypotension, although other causes such as tension pneumothorax, anaphylaxis, and neurogenic shock from high spinal cord injury should be considered (Table 16.12). Cardiogenic shock may occur due to blunt cardiac injury (BCI), tamponade, air embolism, valvular rupture, coronary ischemia, and infarction. BCI may result in subendocardial or subepicardial hemorrhage, intramyocardial hemorrhage, or injury to a branch of coronary artery. BCI often causes conduction disturbances or arrhythmias and may result in right ventricular dysfunction.

Table 16.12 Selected causes of hemodynamic instability and persistent hypotension in aortic trauma

Undetected or underestimated blood loss
Pneumothorax
Hemothorax
Cardiac tamponade
Air embolism
Spinal cord injury
Acidosis
Hypothermia
Hypocalcemia
Blunt cardiac injury with myocardial contusion and right ventricular dysfunction
Pre-existing medical disease (e.g., cardiomyopathy, valvular heart disease)

Tension pneumothorax can result from pulmonary laceration, rupture of the trachea or a major bronchus, esophageal rupture, or from inadequate sealing of an open pneumothorax. Hypoxia, hyperresonance of the chest wall, increased airway pressures, and diminished breath sounds occur. If untreated, obstructive shock follows. Immediate decompression is lifesaving.

High spinal cord lesions cause anatomic sympathectomy. Other clues to support this diagnosis are bradycardia, warm skin, bounding pulses, priapism, and neurologic deficit. Treatment consists of fluids and vasopressors such as phenylephrine or dopamine. Atropine may be necessary for bradycardia.

Hypothermia

Hypothermia is a marker of profound injury. It is often the result of exsanguinating injury and subsequent massive resuscitative effort. Severe hemorrhage causing hypovolemia leads to tissue hypoperfusion, diminished oxygen delivery at the cellular level, and reduced heat generation. The adverse effects of hypothermia (Table 16.13) include arrhythmias, decreased cardiac output, increased systemic vascular resistance, major coagulation derangements, peripheral vasoconstriction, metabolic acidosis, and impaired immune response.[108] Hypothermia slows enzymatic rates of clotting factors and reduces platelet function. Hypothermia also impairs citrate, lactate, and drug metabolism; increases blood viscosity; impairs red blood cell deformability; increases intracellular potassium release; and causes a leftward shift of the oxyhemoglobin dissociation curve.

Temperatures of less than 34.5°C are associated with an increased prevalence of multiorgan dysfunction and increased need for vasopressor and inotropic support. Every effort should be made to avoid hypothermia by increasing ambient temperature (≥28°C), using convective and conductive warmers, and warming all fluids and blood transfusions to 37°C.[109] Evaporation from the respiratory tract can be prevented by use of active airway humidifiers or passive heat and

Table 16.13 Pathophysiological consequences and complications from hypothermia

System affected	Examples
Impaired cardiorespiratory function	• Cardiac depression • Myocardial ischemia • Arrhythmias • Peripheral vasoconstriction • Decreased tissue oxygen delivery • Increased oxygen consumption during rewarming • Blunted response to catecholamines • Increased blood viscosity • Acidosis • Leftward shift of hemoglobin–oxygen dissociation curve
Impaired coagulation	• Decreased function of coagulation factors • Impaired platelet function
Impaired hepatorenal function and decreased drug clearance	• Decreased hepatic blood flow • Decreased clearance of lactic acid • Decreased hepatic metabolism of drugs • Decreased renal blood flow • Cold-induced diuresis
Impaired resistance to infections (pneumonia, sepsis, wound infections) Impaired wound healing.	• Decreased subcutaneous tissue perfusion mediated by vasoconstriction (norepinephrine) • Anti-inflammatory effects and immunosuppression, including reduced T-cell-mediated antibody production and reduced nonspecific oxidative bacterial killing by neutrophils • Decreased collagen deposition

From Soreide and Smith.[109]

moisture exchangers. Effective fluid warmers with high thermal clearances are routinely employed to prevent iatrogenic hypothermia during massive transfusion.

Pain Management

Inadequate treatment of pain after injury is common because pain control is often the last priority in hemodynamically unstable patients.[110] Inadequately treated acute pain after aortic injuries may result in chronic pain syndromes and disability.[111] The effects of pain from penetrating and blunt injuries and the related stress response are almost always detrimental to the patient. The stress response includes hyperglycemia, lipolysis, protein catabolism, increased antidiuretic hormone and catecholamine levels, immunosuppression, and a hypercoagulable state.[112] Untreated pain contributes to the neuroendocrine response with

peripheral inflammation, central sensitization, and release of multiple substances including prostanoids, cytokines, serotonin, bradykinin, hydrogen ions, potassium, and acute phase reactants. Untreated pain can increase adverse effects on normal physiologic functions of the cardiovascular, respiratory, renal, and gastrointestinal systems with resultant hypertension, tachycardia, deep venous thrombosis, pulmonary embolism, immobility, splinting, ventilation-perfusion mismatch, reduced gastrointestinal motility, water and salt retention, hypoxia, and infections.[113] Adequate thoracic pain management fosters earlier rehabilitation and may reduce the incidence of long-term chronic pain syndromes.

Aortic trauma patients frequently present with injuries to multiple areas of the body necessitating flexibility in terms of pain management techniques. For example, it may be necessary to avoid the use of analgesic techniques that reduce the ability to evaluate sensory and motor function.

Issues such as monitoring of central and peripheral neurological function must be considered. Monitoring issues may take priority over advanced pain management techniques.

Analgesics are administered to minimize patient suffering and to improve ventilatory mechanics, allowing patients to breathe more deeply and to cough more effectively (Table 16.14). Adequate pain control diminishes the likelihood of atelectasis, decreases respiratory infections, and prevents episodes of hypoxia that lead to

Table 16.14 Principles of pain management in aortic trauma

DESIRED CHARACTERISTICS OF AN IDEAL ANALGESIC TECHNIQUE IN TRAUMA
Safe
Simple
Predictable
Extended analgesia
Minimal hemodynamic disturbance
Minimal respiratory disturbance
No interference with neurological monitoring
High degree of patient acceptance
Minimal complications
Reduces chronic pain
Economical
Minimal effect on immunity

ADVANTAGES AND LIMITATIONS OF REGIONAL ANESTHESIA/ANALGESIA

Advantages
Opioid sparing/eliminating
Less nausea
Less paralytic ileus
Less immunosuppression
Improved dynamic pain relief
Less blood loss
Lower incidence of thromboembolism
Improved patient satisfaction
Early recovery
Reduced resource utilization
Reduced chronic pain syndromes
Reduced pulmonary morbidity
Reduced cognitive dysfunction
Reduced infective complications
Reduced sedative effect
Economical
Extendable
Smooth transitional analgesia

Limitations
Need for trained personnel
Need for special equipments
Inability to position for neuraxial block
Time required to initiate

(continued)

Table 16.14 (continued)

Failure rate (2–20%)
Nerve injuries (0.5–8%)
Diaphragm and motor weakness
Horner's syndrome
Pneumothorax (0.04–0.15%)
"Masking compartment syndrome"
Epidural spread with paravertebral block
Local anesthetic toxicity
Catheter malfunction (20–25%)
Infection/colonization (1–1.9%/28–57%)
Neuraxial hematoma

PHARMACOLOGICAL ADJUVANTS TO REGIONAL ANALGESIA
Epinephrine
Clonidine
Ketamine
Opioids
Sodium
bicarbonate
Tramadol
Verapamil
Hyaluronidase
Neostigmine
COX 2 inhibitors
Muscle relaxants

COMMONLY USED LOCAL ANESTHETICS AND DOSAGES FOR VARIOUS REGIONAL BLOCKS

Paravertebral block
0.5% 20–25 ml followed by 0.35% ropivacaine or 0.25% bupivacaine 8–10 ml/h

Epidural block
Bupivacaine 0.25% 5–8 ml followed by bupivacaine 0.1% with hydromorphone 10–20 ug/ml; continuous infusion 6–10 ml/h or patient-controlled analgesia 3 ml every 20 min PRN

From Dhir and Ganapathy.[110]

increased requirement for mechanical ventilation. Acute pain control techniques include intercostal nerve blocks, paravertebral block, interpleural catheter, and epidural analgesia.[114]

Intravenous Opioids

Effective analgesia requires recognition and acceptance that relief of pain is an important part of treating trauma patients. Intravenous opioids can be given together with anxiolytics and other adjuncts (multimodal therapy – see below). There is inherent variability in analgesic requirements and frequent dose adjustments are necessary to achieve the desired level of analgesia.

Patient-Controlled Analgesia (PCA)

Intravenous patient-controlled analgesia (IV PCA) is a major improvement over IV infusions in cooperative patients. There is "built-in safety" since the patient can self-administer medication during periods of alertness. The patient also has a sense of control when using IV PCA. Pain and oversedation cycles are reduced using this technique. The technique also is less demanding on nursing resources.

Nerve Blocks

Intercostal nerve blocks have been utilized for many years to alleviate thoracic pain. The technique increases maximal inspiratory flow rates, relieves pain, and improves the ability to cough and breathe deeply. Continuous or single-shot technique can be used. There is a risk of pneumothorax. Rapid vascular absorption of local anesthetics can occur with a risk of toxicity. Paravertebral block can provide intermittent or continuous pain relief in patients with rib fractures together with improved pulmonary function.

Intrapleural Analgesia

An interpleural catheter placed for thoracic pain allows for continuous infusions or intermittent injections to provide prolonged pain relief. The major concerns are that the peak plasma level of local anesthetics is relatively high and pain relief is not consistently achieved. In addition, in patients with thoracostomy tubes, there is a risk of suctioning the injected local anesthetics. This risk is minimized by placing the catheter distant from the thoracostomy tube or delaying the suction of the thoracostomy tube for 15–30 min after injection of the local anesthetic through the interpleural catheter. The use of intrapleural catheters

is patient-position-dependent. The tip of the catheter can migrate in certain patients leading to inadequate analgesia.

Epidural Analgesia

Beneficial Effects

Epidural analgesia improves vital capacity, functional residual capacity (FRC), airway resistance, and dynamic lung compliance after surgery and trauma.[115-118] Patients receiving continuous epidural analgesia have decreased ventilator days, shorter ICU stays, shorter hospitalizations, and decreased incidence of tracheostomy when compared to control-matched groups with similar injury severity indices.[115] Epidural analgesia significantly reduced pain with chest wall excursion compared with PCA and was associated with improved pulmonary function and immune response.[119] Epidural analgesia leads to a lower incidence of respiratory depression, utilizes smaller doses of narcotics, and allows earlier ambulation and discharge when compared to other modes of analgesia. The mortality rates, frequency of respiratory infections, and quality of pain relief reported by the patient are also superior in patients receiving epidural analgesia.[115] Epidural analgesia can be delivered in intermittent boluses, as continuous infusion, and as patient-controlled epidural analgesia. Typically, combinations of low concentrations of long-acting local anesthetics with an opioid provide optimal analgesia and minimum motor block.

Limitations

Factors that preclude the use of epidural analgesia techniques in aortic trauma include insufficient time for insertion of epidural catheter and inadequate positioning for catheter placement (e.g., uncleared spines, pelvic fracture). Patients with associated spinal cord injuries or with coagulopathy are not candidates for epidural analgesia. The use of local anesthetics may produce hypotension and can hinder evaluation of neurologic function. Contraindications to placement of epidural catheters include septicemia, untreated bacteremia, unstable spine, and altered mental status.

Multimodal Approach

There are several nociceptive pathways mediating thoracic pain including the vagus, the phrenic, and intercostal nerves.[120] Other less well-defined pathways may be connected with the autonomic nervous system. Thus, a multimodal (local anesthetics, opioids, acetaminophen, nonsteroidal anti-inflammatory drugs (NSAIDS), alpha 2 agonists, gabapentin, tricyclic antidepressants, ketamine, tramadol, pregabalin) antinociception strategy is optimal for patients with thoracic pain.[121] Local anesthetics are the most effective drugs to block pain. Opioids administered via PCA are extremely valuable as a fall-back in the event of failure of other techniques. Nonsteroidal anti-inflammatory drugs can be used as adjuvants, although the use of NSAIDS is controversial because of gastrointestinal, renal, and bleeding risks. Improvements in intrathecal drug delivery systems and development of additional drugs make this modality appear appropriate for selected patients.

Postoperative Considerations Following Aortic Trauma

Patients sustaining aortic trauma often require postoperative aggressive management of various organ systems. Respiratory insufficiency may be related to ARDS, pneumonia, and pulmonary contusions. Ventilatory management, serial CXR, assessment of chest tube drainage for hemothorax, monitoring and optimization of oxygen delivery, and good pain control are part of the management. Empyema and pneumothorax may complicate the picture. Treatment of head and spinal cord injuries can be challenging, and head injuries are a common cause of mortality in these patients.[122] ICP and CPP monitoring are routine in patients with severe head trauma. Intensive care is also directed toward management of problems such as neuroendocrine response, hyperglycemia, fluid therapy, management of blood transfusion and coagulopathy, central nervous system depression, agitation, and complications of drug abuse. Other nonaortic injuries (e.g., cardiac injury, abdominal, retroperitoneal, orthopedic, and vascular injuries) need further attention. Definitive treatment of spine, pelvic abdominal, and extremity fractures are required. Discharge to a rehabilitation facility is often necessary for optimal recovery of function and long-term care of injuries.

Postoperative complications after cardiac trauma include intracardiac shunts, valvular lesions, ventricular aneurysms, wall motion abnormalities, arrhythmias, and conduction blocks. Retained foreign body, aortocaval, and aortopulmonary fistula may also occur in survivors of penetrating chest trauma.

Specific postaortic trauma complications include ARDS, deep venous thrombosis, multiple organ system failure, and sepsis, the last two being the major late causes of death in trauma. Anticoagulation complicates and may contraindicate the use of epidural analgesia. An inferior vena cava filter may be required.

Key Notes

1. Management of aortic trauma is complex because multiple organ systems may be simultaneously involved. Hypovolemic shock, cardiac failure, head injury, and respiratory compromise may all be present.
2. ATLS principles are followed initially until definitive care of injuries can be provided.
3. Anesthetic care is directed towards restoring hemodynamic function, treating airway problems, providing intraoperative one-lung ventilation during open surgical repair of descending thoracic aorta injuries, facilitating endovascular stenting of aortic injuries, monitoring cerebral oximetry during circulatory arrest for aortic arch repair, maintaining intravascular blood volume, treating coagulopathy, performing operative and ventilatory management, and controlling postoperative pain.
4. The importance of a clear understanding of the pathophysiology of aortic injuries is necessary to optimally manage these challenging patients.

5. Chest CT has become commonplace for the diagnosis of BAI. MRI and TEE may be used in selected circumstances.
6. Urgent repair of thoracic aortic transection in the setting of blunt trauma can be problematic in patients with concomitant traumatic brain injury, pulmonary contusion, cardiac trauma, or other injuries.
7. Endovascular repair has been increasingly shown to be well tolerated with excellent early and midterm results. Endovascular stent grafting avoids the need for thoracotomy, one-lung ventilation, and aortic cross-clamp and is associated with improved mortality and decreased spinal cord ischemia and paraplegia.
8. Epidural analgesia is superior for management of thoracic pain, but may be contraindicated in the setting of trauma due to coagulopathy, hemodynamic instability, abnormal neurologic status, and other factors.

References

1. Besson A, Saegesser F. *Color Atlas of Chest Trauma and Associated Injuries*. Oradell: Medical Economics Books; 1983.
2. Duwayri Y, Abbas J, Cerilli G, Chan E, Nazzal M. Outcome after thoracic aortic injury: experience in a level-1 trauma center. *Ann Vasc Surg*. 2008;22(3):309–313.
3. Richens D, Kotidis K, Neale M, Oakley C, Fails A. Rupture of aorta following road traffic accidents in the United Kingdom 1992–1999: the results of the co-operative crash injury study. *Eur J Cardiothorac Surg*. 2002;23:143–148.
4. Fabian TC, Richardson JD, Croce M, et al. Prospective study of blunt injury: multicenter trial of the American Association for surgery of Trauma. *J Trauma*. 1997;42:374–380.
5. Parmley LF, Mattingly TW, Manion WC, et al. Nonpenetrating traumatic injury of the aorta. *Circulation*. 1958;17:1086–1101.
6. Duan Y, Smith CE, Como JJ. Anesthesia for major cardiothoracic trauma. In: Wilson WC, Grande CM, Hoyt DB, eds. *Trauma: Resuscitation, Anesthesia, and Critical Care*. New York: Informa Healthcare USA, Inc; 2007.
7. Schmoker JD, Lee CH, Taylor RG, et al. A novel model of blunt thoracic aortic injury: a mechanism confirmed? *J Trauma*. 2008;64(4):923–931.
8. Ben-Menachem Y. Rupture of the thoracic aorta by broad side impacts in road traffic and other collisions: further angiographic observations and preliminary autopsy findings. *J Trauma*. 1993;35:363–367.
9. Kodali S, Jamieson WRE, Leia-Stephens M, Miyagishima RT, Janusz MT, Tyers GFO. Traumatic rupture of the thoracic aorta: A 20-year review: 1969–1989. *Circulation*. 1991;84(Suppl III):III40–III46.
10. Hirose H, Moore E. Delayed presentation and rupture of a posttraumatic innominate artery aneurysm: case report and review of the literature. *J Trauma*. 1997;42:1187–1195.
11. Malm JR, Deterling RH. Traumatic aneurysm of the thoracic aorta simulating coarctation. *J Thorac Cardiovasc Surg*. 1960;40:271–278.
12. Bickell WH, Wall MJ, Pepe PE, et al. Immediate versus delayed fluid resuscitation for hypotensive patients with penetrating torso injuries. *N Engl J Med*. 1994;331:1105–1109.
13. Mattox KL, Bickell WH, Pepe PE. Prospective, randomized evaluation of antishock MAST in post traumatic hypotension. *J Trauma*. 1986;26:779–786.
14. American College of Surgeons Committee on Trauma. *Advanced Trauma Life Support for Doctors, Student Course Manual*. 8th ed. Chicago: American College of Surgeons; 2008.
15. Kouchoukos NT, Blackstone EH, Doty DB, Hanley FL, Karp RB. Acute traumatic aortic dissection. In: Kirklin JW, Barrat B, eds. *Cardiac Surgery*. New York: Churchill Livingstone; 1986.
16. Eddy CA, Rush VW, Marchioro T, Ashbaugh D, Verrier ED, Dillard D. Treatment of traumatic rupture of the thoracic aorta. *Arch Surg*. 1990;125:1351–1355.
17. Wall MJ, Storey JH, Mattox KL. Indications for thoracotomy. In: Mattox KL, Feliciano DV, Moore EE, eds. *Trauma*. 4th ed. New York: McGraw-Hill; 2000: 473–482.
18. Aydin NB, Moon MC, Gill I. Cardiac and great vessel trauma. In: Smith CE, ed. *Trauma Anesthesia*. New York: Cambridge University Press; 2008:260–278.
19. Mirvis SE, Bidwell JK, Buddemeyer EU, et al. Value of chest radiography in excluding traumatic aortic rupture. *Radiology*. 1987;163:487–196.
20. Mirvis SE, Shanmuganathan K, Buell J, et al. Use of spiral computed tomography for the assessment of blunt trauma patients with potential aortic injury. *J Trauma*. 1998;45:922–930.
21. Downing SW, Sperling JS, Mirvis SE, et al. Experience with spiral computed tomography as the sole diagnostic method for traumatic aortic rupture. *Ann Thorac Surg*. 2001;72:495–501.
22. Demetriades D, Velmahos GC, Scalea TM, et al. Diagnosis and treatment of blunt thoracic aortic injuries: changing perspectives. *J Trauma*. 2008;64(6): 1415–1418.
23. La Berge JM, Jeffrey RB. Aortic lacerations: fatal complications of thoracic aortography. *Radiology*. 1987;165:367–369.
24. Kram HB, Wohlmuth DA, Appel PL, Shoemaker WC. Clinical and radiographic indications for aortography in blunt chest trauma. *J Vasc Surg*. 1987;6:168–176.

25. Cohn SM, Burns GA, Jaffe C, Milner KA. Exclusion of aortic tear in the unstable trauma patient: the utility of transesophageal echocardiography. *J Trauma.* 1995;39:1087–1090.

26. Ben-Menachem Y. Assessment of blunt aortic-brachiocephalic trauma: should angiography be supplanted by transesophageal echocardiography? *J Trauma.* 1997;42:969–972.

27. Goarin JP, Cluzel P, Gosgnach M, et al. Evaluation of Transesophageal echocardiography for diagnosis of traumatic aortic injury. *Anesthesiology.* 2000;93:1373–1377.

28. Smith MD, Cassidy M, Souther S, et al. Transesophageal echocardiography in the diagnosis of traumatic rupture of the aorta. *N Engl J Med.* 1995;332:356–362.

29. Vignon P, Boncoeur MP, Francois B, et al. Comparison of multiplane transesophageal echocardiography and contrast-enhanced helical CT in the diagnosis of blunt traumatic cardiovascular injuries. *Anesthesiology.* 2001;94:615–622.

30. Fattori R, Celletti F, Bertaccini P, et al. Delayed surgery of traumatic aortic rupture; role of magnetic resonance imaging. *Circulation.* 1996;94:2865–2870.

31. Langanay T, De Latour B, Leguerrier A. Surgical treatment of an acute isthmus traumatic rupture. In: Rousseau H, Verhoye JP, Heautot JF, eds. *Thoracic Aortic Diseases.* 1st ed. Berlin: Springer; 2006: 319–329.

32. Peltz M, Douglass DS, Meyer DM, et al. Hypothermic circulatory arrest for repair of injuries of the thoracic aorta and great vessels. *Interact Cardiovasc Thorac Surg.* 2006;5(5):560–565.

33. Johnston RH Jr, Wall MJ, Mattox KL. Innominate artery trauma: a thirty year experience. *J Vasc Surg.* 1993;17:134–139.

34. Graham JM, Feliciano DV, Mattox KL, Beall AC Jr. Innominate vascular injury. *J Trauma.* 1982;22: 647–655.

35. Von Opell UO, De Groot MK, Zilla P. Traumatic aortic rupture: twenty-year meta analysis of mortality and risk of paraplegia. *Ann Thorac Surg.* 1994;58: 585–593.

36. Jahromi AS, Safar HA, Doobay B, Clina CS. Traumatic rupture of the thoracic aorta: cohort study and systematic review. *J Vasc Surg.* 2001;34:1029–1034.

37. Gleason TG, Benjamin LC. Conventional open repair of descending thoracic aortic aneurysms. *Perspect Vasc Surg Endovasc Ther.* 2007;19:110–121.

38. Kahn RA, Stone ME, Moskowitz DM. Anesthetic consideration for descending thoracic aortic aneurysm repair. *Semin Cardiothorac Vasc Anesth.* 2007;11(3): 205–223.

39. Whitson BA, Nath DS, Knudtson JR, McGonigal MD, Shumway SJ. Is distal aortic perfusion in traumatic thoracic aortic injuries necessary to avoid paraplegic postoperative outcomes? *J Trauma.* 2008;64(1): 115–120.

40. Lebl DR, Dicker RA, Spain DA, Brundage SI. Dramatic shift in the primary management of traumatic thoracic aortic rupture. *Arch Surg.* 2006;141(2):177–180.

41. Downing SW, Cardarelli MG, Sperling J, et al. Heparinless partial cardiopulmonary bypass for the repair of aortic trauma. *J Thorac Cardiovasc Surg.* 2000;120:1104–1111.

42. O'Connor CJ, Rothenberg DM. Anesthetic considerations for descending thoracic aortic surgery: part II. *J Cardiothorac Vasc Anesth.* 1995;9:734–747.

43. Ling E, Arellano R. Systematic overview of the evidence supporting the use of cerebrospinal fluid drainage in thoracoabdominal aneurysm surgery for prevention of paraplegia. *Anesthesiology.* 2000;93: 1115–1122.

44. Katz NM, Blackstone EH, Kirklin JW, Karp RB. Incremental risk factors for spinal cord injury following operation for acute traumatic aortic transection. *J Thorac Cardiovasc Surg.* 1981;81:669–674.

45. Hochheiser GM, Morton JR. Operative technique, paraplegia, and mortality after blunt traumatic aortic injury. *Arch Surg.* 2002;137:434–438.

46. Simpson JI, Eide TR, Newman SB, et al. Trimetaphan versus sodium nitroprusside for the control of proximal hypertension during thoracic aortic cross clamping: the effects on spinal cord ischemia. *Anesth Analg.* 1996;82:68–74.

47. Pierangeli A, Turinetto B, Galli R, Caldarera R, Fattori R, Gavelli G. Delayed treatment of isthmic aortic rupture. *Cardiovasc Surg.* 2000;8:280–283.

48. Langanay T, Verhoye JP, Corbineau H, et al. Surgical treatment of acute traumatic rupture of the thoracic aorta: timing reappraisal. *Eur J Cardiothorac Surg.* 2002;21:282–287.

49. Maggisano R, Nathens A, Alexandrova N. Traumatic rupture of the thoracic aorta: should one always operate immediately? *Ann Vasc Surg.* 1995;9:44–52.

50. Holmes JH, Bloch RD, Hall RA, Carter YM, Karmy-Jones RC. Natural history of traumatic rupture of thoracic aorta managed non-operatively: a longitudinal analysis. *Ann Thorac Surg.* 2002;73:1149–1154.

51. Kato N, Dake MD, Miller DC, et al. Traumatic thoracic aortic aneurysm: treatment with endovascular stent-grafts. *Radiology.* 1997;205(3):657–662.

52. Rousseau H, Soula P, Perreault P, et al. Delayed treatment of traumatic rupture of the thoracic aorta with endoluminal covered stent. *Circulation.* 1999;99(4): 498–504.

53. Kasirajan K, Heffernan D, Langsfeld M. Acute thoracic aortic trauma: a comparison of endoluminal stent grafts with open repair and nonoperative management. *Ann Vasc Surg.* 2003;17:589–595.

54. Peterson BG, Matsumura JS, Morasch MD, West MA, Eskandari MK. Percutaneous endovascular repair of blunt thoracic aortic transection. *J Trauma.* 2005;59(5): 1062–1065.

55. Lachat M, Pfammatter T, Witzke H, et al. Acute traumatic aortic rupture: early stent-graft repair. *Eur J Cardiothorac Surg.* 2002;21(6):959–963.

56. Fattori R, Napoli G, Lovato L, et al. Indications for, timing of, and results of catheter-based treatment of

traumatic injury to the aorta. *AJR Am J Roentgenol.* 2002;179(3):603–609.

57. Alsac JM, Boura B, Desgranges P, et al. Immediate endovascular repair for acute traumatic injuries of the thoracic aorta: a multicenter analysis of 28 cases. *J Vasc Surg.* 2008;48(6):1369–1374.

58. McPhee JT, Asham EH, Rohrer MJ, et al. The midterm results of stent graft treatment of thoracic aortic injuries. *J Surg Res.* 2007;138(2):181–188.

59. Uzieblo M, Sanchez LA, Rubin BG, et al. Endovascular repair of traumatic descending thoracic aortic disruptions: should endovascular therapy become the gold standard? *Vasc Endovasc Surg.* 2004;38:331–337.

60. Marty-Ané CH, Berthet JP, Branchereau P, Mary H, Alric P. Endovascular repair for acute traumatic rupture of the thoracic aorta. *Ann Thorac Surg.* 2003;75:1803–1807.

61. Fayad A. Thoracic endovascular stent graft with a bird's beak sign. *Can J Anaesth.* 2008;55:785–786.

62. Rousseau H, Dambrin C, Marcheix B, et al. Acute traumatic aortic rupture: a comparison of surgical and stent-graft repair. *J Thorac Cardiovasc Surg.* 2005;129(5):1050–1055.

63. Noor N, Sadat U, Hayes PD, Thompson MM, Boyle JR. Management of the left subclavian artery during endovascular repair of the thoracic aorta. *J Endovasc Ther.* 2008;15(2):168–176.

64. Hausegger KA, Oberwalder P, Tiesenhausen K, et al. Intentional left subclavian artery occlusion by thoracic aortic stent-grafts without surgical transposition. *J Endovasc Ther.* 2001;8(5):472–476.

65. Buz S, Zipfel B, Mulahasanovic S, Pasic M, Weng Y, Hetzer R. Conventional surgical repair and endovascular treatment of acute traumatic aortic rupture. *Eur J Cardiothorac Surg.* 2008;33(2):143–149.

66. Day CP, Buckenham TM. Outcomes of endovascular repair of acute thoracic aortic injury: interrogation of the New Zealand thoracic aortic stent database (NZ TAS). *Eur J Vasc Endovasc Surg.* 2008;36(5):530–534.

67. Devitt JH, McLean RF, Koch JP. Anaesthetic management of acute blunt thoracic trauma. *Can J Anaesth.* 1991;38:506–510.

68. Steele EA, Soran D, Marciniak D, Smith CE. Monitoring the trauma patient. In: Smith CE, ed. *Trauma Anesthesia.* New York: Cambridge University Press; 2008:81–100.

69. Morgan BC, Martin WE, Hornbein TF, Crawford EW, Guntheroth WG. Hemodynamic effects of positive pressure ventilation. *Anesthesiology.* 1966;27:584–590.

70. Jardin F, Delorme G, Hardy A, AUvert B, Beuchet A, Bourdarias JP. Reevaluation of hemodynamic consequences of positive pressure ventilation: emphasis on cyclic right ventricular afterloading by mechanical lung inflation. *Anesthesiology.* 1990;72:966–970.

71. Jardin F, Farcot JC, Gueret P, Prost JF, Ozier Y, Bourdarias JP. Cyclical changes in arterial pulse pressure during respiratory support. *Circulation.* 1983;68:266–274.

72. Michard F, Teboul JL. Using heart-lung interactions to assess fluid responsiveness during mechanical ventilation. *Crit Care.* 2000;4:282–289.

73. Coriat P, Vrillon M, Perel A, Baron JF, et al. A comparison of systolic pressure variations and echocardiographic measurements of end-diastolic left ventricular size in patients after aortic surgery. *Anesth Analg.* 1994;78:46–53.

74. Kramer A, Zygun D, Hawes H, Easton P, Ferland A. Pulse pressure variation predicts fluid responsiveness following coronary artery bypass surgery. *Chest.* 2004;126(5):1563–1568.

75. Tavernier B, Makhotine O, Lebuffe G, Dupont J, Scherpereel P. Systolic pressure variation as a guide to fluid therapy in patients with sepsis-induced hypotension. *Anesthesiology.* 1998;89(6):1313–1321.

76. Perel A, Pizov R, Cotev S. The systolic pressure variation is a sensitive indicator of hypovolemia in ventilated dogs subjected to graded hemorrhage. *Anesthesiology.* 1987;67:498–502.

77. Rooke GA, Schwid HA, Shapira Y. The effects of graded hemorrhage and intravascular volume replacement on systolic pressure variation in humans during spontaneous mechanical variation. *Anesth Analg.* 1995;80:925–932.

78. Preisman S, DiSegni E, Vered Z, Perel A. Left ventricular preload and function during graded hemorrhage and retransfusion in pigs: analysis of arterial pressure waveform and correlation with echocardiography. *Br J Anaesth.* 2002;88:716–718.

79. Berkenstadt H, Friedman Z, Preisman S, Keidan I, Livingstone D, Perel A. Pulse pressure and stroke volume variations during severe haemorrhage in ventilated dogs. *Br J Anaesth.* 2005;94(6):721–726.

80. Moomey CB, Fabian TC, Croce MA, et al. Determinants of myocardial performance after blunt chest trauma. *J Trauma.* 1998;45:988–996.

81. Royse C, Royse A. Use of echocardiography and ultrasound in trauma. In: Smith CE, ed. *Trauma Anesthesia.* New York: Cambridge University Press; 2008:514–2.

82. Kneeshaw JD. Transoesophageal echocardiograpgy (TOE) in the operating room. *Br J Anaesth.* 2006;97:77–84.

83. Swaminathan M, Lineberger CK, McCann RL, Mathew JP. The importance of intraoperative transesophageal echocardiography in endovascular repair of thoracic aortic aneurysms. *Anesth Analg.* 2003;97:1566–1572.

84. Dobson G, Petrasek P, Alvarez N. Transesophageal echocardiography enhances endovascular stent placement in traumatic transection of the thoracic aorta. *Can J Anaesth.* 2004;51:9.

85. Deogaonkar A, Gupta R, DeGeorgia M, et al. Bispectral index monitoring correlates with sedation scales in brain-injured patients. *Crit Care Med.* 2004;32:2545–2546.

86. Paul DB, Umamaheswara Rao GS. Correlation of bispectral index with Glasgow coma score in mild and moderate head injuries. *J Clin Monit Comput.* 2006;20:399–404.

87. Bevacqua B, Kazdan D. Is more information better? Intraoperative recall with a Bispectral Index monitor in place. *Anesthesiology*. 2003;99:507–508.

88. Mychaskiw G, Horowitz M, Sachdev V, Heath BJ. Explicit intraoperative recall at a bispectral index of 47. *Anesth Analg*. 2001;92:808–809.

89. Mahla M. Neurologic monitoring. In: Cucchiara RF, ed. *Clinical Neuroanesthesia*. New York: Churchill Livingstone; 1998:125–176.

90. Mahla M, Black S, Cucchiara RF. Neurologic monitoring. In: Miller R, ed. *Miller's Anesthesia*. Philadelphia: Elsevier; 2005:1511–1550.

91. Murkin JM et al. Monitoring brain oxygen saturation during coronary bypass surgery: a randomized, prospective study. *Anesth Analg*. 2007;104:51–58.

92. Dunham CM et al. Correlation of noninvasive cerebral oximetry with cerebral perfusion in the severe heads injured patient: a pilot study. *J Trauma*. 2002;52(1):40–46.

93. Dunham CM et al. Cerebral hypoxia in severely brain injured patients is associated with admission Glasgow Coma Score, CT severity, cerebral perfusion pressure, and survival. *J Trauma*. 2004;56(3):482–491.

94. Rodriguez-Lopez JM, Sanchez-Conde P, Lozano FS, et al. Effects of propofol on the systemic inflammatory response during aortic surgery. *Can J Anaesth*. 2006;53:701–710.

95. Annecke T, Kubitz JC, Kahr S, et al. Effects of sevoflurane and propofol on ischaemia-reperfusion injury after thoracic-aortic occlusion in pigs. *Br J Anaesth*. 2007;98:581–590.

96. Mahoney PH, McFarland CC. Field anesthesia and military injury. In: Smith CE, ed. *Trauma Anesthesia*. New York: Cambridge University Press; 2008:343–359.

97. Buffolo E, Fonseca JHP, Souza JAM, Alves CMR. Revolutionary treatment of aneurysms and dissections of the descending aorta: the endovascular approach. *Ann Thorac Surg*. 2002;74:S1815–S1817.

98. Plaschke K, Boeckler D, Schumacher H, et al. Adenosine-induced cardiac arrest and EEG changes in patients with thoracic aorta endovascular repair. *Br J Anaesth*. 2006;96:310–316.

99. Kahn RA, Marin ML, Hollier L, Parsons R, Griepp R. Induction of ventricular fibrillation to facilitate endovascular stent graft repair of thoracic aortic aneurysms. *Anesthesiology*. 1998;88:534–536.

100. Weigand MA, Motsch J, Bardenheuer HJ. Adenosine-induced transient cardiac arrest for placement of endovascular stent-grafts in the thoracic aorta. *Anesthesiology*. 1998;89:1037.

101. Kanellakos GW, Slinger P. Intraoperative one-ling ventilation for trauma anesthesia. In: Smith CE, ed. *Trauma Anesthesia*. New York: Cambridge University Press; 2008:300–313.

102. Finfer S, Bellomo R, Boyce N, et al. SAFE study investigators: a comparison of albumin and saline for fluid resuscitation in the intensive care unit. *N Engl J Med*. 2004;350(22):2247–2256.

103. Novikov M, Smith CE. Fluid and blood therapy in trauma. In: Smith CE, ed. *Trauma Anesthesia*. New York: Cambridge University Press; 2008:101–120.

104. Practice Guidelines for Perioperative Blood Transfusion and Adjuvant Therapies (Approved by the House of Delegates on October 22, 1995 and last amended on October 25, 2005). An Updated Report by the American Society of Anesthesiologists Task Force on Perioperative Blood Transfusion and Adjuvant therapies. Available at http://www.asahq.org/publicationsAndServices/BCTGuidesFinal.pdf

105. Hardy JF, de Moerloose P, Samama M. and members of the Groupe d'intérêt en Hémostase Périopératoire Massive transfusion and coagulopathy: pathophysiology and implications for clinical management. *Can J Anaesth*. 2004;51:293–310.

106. Naik VN, Mazer CD, Latter DA, et al. Successful treatment using recombinant factor VIIa for severe bleeding post cardiopulmonary bypass. *Can J Anaesth*. 2003;50:599–602.

107. Goskowicz R, Harrell JH, Roth DM. Intraoperative diagnosis of torsion of the left lung after repair of a disruption of the descending thoracic aorta. *Anesthesiology*. 1997;87:164–166.

108. Smith CE, Yamat RA. Avoiding hypothermia in the trauma patient. *Curr Opin Anaesthesiol*. 2000;13:167–174.

109. Soreide E, Smith CE. Hypothermia in trauma. In: Smith CE, ed. *Trauma Anesthesia*. New York: Cambridge University Press; 2008:445–464.

110. Dhir S, Ganapathy S. Trauma and regional anesthesia. In: Smith CE, ed. *Trauma Anesthesia*. New York: Cambridge University Press; 2008:471–498.

111. Ryan D, Tabbaa K. Posttrauma chronic pain. In: Smith CE, ed. *Trauma Anesthesia*. New York: Cambridge University Press; 2008:544–568.

112. Kehlet H. The surgical stress response: should it be prevented? *Can J Surg*. 1991;34:565–567.

113. Rosenberg A, Albert DB, Bernstein RL. Regional anesthesia for orthopaedic trauma. *Probl Anesth*. 1994;8(3):426–444.

114. Orliaguet G, Carli P. Thoracic blocks. In: Rosenberg AD, Grande CM, Bernstein RL, eds. *Pain Management and Regional Anesthesia in Trauma*. London: WB Saunders; 1999:239–251.

115. Kavanagh BP, Katz J, Sandler AN. Pain control after thoracic surgery: a review of current techniques. *Anesthesiology*. 1994;81:737–759.

116. Mackersie RC, Shackford SR, Hoyt DB, et al. Continuous epidural fentanyl analgesia: ventilatory function improvement with routine use in treatment of blunt chest trauma. *J Trauma*. 1987;27:1207–1212.

117. Shulman M, Sandler AN, Bradley JW, et al. Post thoracotomy pain and pulmonary function following epidural and systemic morphine. *Anesthesiology*. 1984;61:569–575.

118. Moon MR, Luchette FA, Gibson SW, et al. Prospective, randomized comparison of epidural versus parenteral opioid analgesia in thoracic trauma. *Ann Surg*. 1999;229:684–692.

119. Grass JA. Surgical outcome: regional anesthesia and analgesia versus general anesthesia. *Anesthesiol Rev.* 1993;10:117–125.
120. Conacher ID. Thoracic anesthesia: post-thoracotomy analgesia. *Anesthesiol Clin N Am.* 2001;19: 611–625.
121. Dhir S, Velayutham V, Ganapathy S. Pharmacologic management of acute pain in trauma. In: Smith CE, ed. *Trauma Anesthesia.* New York: Cambridge University Press; 2008:528–543.
122. Mattox K, Wall MJ. Historical review of blunt injury to the thoracic aorta. *Chest Surg Clin N Am.* 2000;10:167–182.
123. Pretre R, Chilcott M. Blunt trauma to the heart and great vessels. *N Engl J Med.* 1997;336(9): 626–632.
124. Oxorn D, Edelist G, Smith MS. An introduction to transoesophageal echocardiography: II. Clinical applications. *Can J Anaesth.* 1996;43:278–294.
125. Michard F, Teboul JL. Respiratory changes in arterial pressure in mechanically ventilated patients. In: Vincent JL, ed. *Yearbook of Intensive care and Emergency Medicine.* Berlin: Springer; 2000:696–704.
126. Dutton RP. Shock management. In: Smith CE, ed. *Trauma Anesthesia.* New York: Cambridge University Press; 2008:55–68.
127. May TJ, Greilich PE. Cerebral oximetry in cardiac surgery. Society of Cardiovascular Anesthesiologists Newsletter. 2008.
128. Repine TB, Perkins JG, Kauvar DS, Blackborne L. The use of fresh whole blood in massive transfusion. *J Trauma.* 2006;60:S59–S69.

Anesthesia for Adult Congenital Aortic Surgery*

17

Barry D. Kussman and
James A. DiNardo

Congenital Supravalvular Aortic Stenosis

Congenital supravalvular aortic stenosis (SVAS) is a rare form of left ventricular outflow tract (LVOT) obstruction that often is associated with peripheral pulmonary artery stenoses (approximately 40% of patients). Congenital SVAS is an elastin arteriopathy and is most commonly associated with Williams–Beuren syndrome. Williams–Beuren syndrome, commonly referred to as Williams syndrome (WS), is characterized by the presence of SVAS and peripheral pulmonary artery stenoses in association with mental retardation and distinctive elfin facies. It is the result of a microdeletion in the q11.23 region of chromosome 7, which affects several genes, including the elastin gene.[1] SVAS also occurs in a familial autosomal dominant form and in sporadic isolated incidences due to null alleles in the gene encoding for production of elastin; neither of these forms are associated with the extracardiac features of Williams–Beuren syndrome.

* This chapter is intended to be an overview of the anesthetic implications of those unrepaired congenital aortic lesions that are likely to be encountered in an adult population.

B.D. Kussman (✉)
Department of Anesthesiology, Perioperative and Pain Medicine, Children's Hospital Boston and Harvard Medical School, 300 Longwood Avenue, Boston, MA, USA
e-mail: barry.kussman@childrens.harvard.edu

Elastin is responsible for the distensibility of the aorta and large arteries during systole and subsequent recoil during diastole. This allows storage of hydrodynamic energy during systole and its release during diastole, an effect known as the windkessel effect. While loss of aortic distensibility alone is sufficient to elevate left ventricular (LV) afterload, the major impedance to LV ejection is the development of an obstructive aortic lesion. The reduced deposition of elastin in the arterial wall leads to increased proliferation of smooth muscle cells in the media of large arteries and subsequent development of obstructive hyperplastic intimal lesions.[2] A characteristic hourglass narrowing of the aorta develops at the sinotubular junction. In approximately 30% of cases, there is diffuse tubular narrowing of the ascending aorta often extending to the arch and the origin of the brachiocephalic vessels.[3,4] There may also be localized stenosis in the renal and mesenteric arteries.[4]

While peripheral pulmonary artery stenoses are characteristically associated with congenital SVAS, it is not uncommon for central pulmonary artery (pulmonary artery proximal to the hilum) stenoses to exist as well. The natural history of the pulmonary artery lesions is one in which there is a lessening in severity throughout childhood and adolescence.[5,6] Nonetheless, in approximately 40% of patients, severe pulmonary artery stenoses and right ventricular pressure overload exist in conjunction with SVAS and left ventricular pressure overload at the time surgical relief of

K. Subramaniam et al. (eds.), *Anesthesia and Perioperative Care for Aortic Surgery*,
DOI 10.1007/978-0-387-85922-4_17, © Springer Science+Business Media, LLC 2011

SVAS is undertaken.[4] These patients may have right ventricular systolic pressures as high as 200 mmHg and right ventricular to descending aortic pressure ratios as high as 2.0.

The aortic valve itself may also be pathologically involved in congenital SVAS, creating an additional source of LVOT obstruction. The sinotubular junction, the usual location of aortic wall constriction in SVAS, is also the peripheral attachment point of the aortic valve commissures.[7] The sinotubular junction normally expands during systole, allowing the free edge of the leaflets to assume a position parallel to flow during ejection. The narrowed, nondistensible sinotubular junction in SVAS inhibits alignment of the leaflets with blood flow and renders the aortic valve leaflets redundant relative to the size of the aorta. This mechanism is felt to be responsible for the development of the thickened aortic valve leaflets, which have been reported in association with SVAS.[3]

Mechanical impairment of coronary blood flow is a frequent and often unappreciated feature of WS and nonsyndromic SVAS. Adhesion of the right or left aortic leaflet edge to the narrowed sinotubular junction can restrict coronary blood flow into the sinus of Valsalva. It has been suggested that the left coronary sinus of Valsalva is affected more frequently in this process than the right one.[3,5] Cases of total isolation of the left and right coronary artery from the sinus of Valsalva as a result of complete fusion of a leaflet edge to a prominent sinotubular ridge have been reported.[8–10]

The presence of both ostial and diffuse left and right coronary artery stenoses must be considered as well. The etiology of direct coronary artery involvement appears to be multifactorial. The elastin arteriopathy may diffusely involve the coronary arteries, while a thickened aortic wall can directly narrow the coronary ostia.[11] Displacement of the coronary ostia superiorly to a position just below the sinotubular ridge with subsequent obstruction has been reported in three cases of sudden cardiac death.[12] Coronary artery dilation and tortuosity due to exposure of the coronary arteries to high prestenotic pressures may lead to development of accelerated coronary atherosclerosis and coronary aneurysms.[13,14] It should be noted that significant obstruction to coronary blood flow with associated fatal myocardial infarction has been reported in both the presence and the absence of hemodynamically significant SVAS[12,13,15–19]; in other words, although these patients are typically followed and assessed by echocardiography, the possibility of significant coronary obstruction via one or more of the mechanisms outlined can exist independent of the degree of aortic obstruction.

Left and right ventricular hypertrophy induced by outflow tract obstruction is a risk factor for development of subendocardial ischemia. Myocardial oxygen consumption is increased by the mass of the myocardium, the prolonged ejection phase, and a high-pressure isovolumic contraction phase. Myocardial oxygen delivery is compromised by a reduced diastolic interval (prolonged ejection phase), absence of systolic coronary perfusion, particularly in the right ventricle due to elevated right ventricular systolic pressure, elevated LVEDP due to reduced LV compliance, low aortic diastolic pressure due to loss of the windkessel effect, and compression of subendocardial vessels. The presence of obstructed coronary blood flow via any of the mechanisms previously described further increases this risk.

The natural history of SVAS is one of progressive left ventricular pressure overload and concentric hypertrophy complicated by progressive compromise of coronary blood flow. If left untreated, SVAS progresses to produce severe left ventricular dysfunction as a result of chronic pressure overload, myocardial ischemia, and infarction.[13] Additionally, there is a risk for aortic dissection due to high pressure and abnormal aortic wall structure.[13] Surgical intervention is necessary to prevent the development of these sequalae.

Diagnosis

In patients with Williams–Beuren syndrome, the noncardiac features of the syndrome generally bring the patient to medical attention. The extent of SVAS and peripheral pulmonary artery stenoses are initially evaluated with echocardiography. Cardiac catheterization is usually necessary to delineate the etiology and the extent of coronary artery abnormalities. In isolated SVAS, the initial presentation is usually chest pain or syncope.

A unique feature of SVAS is the presence of higher blood pressures in the right as opposed to left upper extremities in some patients. This is felt to be a consequence of the Coanda effect with a greater portion of kinetic energy imparted to the right-sided arch vessels.

Identifying those patients with congenital SVAS at risk for myocardial ischemia is challenging.[20] Echocardiography is useful in assessing ventricular outflow tract gradients, ventricular hypertrophy, and wall motion abnormalities, but is an insensitive method for detecting and delineating compromise of ostial, proximal, and distal coronary blood flow. Of particular concern in this regard is the fact that significant coronary arterial flow impairment can occur in the absence of significant SVAS. Therefore, while the absence of significant SVAS (identified by echocardiographic imaging as "only" minimal or mild LV to aorta pressure gradients) may be reassuring to the clinician, in actuality it does not exclude the possibility that significant impairment of coronary blood flow exists. Cardiac magnetic resonance imaging (CMRI) and computer tomography show increasing promise as noninvasive imaging modalities capable of delineating obstruction to coronary blood flow.[21] However, at present, cardiac catheterization with coronary and aortic angiography remains the gold standard for delineation of aortic leaflet tethering and assessment of coronary artery lumen caliber. Obviously, cardiac catheterization carries its own risks in these patients. Thus, evaluation and risk assessment, particularly as pertains to elective or noncardiac procedures in patients with SVAS, remains problematic.

Treatment

Patients with bilateral outflow tract obstruction and/or those with known coronary blood flow compromise represent a high-risk subset of patients. These patients may require intervention to relieve outflow tract obstruction prior to noncardiac surgical procedures. Percutaneous balloon dilation of congenital SVAS is usually ineffective while outcome following surgery for SVAS is generally good, with 10–20 year survival

of 96% and 77% respectively.[7] As opposed to surgical augmentation of a single aortic sinus (Fig. 17.1a), techniques that provide symmetrical reconstruction of the aortic root (Figs. 17.1b–d)

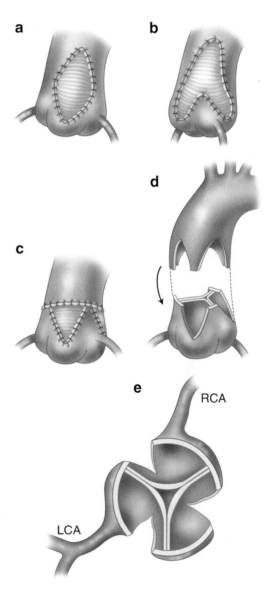

Fig. 17.1 Surgical techniques used for relief of supravalvular aortic stenosis. (**a**), Single diamond or tear drop shaped patch extending into noncoronary sinus. (**b**), Inverted, bifurcated patch extending into noncoronary and right coronary sinuses. (**c**), Transection of aorta with patch insertions in all three sinuses with aortic reanastomosis as described by Brom.[69] (**d**), Transection of the aorta with incisions into all three sinuses with subsequent tailoring and reanastomosis of distal aorta. (**e**), Positions of the three sinus incisions relative to coronary arteries. (Redrawn with permission from Stamm et al. 2001)[3]

result in superior hemodynamics (reduced gradient and prevalence of aortic insufficiency) and reduced mortality rate and need for reoperation.[7] In instances where diffuse tubular hypoplasia of the aorta and arch exists, symmetrical reconstruction of the ascending aorta with extension of the patch to the underside of the aortic arch is necessary. Surgical relief of coronary ostial stenosis may be necessary and long-segment coronary stenosis may require coronary revascularization, usually with an internal thoracic arterial conduit.[7]

Surgical therapy for relief of proximal pulmonary artery obstructions tends to be palliative in that reoperation or subsequent catheter-based intervention is commonly needed.[6] Percutaneous balloon dilation of peripheral pulmonary artery stenoses plays an important role in long-term management of these patients. Balloon dilation of significant peripheral pulmonary artery stenoses is indicated to reduce right ventricular afterload prior to surgical relief of SVAS, regardless of whether surgical relief of more proximal pulmonary artery stenoses is also anticipated.[6] The hypertrophied right ventricle is particularly susceptible to ischemic injury following cardioplegic arrest, so that presurgical reduction of afterload will improve right ventricular function in this setting.

Anesthetic Management

In congenital SVAS, myocardial ischemia has been implicated in the majority of cases of sudden death occurring in conjunction with anesthesia or sedation.[20] Features common to the reported cases are sudden, rapid hemodynamic deterioration associated with hypotension and bradycardia, and a lack of response to aggressive resuscitative measures. It should also be recognized that catheter manipulation during cardiac catheterization can produce hemodynamic instability due to induction of dysrhythmias, exacerbation of outflow tract obstruction, creation of semilunar and atrioventricular valve insufficiency, and exacerbation of compromised coronary blood flow during aortic and coronary angiography. These problems

can of course occur regardless of the sedation or anesthetic technique.[19] Furthermore, while some fatalities during cardiac catheterization have been associated with catheter manipulation, others have occurred before the procedure had begun or after apparently successful completion.

A particularly tenuous myocardial oxygen supply:demand relationship exists in these patients. As previously stated, the incidence of impaired coronary blood flow is often underestimated. As such, all patients with congenital SVAS should be considered at risk for myocardial ischemia and treated accordingly. The anesthetic management of these patients has recently been reviewed.[20] Although there are insufficient data to recommend a specific anesthetic technique, a prudent approach would involve meticulous attention to balancing myocardial oxygen supply and demand. Tachycardia will increase myocardial oxygen consumption while simultaneously reducing diastole and coronary perfusion, with the combination of hypotension and tachycardia being particularly deleterious. In either case, the presence of ventricular hypertrophy will further jeopardize subendocardial perfusion. The anesthetic goals for these patients are summarized in Table 17.1. As with coronary insufficiency patients, the best approach is one that employs a combination of drugs with offsetting hemodynamic effects used judiciously in small doses.

Coarctation of the Aorta

Coarctation of the aorta is a focal narrowing of the aorta. It accounts for 6–8% of all congenital cardiac defects, has a male predominance, and is the most common lesion in patients with Turner syndrome. Almost half of all cases have associated cardiac and noncardiac anomalies, with a bicommissural aortic valve being the most frequent (22–42% of cases).[22] The anatomic pathology is remarkably consistent with a discrete posterior shelf or invagination present just distal to the left subclavian artery opposite the insertion of the ductus arteriosus (juxta-ductal). In some instances, this shelf may be circumferential.

Table 17.1 Anesthetic management goals in patients with supravalvular aortic stenosis (SVAS)

1. Maintain an age-appropriate heart rate
   - Use of vagolytic drugs (atropine, glycopyrrolate) and drugs with sympathomimetic activity (pancuronium, ketamine) should be avoided, particularly in combination
   - The dose of atropine or glycopyrrolate given in conjunction with neostigmine for reversal of neuromuscular blockade should be chosen so as to avoid excessive tachycardia

2. Maintain sinus rhythm
   - Aggressive treatment of supraventricular tachycardia is necessary; cardioversion (regardless of systemic blood pressure) may be preferable to pharmacologic interventions (esmolol, adenosine), which may cause hypotension
   - Treatment of junctional rhythm

3. Maintain preload
   - Agents that increase venous capacitance (propofol, sodium thiopental, inhalation anesthetics) should be used with consideration given to agent-specific dose-related effect
   - In the presence of severe left ventricular hypertrophy, rapid intravascular volume augmentation may cause a precipitous increase in left atrial pressure resulting in pulmonary vascular congestion

4. Maintain contractility
   - Agents with negative inotropic effects (propofol, sodium thiopental, inhalation anesthetics) should be used with consideration given to agent-specific dose-related effect

5. Maintain systemic vascular resistance
   - Agents that reduce systemic vascular resistance (propofol, sodium thiopental, inhalation anesthetics) should be used with consideration to agent-specific dose-related effect
   - Hypotension should be treated aggressively. A pure α-adrenergic agent (phenylephrine) may be most appropriate unless significant bradycardia is also present in which case ephedrine or low-dose epinephrine (0.1–1.0 mcg/kg) is appropriate

6. Avoid increases in pulmonary vascular resistance
   - Avoid hypercarbia and hypoxemia and maintain the lowest mean airway pressures consistent with adequate minute ventilation, particularly in patients with right ventricular outflow tract obstruction

Longer segment coarctation and coarctation of the abdominal aorta are also seen.

It has been postulated that coarctation develops as the result of fetal blood flow patterns, which reduce antegrade aortic blood flow with a proportionate increase in pulmonary artery and ductus arteriosus blood flow. It is, therefore, not surprising that coarctation is associated with aortic valve stenosis or a bicuspid aortic valve, with hypoplasia of other left-sided structures such as the mitral valve and left ventricle, and with hypoplasia of the aortic arch. Hypoplasia of the aortic isthmus (the region of the aortic arch from the left subclavian to the ductus arteriosus) is the isolated aortic arch lesion most commonly associated with coarctation. Ventricular septal defects (VSD), particularly posterior malalignment VSD that cause LVOT obstruction and divert flow from the ascending aorta into the pulmonary artery, are also associated with coarctation. In contrast, coarctation is virtually never found in association with right-sided obstructive lesions. Closure of

the ductus arteriosus may also be associated with constriction of the aorta at the level of the ductus, presumably due to the presence of ductal tissue in this area.[23]

Despite remarkably consistent anatomic pathology, the pathophysiology of coarctation is varied and depends on the severity of the coarctation and the presence of associated lesions (Fig. 17.2). These variations in pathophysiology have led to the use of confusing terms such as infantile and adult coarctation or pre- and post-ductal coarctation, which are of little practical significance. The ductus arteriosus plays a critical role in pathophysiology and presentation will be in infancy for all patients except those capable of tolerating ductal closure without overt hemodynamic compromise. In general, presentation beyond infancy is limited to patients with an isolated coarctation of mild to moderate severity or to those with rapid compensatory collateral formation. In these patients, there is a secondary phase of fibrosis that occurs in the first 2–3 months

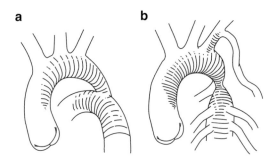

Fig. 17.2 Typical appearances of coarctation of the aorta. (**a**). Coarctation associated with hypoplasia of the aortic isthmus and ductal-dependent perfusion of the descending aorta present at birth. Closure of the ductus arteriosus will likely result in LV afterload mismatch, compromise of systemic perfusion and oxygen delivery, and presentation in infancy. (**b**). Coarctation of the aorta in a patient who has tolerated ductal closure and developed extensive collateralization. Extensive fibrosis in the juxtaductal region in association with growth of the native aorta has produced a discrete hourglass constriction. Presentation will be as a child or young adult

of life. As the child grows and the ligamentum arteriosum continues to fibrose, a thick fibrous shelf forms within the lumen of the aorta.

Diagnosis

Beyond infancy, upper extremity hypertension and/or a murmur is the most common presentation. In the presence of extensive collateral development, it is not at all uncommon for even a severe coarctation to be completely asymptomatic. Symptoms when present include exercise intolerance, headache, chest pain, and lower extremity claudication. Physical examination, however, will reveal elevation of blood pressure in the upper extremities one or two standard deviations above the mean for age. Blood pressure in the arms and legs will generally reveal a significant difference. In the presence of an anomalous right subclavian artery (take-off from the descending aorta distal to the coarctation), the right arm and lower extremity blood pressures will be equal. Femoral pulses will be weak or delayed, but this may be a subtle finding in the presence of extensive collateral development. Murmurs may be due to the coarctation itself, collateral blood

vessels, or associated cardiac defects. The systolic murmur of a narrowed descending thoracic aorta may be best heard along the left paravertebral area between the spine and scapula. Continuous murmurs may be heard along the chest wall due to collateral vessels supplying tissues beyond the coarctation. These collaterals may originate from the internal thoracic, intercostals, subclavian, and/or scapular arteries. Other murmurs can be due to coexistent aortic valve stenosis and/or VSDs.

Electrocardiography may appear normal or display evidence of left ventricular hypertrophy with nonspecific ST-T wave changes. Chest radiography, similarly, may be consistent with increased cardiac size. Rib notching may be seen on chest radiographs in older patients with extensive collateralization. Two-dimensional echocardiography and Doppler evaluations can establish the diagnosis of coarctation and delineate its location and severity as well as define and quantitate additional intracardiac lesions including LVOT obstruction. Magnetic resonance imaging (MRI) can provide high-resolution three-dimensional anatomic reconstruction of the region of coarctation. Specifically, gadolinium-enhanced 3-D MR angiography (MRA) is used to define extracardiac vascular anatomy, in which the signal from blood is particularly high and strongly contrasts with nonvascular structures. Computerized tomography is also useful for the diagnosis of coarctation. Cardiac catheterization is rarely indicated.

Treatment

Treatment of coarctation depends on a number of variables including age, severity, and associated defects. Presentation as an infant generally leads to medical stabilization followed by surgical intervention. The optimal treatment for neonates, infants, and children is currently felt to be complete excision of the area of coarctation and surrounding ductal tissue with end-to-end anastomosis. Alternatively, a reverse subclavian patch repair can be undertaken. In this technique, the left subclavian artery is ligated and transected with the proximal portion of the artery used as a flap to augment the area of coarctation. Following this procedure, left arm pulses will be weak or absent. Dacron patch aortoplasty following resection of the posterior coarctation ridge has also been used; however, this technique is associated with late development of hypertension and aneurysm formation as compared to end-to-end anastomosis.[24] In the case of coarctation associated with a hypoplastic aortic isthmus, complete excision in conjunction with an extended end-to-end or end-to-side anastomosis is recommended.[25] In this circumstance, the descending aorta is anastomosed to the underside of the aortic arch in an end-to-end or end-to-side fashion. It has been argued that resection with extended end-to-end anastomosis should be applied to all infants and young children with coarctation as young age and arch hypoplasia are two important risk factors for recoarctation.[26] Percutaneous balloon angioplasty can be considered as an alternative to reoperation for treatment of recoarctation.[27]

In adults, coarctation resection and a primary end-to-end aortic anastomosis via a left posterolateral thoracotomy is the preferred technique but placement of an interposition graft may be necessary when there is insufficient mobility of the aorta to allow this approach.[28–30] Generally, a clamp and sew technique is used, with use of shunts, left heart bypass, or deep hypothermic circulatory arrest reserved for those patients with complex anatomy or inadequate collateral blood supply.[28,31] Balloon angioplasty and endovascular stent placement to treat adult coarctation are increasingly being employed.[32] Because patients with aortic coarctation are generally young and have hypertension as their sole comorbidity, they are a distinctly different subset than the elderly patient with multiple comorbidities deemed to be high-risk operative candidates who may benefit from a nonoperative approach. Experience to date indicates that while morbidity associated with catheter-based approaches to adult coarctation is similar to a surgical approach, the incidence of restenosis and the need for reintervention is higher following catheter-based techniques.[32]

Anesthetic Management

The anesthetic management of patients for repair of coarctation is not substantially different from those of any proximal descending aortic lesion. Because patients with repaired coarctation may present for additional cardiac or noncardiac surgery, of equal importance to the anesthesiologist is recognition of the long-term consequences of coarctation repair on blood pressure and left ventricular mass.

Persistent arterial hypertension in the absence of recoarctation and regardless of the type of repair is present in as many as one third of repaired coarctation patients in long-term follow-up studies.[29,33–35] In addition, the majority of patients with normal blood pressure at rest show an abnormal blood pressure increase with exercise and activities of daily living.[36] Systolic blood pressure is positively associated with LV mass in this cohort, and elevated systolic blood pressure and LV mass are both important risk factors for late morbidity and mortality from heart failure and coronary and cerebrovascular disease.[34,35,37] While it has been suggested that the risk of developing subsequent hypertension is reduced by repair in the first year of life,[38] more recent series do not support this contention.[39,40]

The etiology of this persistent hypertension is multifactorial. The pulsatility of the post coarctation descending aorta remains reduced following hemodynamically ideal repair.[41] In addition, as compared to the lower body, upper body vascular responses to reactive hyperemia and glyceryl trinitrate are reduced and pulse wave velocity is increased in successfully repaired coarctation patients. This suggests the presence of abnormal smooth muscle relaxation or structural abnormalities of the arterial wall.[35,42] The geometry of the aortic arch following coarctation and distal aortic arch repair is also a determinant of subsequent upper body vascular responses, pulse wave velocity, and left ventricular mass. Anatomy with a high arch height to width ratio (Gothic arch) is associated with impaired vascular response, increased pulse wave velocity, central aortic stiffness, and increased LV mass as compared to anatomy with a lower arch height to width ratio (Crenel and normal Romanesque arch anatomy).[43,44] These

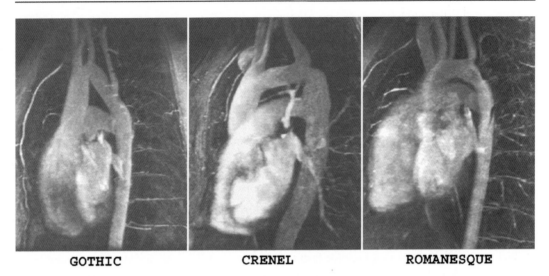

GOTHIC   **CRENEL**   **ROMANESQUE**

Fig. 17.3 Magnetic resonance imaging of the three types of aortic arch anatomy following coarctation repair with primary resection and end-to-to-end or extended end-to-to-end anastomosis. The Gothic arch has the highest height to width ratio while the Romanesque arch (normal arch anatomy) has the lowest; Crenel is intermediate. (Reproduced with permission from: Ou et al. 2007)[43]

anatomies are illustrated in Fig. 17.3. While early repair may be associated with preservation of conduit artery elasticity, vascular reactivity remains impaired.[40] Abnormalities in baroreceptor reflexes and in the renin–angiotensin–aldosterone system have also been implicated as factors in persistent hypertension following successful coarctation repair.[33] Recent evidence suggests that abnormalities in cardiovascular reflexes are already present in neonates with coarctation prior to repair.[45]

Inherent aortic wall abnormalities and persistent hypertension contribute to an increased incidence of cardiovascular complications following successful repair of coarctation. As compared to the general population, these patients are at increased risk for aortic aneurysm and fistula formation, aortic dissections and rupture, premature coronary atherosclerosis, cerebral vascular disease, and endarteritis at the repair site.[29,33] Advanced age and the presence of a bicuspid aortic valve appear to be independent risk factors for aortic complications.[46]

Vascular Rings

A vascular ring is an aortic arch anomaly in which the trachea and esophagus are surrounded completely by vascular structures. Rings are formed by abnormal persistence and/or regression of components of the aortic arch complex. These vascular structures, which need not be patent, can cause compression of the trachea, bronchi, and esophagus. In a vascular sling, tracheal and esophageal compression may be produced without the trachea and oesophagus being completely encircled. Although accounting for less than 1% of all congenital heart defects, vascular rings and slings represent an important source of airway and esophageal obstruction. Approximately 29% of patients have associated intracardiac defects.[47] Table 17.2 lists the vascular anomalies associated with airway and/or esophageal compression and the required surgical approach.[48,49]

The vast majority of patients with a vascular ring have either a double aortic arch with right arch dominance (Fig. 17.4) or a right aortic arch with mirror image branching, an aberrant left subclavian artery, and intact left ligamentum arteriosum (Fig. 17.5).[47–49] A right aortic arch passes rightward and posterior to the trachea while a left aortic arch passes leftward and anterior to the trachea. With mirror image branching, the arch gives off, in order, the common trunk of the left common carotid and left subclavian, the right common carotid, and the right subclavian arteries. With a double aortic arch with

Table 17.2 Classification of vascular rings and slings associated with airway and/or esophageal compression

Lesion	Surgical approach
Double aortic Arch	
• Right arch dominant	Left thoracotomy
• Left arch dominant	Right thoracotomy
• Equal dominance	Left thoracotomy
Right aortic arch	
• Mirror-image branching and aberrant left subclavian artery with left ligamentum arteriosum	Left thoracotomy
• Mirror-image branching and right retro-esophageal ligamentum arteriosum	Left thoracotomy
Left aortic arch	
• Aberrant right subclavian artery with right ligamentum arteriosum	Right thoracotomy
• Right descending aorta and right ligamentum arteriosum	Right thoracotomy
Anomalous innominate artery	Right thoracotomy or median sternotomy
Cervical aortic arch	Median sternotomy
Pulmonary artery sling	Median sternotomy

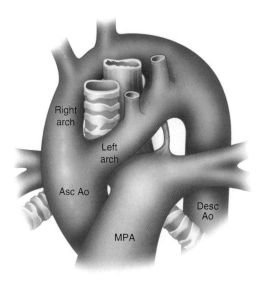

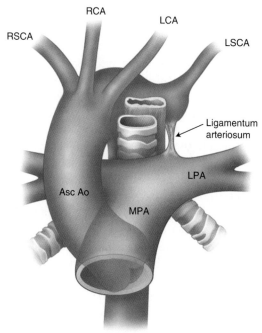

Fig. 17.4 A double aortic arch with right arch dominance creating a vascular ring encircling the trachea and esophagus. The ligamentum arteriosum is seen arising from the underside of the left arch. The vessels arising from the posterior right arch from left to right in the figure are the right carotid and right subclavian arteries. The vessels arising from the anterior left arch from left to right in the figure are the left carotid and left subclavian arteries. In this figure, both arches are patent. The left arch is generally small or atretic distal to the left carotid or left subclavian artery

Fig. 17.5 A right aortic arch with mirror image branching, an aberrant left subclavian artery, and intact left ligamentum arteriosum, creating a vascular ring encircling the trachea and esophagus. (Asc Ao=ascending aorta; *MPA*=main pulmonary artery; *LPA*=left pulmonary artery; *RSCA*=right subclavian artery; *RCA* = right carotid artery; *LCA*=left carotid artery; *LSCA* = left subclavian artery)

right arch dominance, the anteriorly located left aortic arch gives rise to the left carotid and left subclavian arteries. This left arch is generally atretic or severely hypoplastic beyond the origin of either the left carotid or left subclavian artery.

Diagnosis

Vascular rings and slings generally present in childhood with the most common symptoms being inspiratory stridor, dysphagia, wheezing, dyspnea, cough, and recurrent respiratory tract infections.[47] Feeding problems are common. Presentation in adulthood is uncommon and symptoms are often attributed to asthma.[50–52] The development of hypertension and atherosclerotic changes associated with aging may result in exacerbation of symptoms due to development of vascular rigidity, tortuosity, or frank aneurysm formation.

Treatment

The goal of operative repair is to divide the compressive vascular ring, relieve tracheobronchial and/or esophageal compression, and maintain normal perfusion of the aortic arch. The surgical approach to the most common vascular rings is via a left posterolateral thoracotomy; alternately, a video-assisted thoracoscopic approach (VATS) can be utilized. Patients with vascular rings composed of nonpatent vascular structures are considered ideal candidates for VATS.[53] Patients with vascular rings composed of patent vascular structures can be approached with a limited thoracotomy and endoscopic video-assistance. With VATS, four trocars are placed through separate thoracostomies in the posterolateral chest wall. The arch elements are dissected free, and the appropriate ring elements are divided between sutures or vascular clips, with division of any remaining fibrous bands overlying the oesophagus. Advantages of VATS compared to open thoracotomy may include smaller incision(s), improved vision inside the chest cavity, reduced postoperative pain, and reduced risk of chest wall deformity.

Correction for right aortic arch with aberrant left subclavian artery and intact left ligamentum arteriosum involves division of the ligamentum. In circumstances where the diverticulum of Kommerell is large, it may be necessary to excise it as well. Correction for double aortic arch with right arch dominance involves division of the fibrous tissue distal to either the left carotid or subclavian arteries. Bronchoscopy is often performed in conjunction with these repairs to assess the degree to which compression has been relieved and to assess the potential degree of dynamic airway collapse. Long-standing tracheal compression in adult patients may lead to tracheomalacia. Aortopexy, innominate artery suspension, tracheal reconstruction, or stenting may be necessary if symptoms persist following release of the ring.[50,54,55] Chylothorax is an uncommon perioperative complication.

The potential for a variable course and relationship of the recurrent laryngeal nerve (RLN) to the ligamentum arteriosum and descending aorta makes the RLN susceptible to injury during either type of surgical approach to vascular ring. In the largest reported series, there was a 5.3% incidence of unilateral vocal cord paralysis.[56] Intraoperative RLN monitoring for adults has been reported, but a technique for infants and small children has also been described.[57]

Anesthetic Management

The choice of anaesthetic technique will depend on the type of vascular ring, the type and severity of underlying congenital heart disease, and the nature of the planned surgical procedure. Because of airway compression, some advise similar considerations in approaching these patients as for those with anterior mediastinal masses.[58] On the other hand, it is not clear how frequently, if ever, these lesions behave in a fashion that is analogous to anterior mediastinal masses in terms of increased dynamic compression of airway and cardiovascular structures in response to positive pressure ventilation and muscle relaxation. Spontaneous ventilation and avoidance of muscle relaxation may be beneficial in terms of maintaining airway patency during inhalation (radial traction due to negative intrathoracic pressure) and having some degree of active expiratory force generation to overcome obstruction during exhalation. Conversely, agitated breathing and forced exhalation can increase dynamic intrathoracic airway collapse (e.g. tracheomalacia) and airflow turbulence at the site(s) of obstruction. It is, therefore, important to understand the cause, degree, and location of airway compromise in as great a detail as possible. In general, the majority of these patients are best approached by careful induction, assurance of the ability to ventilate with positive pressure, and then muscle relaxation; the application of positive pressure and removal of respiratory effort will usually result in improved airflow. An anaesthetic technique that avoids muscle relaxants is required if RLN monitoring is used.

In most cases with significant airway narrowing, the endotracheal tube should be passed so that it lies proximal to the stenotic segment in order to avoid edema and granulation tissue formation caused by tube impact on the narrowed area. Alternatively, cases of severe collapse may require "stenting" with an endotracheal tube or rigid bronchoscope to ensure adequate ventilation. When not contraindicated by the nature, location, or degree of airway narrowing, the surgical approach (and VATS in particular) may benefit from single-lung ventilation techniques.

Major postoperative issues relate to concurrent cardiac defects and residual airway disorders. Successful tracheal extubation is possible in most patients with isolated vascular rings at the conclusion of the procedure.[59] It is important to remember that successful repair of the ring may not immediately relieve airway obstruction; this may be observed immediately on extubation, or as a remote problem after surgery. Persistent obstruction may be due to residual compression, secondary airway wall instability (malacia), or associated structural anomalies. Tracheomalacia and bronchomalacia are among the commonest problems, can be severe postoperatively, and may persist for months after successful surgery. Both can be exacerbated by posttraumatic edema, other airway lesions, and upper airway obstruction due to sedation or swelling. Prolonged intubation to provide internal stabilization may be required to maintain airway patency in long-segment malacia, but can lead to endoluminal airway complications such as granulation tissue formation. When RLN injury occurs, there is a risk for stridor, hoarseness, and the potential for aspiration.

Patent Ductus Arteriosus

A patent ductus arteriosus (PDA) connects the main pulmonary trunk near the origin of the left pulmonary artery with the proximal descending aorta just distal to the origin of the left subclavian artery (Fig. 17.6). With a large, nonrestrictive PDA, there is little or no pressure gradient across the ductus and the direction and magnitude of shunting is determined by the ratio of pulmonary vascular resistance (PVR) to systemic vascular resistance (SVR). The more restrictive the PDA, the less influential the ratio of PVR:SVR becomes in determining shunt direction and magnitude.

The high PVR present after birth tends to limit the shunt magnitude until PVR begins to decrease. As PVR decreases, a physiologic left-to-right shunt (recirculation of pulmonary venous blood to the pulmonary artery) with increased pulmonary blood flow develops. If the PDA is large and nonrestrictive, pulmonary blood flow will be high and pulmonary artery pressures will be systemic. In this setting, elevated pulmonary artery flow and pressure will eventually produce an elevation in PVR. Eisenmenger's physiology will result with bidirectional shunting (both a physiologic left-to-right and right-to-left shunt) or a pure right-to-left shunt (recirculation of systemic venous blood to the aorta). Adults presenting with PDA generally have a restrictive PDA with subsystemic pulmonary artery pressures and a

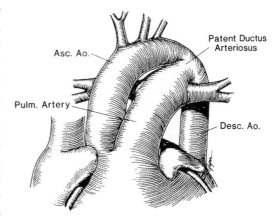

Fig. 17.6 Patent ductus arteriosus. (Asc Ao = ascending aorta; Desc Ao = descending aorta)

pulmonary to systemic blood flow ratio (Q_P:Q_S) <1.5:1. In order for systemic blood flow to be maintained in the presence of a physiologic left-to-right shunt, left ventricular output is increased and a volume load is imposed on the left ventricle. In addition, the increased pulmonary blood flow increases pulmonary venous return and left atrial pressure.

Diagnosis

The murmur associated with continuous left to right flow across the PDA is heard at the first or second left intercostal space and is continuous in nature with a crescendo–decrescendo pattern (loudest in systole, diminished in diastole). Echocardiography typically is used to establish the diagnosis of PDA and to delineate size and direction of blood flow. In addition, the extent of left ventricular volume overload can be determined and indirect assessment of pulmonary artery pressures can be made. Echocardiography can also be used to quantify Q_P:Q_S. In the absence of other cardiac lesions and in the presence of left to right shunting, volumetric measurements at the mitral valve or left ventricular outflow tract will yield Q_P (total volume traversing the pulmonary artery and delivered to the pulmonary veins) while volumetric measurements at the tricuspid valve or right ventricular outflow tract will yield Q_S (total volume traversing the aorta and delivered to the systemic veins). Recently, use of the proximal isovelocity surface area (PISA) method to directly quantify PDA shunt volume has been described.[60] MRI can provide high-resolution three-dimensional anatomic reconstruction of the region of the PDA. Cardiac catheterization is not indicated unless there is concern that significantly elevated PVR is present.

Treatment

Closure of the PDA was the first "cardiac" operation successfully performed by Robert Gross at Children's Hospital Boston in 1938. The usual surgical approach is via a left thoracotomy or via

VATS. The ductus is either ligated or ligated and transected. The left pulmonary artery, left main stem bronchus, and descending aorta are at risk of inadvertent ligation if the PDA is misidentified. Injury to the recurrent laryngeal nerve is also possible. In some adults, calcification and friability of the aorta and the PDA may preclude ligation. In this circumstance, a median sternotomy and CPB is necessary. The preferred technique is closure of the ductal orifice via a transpulmonary artery approach using either a patch, a purse string, or pledgeted sutures.[61–63] With this approach, a balloon-tipped catheter is used to occlude the aortic end of the ductus to facilitate exposure by preventing back-bleeding (Fig. 17.7). Rarely, deep hypothermic circulatory arrest is utilized to facilitate exposure without use of balloon occlusion.[64] Some patients with Eisenmenger's physiology are not candidates for closure as removal of the right-to-left "pop-off" results in right ventricular failure and low cardiac output syndrome.

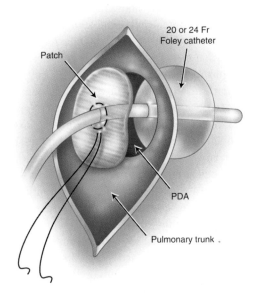

Fig. 17.7 Illustration of transpulmonary artery approach to PDA. A balloon-tip catheter is passed through a patch via a purse string and used to occlude the PDA while on cardiopulmonary bypass. Once the patch is sewn in place, the balloon is deflated, the catheter is removed, and the purse string closed. (Redrawn with permission from Toda et al. 2000)[61]

Table 17.3 Anesthetic management goals in patients with PDA

1. Maintain heart rate, contractility, and preload to maintain cardiac output. A reduction in cardiac output may compromise systemic perfusion, despite a relatively high pulmonary blood flow.

2. Avoid decreases in the PVR:SVR ratio. The increase in pulmonary blood flow that accompanies a reduced PVR:SVR ratio necessitates an increase in cardiac output to maintain systemic blood flow.

3. Avoid large increases in the PVR:SVR ratio. An increase may result in production of a right-to-left shunt.

4. In instances in which a right-to-left shunt exists, ventilatory measures to decrease PVR should be used. In addition, SVR must be maintained or increased. These measures will reduce the magnitude of the right-to-left shunt.

5. Control of ventilation with manipulation of PaO_2, $PaCO_2$, pH, and lung volumes are the best methods for altering PVR independently of SVR. PVR is lowest when lung volumes are at or near FRC. A combination of a high inspired FiO_2, a PaO_2 higher than 60 mmHg, a $PaCO_2$ of 30–35 mmHg, a pH of 7.50–7.60, and low inspiratory pressures without high levels of PEEP, will produce reliable reductions in PVR. Conversely, a reduced FiO_2, a PaO_2 of 50–60 mmHg, a $PaCO_2$ of 45–55 mmHg, and the application of PEEP, can be used to increase PVR.

PDA = patent ductus arteriosus; PVR = pulmonary vascular resistance; SVR = systemic vascular resistance; FRC = functional residual capacity.

Both percutaneous device closure and covered stent placement in the aorta have been used as nonoperative approaches to PDA.[65,66] In patients with Eisenmenger's physiology, percutaneous device closure offers the advantage of assessing hemodynamics immediately following test balloon occlusion of the PDA prior to definitive closure.[67,68] Percutaneous device or stent placement can be complicated by dislodgement of the hardware downstream into the pulmonary artery or aorta; retrieval may require surgical intervention.

Anesthetic Management

The anesthetic management goals are summarized in Table 17.3. There are a few additional considerations. Patients undergoing ligation via VATS or thoracotomy will benefit from single-lung ventilation techniques. Blood pressure should be monitored in an upper and lower extremity. The right arm is preferable to the left arm because the surgeon may have to place a clamp on the aorta if control of the aortic end of the PDA is lost during dissection or ligation. Consideration should also be given to use of cerebral near-infrared spectroscopy (NIRS) to monitor cerebral perfusion if clamping is likely to compromise left carotid blood flow. In patients with a large left to right shunt, there will be an increase in aortic diastolic blood pressure following ligation due to cessation of runoff of

blood into the pulmonary circulation. An upper and lower extremity blood pressure should be compared following ligation to assure that a coarctation has not been created.

Key Notes

1. In patients with SVAS, the risk of sudden death related to procedural sedation/anesthesia is underestimated. All patients with congenital SVAS should be considered at risk for myocardial ischemia and treated accordingly. SVAS patients with concomitant right ventricular outflow tract obstruction are a particular risk.

2. Adults with successfully repaired coarctation of the aorta can be expected to have systemic hypertension due to both anatomic abnormalities of the aorta and impaired vascular reactivity.

3. The vast majority of patients with a vascular ring have either a double aortic arch with right arch dominance or a right aortic arch with mirror image branching, an aberrant left subclavian artery, and intact left ligamentum arteriosum. Many of these patients will have associated tracheomalacia that may be slow to resolve following successful surgery.

4. Patients with PDA will have right ventricular volume overload, the severity of which parallels the magnitude of the physiologic

left-to-right shunt. Some adult patients will require PDA closure on CPB due to calcification of the aorta or aortic atheromatous disease.

References

1. Urban Z, Peyrol S, Plauchu H, et al. Elastin gene deletions in Williams syndrome patients result in altered deposition of elastic fibers in skin and a subclinical dermal phenotype. *Pediatr Dermatol.* 2000;17:12–20.

2. Urban Z, Zhang J, Davis EC, et al. Supravalvular aortic stenosis: genetic and molecular dissection of a complex mutation in the elastin gene. *Hum Genet.* 2001;109:512–520.

3. Stamm C, Li J, Ho SY, Redington AN, Anderson RH. The aortic root in supravalvular aortic stenosis: the potential surgical relevance of morphologic findings. *J Thorac Cardiovasc Surg.* 1997;114:16–24.

4. Stamm C, Friehs I, Ho SY, Moran AM, Jonas RA, del Nido PJ. Congenital supravalvar aortic stenosis: a simple lesion? *Eur J Cardiothorac Surg.* 2001;19: 195–202.

5. Kim YM, Yoo SJ, Choi JY, Kim SH, Bae EJ, Lee YT. Natural course of supravalvar aortic stenosis and peripheral pulmonary arterial stenosis in Williams' syndrome. *Cardiol Young.* 1999;9:37–41.

6. Stamm C, Friehs I, Moran AM, et al. Surgery for bilateral outflow tract obstruction in elastin arteriopathy. *J Thorac Cardiovasc Surg.* 2000;120:755–763.

7. Stamm C, Kreutzer C, Zurakowski D, et al. Forty-one years of surgical experience with congenital supravalvular aortic stenosis. *J Thorac Cardiovasc Surg.* 1999;118:874–885.

8. Martin MM, Lemmer JH Jr, Shaffer E, Dick M 2nd, Bove EL. Obstruction to left coronary artery blood flow secondary to obliteration of the coronary ostium in supravalvular aortic stenosis. *Ann Thorac Surg.* 1988;45:16–20.

9. Thiene G, Ho SY. Aortic root pathology and sudden death in youth: review of anatomical varieties. *Appl Pathol.* 1986;4:237–245.

10. Sun CC, Jacot J, Brenner JI. Sudden death in supravalvular aortic stenosis: fusion of a coronary leaflet to the sinus ridge, dysplasia and stenosis of aortic and pulmonic valves. *Pediatr Pathol.* 1992;12: 751–759.

11. Matsuda H, Miyamoto Y, Takahashi T, Kadoba K, Nakano S, Sano T. Extended aortic and left main coronary angioplasty with a single pericardial patch in a patient with Williams syndrome. *Ann Thorac Surg.* 1991;52:1331–1333.

12. Bird LM, Billman GF, Lacro RV, et al. Sudden death in Williams syndrome: report of ten cases. *J Pediatr.* 1996;129:926–931.

13. Van Son JA, Edwards WD, Danielson GK. Pathology of coronary arteries, myocardium, and great arteries in supravalvular aortic stenosis. Report of five cases with implications for surgical treatment. *J Thorac Cardiovasc Surg.* 1994;108:21–28.

14. Mignosa C, Agati S, Di Stefano S, et al. Dysphagia: an unusual presentation of giant aneurysm of the right coronary artery and supravalvular aortic stenosis in Williams syndrome. *J Thorac Cardiovasc Surg.* 2004;128:946–948.

15. Terhune PE, Buchino JJ, Rees AH. Myocardial infarction associated with supravalvular aortic stenosis. *J Pediatr.* 1985;106:251–254.

16. Conway EE Jr, Noonan J, Marion RW, Steeg CN. Myocardial infarction leading to sudden death in the Williams syndrome: report of three cases. *J Pediatr.* 1990;117:593–595.

17. van Pelt NC, Wilson NJ, Lear G. Severe coronary artery disease in the absence of supravalvular stenosis in a patient with Williams syndrome. *Pediatr Cardiol.* 2005;26:665–667.

18. Bonnet D, Cormier V, Villain E, Bonhoeffer P, Kachaner J. Progressive left main coronary artery obstruction leading to myocardial infarction in a child with Williams syndrome. *Eur J Pediatr.* 1997;156:751–753.

19. Geggel RL, Gauvreau K, Lock JE. Balloon dilation angioplasty of peripheral pulmonary stenosis associated with Williams syndrome. *Circulation.* 2001;103: 2165–2170.

20. Burch TM, McGowan FX Jr, Kussman BD, Powell AJ, DiNardo JA. Congenital supravalvular aortic stenosis and sudden death associated with anesthesia: what is the mystery? *Anesth Analg.* 2008;107:1848–1854.

21. Park JH, Kim HS, Yong Jin G, Joo CU, Ko JK: Demonstration of peripheral pulmonary stenosis and supravalvular aortic stenosis by different cardiac imaging modalities in a patient with Williams syndrome - usefulness of noninvasive imaging studies. Int J Cardiol 2007

22. Aboulhosn J, Child JS. Left ventricular outflow obstruction: subaortic stenosis, bicuspid aortic valve, supravalvar aortic stenosis, and coarctation of the aorta. *Circulation.* 2006;114:2412–2422.

23. Liberman L, Gersony WM, Flynn PA, Lamberti JJ, Cooper RS, Stare TJ. Effectiveness of prostaglandin E1 in relieving obstruction in coarctation of the aorta without opening the ductus arteriosus. *Pediatr Cardiol.* 2004;25:49–52.

24. Walhout RJ, Lekkerkerker JC, Oron GH, Hitchcock FJ, Meijboom EJ, Bennink GB. Comparison of polytetrafluoroethylene patch aortoplasty and end-to-end anastomosis for coarctation of the aorta. *J Thorac Cardiovasc Surg.* 2003;126:521–528.

25. Backer CL. Coarctation: the search for the Holy Grail. *J Thorac Cardiovasc Surg.* 2003;126:329–331.

26. Dodge-Khatami A, Backer CL, Mavroudis C. Risk factors for recoarctation and results of reoperation: a 40-year review. *J Card Surg.* 2000;15:369–377.

27. Zoghbi J, Serraf A, Mohammadi S, et al. Is surgical intervention still indicated in recurrent aortic arch obstruction? *J Thorac Cardiovasc Surg.* 2004;127: 203–212.

28. Carr JA, Amato JJ, Higgins RS. Long-term results of surgical coarctectomy in the adolescent and young adult with 18-year follow-up. *Ann Thorac Surg.* 2005;79:1950–1955. discussion 1955–6.

29. Hager A, Kanz S, Kaemmerer H, Schreiber C, Hess J. Coarctation long-term assessment (COALA): significance of arterial hypertension in a cohort of 404 patients up to 27 years after surgical repair of isolated coarctation of the aorta, even in the absence of restenosis and prosthetic material. *J Thorac Cardiovasc Surg.* 2007;134:738–745.

30. Duara R, Theodore S, Sarma PS, Unnikrishnan M, Neelakandhan KS. Correction of coarctation of aorta in adult patients–impact of corrective procedure on long-term recoarctation and systolic hypertension. *Thorac Cardiovasc Surg.* 2008;56:83–86.

31. Gudbjartsson T, Mathur M, Mihaljevic T, Aklog L, Byrne JG, Cohn LH. Hypothermic circulatory arrest for the surgical treatment of complicated adult coarctation of the aorta. *J Am Coll Cardiol.* 2003;41:849–851.

32. Carr JA. The results of catheter-based therapy compared with surgical repair of adult aortic coarctation. *J Am Coll Cardiol.* 2006;47:1101–1107.

33. Rosenthal E. Coarctation of the aorta from fetus to adult: curable condition or life long disease process? *Heart.* 2005;91:1495–1502.

34. Toro-Salazar OH, Steinberger J, Thomas W, Rocchini AP, Carpenter B, Moller JH. Long-term follow-up of patients after coarctation of the aorta repair. *Am J Cardiol.* 2002;89:541–547.

35. de Divitiis M, Pilla C, Kattenhorn M, et al. Ambulatory blood pressure, left ventricular mass, and conduit artery function late after successful repair of coarctation of the aorta. *J Am Coll Cardiol.* 2003;41: 2259–2265.

36. Hauser M, Kuehn A, Wilson N. Abnormal responses for blood pressure in children and adults with surgically corrected aortic coarctation. *Cardiol Young.* 2000;10:353–357.

37. Ou P, Celermajer DS, Jolivet O, et al. Increased central aortic stiffness and left ventricular mass in normotensive young subjects after successful coarctation repair. *Am Heart J.* 2008;155:187–193.

38. Seirafi PA, Warner KG, Geggel RL, Payne DD, Cleveland RJ. Repair of coarctation of the aorta during infancy minimizes the risk of late hypertension. *Ann Thorac Surg.* 1998;66:1378–1382.

39. O'Sullivan JJ, Derrick G, Darnell R. Prevalence of hypertension in children after early repair of coarctation of the aorta: a cohort study using casual and 24 hour blood pressure measurement. *Heart.* 2002;88: 163–166.

40. de Divitiis M, Pilla C, Kattenhorn M, et al. Vascular dysfunction after repair of coarctation of the aorta: impact of early surgery. *Circulation.* 2001;104: I165–I170.

41. Pfammatter JP, Berdat P, Carrel T. Impaired poststenotic aortic pulsatility after hemodynamically ideal coarctation repair in children. *Pediatr Cardiol.* 2004;25:495–499.

42. Murakami T, Takeda A. Enhanced aortic pressure wave reflection in patients after repair of aortic coarctation. *Ann Thorac Surg.* 2005;80:995–999.

43. Ou P, Celermajer DS, Mousseaux E, et al. Vascular remodeling after "successful" repair of coarctation: impact of aortic arch geometry. *J Am Coll Cardiol.* 2007;49:883–890.

44. Ou P, Celermajer DS, Raisky O, et al. Angular (Gothic) aortic arch leads to enhanced systolic wave reflection, central aortic stiffness, and increased left ventricular mass late after aortic coarctation repair: evaluation with magnetic resonance flow mapping. *J Thorac Cardiovasc Surg.* 2008;135:62–68.

45. Polson JW, McCallion N, Waki H, et al. Evidence for cardiovascular autonomic dysfunction in neonates with coarctation of the aorta. *Circulation.* 2006;113: 2844–2850.

46. Oliver JM, Gallego P, Gonzalez A, Aroca A, Bret M, Mesa JM. Risk factors for aortic complications in adults with coarctation of the aorta. *J Am Coll Cardiol.* 2004;44:1641–1647.

47. Humphrey C, Duncan K, Fletcher S. Decade of experience with vascular rings at a single institution. *Pediatrics.* 2006;117:e903–e908.

48. Kussman BD, Geva T, McGowan FX. Cardiovascular causes of airway compression. *Paediatr Anaesth.* 2004;14:60–74.

49. Dodge-Khatami A, Tulevski II, Hitchcock JF, de Mol BA, Bennink GB. Vascular rings and pulmonary arterial sling: from respiratory collapse to surgical cure, with emphasis on judicious imaging in the hi-tech era. *Cardiol Young.* 2002;12:96–104.

50. Hardin RE, Brevetti GR, Sanusi M, et al. Treatment of symptomatic vascular rings in the elderly. *Tex Heart Inst J.* 2005;32:411–415.

51. Hickey EJ, Khan A, Anderson D, Lang-Lazdunski L. Complete vascular ring presenting in adulthood: an unusual management dilemma. *J Thorac Cardiovasc Surg.* 2007;134:235–236.

52. Kafka H, Uebing A, Mohiaddin R. Adult presentation with vascular ring due to double aortic arch. *Congenit Heart Dis.* 2006;1:346–350.

53. Burke RP. Video-assisted endoscopy for congenital heart repair. *Semin Thorac Cardiovasc Surg Pediatr Card Surg Annu.* 2001;4:208–215.

54. van Son JA, Julsrud PR, Hagler DJ, et al. Surgical treatment of vascular rings: the Mayo clinic experience. *Mayo Clin Proc.* 1993;68:1056–1063.

55. Grillo HC, Wright CD. Tracheal compression with "hairpin" right aortic arch: management by aortic division and aortopexy by right thoracotomy guided by intraoperative bronchoscopy. *Ann Thorac Surg.* 2007;83:1152–1157.

56. Geva T, Keane JF, Mora BN, Burke RP, del Nido PJ. Video-assisted thoracoscopic vascular ring division in infants and children. *Heart Surg Forum.* 2002;5:S195.

57. Odegard KC, Kirse DJ, del Nido PJ, et al. Intraoperative recurrent laryngeal nerve monitoring during video-assisted throracoscopic surgery for patent ductus arteriosus. *J Cardiothorac Vasc Anesth.* 2000;14:562–564.

58. Pullerits J, Holzman R. Anaesthesia for patients with mediastinal masses. *Can J Anaesth.* 1989;36:681–688.

59. Roesler M, De Leval M, Chrispin A, Stark J. Surgical management of vascular ring. *Ann Surg.* 1983;197: 139–146.

60. Kronzon I, Tunick PA, Rosenzweig BP. Quantification of left-to-right shunt in patent ductus arteriosus with the PISA method. *J Am Soc Echocardiogr.* 2002;15: 376–378.

61. Toda R, Moriyama Y, Yamashita M, Iguro Y, Matsumoto H, Yotsumoto G. Operation for adult patent ductus arteriosus using cardiopulmonary bypass. *Ann Thorac Surg.* 2000;70:1935–1937.

62. Inaba H, Higuchi K, Koseni K, Osawa H, Kinoshita O. Surgical closure of adult patent ductus arteriosus using a pursestring suture. *Asian Cardiovasc Thorac Ann.* 2008;16:59–61.

63. Tekin Y, Ozer S, Murat B, Hulusi UM, Timucin ON. Closure of adult patent ductus arteriosus under cardiopulmonary bypass by using foley balloon catheter. *J Card Surg.* 2007;22:219–220.

64. Gurcun U, Boga M, Badak MI, Ozkisacik EA, Discigil B. Transpulmonary surgical closure of patent ductus arteriosus with hypothermic circulatory arrest in an adult patient. *Tex Heart Inst J.* 2005;32:88–90.

65. Wang JK, Wu MH, Hwang JJ, Chiang FT, Lin MT, Lue HC. Transcatheter closure of moderate to large patent ductus arteriosus with the Amplatzer duct occluder. *Catheter Cardiovasc Interv.* 2007;69: 572–578.

66. Ozmen J, Granger EK, Robinson D, White GH, Wilson M. Operation for adult patent ductus arteriosus using an aortic stent-graft technique. *Heart Lung Circ.* 2005;14:54–57.

67. Hokanson JS, Gimelli G, Bass JL. Percutaneous closure of a large PDA in a 35-year-old man with elevated pulmonary vascular resistance. *Congenit Heart Dis.* 2008;3:149–154.

68. Yan C, Zhao S, Jiang S, et al. Transcatheter closure of patent ductus arteriosus with severe pulmonary arterial hypertension in adults. *Heart.* 2007;93: 514–518.

69. Hazekamp MG, Kappetein AP, Schoof PH, et al. Brom's three-patch technique for repair of supravalvular aortic stenosis. *J Thorac Cardiovasc Surg.* 1999;118:252–258.

Atherosclerosis of the Aorta and Prevention of Neurological Dysfunction After Cardiac Surgery

18

Fellery de Lange, G. Burkhard Mackensen, and Madhav Swaminathan

Introduction

On May 6, 1953, John H Gibbon Jr., a Philadelphia surgeon, performed the world's first successful open heart procedure in which total heart–lung bypass was employed.[1] Since that time, aortic manipulation and postoperative neurological complications have coexisted. Aortic atherosclerosis remains a significant marker of coronary artery disease, perioperative vascular events, stroke, and even renal dysfunction. Although cardiac surgery is unique in that manipulation of the ascending aorta is almost routine, surgical handling of a diseased aorta is not always without risk.

The early days of valve replacement surgery were marked by frequent and severe cerebral complications. Fatal ischemic brain injury was observed in 9–14% of patients.[2-4] However, variations in methodology were responsible for large differences in the incidence of central nervous system (CNS) complications.[5] Prospective studies reported that postoperative CNS complications were common and manifest in over 60% of patients, whereas retrospective studies reported cerebral complications detectable in as little as 1–6% of patients.[6-9] Mechanisms contributing to those complications were thought to be mainly cerebral hypoperfusion as well as macro- and microembolizations of air, particulate matter, or aggregated blood elements.[5] However, despite advances in surgical and perfusion techniques, neurological complications after cardiac surgery remained a clinically relevant problem.

In 1996, halfway into what was later known as "the decade of the brain,"[10] Roach *et al.* published the results of a prospective observational study on adverse cerebral outcomes after coronary artery bypass surgery (CABG).[11] They reported a 6.1% incidence of adverse cerebral outcomes (coma, stroke, transient ischemic attacks – TIAs, seizures, or cognitive deficits). This study led to widespread recognition of a problem that had been described in similar settings since the early 1980s.[12,13] In the current era, these complications mainly present as deficits in memory and learning, and are often defined as postoperative neurocognitive deficits (POCD) that may exist in a large proportion of patients undergoing cardiac surgery.[14] The spectrum of neurological dysfunction after cardiac surgery therefore ranges from ischemic stroke to the more subtle POCD. Atherosclerotic disease of the aorta is considered one of the most important etiologic risk factors common to all types of neurological dysfunctions.

M. Swaminathan (✉)
Department of Anesthesiology, Duke University Medical Center, Durham, NC, USA
e-mail: swami001@mc.duke.edu

K. Subramaniam et al. (eds.), *Anesthesia and Perioperative Care for Aortic Surgery*,
DOI 10.1007/978-0-387-85922-4_18, © Springer Science+Business Media, LLC 2011

Neurological Dysfunction After Cardiac Surgery

Atherosclerotic disease of the aorta is strongly associated with neurological complications after cardiac surgery (Fig. 18.1). Both stroke and POCD can be devastating for the patient and their family, and have major implications for quality of life and hospital resource utilization. The relationship between aortic atheroma and stroke following cardiac surgery has been confirmed in several studies.[15–17] The location of atheroma in separate regions within the ascending aorta have also been evaluated in their association with stroke.[17] From a mechanistic viewpoint, the relationship is simple – atheroma may be detached from surgical manipulation for cannulation, cross-clamping and aorto-coronary anastomoses, and get redirected to the cerebral circulation where they cause ischemic complications. However, the relationship between aortic atherosclerosis and POCD is more complex.

The incidence of POCD after cardiac surgery varies between 20% and 80%, depending on the definition used, population studied, tests used to evaluate POCD, and the timing of the evaluation after surgery.[18] In a longitudinal study by the Neurological Outcomes Research Group at our institution, the incidence of POCD after CABG was found to be 53% at discharge, 36% at 6 weeks after operation, and 24% at 6 months.[18] Importantly, neurocognitive decline significantly reduced quality of life after surgery, which may have important social and financial implications, again highlighting the importance of preventing this complication.[19]

While the etiology of postoperative stroke has been established, the causative factors for POCD are less clearly defined. Some known risk factors for POCD after cardiac surgery include advanced age, lower level of education, apolipoprotein E4 genotype, atrial fibrillation, rate of rewarming after hypothermic cardiopulmonary bypass (CPB), and postoperative hyperthermia.[20] A major mechanism implicated in POCD after cardiac surgery is multiple brain microemboli, and a correlation exists between atherosclerotic aortic disease and the number of cerebral emboli detected by transcranial Doppler (TCD) (Fig. 18.2).[21] Some studies have reported a correlation between degree of aortic atheroma burden and incidence of POCD,[22] while others have not confirmed such an association.[23]

Several large studies have grouped adverse cerebral outcomes after cardiac surgery into type I (death to stroke or hypoxic encephalopathy, nonfatal stroke, TIA, or stupor or coma at time of discharge) or type II (decline in intellectual function, memory deficit, or seizures) outcomes. Roach *et al.* reported a 3.1% and 3.0% incidence of both

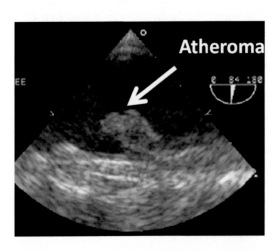

Fig. 18.1 Intraoperative transesophageal echocardiographic view of the descending aorta in long axis demonstrating a large intraluminal atheroma

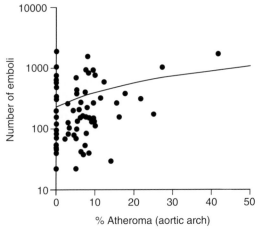

Fig. 18.2 Relationship between atheroma burden in the aortic arch and number of emboli detected by transcranial Doppler (Permission obtained from Mackensen et al.[21])

outcomes, respectively, after CABG surgery. In a study examining patients undergoing intracardiac procedures combined with CABG, Wolman found adverse cerebral outcomes in 16% of patients, being nearly equally divided between type I (8.4%) and type II outcomes (7.3%).[24] Their group also showed that resource utilization was significantly increased with this complication. Considering the large number of cardiac surgical procedures performed worldwide, the implications of these adverse events on healthcare stay and costs are significant. As an example, estimated costs for patients with stroke after CABG surgery exceed $2–4 billion annually worldwide.[11]

Several patient factors for neurological dysfunction have been identified over the years (Table 18.1). While some are more specific to type I outcomes (proximal aortic atherosclerosis, history of neurologic disease, age of 70 or more, history of hypertension, pulmonary disease, diabetes mellitus, and unstable angina), other risk factors are more common in type II complications (prior cardiac surgery, dysrhythmias, excessive alcohol consumption, history of peripheral vascular disease, pulmonary disease, age and hypertension).[11] In addition, Newman et al. identified older age, lower level of education, and evidence of cognitive decline at discharge as predictors of cognitive decline 5 years after CABG surgery.[18] A relatively recent development is the finding that certain genetic variations may increase susceptibility for cardiac surgery-associated

Table 18.1 Preoperative patient factors increasing the risk of postoperative neurologic dysfunction after cardiac surgery

Older age
Obesity
Advanced proximal aortic atherosclerosis with risk of cerebral embolism
Cerebrovascular disease
History of neurologic disease (stroke, transient ischemic attack, or depression)
Other systemic illnesses (Hypertension, diabetes, renal insufficiency, chronic pulmonary disease, coronary artery disease, peripheral vascular disease)
Hypercoagulability
Lower education level and lower baseline cognition
Presence of CRP1059G/SELP1087G polymorphisms

adverse cerebral outcomes. Mathew and colleagues have shown that certain platelet glycoprotein polymorphisms and P-selectin and C reactive protein variants predispose individuals to POCD after CABG surgery.[25,26]

In the following text, a select few factors proposed as primary causes of adverse cerebral outcomes will be briefly discussed. These are important, in that they may represent modifiable factors in our efforts to prevent neurological complications after cardiac surgery.

Microemboli

Microemboli are defined as emboli less than 200 μm in size. Microembolization of gas or particulate material into the cerebral circulation can result in focal ischemia with devastating effects. Particulate material mostly consists of aortic atheroma, thrombus, or other debris from the surgical area, released during aortic manipulation, for instance, during cannulation or cross-clamping.[27] During CPB, the pulmonary vascular bed that under normal conditions functions as a natural filter between the venous and arterial circulation, is removed. At the end of the 1980s, evidence accumulated that bubble oxygenators – compared to membrane oxygenators – produce large quantities of microbubbles that can be detected in cerebral and carotid arteries when compared to membrane oxygenators.[28,29] As a result, bubble oxygenators were slowly replaced by membrane oxygenators, and in modern cardiac surgery, these are now the standard of care. The change in oxygenator type is an excellent example of how research in neurological outcomes prompted a relevant change in clinical practice.

Cognitive decline after cardiac surgery has also been related to the cerebral microembolic load during CPB and the length of CPB and aortic cross-clamp times.[30,31] Katz and colleagues showed a relationship between the severity of protruding aortic arch atheroma and the incidence of stroke.[15] The severity of aortic atheromatous disease in the descending aorta as diagnosed by transesophageal echocardiography (TEE) has

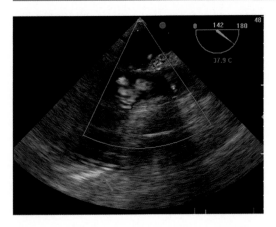

Fig. 18.3 Air in the left ventricular cavity during de-airing after open cardiac procedure in the mid-esophageal long axis view. Air can be seen as a bright echogenic mobile mass (*arrow*) with significant acoustic drop-out. The mass quickly dissipates into micro-bubbles that escape through the aortic valve and may be vented out or embolize into the cerebral circulation

also been shown to be a predictor for stroke in CABG surgery.[16] Even outside the setting of cardiac surgery, significant thoracic aortic plaques (>4 mm) are found to be an independent risk factor for ischemic stroke and patients suffering from a stroke may now routinely undergo TEE examinations to monitor the progress of their atheromatous disease.[32,33]

A postmortem study examining brains of patients who died shortly after surgery using CPB revealed small capillary arteriolar dilatations (SCADs). These SCADs occur in large numbers and are thought to be the result of microembolization of lipids.[34,35] Non particulate emboli are mostly gaseous in composition and are often introduced into the circulation during cannulation or insufficient de-airing after open-chamber procedures (Fig. 18.3).[36]

Hypoperfusion

Hypoperfusion, as a result of generalized hypotension, is also considered an important etiologic factor. Hypotension may also be associated with increased incidence of stroke, especially when it occurs in combination with severe atheromatous disease of the descending aorta.[16] Several studies

have identified prolonged hypotension as a risk factor for adverse cerebral outcomes.[11,37] In a randomized trial, Gold et al. showed that a higher MAP (80–100 mmHg) during bypass improves outcomes in long- and short-term follow-up when compared to low MAP (50–60 mmHg).[38]

Temperature Management

Animal studies have repeatedly demonstrated the beneficial effect of hypothermia in experimental cerebral ischemia.[39–41] However, in the clinical setting, its neuroprotective effects remain unclear. A large number of clinical trials have failed to demonstrate any benefits of hypothermia for the prevention of postoperative neurologic and neurocognitive deficits.[42–44] One possible explanation for the lack of difference in the various "hypothermia versus normothermia" studies is that all of the hypothermic patients eventually had to undergo rewarming. The rewarming process itself may have mitigated any benefit related to hypothermia by causing an "overshoot" in cerebral temperature during rewarming and relative cerebral hyperthermia.[45] During active rewarming, harmful cerebral hyperthermia might occur as the perfusate temperature often is 4–6°C higher than the nasopharyngeal temperature. While the impact of delayed rewarming (and thus hypothermia itself) on cognitive outcome from CPB has been demonstrated to provide benefit both experimentally as well as clinically,[46,47] this paradigm recently has been challenged. Boodhwani et al.[48] performed a randomized double-blind trial in 262 patients to examine the effects of sustained mild hypothermia (34°C) versus normothermia (37°C) on POCD after CABG surgery. This study found that mild intraoperative hypothermia did not decrease the incidence of neurocognitive deficits as measured 3 months postoperatively. This conclusion was supported by another report of a 5-year follow-up by Nathan et al. who found benefit from delayed rewarming as late as 3 months.[49] However, after 5 years, efforts to identify benefit were inconclusive.[50]

Collectively, these studies indicate an adverse effect from rapid rewarming and cerebral hyperthermia. Therefore, in light of experimental evidence showing that very small differences in temperature may significantly alter outcomes following cerebral ischemia, hyperthermia in the setting of cardiac surgery should be avoided.[51]

Inflammation

The conduct of CPB is associated with an enhanced systemic inflammatory response. Contact of blood components with the nonendothelialized artificial surfaces of the circuit, along with the reaction to tissue injury due to surgery itself, possible endotoxemia from the gut, and the inevitable ischemia-perfusion injury of heart and lungs all lead to activation of leukocytes, endothelial cells, and coagulation cascades. This leads to leukocyte extravasation, lipid peroxidation, cell death, and organ dysfunction.[52,53] However, evidence for this sequence of events in humans is indirect (measurement of cytokine levels) or extrapolated from animal studies. In a rat model of CPB, Hindman et al. showed that bypass induces upregulation of the proinflammatory cyclooxygenase-2 gene in the brain.[54] In rats, it was also shown that CPB *per se* induces apoptosis-related caspases in the brain,[55] but direct evidence of a relationship between inflammation and outcomes remains unclear.

Westaby et al. found no correlation between inflammation and neurologic outcomes in CABG patients.[56] Interestingly however, studies suggest that genetic variability associated with inflammatory pathways, like certain interleukin (IL-6) and C-reactive protein (CRP) polymorphisms, are significantly associated with postoperative stroke.[25,57] In more recent work, we have also identified single-nucleotide polymorphism of P-selectin and CRP genes that modulate susceptibility to cognitive decline after cardiac surgery. In 513 patients, logistic regression revealed that in addition to age, baseline cognition, and years of education, a CRP 1059 G/C SNP and an SELP (P-selectin) 1087 G/A SNP were significantly associated with postoperative cognitive decline.[25] Functionally, these CRP

and SELP SNPs were associated with reductions in serum CRP and platelet activation, respectively, suggesting that therapies aimed at reducing the perioperative inflammatory and prothrombotic state may be beneficial. In summary, these findings suggest that specific genes modulate the incidence and variability of cerebral injury after cardiac surgery.

Echocardiographic Assessment of Atheromatous Disease

The high risk of neurological dysfunction associated with aortic atherosclerosis is a compelling argument for routine atheroma screening of the thoracic aorta during cardiac surgery.[58] Practice guidelines published by the American College of Cardiology/American Heart Association/American Society of Echocardiography consider the use of TEE for cardiac surgery utilizing CPB a class IIA indication for the assessment of aortic atheroma.[59,60]

The anatomical proximity of the aorta with the esophagus makes TEE an ideal imaging modality for the thoracic aorta. Echocardiographic views must keep the relationship between the esophagus and the aorta in perspective at all times. Since the aorta and TEE probe are in proximity, high-resolution images can be acquired at an imaging depth of about 5–7 cm in most adult patients. This imaging depth also provides adequate spatial resolution to measure atheroma burden in the aorta. Detailed TEE examination of aorta is described in the chapter on echocardiography of aorta.

The thoracic aorta can be divided into six zones corresponding to potential manipulations during cardiac surgery. Zone 1 (proximal ascending) is the site of aortotomy for valve replacement. Zone 2 (mid ascending) is the site of proximal anastomosis of coronary grafts. Zone 3 (distal ascending) is the site of antegrade cardioplegia cannulation and aortic cross-clamping. Zone 4 (proximal arch) is the site of aortic cannulation. Zone 5 (distal arch) is not manipulated directly but can be affected by jet stream of CPB flow and prone for sand blasting effect of

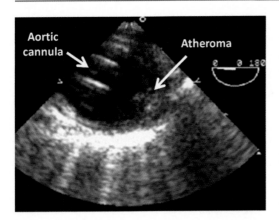

Fig. 18.4 Upper esophageal view of the junction of the distal aortic arch and descending aorta demonstrating the proximity of the aortic cannula to a large atheroma located on the opposite wall

atheromas from the aortic cannula tip (Fig. 18.4).[61] Zone 6 is the proximal descending aorta and is the position of correctly placed IABP. Zones 3 and 4, the sites of important manipulations during cardiac surgery, are difficult to visualize using TEE because of the so-called "blind-spot." At this level, the air-filled trachea and left main bronchus are interposed between the esophagus and the ascending aorta and therefore echocardiographic visualization with TEE becomes difficult.[62] A meta-analysis published in 2008 showed that conventional TEE is not sufficiently capable of adequately assessing the ascending aorta for clinically relevant atherosclerosis.[63] The low sensitivity of TEE (21%) implies that in case of a negative TEE result, further verification by additional testing using an alternate technique may be indicated.

Some of these alternate techniques include a novel saline-filled balloon catheter that replaces the air in the trachea, and epiaortic ultrasound imaging.

A-View Catheter

The newly introduced A-view catheter (Cordatec Inc., Zoersel, Belgium) uses a saline-filled balloon catheter to replace the air in the trachea to overcome the "blind spot of TEE."[64,65] The saline creates an ultrasound conducting medium through

which imaging of the distal ascending aorta is feasible. After several minutes of preoxygenation, the catheter is gently introduced through the endotracheal tube into the trachea and left main bronchus of the patient and filled with sterile saline. The A-view catheter exhibited good agreement when compared to epiaortic ultrasound (EAU) in detecting plaque presence, but performed poorly with regard to plaque-size measurements. This catheter might prove to be a quick and reliable technique to assess atheromatous disease when epiaortic scanning is unavailable (closed chest) or considered a risk (e.g., introduction of infection?) and may also prove to be very suitable in perioperative assessment of dissections. A prospective randomized trial that examines the usefulness of the A-view catheter to assess the severity of atheromatous disease of the ascending aorta as compared to regular epiaortic scanning and surgical palpation of the aorta is ongoing in the Netherlands (personal communication, Dr. A. Nierich).

Epiaortic Ultrasound

Although still not routinely applied in all settings, EAU has consistently been shown to be superior in localizing atheromatous disease when compared to direct surgical palpation. Marshall et al. showed that when digital palpation identified 24% of CABG patients with atherosclerotic disease in the ascending aorta, EAU identified 58% of the study population with atheromatous disease.[66] In a recent study, 12% of patients were determined to have atheromatous disease with digital palpation compared with 20% on TEE and 53% by EAU.[67] Palpation therefore seems to underestimate the presence of atherosclerotic disease in the ascending aorta, while EAU appears to currently be the best imaging modality for determining severity of atheromatous disease in the ascending aorta intraoperatively. Detailed description of the technique are provided in a recent ASE/SCA guidelines document that features intraoperative EAU (Fig. 18.5).[68]

The ASE/SCA guidelines for EAU recommend a minimum of five views, starting from the

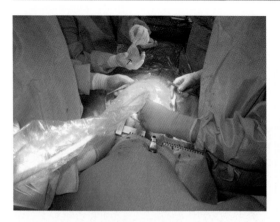

Fig. 18.5 Technique of epiaortic ultrasound examination of the ascending aorta. Picture shows the surgeon placing the epiaortic probe covered in the sterile sheath directly on the aorta. A saline standoff (*arrow*) can be placed between the aorta and the probe for the better visualization of the anterior wall of aorta. Anesthesiologist looks at the echocardiography machine screen and interprets the aortic pathology

sinotubular junction and extending up to the origin of the innominate artery and the aortic arch. Each of the proximal, mid and distal segments in short axis should be obtained along with a long axis image of the ascending aorta and a long axis view of the aortic arch including all three major vessels (Fig. 18.6a and 18.6b). It is imperative that all pertinent findings should be reported to the surgical team before manipulation of the aorta as this knowledge will enable the surgeon to optimize surgical technique for the individual patient and reduce the risk of stroke.

3D TEE

A relatively new development in ultrasound technology, real-time three-dimensional TEE (RT-3D-TEE), may provide more detailed information on the extent and location of atheromatous disease. It also allows for volumetric imaging of atherosclerotic plaque. While a live 3D slice is easier to obtain, a live 3D zoom image or a full volume loop allow offline volumetric assessment. The limitations of imaging the distal ascending aorta, however, remain with RT-3D-TEE. Some of these may be overcome with 3D epiaortic imaging. While real-time 3D ultrasound images can be

acquired using a 3D surface probe, these are subject to the same pros and cons as 2D epiaortic imaging. Another disadvantage could be the relatively lower imaging resolution when using a 4 MHz 3D probe compared to the superior resolution from the more typical 10–12 MHz 2D surface probes. Some authors have described the use of live 3D imaging for the identification and localization of plaque and correlating this with the proposed surgical entry sites. The full-volume mode was then used to evaluate the proposed sites completely and to ensure that no plaques were missed at those sites during the live 3D scanning.[69] A case series using RT-3D EAU showed that 3D was better in displaying diffusely dispersed plaques. Another advantage of 3D epiaortic scan might be the inclusion of discernable landmarks within the aorta like the AV to clarify the relative position of the plaque.[70] To our knowledge, no grading scale specific to 3D assessment of aortic atheroma has been described so far.

Grading of Atheroma

Several investigators have attempted to objectively define the risk of postoperative complications with aortic atheromatous disease. Grading systems have evolved to categorize atheromatous plaques based on physical appearance during perioperative ultrasound imaging.

The appearance of an atheroma primarily determines its prognostic value. An ideal grading system must take several factors into consideration. First, a smooth intimal surface poses less risk compared to irregular intimal thickening. Second, protruding atheromas carry a higher risk compared to simple intimal thickening. Third, atheromas with mobile elements have the highest risk and must receive special attention. Complex plaques with calcification and/or ulcerations also carry a higher risk of detachment and embolization. They may represent a more severe form of generalized atherosclerosis and are strongly associated with adverse outcome.

Location of the atheroma is another important consideration in determining the risk of adverse outcome. Investigators attempting to quantify

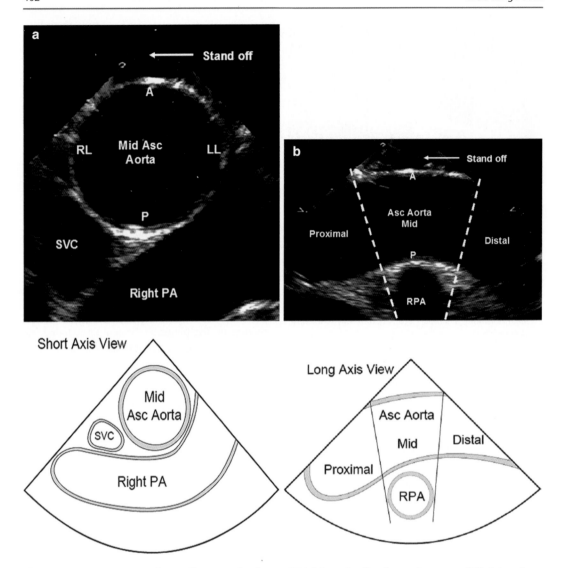

Fig. 18.6 Epiaortic image of ascending aorta in short axis (18.6a) and long axis (18.6b) obtained with phased array transducer. *A* anterior, *P* posterior, *RL* right lateral, *LL* left lateral walls of ascending aorta, *RPA* right pulmonary artery, *SVC* superior vena cava (Reprinted with permission from Glas et al.[68])

risk of aortic atheroma have done so using various techniques (epiaortic ultrasound, biplane TEE, grayscale density) in different locations (ascending, arch, and descending aorta). The alteration of surgical technique after detection of atheromatous disease also confounds risk assessment. However, if an atheroma of any grade greater than simple intimal thickening is detected in a manipulation zone by epiaortic ultrasound, a suitable alternate location is usually explored.

There is considerable variability between qualitative and quantitative interpretation of atheroma. There is no uniform definition of irregularity of surface, echocardiographic appearance of ulcerated plaques, calcified lesions, or grayscale intensity. Therefore, these features cannot be universally applied to a common grading protocol. For instance, grayscale intensity of an atheromatous lesion can be altered by the machine operator, while the distinction between a calcified plaque versus a densely fibrotic one may not be simple. On the other hand, size and mobility are objective criteria that are less subject to variability in interpretation.

Several grading protocols have been described (Table 18.2). These studies have used TEE in different patient populations and categorized atheromas in various locations in the thoracic aorta. They are common in that they have attempted to use atheroma grades to predict mortality, stroke, or other embolic phenomena.

Kronzon and associates introduced a widely used grading protocol in 1992.[15] They classified atheromas based on intraoperative TEE in any location in the aorta. They also correlated the grade or severity of atheroma with postoperative stroke. They found a highly significant association between mobile plaques and stroke and concluded that aortic manipulation during surgery played an important role in detachment of these mobile atheromas.

The French Study of Aortic Plaques in Stroke Group classified atherosclerotic plaques in the aorta based on the maximal size of plaque in the "far wall" of the image in 250 patients with history of stroke compared with 250 controls.[33] They did not separately classify plaques with a mobile element, but did find that plaques greater than 4 mm in thickness were strongly associated with cerebral infarction. Ferrari and colleagues adapted the grading system from the French group and classified mobile atheroma separately.[71] These investigators also found a strong association between mobile atheroma (referred to as aortic debris) and mortality or embolic events.

In an analysis of 104 of 3,661 patients undergoing CABG determined to have mobile aortic plaques on TEE examination, Trehan et al. reported one incident of postoperative stroke.[72] Significantly, surgical technique was modified when a mobile plaque was observed in order to reduce the risk of an adverse neurological outcome.

Almost all studies have reported a strong association between higher grades of atheroma and adverse outcome (Table 18.3). This association is particularly strong when the atheroma has a mobile element to it. Although mobile atheromas represent a severe form of atherosclerosis, other

versions of the same disease process may exist. These are termed as "complex" plaques with calcification, ulceration, or thrombosis. Each of these lesions also represents severe atherosclerotic disease that is associated with adverse neurological outcome.

A common feature of studies on aortic atheroma and outcome has been a universal admission of TEE being a poor modality for imaging the proximal-mid aortic arch. The anatomical interposition of an air-filled trachea between this portion of the aorta and the esophagus makes TEE imaging difficult. Another limitation of TEE is that by only using maximal height of an atheroma, the atheroma "burden" of more extensive plaques may be underestimated. Some investigators have attempted to overcome this limitation by using area of atheroma to represent total atheroma burden (Fig. 18.7).[21] This, however, is a continuous measure rather than a categorical one and cannot be extrapolated to currently used grading systems. In addition, area measurements of atheroma burden are made using specialized software and are usually analyzed "offline." This does not enable instantaneous decision-making in the operating room, and therefore is not typically used for preventive surgical strategies.

A systematic analysis of grading systems in published literature revealed nine unique categorical grading systems. Of these, two grading systems[15,73] were used in 17 studies involving 10,300 cardiac surgery patients from 1992 to 2005 (Table 18.3). The remaining grading systems were not validated by other investigators. Two distinct features were clear. Mobile atheromas confer the highest risk of adverse neurological outcome regardless of size. A comparison of outcomes between patients who have atheromas less than 5 mm and less than 3 mm is not feasible, since studies that grouped atheromas less than 5 mm also included cases with atheromas less than 3 mm.

The American Society of Echocardiography (ASE) and the Society of Cardiovascular Anesthesiologists (SCA) have published recommendations for atheroma grading as part of the guideline document on epiaortic ultrasound.[68]

Table 18.2 Grading protocols for aortic atheromatous disease

Reference	Grades	Description of grades	Population studied	Outcome
Katz et al.[15]	I	Normal to mild intimal thickening	Cardiac surgery (n=130)	Stroke
	II	Severe intimal thickening without protruding atheroma		
	III	Atheroma protruding <5 mm into lumen		
	IV	Atheroma protruding ≥5 mm into lumen		
	V	Any thickness with mobile component(s)		
Amarenco et al.[33]	I	<1 mm	Stroke (n=250) vs. Controls (n=250)	Stroke[a]
	II	1–1.9 mm		
	III	2–2.9 mm		
	IV	3–3.9 mm		
	V	≥4 mm		
Davila-Roman et al.[97]	None	No identifiable intimal thickening	CABG Surgery (n=44)	Agreement between two ultrasound techniques[b]
	Mild	<3.0 mm intimal thickening without irregularities		
	Moderate	≥3.0 mm intimal thickening with diffuse irregularities and/or calcification		
	Severe	>5.0 mm intimal thickening and one or more of – protruding debris or thrombus, calcification, or ulcerated plaque		
Acarturk et al.[98]	I	Smooth internal surface without lumen irregularities or increased echodensity	Coronary angiography (n=60)	Coronary artery disease severity
	II	Increased echodensity of intima without lumen irregularity or thickening		
	III	Increased echodensity of intima with well-defined atheroma <3 mm		
	IV	Atheroma ≥3 mm		
	V	Mobile atheroma		
Ferrari et al.[71]	I	Plaque with a thickness ranging from 1 to 3.9 mm	Patients referred for TEE exam (n=1,112)	Mortality, embolic events[c]
	II	Plaque of more than 4 mm in thickness		
	III	Any plaque, whatever its thickness, with an obvious mobile component (aortic debris)		
Blackshear et al.[99]	Simple	Sessile plaque <4.0 mm	Atrial fibrillation (n=786)	Descriptive study[d]
	Complex	Plaque ≥4.0 mm with ulceration, pedunculation, or mobile elements		
Trehan et al.[72]	I	Simple smooth-surfaced plaques, focal increase in echo density, and thickening of intima extending less than 5 mm into the aortic lumen	CABG Surgery (n=3,660)	Stroke, embolic events[e]
	II	Marked irregularity of intimal surface, focal increase in echo density, and thickening of adjoining intima with overlying shaggy echogenic material extending more than 5 mm into aortic lumen.		
	III	Plaques with a mobile element		

Nohara et al.[100]			CABG Surgery (n = 314)	Stroke, embolic events[f]
	I	Normal or thickening of the intima extending less than 3 mm into the aortic lumen		
	II	Smooth-surfaced plaques and thickening of the intima extending more than 3 mm into the aortic lumen.		
	III	Marked irregularity of the intimal surface and thickening of the intima extending more than 3 mm into the aortic lumen		
	IV	Plaque with a mobile element		

CABG coronary artery bypass graft surgery, *TEE* transesophageal echocardiography

[a] TEE findings in 250 patients admitted with stroke were compared to 250 controls

[b] Atheroma grade was compared between biplane TEE and epiaortic ultrasound in all patients studied

[c] Aortic atheromas were found and graded in 12% of the 1,112 patients referred for a TEE exam for several reasons including history of stroke. The grading system was adapted from the earlier study by Amarenco.[33]

[d] Stroke Prevention in Atrial Fibrillation (SPAF) III trial including 382 patients at high risk and 404 patients at low risk for stroke. All patients had atrial fibrillation

[e] From the population 3,660 CABG surgery patients, only those with mobile or grade 3 atheromas (104 or 2.8%) were included for outcome analysis

[f] Atheromas were studied in context of gray-scale echodensity rather than size alone

Table 18.3 Grades of aortic atheromatous disease and their relation to adverse outcomes after cardiac surgery

Reference grading system	Subsequent studies	Study summary	Study population	Total N
Katz et al.[15]	Katz[15]	5/130 patients had stroke; 3 with grade V, 1 with grade III, and 1 with grade I disease	N = 130	2,807
	Sharony,[101]	Grade IV/V disease had OPCAB vs. grade I-III disease had OPCAB; found decreased mortality and stroke prevalence	N = 281	
	Sharony[102]	Grade IV/V disease patients. OPCAB vs. CBP-CAB; found decreased hospital mortality, decreased stroke rate, and freedom from all complications and hospital death	N = 235	
	Ribakove[103]	Grade IV/V disease patients had increased incidence of stroke	N = 97	
	Barbut[104]	Mobile plaque present in 60% of patients who had a stroke	N = 84	
	Hartman[16]	Grade III-V disease was associated with stroke at 1-week post-op. Incidence of stroke according to atheroma severity; Grade III [2/39(5.5%)], Grade IV [2/19 (10.5%)], Grade V [5/11(45.5%)]. Atheroma grade also predicted the 6 month outcome of stroke and death	N = 189	
	Choudhary[105]	Grade V disease present in 2/126 patients who had a stroke	N = 126	
	Vogt[106]	Grade IV/V disease patients underwent complete thromboendarterctomy of ascending aorta and transverse arch under DHCA	N = 22	
	Grossi[107]	Grade IV/V disease, comparing OPCAB vs. CBP-CAB; decreased hospital mortality and stroke	N = 913	
	Gold[74]	Grade IV/V for OP-CAB vs. Grade I-III for CBP-CAB; no hospital or 30 day mortality in OP-CAB group	N = 500	
Davila-Roman et al.[97]	Bolotin[108]	Moderate–severe atheroma in ascending aorta warranted change in surgical technique (OPCAB). No stroke in OPCAB group vs. 5/80 in CBP-CAB group	N = 105	7,493
	Hogue[109]	Ascending atherosclerosis is independent risk factor for stroke (does not differentiate between grades)	N = 2,972	
	Davila-Roman[110]	1.5-fold increase in incidence of both neurological events and mortality as severity of atheroma increased from mild-moderate, and 3-fold increase of both as severity increased from normal-mild to severe	N = 1,957	
	Hangler[111]	Severe lesions stratified to "no touch" techniques; stroke rates demonstrated a potentially positive effect of operative strategies concerning stroke caused by aortic manipulation	N = 352	
	Wareing[112]	Modification of surgical technique based on Severe grade disease. No strokes in modified group (68/500). 5 strokes in patients with mild or no disease.	N = 500	
	Bonatti[113]	Severe disease with "beating heart" surgery. No perioperative strokes.	N = 407	
	Wareing[80]	Modification of surgical technique with Moderate to Severe disease. 8/231 had stroke compared to 11/969 in None-Mild disease	N = 1,200	
Royse et al.[114]	Royse[114]	Moderate and severe atheroma warranted change in surgical technique in 13/14 patients; no postoperative strokes in this group	N = 68	115
	Royse[75]	Avoidance of atheroma at by echocardiography versus manual palpation combined with Y Grafting. Late (57±2 days) neuropsychological decline less in epiaortic screening (3.8% vs. 38.1%)	N = 47	

Study	Reference	Findings	N	Total
Trehan et al.[115]	Trehan[115]	Grade II/III disease in proximal two thirds ascending aorta warranted surgical modification. Clear reduction in stroke risk in this group with surgical modification	N=6,138	10,590
	Trehan[72]	Mobile atheromas warranted surgical modification. No stroke in patients who had OPCAB: 0.96% in rest of group vs. remaining population (without mobile atheromas) of 0.4%	N=3,660	
	Trehan[116]	Grade II/III disease warranted surgical modification. No perioperative stroke in this group vs. 0.76% for overall group	N=792	
Nohara et al.[100]	N/A	Grade III–V lesions studied with gray-scale median (GSM) to measure plaque density. GSM <100 58.3% stroke rate vs. GSM >100 stroke rate of 3.6%	N=315	315
Nicolosi et al.[117]	N/A	Cumulative score for severity and location of atheromatous disease. Modifications of surgical technique for higher-grade scores in 18 patients, with one perioperative stroke vs. one perioperative stroke in rest of the group	N=89	89
van der Linden et al.[17]	N/A	Atheromatous disease >0.5 mm and/or calcification in ascending aorta. Stroke rate 8.7% for patients with above lesions vs. 1.8% without	N=921	921
Djaiani et al.[118]	N/A	Grade 1–3 disease (>2 mm or mobile), 8/50 had new ischemic brain lesions, all in this "high-risk" group	N=50	50
Kumral et al.[119]	N/A	Grade II/III disease (>1.5 mm with/without mobile component or calcification), increased the risk of perioperative stroke and higher incidence of microembolic signals	N=69	69
				15,404

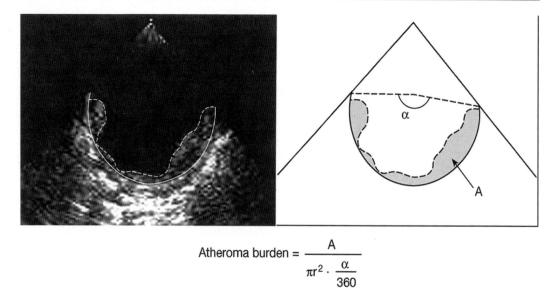

$$\text{Atheroma burden} = \frac{A}{\pi r^2 \cdot \dfrac{\alpha}{360}}$$

Fig. 18.7 Atheroma burden estimation using the technique described by Mackensen et al. (Permission obtained from Mackensen et al.[21])

Strategies for Preventing Neurological Dysfunction

Multiple strategies exist that can be utilized to minimize embolization of atheromatous material liberated from the aortic wall to the cerebral circulation. As outlined above, the use of TEE and epiaortic scanning facilitates a "knowledgeable avoidance" of the atheromatous ascending aorta with respect to cannulation, clamping, and anastomosis placement.[74–76] Optimal placement of the aortic cannula in an area relatively devoid of plaque,[61,75] and the use of specialized cannulae with optimal hydrodynamics and less "sandblasting" effects can also be considered to decrease embolization of the plaque.[77] Cannulation of the axillary artery for patients with extensive aortic plaque may also be beneficial and is used by many centers as an alternative approach.[78] Without question, patients with severe atheromatous burden in the aortic arch are at highest risk for the development of perioperative stroke. However, endarterectomy of the aortic arch does not appear to be a suitable approach to prevent embolization of atheromatous material during surgery in these patients. In fact,

the opposite is the case as it has been shown to increase the risk of serious embolization significantly. In a subgroup of 43 patients that were part of a larger study of cardiac surgery patients with severe aortic arch plaque, aortic arch endarterectomy was performed to prevent perioperative stroke. Of note, the stroke rate was nearly three times higher (34.9%) if an endarterectomy was done just before the onset of cardiac surgery than if an endarterectomy was not performed.[79] Manipulation of the diseased aorta may have resulted in embolization of debris or the disruption of the intimal surface may have resulted in formation of new thrombus that subsequently became dislodged. Ascending aortic replacement has also been reported in patients with moderate to severe plaque in the ascending aorta without postoperative stroke.[80] The conflicting data and the lack of a large randomized trial comparing these rather aggressive interventions with a standard approach indicate more conservative alterations of the surgical technique. These include the change of the aortic cannulation site, the use of an axillary or femoral cannulation site, or the conduct of single aortic cross-clamping fibrillatory arrest. Other strategies to reduce manipulation of the

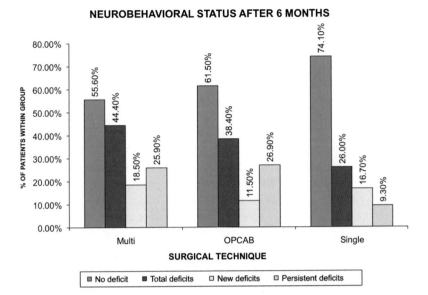

Fig. 18.8 Neurobehavioral status at 6 months. $p=0.179$ by Fisher's exact test. Neuropsychological deficits in all three groups up to 6 months. At 6 weeks and 6 months, patients assigned to the single clamp technique had a significantly lower incidence of neurocognitive deficits than those treated with multiple clamp technique. Patients undergoing off-pump surgery were not different from those with reduced aortic manipulation suggesting that the surgical technique may indeed play a primary role. Multi = multiple aortic cross-clamp; *OPCAB* = off-pump coronary artery bypass grafting; Single = single aortic cross-clamp (Reproduced with permission from Hammon et al.[82])

diseased aorta include the use of all arterial grafts such as internal mammary arteries, single aortic cross-clamping, or off-pump cardiac surgery with the use of an aortic side-clamp only.[81] Using a single aortic cross-clamp application, Hammon et al. have demonstrated that minimizing manipulation of the ascending aorta can significantly reduce postoperative cognitive loss (Fig. 18.8).[82]

Specialized cannulae that contain filtering technologies have been developed and while they have been shown to be safe and effective with an emboli capture rate of up to 97%, a multicenter randomized trial showed no difference in stroke, transient ischemic attack, or mortality rates in the filtered versus the nonfiltered group.

Although it may seem reasonable to assume that the elimination of CPB with off-pump coronary bypass surgery (OPCAB) would reduce some of the cerebral injury associated with aortic atherosclerosis, other mechanisms of cerebral injury remain and cognitive dysfunction is well documented in OPCAB patients.[83] In fact, a randomized controlled trial of off-pump versus on-pump cardiac surgery reported an incidence of 30.8% of cognitive decline at 12 months in the off-pump group.[83,84] The reason for this may be explained by the complex underlying pathophysiology. OPCAB, with its continued use of sternotomy, heparin administration, and wide hemodynamic swings activates the inflammatory processes that play a role in mediating cardiac surgery-related cerebral injury.[85] Traditional embolic theories are also still valid, as ascending aortic manipulation with the resultant particulate embolization is still commonly used. In addition, hemodynamic compromise due to manipulation of the heart has been associated with significant jugular venous desaturation,[86] which in turn is associated with cognitive decline.[87]

With a recent meta-analysis concluding that graft patency in OPCAB is inferior to that in on-pump CPB,[88] there is increasing interest in determining the effect of OPCAB on neurological outcome. The largest trial to date comparing OPCAB to conventional on-pump CABG surgery failed to show a difference in stroke rate or neurocognitive outcome in low-risk patients at 1 year and 5 years after surgery.[83,84] Al-Ruzzeh et al. re-examined the potential benefit of OPCAB in a more recent study ($n = 168$) that better controlled for some of the aortic manipulative limitations.[89] They demonstrated better neurocognitive function in the OPCAB group at both 6 weeks and 6 months postoperatively, without any compromise in coronary angiographic outcome in the OPCAB group. A meta-analysis performed by Wijeysundera et al. assessed the effects of OPCAB surgery on mortality and morbidity, and included 37 randomized controlled trials and 22 risk-adjusted observational studies. While observational studies showed OPCAB to be associated with a reduced stroke rate (OR 0.62; 95% CI 0.55–0.69), the randomized controlled trials did not show a statistically significant reduction (OR 0.52; 95% CI 0.25–1.05).[90] Results of further prospective studies will not only help to clarify whether OPCAB procedures will lower neurological complications, but also in which patient population this procedure should be optimally targeted. Are high-risk neurologic patients the best choice for OPCAB, where a compromise of potentially incomplete adequate revascularization may be made in order to prevent debilitating stroke? Or should we perform OPCAB procedures predominantly in younger patients, in whom the risk of neurological complications is lower, but who would gain from the longer graft patency from conventional CABG?

As outlined above, there are multiple sources of emboli, both particulate and gaseous, during the normal conduct of CPB. The CPB circuit itself contributes to this load through the generation of particulate emboli in the form of platelet–fibrin aggregates and other debris produced within the circuit. Shed blood that is returned to the venous reservoir from the surgical field via cardiotomy suction has been identified as a major contributing factor as it adds to the embolic load by increasing thrombin and platelet activation,[91] levels of lipid microparticles, as well as other cellular debris.[34,92] Due to its small size and deformability, most of this material will unfortunately pass through standard arterial line filters. Despite evidence that leukocyte-depleting filters may reduce cerebral microemboli during CPB based on transcranial Doppler measurements, this resulted only in a trend toward improved neuropsychological outcome in the filtered group.[93] There is also

evidence that lipid microparticles may embolize into the cerebral circulation as they can be found in cerebral vasculature after cardiac surgery.[94] Two recent prospective randomized double-blind trials investigated the effect of blood processing via a cell-saver system as opposed to cardiotomy suction on cognitive outcome after cardiac surgery. Rubens et al. who included 264 patients undergoing CABG and/or aortic valve surgery reported no clinical evidence of a beneficial effect on postoperative cognition.[95] In the second trial that also compared the use of cell-saver with cardiotomy suction (defined as control), processing shed blood resulted in a significant reduction in postoperative neurocognitive dysfunction after CABG surgery in the elderly.[96] Importantly, there were significant differences in the study design of these two trials that may have contributed to the conflicting results. Among others, these include differences in the definition of cognitive decline and the use of two very different cell-saver systems with uniquely diverse processing capabilities. Further, both trials demonstrated an increase in bleeding and transfusion, a risk that may outweigh any potential benefit of this technique and may be due to a reduction of both platelet and coagulation factors.

Neurological Dysfunction After Aortic Surgery

Patients undergoing aortic surgery are at a higher risk for the development of postoperative neurologic dysfunction than any other cardiac surgery. Manipulation of the diseased aorta, which is unavoidable in these patients, and the use of hypothermic circulatory arrest predispose them to the higher incidence of stroke and POCD. Risk is highest with aortic arch surgery (up to 30%), but neurological deficits are not uncommon following ascending aortic (1.8–5.9%), descending thoracic aortic (6%), and endovascular aortic surgery (2.3–8.7%). In addition to preoperative patient factors (Table 18.1), numerous perioperative risk factors have been identified (Table 18.4). Neurological complications after aortic surgery may range from transient reversible dysfunction (delirium, confusion, agitation, lethargy) to serious permanent

Table 18.4 Perioperative risk factors for postoperative neurological dysfunction after aortic surgery

Intraoperative	Postoperative
Surgery involving aortic arch	Reduced oxygen delivery (cardiac failure, respiratory failure, and multiorgan failure)
Urgent and emergency surgery (dissections and ruptured aneurysms)	Hemodynamic instability
Complex and prolonged repairs (prolonged bypass and cross-clamp time)	Hyperthermia
Blood loss and hemodynamic instability (hypotension)	Hyperglycemia
Long circulatory arrest time with inadequate cerebral perfusion	Atrial fibrillation
Hyperglycemia	
Rapid rewarming	

deficits. Permanent dysfunction can be focal (stroke) or global (extended encephalopathy, coma, psychosis, parkinsonism, and gait disturbances). In addition, patients who developed transient dysfunction are more prone for persistent long-term cognitive dysfunction. While it is well known that prolonged circulatory arrest time is a major risk factor for neurological dysfunction, the impact of antegrade and retrograde cerebral perfusion in preventing the stroke and cognitive dysfunction is not clear. Antegrade cerebral perfusion should be considered, when the circulatory arrest time is more than 30 min based on the evidence from the available literature. However, there is a clear need for future research on strategies to improve neurological outcomes after aortic surgery.

Key Notes

1. Neurological injury after any cardiac surgery can be of two types: Type 1 injury is caused by macroembolization leading to cerebral infarction and stroke. Type 2 injury or transient neurologic dysfunction is multifactorial. While several risk factors have been identified as important "players" in the etiology of neurological injury, it is clear that micro and macroembolization from atherosclerosis of the aorta represents the most important risk factor that is strongly associated with adverse neurological outcomes after cardiac surgery including aortic surgery.

2. Initial neuronal damage caused by ischemia/hypoperfusion (atheroembolization, hypotension, rapid rewarming, prolonged hypothermic circulatory arrest, etc.) initiates cascade of events leading to ischemic reperfusion injury. Neurotransmitters (e.g., glutamate), apoptosis, calcium, oxygen free radicals, nitric oxide, and inflammatory mediators are involved in ischemia reperfusion injury. While experimental studies on pharmacologic agents are targeted at these mechanisms to reduce neuronal injury, no such drug with proven efficacy is available for clinical use. Therefore, prevention of ischemic injury should be given priority. Efforts must be made to diagnose atheromatous aortic disease, and apply strategies to prevent embolization. In addition, adequate perfusion pressure and oxygen delivery should be ensured to prevent neurological compromise.

3. Evaluation for atherosclerotic disease of aorta and its branches should include palpation of pulses, blood pressure measurement in both arms, duplex ultrasonography of carotid and subclavian vessels, and chest roentgenography (calcifications). Preoperative computerized tomographic angiography (CTA), magnetic resonance imaging (MRA), transthoracic echocardiography, and aortography, if available, should be reviewed for possible atheromatous aortic disease.

4. Intraoperatively, TEE is used to evaluate the extent and severity of atheromatous disease. TEE evaluation of the distal ascending aorta is difficult because air-filled trachea and left main bronchus are interposed between the esophagus and the distal ascending aorta. A-view catheter and the epiaortic ultrasound can be utilized to define atheromas at distal ascending aorta and proximal arch. Epiaortic scanning is superior to surgical palpation of the aorta in localizing atheromatous aortic disease.

5. Several grading systems exist to define the echocardiographic severity of atheromatous disease. Higher-grade atheromas with mobile elements are associated with adverse neurological events.

6. The use of TEE and epiaortic scanning facilitates a "knowledgeable avoidance" of the atheromatous aorta during cardiac surgical procedure. Such modifications of the surgical procedure include the use of alternate cannulation sites (axillary), single clamp technique, off pump internal mammary arterial grafts only, off pump with side clamp only, the use of special cannulae with emboli-filtering technologies, and replacement of aorta in case of severe calcific atheromatous aortic disease.

7. Neurological dysfunction after aortic surgery is associated with increased hospital mortality and morbidity, increased length of intensive care unit and hospital stay, and poor quality of life in discharged patients. While there is a need for more evidence-based guidelines, a multimodal strategy utilizing hypothermia, cerebral perfusion, cerebral monitoring, and pharmacologic agents should be adapted to reduce the incidence of neurologic deficits after aortic surgery.

References

1. DeBakey ME. John Gibbon and the heart-lung machine: a personal encounter and his import for cardiovascular surgery. *Ann Thorac Surg.* 2003;76: S2188–2194.
2. Gilman S. Cerebral disorders after open-heart operations. *N Engl J Med.* 1965;272:489–498.
3. Javid H, Tufo HM, Najafi H, Dye WS, Hunter JA, Julian OC. Neurological abnormalities following open-heart surgery. *J Thorac Cardiovasc Surg.* 1969; 58:502–509.
4. Tufo HM, Ostfeld AM, Shekelle R. Central nervous system dysfunction following open-heart surgery. *J Am Med Assoc.* 1970;212:1333–1340.
5. Sotaniemi KA. Prevalence and causes of cerebral complications in cardiac surgery. In: Willner AE, ed. *Cerebral Damage Before and After Cardiac Surgery.* Dordrecht: Kluwer Academic Publishers; 1993:37–46.
6. Branthwaite MA. Prevention of neurological damage during open-heart surgery. *Thorax.* 1975;30:258–261.
7. Coffey CE, Massey EW, Roberts KB, Curtis S, Jones RH, Pryor DB. Natural history of cerebral complications of coronary artery bypass graft surgery. *Neurology.* 1983;33:1416–1421.
8. Shaw PJ, Bates D, Cartlidge NE, et al. Neurologic and neuropsychological morbidity following major surgery: comparison of coronary artery bypass and peripheral vascular surgery. *Stroke.* 1987;18:700–707.
9. Sotaniemi KA, Mononen H, Hokkanen TE. Long-term cerebral outcome after open-heart surgery. A five-year neuropsychological follow-up study. *Stroke.* 1986;17:410–416.
10. Hindman BJ, Todd MM. Improving neurologic outcome after cardiac surgery. *Anesthesiology.* 1999;90:1243–1247.
11. Roach GW, Kanchuger M, Mangano CM, et al. Adverse cerebral outcomes after coronary bypass surgery. Multicenter study of perioperative Ischemia research group and the Ischemia research and education foundation investigators. *N Engl J Med.* 1996;335:1857–1863.
12. Breuer AC, Furlan AJ, Hanson MR, et al. Central nervous system complications of coronary artery bypass graft surgery: prospective analysis of 421 patients. *Stroke.* 1983;14:682–687.
13. Sotaniemi KA. Cerebral outcome after extracorporeal circulation. Comparison between prospective and retrospective evaluations. *Arch Neurol.* 1983;40:75–77.
14. van Dijk D, Keizer AM, Diephuis JC, Durand C, Vos LJ, Hijman R. Neurocognitive dysfunction after coronary artery bypass surgery: a systematic review. *J Thorac Cardiovasc Surg.* 2000;120:632–639.
15. Katz ES, Tunick PA, Rusinek H, Ribakove G, Spencer FC, Kronzon I. Protruding aortic atheromas predict stroke in elderly patients undergoing cardiopulmonary bypass: experience with intraoperative transesophageal echocardiography. *J Am Coll Cardiol.* 1992;20:70–77.
16. Hartman GS, Yao FS, Bruefach M 3rd, et al. Severity of aortic atheromatous disease diagnosed by transesophageal echocardiography predicts stroke and other outcomes associated with coronary artery surgery: a prospective study. *Anesth Analg.* 1996;83:701–708.
17. van der Linden J, Hadjinikolaou L, Bergman P, Lindblom D. Postoperative stroke in cardiac surgery is related to the location and extent of atherosclerotic disease in the ascending aorta. *J Am Coll Cardiol.* 2001;38:131–135.
18. Newman MF, Kirchner JL, Phillips-Bute B, et al. Longitudinal assessment of neurocognitive function after coronary-artery bypass surgery. *N Engl J Med.* 2001;344:395–402.
19. Newman MF, Grocott HP, Mathew JP, et al. Report of the substudy assessing the impact of neurocognitive function on quality of life 5 years after cardiac surgery. *Stroke.* 2001;32:2874–2881.
20. Stanley TO, Mackensen GB, Grocott HP, et al. The impact of postoperative atrial fibrillation on neurocognitive outcome after coronary artery bypass graft surgery. *Anesth Analg.* 2002;94:290–295.
21. Mackensen GB, Ti LK, Phillips-Bute BG, Mathew JP, Newman MF, Grocott HP. Cerebral embolization

during cardiac surgery: impact of aortic atheroma burden. *Br J Anaesth*. 2003;91:656–661.
22. Goto T, Baba T, Yoshitake A, Shibata Y, Ura M, Sakata R. Craniocervical and aortic atherosclerosis as neurologic risk factors in coronary surgery. *Ann Thorac Surg*. 2000;69:834–840.
23. Bar-Yosef S, Anders M, Mackensen GB, et al. Aortic atheroma burden and cognitive dysfunction after coronary artery bypass graft surgery. *Ann Thorac Surg*. 2004;78:1556–1562. discussion 1562–1553.
24. Wolman RL, Nussmeier NA, Aggarwal A, et al. Cerebral injury after cardiac surgery: identification of a group at extraordinary risk. Multicenter study of perioperative Ischemia research group (McSPI) and the Ischemia research education foundation (IREF) investigators. *Stroke*. 1999;30:514–522.
25. Mathew JP, Podgoreanu MV, Grocott HP, et al. Genetic variants in P-selectin and C-reactive protein influence susceptibility to cognitive decline after cardiac surgery. *J Am Coll Cardiol*. 2007;49:1934–1942.
26. Mathew JP, Rinder CS, Howe JG, et al. Platelet PlA2 polymorphism enhances risk of neurocognitive decline after cardiopulmonary bypass. Multicenter study of perioperative Ischemia (McSPI) research group. *Ann Thorac Surg*. 2001;71:663–666.
27. Mullges W, Franke D, Reents W, Babin-Ebell J. Brain microembolic counts during extracorporeal circulation depend on aortic cannula position. *Ultrasound Med Biol*. 2001;27:933–936.
28. Blauth C, Smith P, Newman S, et al. Retinal microembolism and neuropsychological deficit following clinical cardiopulmonary bypass: comparison of a membrane and a bubble oxygenator. A preliminary communication. *Eur J Cardiothorac Surg*. 1989;3:135–138.
29. Deverall PB, Padayachee TS, Parsons S, Theobold R, Battistessa SA. Ultrasound detection of micro-emboli in the middle cerebral artery during cardiopulmonary bypass surgery. *Eur J Cardiothorac Surg*. 1988;2:256–260.
30. Brown WR, Moody DM, Challa VR, Stump DA, Hammon JW. Longer duration of cardiopulmonary bypass is associated with greater numbers of cerebral microemboli. *Stroke*. 2000;31:707–713.
31. Pugsley W, Klinger L, Paschalis C, Treasure T, Harrison M, Newman S. The impact of microemboli during cardiopulmonary bypass on neuropsychological functioning. *Stroke*. 1994;25:1393–1399.
32. Davila-Roman VG, Murphy SF, Nickerson NJ, Kouchoukos NT, Schechtman KB, Barzilai B. Atherosclerosis of the ascending aorta is an independent predictor of long-term neurologic events and mortality. *J Am Coll Cardiol*. 1999;33:1308–1316.
33. Amarenco P, Cohen A, Tzourio C, et al. Atherosclerotic disease of the aortic arch and the risk of ischemic stroke. *N Engl J Med*. 1994;331:1474–1479.
34. Brooker RF, Brown WR, Moody DM, et al. Cardiotomy suction: a major source of brain lipid emboli during cardiopulmonary bypass. *Ann Thorac Surg*. 1998;65:1651–1655.
35. Moody DM, Brown WR, Challa VR, Stump DA, Reboussin DM, Legault C. Brain microemboli associated with cardiopulmonary bypass: a histologic and magnetic resonance imaging study. *Ann Thorac Surg*. 1995;59:1304–1307.
36. Taylor RL, Borger MA, Weisel RD, Fedorko L, Feindel CM. Cerebral microemboli during cardiopulmonary bypass: increased emboli during perfusionist interventions. *Ann Thorac Surg*. 1999;68:89–93.
37. Selim M. Perioperative stroke. *N Engl J Med*. 2007;356:706–713.
38. Gold JP, Charlson ME, Williams-Russo P, et al. Improvement of outcomes after coronary artery bypass. A randomized trial comparing intraoperative high versus low mean arterial pressure. *J Thorac Cardiovasc Surg*. 1995;110:1302–1311.
39. Barone FC, Feuerstein GZ, White RF. Brain cooling during transient focal ischemia provides complete neuroprotection. *Neurosci Biobehav Rev*. 1997;21:31–44.
40. Busto R, Dietrich WD, Globus MY, Scheinberg P, Ginsberg MD. Small differences in intraischemic brain temperature critically determine the extent of ischemic neuronal injury. *J Cereb Blood Flow Metab*. 1987;7:729–738.
41. Minamisawa H, Nordstrom CH, Smith ML, Siesjo BK. The influence of mild body and brain hypothermia on ischemic brain damage. *J Cereb Blood Flow Metab*. 1990;10:365–374.
42. Randomised trial of normothermic versus hypothermic coronary bypass surgery. The warm heart investigators. *Lancet*. 1994;343:559–563.
43. Grigore AM, Mathew J, Grocott HP, et al. Prospective randomized trial of normothermic versus hypothermic cardiopulmonary bypass on cognitive function after coronary artery bypass graft surgery. *Anesthesiology*. 2001;95:1110–1119.
44. McLean RF, Wong BI, Naylor CD, et al. Cardiopulmonary bypass, temperature, and central nervous system dysfunction. *Circulation*. 1994;90:II250–255.
45. Grocott HP, Mackensen GB, Grigore AM, et al. Postoperative hyperthermia is associated with cognitive dysfunction after coronary artery bypass graft surgery. *Stroke*. 2002;33:537–541.
46. de Lange F, Yoshitani K, Proia AD, Mackensen GB, Grocott HP. Perfluorocarbon administration during cardiopulmonary bypass in rats: an inflammatory link to adverse outcome? *Anesth Analg*. 2008;106:24–31.
47. Grigore AM, Grocott HP, Mathew JP, et al. The rewarming rate and increased peak temperature alter neurocognitive outcome after cardiac surgery. *Anesth Analg*. 2002;94:4–10.
48. Boodhwani M, Rubens F, Wozny D, Rodriguez R, Nathan HJ. Effects of sustained mild hypothermia on neurocognitive function after coronary artery bypass surgery: a randomized, double-blind study. *J Thorac Cardiovasc Surg*. 2007;134:1443–1450.
49. Nathan HJ, Wells GA, Munson JL, Wozny D. Neuroprotective effect of mild hypothermia in patients undergoing coronary artery surgery with cardiopulmonary bypass: a randomized trial. *Circulation*. 2001;104(12 Suppl 1):I85–91.

50. Nathan HJ, Rodriguez R, Wozny D, et al. Neuroprotective effect of mild hypothermia in patients undergoing coronary artery surgery with cardiopulmonary bypass: five-year follow-up of a randomized trial. *J Thorac Cardiovasc Surg.* 2007;133:1206–1211.

51. Warner DS, McFarlane C, Todd MM, Ludwig P, McAllister AM. Sevoflurane and halothane reduce focal ischemic brain damage in the rat. Possible influence on thermoregulation. *Anesthesiology.* 1993;79:985–992.

52. Hall RI, Smith MS, Rocker G. The systemic inflammatory response to cardiopulmonary bypass: pathophysiological, therapeutic, and pharmacological considerations. *Anesth Analg.* 1997;85:766–782.

53. Paparella D, Yau TM, Young E. Cardiopulmonary bypass induced inflammation: pathophysiology and treatment. An update. *Eur J Cardiothorac Surg.* 2002;21:232–244.

54. Hindman BJ, Moore SA, Cutkomp J, et al. Brain expression of inducible cyclooxygenase 2 messenger RNA in rats undergoing cardiopulmonary bypass. *Anesthesiology.* 2001;95:1380–1388.

55. Sato Y, Laskowitz DT, Bennett ER, Newman MF, Warner DS, Grocott HP. Differential cerebral gene expression during cardiopulmonary bypass in the rat: evidence for apoptosis? *Anesth Analg.* 2002;94:1389–1394.

56. Westaby S. Organ dysfunction after cardiopulmonary bypass. A systemic inflammatory reaction initiated by the extracorporeal circuit. *Intensive Care Med.* 1987;13:89–95.

57. Grocott HP, Newman MF, El-Moalem H, Bainbridge D, Butler A, Laskowitz DT. Apolipoprotein E genotype differentially influences the proinflammatory and anti-inflammatory response to cardiopulmonary bypass. *J Thorac Cardiovasc Surg.* 2001;122:622–623.

58. Whitley WS, Glas KE. An argument for routine ultrasound screening of the thoracic aorta in the cardiac surgery population. *Semin Cardiothorac Vasc Anesth.* 2008;12:290–297.

59. Cheitlin MD, Armstrong WF, Aurigemma GP, et al. ACC/AHA/ASE 2003 guideline update for the clinical application of echocardiography: summary article: a report of the American college of cardiology/American heart association task force on practice guidelines (ACC/AHA/ASE committee to update the 1997 guidelines for the clinical application of echocardiography). *Circulation.* 2003;108:1146–1162.

60. Shanewise JS, Cheung AT, Aronson S, et al. ASE/SCA guidelines for performing a comprehensive intraoperative multiplane transesophageal echocardiography examination: recommendations of the American society of echocardiography council for intraoperative echocardiography and the society of cardiovascular anesthesiologists task force for certification in perioperative transesophageal echocardiography. *Anesth Analg.* 1999;89:870–884.

61. Swaminathan M, Grocott HP, Mackensen GB, Podgoreanu MV, Glower DD, Mathew JP. The "sandblasting" effect of aortic cannula on arch atheroma

during cardiopulmonary bypass. *Anesth Analg.* 2007;104:1350–1351.

62. Konstadt SN, Reich DL, Quintana C, Levy M. The ascending aorta: how much does transesophageal echocardiography see? *Anesth Analg.* 1994;78:240–244.

63. Van Zaane B, Zuithoff NP, Reitsma JB, Bax L, Nierich AP, Moons KG. Meta-analysis of the diagnostic accuracy of transesophageal echocardiography for assessment of atherosclerosis in the ascending aorta in patients undergoing cardiac surgery. *Acta Anaesthesiol Scand.* 2008;52:1179–1187.

64. Nierich AP, van Zaane B, Buhre WF, Coddens J, Spanjersberg AJ, Moons KG. Visualization of the distal ascending aorta with A-Mode transesophageal echocardiography. *J Cardiothorac Vasc Anesth.* 2008; 22:766–773.

65. Van Zaane B, Nierich AP, Buhre WF, Brandon Bravo Bruinsma GJ, Moons KG. Resolving the blind spot of transoesophageal echocardiography: a new diagnostic device for visualizing the ascending aorta in cardiac surgery. *Br J Anaesth.* 2007;98:434–441.

66. Marshall WG Jr, Barzilai B, Kouchoukos NT, Saffitz J. Intraoperative ultrasonic imaging of the ascending aorta. *Ann Thorac Surg.* 1989;48:339–344.

67. Suvarna S, Smith A, Stygall J, et al. An intraoperative assessment of the ascending aorta: a comparison of digital palpation, transesophageal echocardiography, and epiaortic ultrasonography. *J Cardiothorac Vasc Anesth.* 2007;21:805–809.

68. Glas KE, Swaminathan M, Reeves ST, et al. Guidelines for the performance of a comprehensive intraoperative epiaortic ultrasonographic examination: recommendations of the American society of echocardiography and the society of cardiovascular anesthesiologists; endorsed by the society of thoracic surgeons. *J Am Soc Echocardiogr.* 2007;20:1227–1235.

69. Bainbridge D. 3-D imaging for aortic plaque assessment. *Semin Cardiothorac Vasc Anesth.* 2005;9:163–165.

70. Bainbridge DT, Murkin JM, Menkis A, Kiaii B. The use of 3D epiaortic scanning to enhance evaluation of atherosclerotic plaque in the ascending aorta: a case series. *Heart Surg Forum.* 2004;7:E636–638.

71. Ferrari E, Vidal R, Chevallier T, Baudouy M. Atherosclerosis of the thoracic aorta and aortic debris as a marker of poor prognosis: benefit of oral anticoagulants. *J Am Coll Cardiol.* 1999;33:1317–1322.

72. Trehan N, Mishra M, Kasliwal RR, Mishra A. Reduced neurological injury during CABG in patients with mobile aortic atheromas: a five-year follow-up study. *Ann Thorac Surg.* 2000;70:1558–1564.

73. Davila-Roman VG, Barzilai B, Wareing TH, Murphy SF, Schechtman KB, Kouchoukos NT. Atherosclerosis of the ascending aorta. Prevalence and role as an independent predictor of cerebrovascular events in cardiac patients. *Stroke.* 1994;25:2010–2016.

74. Gold JP, Torres KE, Maldarelli W, Zhuravlev I, Condit D, Wasnick J. Improving outcomes in coronary surgery: the impact of echo-directed aortic cannulation

and perioperative hemodynamic management in 500 patients. *Ann Thorac Surg.* 2004;78:1579–1585.

75. Royse AG, Royse CF, Ajani AE, et al. Reduced neuropsychological dysfunction using epiaortic echocardiography and the exclusive Y graft. *Ann Thorac Surg.* 2000;69:1431–1438.

76. Glas KE, Swaminathan M, Reeves ST, et al. Guidelines for the performance of a comprehensive intraoperative epiaortic ultrasonographic examination: recommendations of the American society of echocardiography and the society of cardiovascular anesthesiologists; endorsed by the society of thoracic surgeons. *J Am Soc Echocardiogr.* 2007; 20:1227–1235.

77. Scharfschwerdt M, Richter A, Boehmer K, Repenning D, Sievers HH. Improved hydrodynamics of a new aortic cannula with a novel tip design. *Perfusion.* 2004;19:193–197.

78. Sabik JF, Lytle BW, McCarthy PM, Cosgrove DM. Axillary artery: an alternative site of arterial cannulation for patients with extensive aortic and peripheral vascular disease. *J Thorac Cardiovasc Surg.* 1995;109:885–890.

79. Stern A, Tunick PA, Culliford AT, et al. Protruding aortic arch atheromas: risk of stroke during heart surgery with and without aortic arch endarterectomy. *Am Heart J.* 1999;138:746–752.

80. Wareing TH, Davila-Roman VG, Daily BB, et al. Strategy for the reduction of stroke incidence in cardiac surgical patients. *Ann Thorac Surg.* 1993;55:1400–1407.

81. Murkin JM, Boyd WD, Ganapathy S, Adams SJ, Peterson RC. Beating heart surgery: why expect less central nervous system morbidity? *Ann Thorac Surg.* 1999;68:1498–1501.

82. Hammon JW, Stump DA, Butterworth JF, et al. Coronary artery bypass grafting with single cross clamp results in fewer persistent neuropsychological deficits than multiple clamp or off pump coronary artery bypass grafting. *Ann Thorac Surg.* 2007;84:1174–1179.

83. Van Dijk D, Jansen EW, Hijman R, et al. Cognitive outcome after off-pump and on-pump coronary artery bypass graft surgery: a randomized trial. *JAMAJ Am Med Assoc.* 2002;287:1405–1412.

84. van Dijk D, Spoor M, Hijman R, et al. Cognitive and cardiac outcomes 5 years after off-pump vs on-pump coronary artery bypass graft surgery. *J Am Med Assoc.* 2007;297:701–708.

85. McBride WT, Armstrong MA, McMurray TJ. An investigation of the effects of heparin, low molecular weight heparin, protamine, and fentanyl on the balance of pro- and anti-inflammatory cytokines in in-vitro monocyte cultures. *Anaesthesia.* 1996;51:634–640.

86. Diephuis JC, Moons KG, Nierich AN, Bruens M, van Dijk D, Kalkman CJ. Jugular bulb desaturation during coronary artery surgery: a comparison of off-pump and on-pump procedures. *Br J Anaesth.* 2005; 94:715–720.

87. Croughwell ND, Newman MF, Blumenthal JA, et al. Jugular bulb saturation and cognitive dysfunction after cardiopulmonary bypass. *Ann Thorac Surg.* 1994;58:1702–1708.

88. Takagi H, Kato T, Umemoto T. Off-pump coronary artery bypass sacrifices graft patency. *J Thorac Cardiovasc Surg.* 2007;133:1394–1395.

89. Al-Ruzzeh S, George S, Bustami M, et al. Effect of off-pump coronary artery bypass surgery on clinical, angiographic, neurocognitive, and quality of life outcomes: randomised controlled trial. *BMJ (Clinical research edBri Med J.* 2006;332:1365.

90. Wijeysundera DN, Beattie WS, Djaiani G, et al. Off-pump coronary artery surgery for reducing mortality and morbidity: meta-analysis of randomized and observational studies. *J Am Coll Cardiol.* 2005;46: 872–882.

91. Aldea GS, Soltow LO, Chandler WL, et al. Limitation of thrombin generation, platelet activation, and inflammation by elimination of cardiotomy suction in patients undergoing coronary artery bypass grafting treated with heparin-bonded circuits. *J Thorac Cardiovasc Surg.* 2002;123:742–755.

92. Kincaid EH, Jones TJ, Stump DA, et al. Processing scavenged blood with a cell saver reduces cerebral lipid microembolization. *Ann Thorac Surg.* 2000;70: 1296–1300.

93. Whitaker DC, Newman SP, Stygall J, Hope-Wynne C, Harrison MJ, Walesby RK. The effect of leucocyte-depleting arterial line filters on cerebral microemboli and neuropsychological outcome following coronary artery bypass surgery. *Eur J Cardiothorac Surg.* 2004;25:267–274.

94. Challa VR, Lovell MA, Moody DM, Brown WR, Reboussin DM, Markesbery WR. Laser microprobe mass spectrometric study of aluminum and silicon in brain emboli related to cardiac surgery. *J Neuropathol Exp Neurol.* 1998;57:140–147.

95. Rubens FD, Boodhwani M, Mesana T, Wozny D, Wells G, Nathan HJ. The cardiotomy trial: a randomized, double-blind study to assess the effect of processing of shed blood during cardiopulmonary bypass on transfusion and neurocognitive function. *Circulation.* 2007;116(11 Suppl):I89–97.

96. Djaiani G, Fedorko L, Borger MA, et al. Continuous-flow cell saver reduces cognitive decline in elderly patients after coronary bypass surgery. *Circulation.* 2007;116:1888–1895.

97. Davila-Roman VG, Phillips KJ, Daily BB, Davila RM, Kouchoukos NT, Barzilai B. Intraoperative transesophageal echocardiography and epiaortic ultrasound for assessment of atherosclerosis of the thoracic aorta. *J Am Coll Cardiol.* 1996;28:942–947.

98. Acarturk E, Demir M, Kanadasi M. Aortic atherosclerosis is a marker for significant coronary artery disease. *Jpn Heart J.* 1999;40:775–781.

99. Blackshear JL, Pearce LA, Hart RG, et al. Aortic plaque in atrial fibrillation: prevalence, predictors, and thromboembolic implications. *Stroke.* 1999;30:834–840.

100. Nohara H, Shida T, Mukohara N, Obo H, Higami T. Ultrasonic plaque density of aortic atheroma and stroke in patients undergoing on-pump coronary bypass surgery. *Ann Thorac Cardiovasc Surg.* 2004;10:235–240.

101. Sharony R, Grossi EA, Saunders PC, et al. Propensity case-matched analysis of off-pump coronary artery bypass grafting in patients with atheromatous aortic disease. *J Thorac Cardiovasc Surg.* 2004;127:406–413.

102. Sharony R, Bizekis CS, Kanchuger M, et al. Off-pump coronary artery bypass grafting reduces mortality and stroke in patients with atheromatous aortas: a case control study. *Circulation.* 2003;108(Suppl 1): II15–20.

103. Ribakove GH, Katz ES, Galloway AC, et al. Surgical implications of transesophageal echocardiography to grade the atheromatous aortic arch. *Ann Thorac Surg.* 1992;53:758–761.

104. Barbut D, Lo YW, Hartman GS, et al. Aortic atheroma is related to outcome but not numbers of emboli during coronary bypass. *Ann Thorac Surg.* 1997;64: 454–459.

105. Choudhary SK, Bhan A, Sharma R, et al. Aortic atherosclerosis and perioperative stroke in patients undergoing coronary artery bypass: role of intraoperative transesophageal echocardiography. *Int J Cardiol.* 1997;61:31–38.

106. Vogt PR, Hauser M, Schwarz U, et al. Complete thromboendarterectomy of the calcified ascending aorta and aortic arch. *Ann Thorac Surg.* 1999;67: 457–461.

107. Grossi EA, Bizekis CS, Sharony R, et al. Routine intraoperative transesophageal echocardiography identifies patients with atheromatous aortas: impact on "off-pump" coronary artery bypass and perioperative stroke. *J Am Soc Echocardiogr.* 2003;16:751–755.

108. Bolotin G, Domany Y, de Perini L, et al. Use of intraoperative epiaortic ultrasonography to delineate aortic atheroma. *Chest.* 2005;127:60–65.

109. Hogue CW Jr, Murphy SF, Schechtman KB, Davila-Roman VG. Risk factors for early or delayed stroke after cardiac surgery. *Circulation.* 1999;100: 642–647.

110. Davila-Roman VG, Kouchoukos NT, Schechtman KB, Barzilai B. Atherosclerosis of the ascending aorta is a predictor of renal dysfunction after cardiac operations. *J Thorac Cardiovasc Surg.* 1999;117:111–116.

111. Hangler HB, Nagele G, Danzmayr M, et al. Modification of surgical technique for ascending aortic atherosclerosis: impact on stroke reduction in coronary artery bypass grafting. *J Thorac Cardiovasc Surg.* 2003;126:391–400.

112. Kouchoukos NT, Wareing TH, Daily BB, Murphy SF. Management of the severely atherosclerotic aorta during cardiac operations. *J Card Surg.* 1994;9: 490–494.

113. Bonatti J, Nagele G, Hangler H, et al. Extraanatomical coronary artery bypass grafts on the beating heart for management of the severely atherosclerotic ascending aorta. *Heart Surg Forum.* 2002;5(Suppl 4):S272–281.

114. Royse C, Royse A, Blake D, Grigg L. Assessment of thoracic aortic atheroma by echocardiography: a new classification and estimation of risk of dislodging atheroma during three surgical techniques. *Ann Thorac Cardiovasc Surg.* 1998;4:72–77.

115. Trehan N, Mishra M, Kasliwal RR, Mishra A. Surgical strategies in patients at high risk for stroke undergoing coronary artery bypass grafting. *Ann Thorac Surg.* 2000;70:1037–1045.

116. Trehan N, Mishra M, Dhole S, Mishra A, Karlekar A, Kohli VM. Significantly reduced incidence of stroke during coronary artery bypass grafting using transesophageal echocardiography. *Eur J Cardiothorac Surg.* 1997;11:234–242.

117. Nicolosi AC, Aggarwal A, Almassi GH, Olinger GN. Intraoperative epiaortic ultrasound during cardiac surgery. *J Card Surg.* 1996;11:49–55.

118. Djaiani G, Fedorko L, Borger M, et al. Mild to moderate atheromatous disease of the thoracic aorta and new ischemic brain lesions after conventional coronary artery bypass graft surgery. *Stroke.* 2004;35: e356–358.

119. Kumral E, Balkir K, Uzuner N, Evyapan D, Nalbantgil S. Microembolic signal detection in patients with symptomatic and asymptomatic lone atrial fibrillation. *Cerebrovasc Dis.* 2001;12:192–196.

Postoperative Care After Aortic Surgery

19

Elnazeer O. Ahmed and Davy C. Cheng

Introduction

Patients undergoing aortic surgery are generally high-risk patients, with high prevalence of generalized atherosclerotic cardiovascular involvement, hypertension, heart disease, cerebrovascular disease, renal impairment, and diabetes, which further complicate the postoperative course. There are over 10,000 aortic aneurysm surgeries performed in the US (2008, STS), and majority is ascending aortic surgery. The goals of postoperative care of these patients are, consequently, to minimize the risk of potentially severe complications by maintaining the following:

- Serial clinical examination and high clinical index of suspicion of potential complications in relation to the aortic aneurysm disease (ascending, arch, descending, and thoracoabdominal)
- Adequate cardiac index (CI) and well-controlled blood pressure
- Monitoring for cardiovascular and neurological parameters
- Adequate oxygenation and respiratory function
- Attention to hemostatic function
- Adequate urine output
- Adequate analgesia

E.O. Ahmed (✉)
Department of Cardiac Surgery, London Health Sciences Centre, London, ON, Canada
e-mail: drnazeer@hotmail.com

Patients undergoing open aortic surgery require admission to a high-dependency unit with a nurse to patient ratio of at least 1:1.

Specific Aortic Surgery Considerations

Aortic Root and Ascending Aorta

Surgery involving the ascending aorta with coronary re-implantation can be complicated specifically by:

Coronary insufficiency secondary to kinking of the coronary stems or embolization of bioglue material, which may be used for hemostasis in these procedures.

Heart blocks due to the potentially vulnerable bundle of HIS in aortic root procedures.

Discussion with the surgeons regarding technical concerns is important, should any coronary insufficiency occur. Suspicion of coronary compromise should be immediately evaluated by coronary angiography or reoperations. Pacing wires function should be checked in aortic root procedures.

Aortic Arch Surgery

Surgery on the aortic arch involves placing the patient in deep hypothermic circulatory arrest (DHCA). Particular concerns of these patients:

Hypothermia: To avoid the deleterious effects of hypothermia, the patient should be restored to

K. Subramaniam et al. (eds.), *Anesthesia and Perioperative Care for Aortic Surgery*,
DOI 10.1007/978-0-387-85922-4_19, © Springer Science+Business Media, LLC 2011

normothermia gradually. Rapid rewarming may lead to hypotension, hence it is important to have afterload restoration with adequate volume replacement.

Bleeding: Coagulopathy can be a challenging problem in these patients. 2.4–11.1% may require re-exploration for bleeding.[1] Factor VIIa (2.4–4.8 mg) can be considered in difficult cases.

Neurological complications: Stroke complicates 21.7% of aortic arch aneurysm surgery.[1] It results from embolization of atherosclerotic debris leading to focal deficits, or microemboli of air or debris leading to diffuse brain injury.

Descending Thoracic and Thoracoabdominal Aortic Surgery

Paraplegia is a devastating complication of thoracoabdominal aortic surgery. Other rare complications include recurrent laryngeal nerve palsy and chylothorax.

Spinal cord ischemia and paraplegia. It is the most feared complication resulting from interruption of spinal cord blood supply during aortic clamping. Incidence varies substantially from 4% to 32%.[2] Delayed paraplegia accounts for up to 30% of paraplegia cases. Postoperative preventive measures such as maintenance of adequate mean perfusion pressure should start in the operating room and continued in the postoperative period.

Cerebrospinal Fluid (CSF) Drainage

Clamping the ascending aorta results in increased proximal hypertension that elevates the cerebrospinal fluid pressure and decreases distal spinal perfusion pressure. CSF drainage to maintain a CSF pressure ≤ 10 mmHg ameliorates spinal cord ischemia and possibly removes the negative neurotrophic factors that accumulate in the CSF during the ischemic period. Studies have shown that CSF drainage substantially decreases the incidence of paraplegia.[3]

Method of CSF Drainage

CSF drainage is commenced in the operating room and continued in the ICU for 72 h.

- An 18 G intrathecal catheter is placed through the L_4–L_5 intervertebral space.

- The catheter is connected to an external drainage system under sterile precautions via a three-way stopcock. This drainage system has a scale and a collecting chamber.
- The 3rd port of the stopcock is connected through a transducer to a bed side monitor.
- CSF pressure is maintained at **10 mmHg**. If the pressure is higher, then the CSF is allowed to drain in the drip chamber and the pressure is reassessed by closing the stopcock towards the draining port. The drainage limit should be kept **<10–15 mls/h.**
- The process can be repeated until the target CSF pressure is obtained.
- Send samples daily for microbiology. Insertion site should be kept dry.
- Maintain a closed system and keep the connections tight.

Recurrent laryngeal nerve palsy. Reported to occur in 8.6% of descending thoracic aneurysm surgery. It results in hoarseness and impaired phonation. Direct laryngoscopy should be performed if these symptoms persist >2 weeks. There is a risk of aspiration pneumonitis.

Chylothorax. It is an infrequent but serious complication of thoracic aneurysm surgery. It complicates 0.5–2% of cases. The chest drainage turns milky when the patient is on enteral feeding. It can present as pleural effusion when the chest tube is already removed. Biochemical analysis reveals a triglyceride level >100 mg/dl. Cell count shows lymphocyte predominance $(3.5–75 \times 10^6/\text{ml})$. Sudan III staining reveals fat globules (chylomicrons). Management of chylothorax includes instituting TPN and drainage. Refractory cases are managed by surgical intervention.

Patient's Admission to the Postoperative Intensive Care Unit

There should be a smooth transition of care from the OR team to the postoperative recovery unit.[4]
- Obtain a comprehensive report from the anesthesiologist (Table 19.1).
- Obtain a full surgical report from the surgeon.
- TEE report from OR including the correlation of the hemodynamic parameters, with adequacy

Table 19.1 Anesthesia report

- Preoperative history
- Surgical procedure and procedural issues such as second pump run, uncontrolled hemorrhage and unidentified surgical bleeder, aortic valve incompetence, etc.
- Anesthesia technical issues such as difficult intubation, line insertion, etc.
- Anesthetic regimen used
- TEE findings
- Metabolic and gas-exchange issues; K+, glucose, Alveolar-arterial gradients
- Coagulation pharmacotherapy (protamine, tranexamic acid, DDAVP)
- Blood products use

of cardiac volumes, e.g. the optimum pulmonary diastolic pressure (PAD) to guide postoperative fluid management.

- A thorough physical examination should be undertaken. This should be a head-to-toe documentation of the baseline findings, including the pupillary size and reaction to light, peripheral pulses, abdomen, and skin temperature, urine output, and chest tube output.
- Establish the invasive monitoring tools provided from OR, e.g. Swan – Ganz catheter, arterial lines, epidural catheters for patient-controlled analgesia (PCA), intrathecal catheter for CSF drainage.
- Obtain baseline complete blood count (CBC), arterial blood gas (ABG), serum electrolytes, coagulation profile (prothrombin time (PT) and partial thromboplastin time (PTT)), and other blood biochemical tests (e.g., serum creatinine).
- Assess initial chest radiograph systematically for the position of central venous lines, chest and mediastinal tubes, lung and pleural space condition, and cardiac and mediastinal outline.

Hemodynamic Monitoring and Management

Blood Pressure Control

Invasive monitoring should be used for blood pressure and cardiac indices. Blood pressure should be obtained in upper limbs and lower

limbs and on both sides and the difference should be noted. Initial target systolic blood pressure should be 90–110 mmHg. *Begin with adequate analgesia and sedation to prevent surges in blood pressure.* Beta-blockers are the preferred initial agents to decrease the force of myocardial contraction and heart rate (dP/dt); however, an alternative agent should be used in asthmatic patients. Use of nitroglycerin and nitroprusside could precipitate undesired reflex tachycardia.[5]

Pharmacological agents used to control hypertension:

1. **Nitroglycerin (NTG)**
   NTG is a vasodilator. It lowers the blood pressure by decreasing the preload. Hypovolemia should be corrected to prevent reflex tachycardia.
   Dose: **0.1–10 mcg/kg/min**. Administration of the drug should be through a non-polyvinylchloride tubing, which may adsorb 80% of the drug.
   Adverse reactions include reflex tachycardia and methemoglobinemia (metHb > 1% of total hemoglobin). Methemoglobinemia interferes with oxygen transport and it is managed by drug withdrawal or methylene blue (1% solution) 1 mg/kg.

2. **Sodium nitroprusside (Nipride)**
   Nipride decreases blood pressure by causing arterial smooth muscle relaxation and a lesser effect on venous capacitance resulting in a decreased systemic vascular resistance (SVR) and pulmonary vascular resistance (PVR).
   Dose: **0.1–8 mcg/kg/min**. It should be protected from light to prevent metabolic breakdown.
   Continuous blood pressure monitoring is essential.
   Adverse effects include:
   a. Reflex tachycardia is minimized by optimizing the preload.
   b. Hypoxia: ventilation perfusion mismatch occurs as a result of inhibition of hypoxic vasoconstriction
   c. Myocardial ischemia results from shunting blood away from the ischemic zones.
   d. Cyanide toxicity: Occurs when doses in excess of 1 mg/kg are given over less than 12–24 h. Hepatic dysfunction is a risk

factor. It is manifested by metabolic acidosis and high mixed oxygen saturations (cytotoxic anoxia). Treatment consists of drug withdrawal and sodium thiosulfate, 150 mg/ kg over 10 min. Metabolic acidosis is treated with IV sodium bicarbonate.

e. Spinal cord ischemia: There is a potential for decreased spinal cord perfusion pressure (animal studies). Vigilance should be exercised and high doses of nipride should be avoided.

3. **Beta-blockers**

Beta-blockers reduce the force of myocardial contraction and slow the heart rate (dp/dt); hence, it is a preferred drug in the settings of aortic aneurysm surgery.

a. Labetolol: It is a nonselective α- and β-blocker. Can be given in bolus of 0.25 mg/ kg over 2 min (about 5 mg every 5–10 min) or infusion at a rate of 1–4 mg/ min titrated to effect.

b. Esmolol: It is a cardio-selective ultrashort acting β-blocker and should be avoided in patients with marginal cardiac indices (CI ≤ 2.2 l/min/m²) because of its negative inotropic effect. It can be used in asthmatic patients because of its cardio-selectivity. The recommended initial dose is 0.25 mg/ kg load over 1 min, followed by 50–100 mcg/kg/min infusion.

4. **Calcium channel blockers**

These are alternative agents for patients of bronchial asthma. Their use is limited by their negative inotropic effect or the prolonged duration of action (nicardipine) that is not desired in hemodynamically unstable patients.

Coagulation and Bleeding Management

1. The postoperative blood drainage can be approached through addressing the following:
   a. Frequent assessment of chest tube output
   b. Establish surgical versus coagulopathy related bleeding? (Table 19.2)
   c. Is there any associated hemodynamic instability? What are the filling pressures?
   d. Are the drainage tubes patent?
   e. Does the patient need re-exploration?

Table 19.2 Etiology of postoperative bleeding

1) Surgical
2) Coagulopathy:
   – Anticoagulation (e.g. heparin rebound)
   – Thrombocytopenia and platelet dysfunction
   – Hypertension
   – Clotting factors depletion
   – Hypothermia
   – Fibrinolysis

2. Generally, patients drain less than **2 ml/kg or 100 ml/h** in the immediate postoperative phase with a trend towards a tapering amount of drainage.

3. Treat low cardiac preload by volume infusion. Generally, transfuse packed cells when hematocrit drops below 26%.

4. Treat coagulopathy guided by traditional laboratory studies (PT, PTT, and platelet counts) or point of care coagulation studies such as thromboelastogram. The latter provide a qualitative assessment of coagulation deficiency with distinct contours.
   a. A high PTT is treated by protamine 50 mg IV infusion over 10–15 min.
   b. High PT and INR are corrected by 2–6 units of fresh frozen plasma (FFP) infusion.
   c. Thrombocytopenia of <50,000 is corrected by platelet transfusion (1–2 adult units)
   d. Hypofibrinogenemia 150 mg/dl is treated with cryoprecipitate one unit/10 kg.
   e. Suspected platelet dysfunction (renal failure and NSAIDs) can be treated by desmopressin (DDAVP) 20 mcg IV over 20 min.
   f. Hypocalcemia is treated by 1 g calcium chlorine or calcium gluconate IV infusion over 30 min.

5. Cardiac tamponade should be suspected if drainage of bleeding suddenly ceases with dropping cardiac index, equalization of diastolic pressures, and reduced urine output. TEE can be helpful in these settings, but it should not delay timely surgical re-exploration.

6. Guidelines for re-exploration include bleeding >400 ml in the first hour, >300 ml/h for 2–3 h, or 200 ml/h for 4 h.[5]

7. Emergency re-exploration in the intensive care unit (ICU) is indicated for patients in pre-arrest

or arrest situation (exsanguinations or tamponade). Attending ICU team should be familiar with the technical aspects of this life-saving procedure.

Temperature Management

1. Hypothermia (<36°C) can result in adverse postoperative complications (Table 19.3). Treatment consists of warming blankets, forced air warming systems, and warming IV fluids.
2. Rewarming the patient may be accompanied by profound vasodilatation and hypotension; therefore, adequate volume infusion may be needed to maintain cardiac filling pressure.

Analgesia and Sedation Management

Most aortic surgery patients arrive in the ICU while still under the effect of anesthesia. The subsequent plan for sedation and analgesia depends primarily on the hemodynamic status and the potential for early extubation. When adequately addressed, postoperative analgesia and sedation decrease the stress load and the risk of stress-associated complications.[6–8]

a. As a general rule, short-acting agents for sedation and analgesia are used for stable patients with anticipated early extubation.
b. Propofol infusion 1–2 mg/kg/h is used for sedation.
c. Analgesia: Narcotics boluses, e.g. morphine 2–4 mg IV every 5 min as required, or fentanyl infusion 12.5–25 mcg/h can be used. Infusion is continued after extubation. This approach is avoided in overly sedated patients.

Table 19.3 Complications of hypothermia

- Ventricular arrhythmia
- Coagulopathy and bleeding
- Hypertension
- Shivering and increased O_2 consumption
- Increase SVR and decrease CI
- Delayed extubation

d. Nonsteroidal anti-inflammatory agents are helpful, provided they are not contraindicated by peptic ulcer disease or renal dysfunction. Ketorolac 15–30 mg IV can be used for breakthrough pains. Indomethacin 50 mg can also be used before discontinuation of sedation and extubation.
e. Patients requiring prolonged ventilation due to hemodynamic status may be sedated with longer acting agents. Midazolam 1–4 mg/h combined with morphine infusion. Fentanyl infusion (25–200 mcg/h) provides both analgesia and sedation.
f. Thoracic Epidural Analgesia (TEA) is a useful method of analgesia for thoracotomy patients. It is associated with decreased postoperative respiratory failure. However, patients who are coming from the operating room (OR) with epidural catheters and have been anticoagulated should be monitored for leg motor deficits secondary to epidural hematomas and infection. Analgesia can be provided using a combination of a local anesthetic and a narcotic (morphine or fentanyl 4 mcg/ml and bupivacaine 0.05%). The major side effects include itching, hypotension, and nausea.

Ventilation and Fast Track Management

Nearly all patients after midline sternotomy or thoracotomy have some degree of respiratory insufficiency (14%), which is well tolerated in most of the cases. Patients after thoracoabdominal aortic surgery are at particularly high risk of pulmonary complications (20–30%). Fast tracking has been successful in open heart surgery patients, including aortic surgery patients, and has sizeable economic benefits when a good clinical judgment is exercised.[9-12]

1. **Early Extubation**

   On arrival to the ICU, the patient, after an uncomplicated aortic surgery that is not unduly prolonged, should have an initial evaluation to ensure hemodynamic stability, normothermia, and absence of bleeding. Early extubation within the first 10–12 h after uncomplicated aortic surgery should always be the aim, as this has been shown to reduce pulmonary complications, encourage earlier mobilization, and is associated with shorter length of hospital stay.

Extubation Criteria

a. Patient is fully awake and obeys command
b. Stable hemodynamics (i.e. cardiac index > 2.2 l/min/m² on minimal or no inotropic support and absent arrhythmias)
c. Bleeding ≤ 50 mls/h
d. Normal ABG on minimal ventilatory settings (i.e. Pressure support ≤ 5 mmHg, PEEP ≤ 5 mmHg, and FiO2 ≤ 0.5)
e. Acceptable respiratory mechanics: Spontaneous respiratory rate ≤ 24/min; Negative inspiratory force (NIF) ≥ 20 mmHg; Vital capacity ≥ 10 ml/kg.

2. **Acute respiratory failure**

Acute respiratory failure is characterized by hypoxia ($PaO_2 \leq 60$ mmHg) and hypercapnia ($PaCO_2 \geq 50$ mmHg), either of them may occur in isolation. Patients become agitated if awake, can have arrhythmias, or even go in cardiorespiratory arrest. Ten to eighteen percent of patients may require prolonged ventilation. The etiology can be a single factor or multifactorial (Table 19.4).

3. **Management**

a. Clinical assessment
b. Manual ventilation with high FiO_2. Increase PEEP when the patient is back on the ventilator.
c. Ensure optimum hemodynamics.
d. Treat mechanical causes by addressing pneumothorax and significant pleural effusions

Table 19.4 Differential diagnosis of acute respiratory insufficiency

- Mechanical: Ventilator malfunction, endotracheal tube displacement
- Low cardiac output states and pulmonary edema
- Pleural problem: Tension pneumothorax and pleural effusion
- Pre-existing COPD, air space disease, and atelectasis
- Transfusion-related acute lung injury (TRALI)
- Acute respiratory distress syndrome (ARDS)
- Medications, e.g. sodium nitroprusside
- Pulmonary embolism
- Pain

e. Bronchodilators for bronchspasm in asthmatics and chronic obstructive pulmonary disease (COPD) patients
f. Bronchoscopy for lung collapse failing to percussion therapy
g. Antibiotics for pneumonia
h. Discontinue nitroprusside in hypoxic patients as it may cause ventilation perfusion mismatch and shunting

4. **Postoperative Preventive Measures**

a. Adequate analgesia. The use of epidural analgesia in thoracotomy patients can reduce the incidence of respiratory morbidity
b. Early extubation strategy
c. Minimize blood transfusion and lowering the threshold for early re-exploration for bleeding patients
d. Adequate bronchodilator therapy for COPD patients
e. Diuretics in volume overloaded and congestive heart failure (CHF) patients
f. Patient education
g. Physiotherapy and incentive spirometry

Myocardial Complications

1. **Incidence:** Coronary insufficiency complicates 2.5% of ascending aortic aneurysm surgery and it is the most common cause of death after vascular surgery.

2. **Mechanism:** In the context of aortic root and ascending aortic surgery, technical problems related to coronary re-implantation should be kept in mind. Increased myocardial oxygen demand, pre-existing coronary artery disease, postoperative hypercoagulopathy, cessation of antiplatelet medications prior to surgery, perioperative tachycardia, and hypotension are other etiologic factors for myocardial ischemia (MI).

3. **Presentation and diagnosis**

Patient in the immediate postoperative phase is kept under continuous surveillance in anticipation of occurrence of this complication.

a. Hemodynamic instability: Low cardiac output syndrome (CI ≤ 2.2 l/min/m²). Arrhythmias, Hypotension.

b. ECG changes: ST segment elevation, new onset Q waves, and new left bundle branch block (LBBB).

c. Elevated cardiac enzymes: Creatinine kinase (CK-MB) levels exceeding five times the upper limit of normal. Troponin I in excess of 15 mcg/l. Troponin I peaks at 12 h and returns to normal in 24 h.

d. Echocardiography may reveal new regional wall motion abnormalities and decrease in the left ventricular ejection fraction (LVEF).

4. Management

a. Arrhythmias should be treated by electrical cardioversion if unstable. Amiodarone is the drug of choice when pharmacotherapy is indicated. The ACLS algorithms should be followed.

b. Optimize CI by optimizing the preload, afterload, and contractility. Excessive fluid administration may compromise cardiac function (Laplace law) as well as pulmonary function. The cardiac contractility may be enhanced by the use of milrinone (50 mcg/kg loading dose) in addition to the other inotropes.

c. Intra-aortic balloon pump (IABP) can be used with great caution and should be avoided in the presence of complicated aortic dissection or severe peripheral vascular disease.

d. Sinus tachycardia poses a particular management challenge, being a compensatory mechanism to low cardiac output and at the same time being deleterious to the myocardium.

e. Commence antiangina medication, e.g. nitroglycerin and heparin infusion, if the blood pressure allows and no ongoing bleeding.

f. Cardiac catheterization and reoperation: Perioperative MI should be evaluated by coronary angiography with or without reoperation.

Neurological Complications

Stroke is a dreaded complication of aortic surgery. Type I neurologic dysfunction involves focal neurological deficit, while type II is a manifestation of diffuse brain insult.

1. Incidence: Stroke complicates 1.8–5.9% of ascending aortic aneurysm surgery and up to 21.7% of aortic arch surgery.[1,13] Particulate embolism from the aorta is the most common cause of stroke.

2. Postoperative assessment: Stroke can occur early or late. The early stroke manifests in the first 24 h by any one or combination of the following:

a. Nonawakening patient

b. Focal neurological deficit

c. Severe confusion and combativeness

d. Seizures

These patients should be evaluated by thorough clinical examination, electroencephalography (EEG), computerized tomographic scan (CT), or magnetic resonance imaging (MRI) of the brain. Imaging helps to rule out hemorrhagic stroke, which alters the plan of management.

3. Management

a. Aim at preventing secondary brain injury by maintaining adequate oxygenation, perfusion pressure, and normoglycemia

b. Heparin improves the microcirculation. The possibility of hemorrhagic transformation should be kept in mind when deciding about anticoagulation

c. Antiplatelets therapy: Aspirin and clopidogrel

d. Interventional neuroradiology is a promising field and should be involved in the evaluation of acute stroke patients

e. Early rehabilitation

Renal Complications

1. Incidence: Acute renal insufficiency complicates 6–18% of thoracoabdominal aortic aneurysm surgery, 30% of these require hemodialysis. The incidence is lower for the arch surgery (4.6%) and descending thoracic aorta (3–5%).

2. Etiology: Renal failure in aortic surgery patients can be precipitated by these additional mechanisms:

a. Renal ischemia secondary to suprarenal aortic cross-clamp

b. Atheroembolization
c. Dissection involving renal arteries
d. Rhabdomyolysis with myoglobinuria
e. Low cardiac output states

3. **Assessment**
   a. Monitor urine output on hourly basis. Oliguria (urine output ≤ 0.5 ml/h) is a sign of poor tissue perfusion. The majority of renal failure cases are nonoliguric.
   b. Calculate creatinine clearance as it parallels the glomerular filtration rate (GFR), which is a better indicator of renal function compared to serum creatinine. A 2 h urine sample is analyzed for creatinine. It is calculated using the following formula:
      - Ccr (ml/min) = Ucr (mg/dl) × V (ml)/Pcr (mg/dl) × time (min) [where Ucr = urine creatinine, V = total volume of urine collected, Pcr = plasma creatinine]
      - The normal value is 120 ml/min. Levels of 15–25 ml/min occur in acute tubular necrosis (ATN).
   c. Establish prerenal from ATN based on clinical judgment and biochemical parameters depicted in Table 19.5.
   d. Renal ultrasound

4. **Management of acute oliguric renal failure**
   a. Assess urinary catheter for patency
   b. Optimize hemodynamic parameters: Ensure adequate filling pressures, adequate perfusion pressure, and CI > 2.2 l/min/m²
   c. Persistence of oliguria after optimizing hemodynamics requires a trial of diuresis. Furosemide 10–100 mg IV (incremental doses up to 500 mg can be given) or 10–40 mg/h infusion. The use of diuretics does not alter the natural history of ATN, but it can convert oliguric renal failure into

nonoliguric renal failure, which may ameliorate pulmonary congestion
   d. Renal dose of dopamine (1–5 mcg/kg/min) is worth trying in spite of the lack of satisfactory evidence to support it. It does not prevent occurrence of ATN nor does it alter its duration. Like furosemide, it can convert oliguric renal failure into nonoliguric renal failure, thus improving respiratory function
   e. Renal replacement therapy

5. **Management of acute or chronic renal insufficiency**
   a. Maintain adequate perfusion pressure. It should be higher in hypertensive patients
   b. Fluid balance should be maintained. The intake should be equal to the output plus additional 500 ml for insensible losses
   c. Monitor electrolyte levels. Treat hyperkalemia (K+ > 6.0) by 1 g Ca-gluconate IV over 15 min to stabilize the cell membranes. Shift potassium into the cells by administering 50 ml of 50% Dextrose plus 10 units regular insulin. Give Kayexalate (Sodium Polystyrene) 30 g in 50 ml sorbitol PO or PR every 6 h. Each gram of resin removes up to 1 meq of K+
   d. Avoid nephrotoxic medications, e.g. aminoglycosides, nonsteroidal anti-inflammatory drugs (NSAIDS), Angiotensin-converting enzyme inhibitors (ACEI), and adjust doses for renal excreted medications
   e. Nutrition: protein should not be restricted in patients on hemodialysis. Nondialysis patients should have low protein diet (0.5–0.8 g/kg/D)
   f. Renal replacement therapy (Dialysis)

6. **Renal Replacement Therapy**
   a. **Indications**
      - Volume overload
      - Metabolic acidosis
      - Refractory hyperkalemia
      - Uremic symptoms
      - Space creation for nutrition and medication administration
   b. **Methods**
      - Intermittent hemodialysis: Used for hemodynamically stable patients. It takes 3–4 h per session. It is the most effective in fluid and solute removal

Table 19.5 Distinction between prerenal azotemia and ATN

Test	Prerenal	ATN
Urine Osmolality	>500	<350
Urine sodium	<20	>40
FENa (5%)	<1	>1

FENa Fractional excretion of sodium, *ATN* Acute tubular necrosis.

- Continuous hemodialysis/hemofiltration (Continuous venovenous hemodialysis CVVHD, and Continuous venoarterial hemodialysis CAVHD). CVVHD is most commonly used for hemodynamically unstable patients. It requires some form of anticoagulation. CAVHD requires arterial access and it is rarely used
- Peritoneal dialysis (PD) requires no anticoagulation. It is hemodynamically well tolerated, but is not tolerated by patients in respiratory compromise

Gastrointestinal Complications

1. **Stress ulcer prophylaxis:** Sucralfate 1 g every 6 h or ranitidine 50 mg IV every 8 h can be used in routine patients, whereas patients with a pre-existing history of peptic ulcer disease should have a proton pump inhibitor (PPI) prescribed.
2. **Feeding:** Early enteral feeding should be the aim in all patients, starting with water sips or green tea on the first postoperative day and gradually advanced to normal daily diet.
3. **Anticipation of visceral malperfusion:** This is an important consideration in the postoperative care of aortic aneurysm surgery patients, especially in the acute aortic dissection settings. Mesenteric ischemia can be occult for hours before the diagnosis is made. Mesenteric ischemia results from intraoperative hypotension, thrombosis, embolization, or involvement of mesenteric vessels in dissection leading to their occlusion or becoming supplied by a no flow false lumen.
   a. **Features indicating mesenteric ischemia**
   - Bloody diarrhea
   - Intense abdominal pain
   - Leucocytosis
   - Fever
   - Increased nasogastric tube output
   - Refractory lactic acidosis
   - Tachycardia
   - Peritoneal signs indicate perforation
   b. **Diagnostic tests and management**
   - Given the high mortality related to this complication, patients should have

aggressive workup and hasty intervention. CT angiography can be negative for mesenteric occlusion in cases of nonocclusive mesenteric ischemia. Radiological findings include bowel wall thickening, pneumatosis intestinalis, portal venous gas, and arterial or venous occlusion.
- The best diagnostic test should be timely exploratory laparotomy.
- Fenestration, stenting, or revascularization procedure may be required in dissection cases.[14]

References

1. Cohn LH, Rizzo RJ, Adams DH, et al. Reduced mortality and morbidity for ascending aortic aneurysm resection regardless of cause. *Ann Thorac Surg.* 1996;62:463.
2. Pannetan JM, Hollier LH. Basic data underlying clinical decision making. *Ann Vasc Surg.* 1995;9:503.
3. Cina CS, Abouzahr L, Arena GO, et al. Cerebrospinal fluid drainage to prevent paraplegia during thoracic and thoracoabdominal aortic aneurysm surgery. A systematic review and meta-analysis. *J Vasc Surg.* 2004;40:36.
4. Cheng DC, Bainbridge D. Postoperative cardiac surgery recovery and outcomes. In: Kaplan JA, Reich DL, Lake CL, Konstadt SN, eds. *Cardiac Anesthesia.* 5th ed. Philadelphia: Elsevier; 2006:1043–1060.
5. Bojar R. Synopsis of adult cardiac surgical disease. In: *Manual of Perioperative Care in Adult Cardiac Surgery Patients.* 4th ed. Massachusetts: Blackwell; 2004:33–40.
6. Her C, Kizleshteyn G, Walker V, et al. Combined epidural and general anesthesia for abdominal aortic surgery. *J Cardiothorac Anesth.* 1990;4:552–557.
7. Meade MO, Guyatt G, Butler R, et al. Trials comparing early versus late extubation following cardiovascular surgery. *Chest.* 2001;120:445S–453S.
8. Wennberg E, Haljamae H. Postoperative care of the vascular surgery patient. *Curr Anaesth Crit Care.* 1999;10:207–214.
9. Cheng D, Karski J, Peniston C, et al. Early tracheal extubation after coronary artery bypass graft surgery reduces cost and improves resource use. A prospective randomized controlled trial. *Anesthesiology.* 1996;85:1300–1310.
10. Bainbridge D, Cheng DC. Routine cardiac surgery recovery care: extubation to discharge. In: Cheng DC, David TE, eds. *Perioperative Care in Cardiac Anesthesia and Surgery.* 1st ed. Philadelphia: Lippincott Williams & Wilkins; 2006:341–345.
11. Cheng DC. Fast-track cardiac surgery. In: Kirby RR, Gravenstein N, Lobato EB, eds. *Complications in*

Anesthesiology. 2nd ed. Philadelphia: Saunders Elsevier; 2007:356–360.

12. Oxelbark S, Bengtsson L, Eggersen M, Kopp J, Pedersen J, Sanchez R. Fast track as a routine for open heart surgery. *Eur J Cardiothorac Surg*. 2001; 19:460–463.

13. Crawford ES, Svensson LG, Coselli L, et al. Surgical treatment of aneurysm and/or dissection of the ascending aorta, transverse aortic arch, and ascending aorta and transverse aortic arch. Factors influencing survival in 717 patients. *Thorac Cardiovasc Surg*. 1989; 98:659–673.

14. William DM, Lee YD, Hamilton BH, et al. The dissected aorta: percutaneous treatment of ischemic complications- principles and results. *J Vasc Interv Radiol*. 1997;8:605–625.

Index

K. Subramaniam et al. (eds.), *Anesthesia and Perioperative Care for Aortic Surgery*,
DOI 10.1007/978-0-387-85922-4, © Springer Science+Business Media, LLC 2011

Hensley, F.A. Jr., 155
Hertzer, N.R., 307
Hess, K.R., 228
Hickey, P.R., 158
Higami, T., 403, 405
Hinchliffe, R., 306
Hindman, B.J., 397
Hiramatsu, T., 151
Hlatky, M.A., 42
Hnath, J.C., 290
Hoeft, A., 175
Hogue, C.W. Jr., 134, 404
Hollier, L., 363
Holt, P.J., 306
Holzknecht, N., 52
Ho, S.Y., 379
Howard, G., 311
Hsu, R.C., 255
Hu, B.S., 52
Hughes, C., 327
Hughes, G.C., 289
Husain, A.M., 289
Hutschala, D., 127
Hu, Y., 176
Hynninen, M., 307
Hypothermic cerebral protection
　cooling
　　brain damage, 150
　　topical and surface, 150
　deliberate postoperative hypothermia, 150–151
　DHCA and extracerebral organs dysfunction, 149
　grades, 146
　mechanisms
　　cardiac surgery, 146, 156
　　$CMRO_2$, 147
　　temperature effect, metabollic rate, 147, 148
　　VO_2, 146–147
　moderate hypothermia and aortic surgery
　　favorable outcomes, 148
　　non-randomized study, 148–149
　　oxygen metabolism, 148
　　spinal cord and extracerebral organs, 149
　postoperative neurologic dysfunction
　　inflammatory mediators and vasoactive sub-
　　　stances, 149
　　ischemia and reperfusion, 149
　　neurological injury, 149
　profound hypothermia and hibernation, 147–148
　rewarming and reperfusion, 150
　temperature management and monitoring
　　bypass circuit, 150
　　rapid rewarming, 149

I

Iguro, Y., 388
Ihaya, A., 159
Imai, K., 71, 187
IMH. *See* Intramural hematoma
Inflammatory aortic disease
　infectious, 126

noninfectious, 126
syphilis, 125
Intermittent hemodialysis, 422
Intermittent perfusion
　DHCA, 159
　flow rate, 159
　timing, 159
International Registry of Aortic Dissection (IRAD), 17,
　　102, 103
Intimal tear
　endograft exclusion procedures, 65
　pulse wave Doppler, 65
　sinuses of valsalva, 65
Intramural hematoma (IMH)
　echolucency, ascending aorta, 77
　evolution, 21–22
　intimal tears, 76
　occurence, 76
　surgical intervention, 77
　type A and B disease, 32
Intraoperative TEE, aortic aneurysm surgery
　complications, 80
　pseudoaneurysms, 80
Intravascular ultrasound (IVUS), 85–86, 91
Invasive monitoring, traumatic aortic injury
　CVP, 359
　PPV, 358
　SPV, 359
IRAD. *See* International registry of aortic dissection
Irwin, M.G., 176

J

Jacobs, M.J., 228
Jaggers, J.J., 157, 159
Javerliat, I., 305
Johnston, W.E., 311, 314
Joist, J.H., 134
Jonas, R.A., 154, 379
Joseph, J., 42
Joshua, A.B., 280
Jugular venous oxygen saturation ($SJVO_2$)
　and $CMRO_2$, 183
　SACP monitoring, 183
　wall-artifact, 183
Junoven, T., 33

K

Kabbani, L., 261
Kahn, R.A., 363
Kaji, S., 33
Kakisis, J.D., 306
Kaluza, G.L., 42
Kamiya, H., 148
Kanadasi, M., 402
Kanchuger, M., 393, 394
Karp, R.B., 218
Kasliwal, R.R., 401, 402, 405
Katz, E.S., 395, 402, 404
Kauvar, D.S., 366

Printed in the United States of America